UNCOMMON PROBLEMS IN INTENSIVE CARE

To Tom, Jacqueline and John, to whom writing a book should mean weaving a tale of high adventure rather than constructing a catalogue of boring nostrums. Paternal apologies for the disappointment, but perhaps next time . . .

UNCOMMON PROBLEMS IN INTENSIVE CARE

J.F. Cade MD, PhD, FRACP, FANZCA, FFICANZCA, FCCP

Director of Intensive Care, The Royal Melbourne Hospital
& Professorial Fellow, University of Melbourne

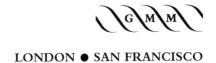

LONDON ● SAN FRANCISCO

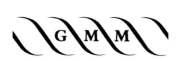

© 2002

Greenwich Medical Media Limited
137 Euston Road
London
NW1 2AA

ISBN 184 1100919

First published 2002

Visit our website at: www.greenwich-medical.co.uk

Distributed worldwide by Plymbridge Distributors Ltd
Typeset by Servis Filmsetting Ltd, Manchester, England
Printed by MPG Books Ltd, Bodmin, Cornwall, UK

Contents

A

Abciximab 1
Abortion 1
Acanthosis nigricans 1
Acetazolamide 1
Acetylsalicylic acid 1
Achlorhydria 1
Acidosis, renal tubular 2
Acquired immunodeficiency syndrome 2
Acromegaly 3
ACTH 4
Actinomycosis 4
Acute brain syndrome 4
Acute fatty liver of pregnancy 4
Acute lung irritation 5
Acute pulmonary oedema 5
Acute respiratory distress syndrome 7
Acyclovir 7
Addison's disease 8
Adenosine 8
Adrenal insufficiency 9
Adrenocorticotropic hormone 10
Adult respiratory distress syndrome 11
Agammaglobulinaemia 11
Agranulocytosis 11
AIDS 11
Air embolism 11
Alcohol, methyl 11
Aldosterone 11
Alkaloids 12
Allergic bronchopulmonary aspergillosis 12
Allergic granulomatosis and angiitis 12
Alopecia 12
Alpha-fetoprotein 13
Alpha$_1$-antitrypsin deficiency 13
Altitude 14
Aluminium 14
Alveolar hypoventilation 16
Alzheimer's disease 16

Amanita 16
Amenorrhoea 16
Aminoaciduria 16
Aminocaproic acid 16
Ammonia 16
Amnesia 16
Amniotic fluid embolism 17
Amoebiasis 17
Amphetamines 18
Amyloid 20
Amyotrophic lateral sclerosis 20
Anaemia 20
Anaphylaxis 24
ANCA 24
Aneurysms, mycotic 24
Angiodysplasia 24
Angioedema 24
Angiotensin 24
Angiotensin-converting enzyme 25
Animal bites 25
Ankylosing spondylitis 25
Anorectal infections 27
Anorectic agents 27
Anorexia nervosa 27
Anthrax 27
Antibiotic-associated colitis 28
Anticardiolipin antibody 28
Anticholinergic (cholinolytic) agents 28
Anticholinesterases 29
Antidiuretic hormone 30
Antinuclear antibodies 30
Antiphospholipid syndrome 30
Antiprotease 32
Antithrombin III 32
Aortic coarctation 33
Aortic dissection 33
Aplastic anaemia 34
ARDS 34
Arnold-Chiari malformation 34

Arsenic 35
Arteriovenous malformations 36
Arteritis 37
Arthritis 38
Arthropathies 39
Arthus reaction 39
Asbestos 39
Aspergillosis 40
Aspiration 41
Aspirin 41
Asthma 42
Asthmatic pulmonary eosinophilia 44
Atrial natriuretic factor 44
Autacoids 44
Auto-erythrocyte purpura 44
Autoimmune disorders 44

B
Bacillary angiomatosis 46
Bacillary peliosis hepatis 46
Bacitracin 46
BAL 46
Barotrauma 46
Basophilia 46
Bat bites 47
Bathing 47
Bed rest 47
Bee stings 47
Behçet's syndrome 47
Bell's palsy 48
Bence Jones protein 49
Benign intracranial hypertension 49
Beriberi 49
Beryllium 50
Beta$_2$-microglobulin 50
Biliary cirrhosis 50
Bioterrorism 51
Bird fancier's lung 51
Bismuth 51
Bites and stings 51
Bleomycin 56
Blisters 56
Boerhaave's syndrome 56
Botulism 56
Bovine spongiform encephalopathy 57
Bromocriptine 57
Bronchiectasis 57
Bronchiolitis obliterans 58

Bronchocentric granulomatosis 58
Brucellosis 58
Budd-Chiari syndrome 59
Bullae 59
Burns, respiratory complications 59
Byssinosis 61

C
Cadmium 62
Calcitonin 62
Calcium 63
Calcium disodium edetate 63
Cancer 63
Cancer complications 64
Carbon monoxide 65
Carbon tetrachloride 66
Carbonic anhydrase inhibitors 67
Carboxyhaemoglobin 67
Carcinoembryonic antigen 68
Carcinoid syndrome 68
Cardiac tumours 69
Cardiomyopathies 70
Cardiovascular diseases 73
Cat bites 74
Cat-scratch disease 74
Cavitation 76
Cellulitis 77
Central pontine myelinolysis 77
Cerebellar degeneration 78
Cerebral arterial gas embolism 78
Cerebral arteritis 78
Charcot-Marie-Tooth disease 78
Chelating agents 78
Chemical poisoning 81
Chest wall disorders 82
Chinese restaurant syndrome 82
Chlorine 82
Cholangitis 83
Cholera 83
Cholestasis 84
Cholinergic agonists 84
Cholinergic crisis 85
Christmas disease 85
Chromium 85
Chronic fatigue syndrome 85
Churg–Strauss syndrome 85
Chylothorax 86
Ciguatera 86

vi

Clostridial infections 87
Clostridium difficile 88
Coagulation disorders 88
Cocaine 89
Cold 90
Cold agglutinin disease 90
Colitis 90
Complement deficiency 91
Conjunctivitis 92
Conn's syndrome 93
Copper 94
Costochondritis 94
CREST syndrome 95
Creutzfeldt-Jakob disease 95
Cricoarytenoid arthritis 96
Critical illness myopathy 96
Critical illness polyneuropathy 96
Crohn's disease 96
Cryoglobulinaemia 97
Cryptococcosis 97
Cushing's syndrome 97
Cyanide 99
Cystic fibrosis 100
Cytomegalovirus 101

D
Dantrolene 103
Decompression sickness 103
Delirium 103
Dementia 103
Demyelinating diseases 104
Dengue 105
Dermatitis 105
Dermatology 106
Dermatomyositis 107
Desferrioxamine 107
Desmopressin 107
Diaphragm 108
Diarrhoea 108
Diffuse fibrosing alveolitis 110
Digoxin-specific antibody 112
Dimercaprol 113
Dioxins 113
Diphtheria 113
Dissecting aneurysm 114
Disseminated intravascular
  coagulation 114
Diving 114

Dog bites 115
Drowning 115
Drug allergy 117
Drug fever 118
Drug-drug interactions 118
Drugs 119
Drugs and the kidney 121
Drugs and the lung 122
Dysentery 124
Dysphagia 124
Dysproteinaemias 124

E
Eaton Lambert syndrome 125
Ebola haemorrhagic fever 125
Echinacea 125
Echinococcosis 125
Ecstasy 126
Ecthyma 126
Ectopic hormone production 126
EDTA 126
Eisenmenger syndrome 126
Embolism, air 127
Emphysema 127
Empyema 127
Encephalitis 127
Encephalopathy 127
Endarteritis 128
Endocarditis 128
Endocrinology 131
Enterocolitis 133
Enteropathogenic E. coli 133
Envenomation 133
Environment 133
Eosinopenia 133
Eosinophilia 134
Eosinophilia and lung infiltration 134
Eosinophilic granuloma 136
Eosinophilic pneumonia 136
Epidermolysis bullosa 136
Epididymitis 136
Epidural abscess 136
Epstein–Barr virus 137
Ergot 138
Erysipelas 138
Erythema marginatum 138
Erythema migrans 139
Erythema multiforme 139

Erythema nodosum 139
Erythrocytosis 139
Erythromelalgia 139
Ethylene glycol 140
Euthryoid sick syndrome 141
Exfoliative dermatitis 142
Exophthalmos 143
Exotic pneumonia 143
Extrinsic allergic alveolitis 143

F
Factitious disorders 144
Familial hypocalciuric hypercalcaemia 144
Fanconi's syndrome 144
Farmer's lung 144
Fasciitis 144
Felty's syndrome 144
Fetal haemoglobin 145
Fever 145
Fever of unknown origin 145
Fibrinolysis 145
Fish envenomation 146
Flushing 146
Folic acid deficiency 147
Folliculitis 147
Food poisoning 147
Formaldehyde 148
Fournier's gangrene 148
Friedreich's ataxia 148
Frostbite 148
Furunculosis 149

G
Gamma-hydroxybutyric acid 150
Ganciclovir 150
Gangrene 150
Gas gangrene 151
Gas in soft tissues 152
Gastric emptying 152
Gastrinoma 152
Gastroenteritis 152
Gastroenterology 152
Germ warfare 153
Giant cell arteritis 153
Gingivitis 153
Glomerular disease 153
Glossitis 154
Glucagonoma 154

Glucose-6-phosphate dehydrogenase
    deficiency 155
Glycogen storage diseases 156
Goodpasture's syndrome 156
Gout 157
Graves' disease 158
Growth hormone 158
Guillain–Barré syndrome 158

H
Haemangioma 159
Haematology 159
Haematuria 161
Haemochromatosis 161
Haemodilution 163
Heamoglobin disorders 163
Haemoglobinopathy 165
Haemogloninuria 165
Haemolysis 165
Haemolytic–uraemic syndromes 165
Haemophilia 167
Haemoptysis 167
Haemostasis 168
Hamman–Rich syndrome 168
Hand–Schüller–Christian disease 168
Hantavirus 168
Heat 168
Heat cramps 169
Heat exhaustion 169
Heat rash 169
Heat shock proteins 169
Heat stroke 170
Heavy chains 171
Heavy metal poisoning 171
HELLP syndrome 171
Hemianopia 172
Henoch–Schonlein purpura 172
Heparin 172
Hepatic diseases 173
Hepatic necrosis 174
Hepatic vein thrombosis 174
Hepatitis 174
Hepatocellular carcinoma 177
Hepatoma 177
Hepatopulmonary syndrome 178
Hereditary haemorrhagic telangiectasia 179
Herpesviruses 179
High altitude 179

Hirsutism 181
Histiocytosis X 181
Histocompitability complex 182
Histoplasmosis 183
Horner's syndrome 183
Hot tubs 184
Human bites 184
Hydatid disease 184
Hydrocephalus 184
Hydrogen sulfide 184
Hyperbaric oxygen 184
Hypercalcaemia 184
Hyperparathyroidism 186
Hyperphosphataemia 188
Hypersensitivity pneumonitis 188
Hypersplenism 189
Hyperthermia 189
Hyperthyroidism 189
Hypertrichosis 191
Hyperuricaemia 191
Hyperviscosity 191
Hypocalcaemia 191
Hypoglycaemia 192
Hypokalaemia 192
Hyponatraemia 192
Hypoparathyroidism 192
Hypophosphataemia 193
Hypothermia 194
Hypothyroidism 195

I

Idiopathic pulmonary fibrosis 197
Idiopathic pulmonary haemosiderosis 197
Idiopathic thrombocytopenic
    purpura 197
Immotile cilia syndrome 197
Immune complex disease 197
Immunodeficiency 199
Immunology 200
Infections 201
Inflammatory bowel disease 203
Inhalation injury 205
Insect bites and stings 205
Interstitial lung disease 205
Interstitial nephritis 206
Interstitial pneumonitis 206
Iron 206
Iron overload disease 207

Irritable bowel syndrome 207
Islet cell tumour 207

J

Jarisch–Herxheimer reaction 209
Jellyfish envenomation 209

K

Kaposi's sarcoma 210
Kartagener's syndrome 210
Korsakoff syndrome 210
Kyphoscoliosis 210

L

Lactase Deficiency 211
Lactic acidosis 211
Lassa fever 212
Lateral medullary syndrome 213
Lead 213
Leptospirosis 214
Leukocytoclastic vasculitis 214
Leukoencephalopathy 214
Lewisite 214
Lice 215
Light chains 215
Lightning 215
Liquorice 215
Listeriosis 216
Lithium 216
Livedo reticularis 218
Liver abscess 218
Loeffler's syndrome 219
Lung tumours 219
Lupus anticoagulant 220
Lyme disease 220
Lymphadenopathy 221
Lymphocytosis 221
Lymphomatoid granulomatosis 222
Lymphopenia 222
Lyssavirus 222

M

Magnesium 223
Malabsorption 224
Malaria 225
Malignant hyperthermia 226
Mallory–Weiss syndrome 227
Manganese 227

ix

Marfan's syndrome 228
Marine vertebrate and invertebrate
    stings 228
Mast cells 228
Mastocytosis 228
Mediastinal diseases 228
Mediastinitis 230
Mediterranean fever 230
Medullary sponge kidney 230
Medullary thyroid cancer 230
Megaloblastic anaemia 230
Melatonin 231
Meleney's progressive synergistic
    gangrene 231
Melioidosis 231
Mendelson's syndrome 232
Meningococcaemia 232
Meningoencephalitis 232
Mercury 232
Mesothelioma 233
Metabolic acidosis 233
Metabolism and nutrition 233
Methaemoglobinaemia 234
Methanol 235
Methylene blue 236
Microangiopathic haemolysis 237
Miller Fisher syndrome 237
Mites 237
Mixed connective tissue disease 237
Monkey bites 238
Monosodium glutamate 238
Motor neurone disease 238
Mouth diseases 238
Multifocal motor neuropathy 240
Multiple endocrine neoplasia 240
Multiple myeloma 241
Multiple sclerosis 243
Muscular dystrophies 244
Mushroom poisoning 245
Mustards 246
Myasthenia gravis 246
Mycetism 248
Mycetoma 248
Mycoplasma hominis 248
Mycoplasma pneumoniae 248
Mycotic aneurysms 248
Myelitis 248
Myelopathy 248

Myoglobinuria 248
Myopathy 248
Myositis 249
Myotonia 250
Myxoedema 250
Myxoma 250

N
Nails 251
Necrolytic migratory erythema 251
Necrotizing cutaneous mucormycosis 251
Necrotizing pneumonia 251
Nephrolithiasis 251
Nephrology 252
Nephrotic syndrome 254
Neural tube defects 254
Neurofibromatosis 254
Neuroleptic malignant syndrome 254
Neurology 255
Neuropathy 257
Neutropenia 261
Neutrophilia 262
Non-respiratory thoracic disorders 263
Norwalk virus 263
Nutrition 263

O
Obstetrics and gynaecology 264
Occupational lung diseases 265
Octreotide 267
Oncofetal antigen 267
Ophthalmoplegia 267
Optic neuritis 267
Orchitis 267
Organophosphates 267
Osler–Weber–Rendu disease 267
Ovarian hyperstimulation syndrome 267
Oxytocin 268

P
Paget's disease 269
Palmar erythema 270
Pancreatitis 270
Pancytopenia 270
Papilloedema 271
Paragonimiasis 271
Paraneoplastic syndromes 271
Paraquat 273

x

Parotitis 274
Paroxysmal nocturnal haemoglobinuria 274
Pediculosis 274
Pelvic inflammatory disease 274
Pemphigus 274
Penicillamine 275
Periodic breathing 275
Periodic paralysis 275
Pernicious anaemia 275
Peroneal muscular atrophy 275
Petechiae 275
Peutz–Jeghers syndrome 276
Phaeochromocytoma 276
Phosgene 277
Phrenic nerve 277
Phthiriasis 277
Physical exposure 277
Pigmentation disorders 277
Pituitary 278
Pituitary apoplexy 279
Placental abruption 279
Plasmacytoma 279
Plasminogen 279
Platelet function defects 279
Pleural cavity 280
Plumbism 284
Plummer–Vinson syndrome 284
Pneumatosis coli 284
Pneunoconiosis 284
Pneumomediastinum 284
Pneumonia, exotic 284
Pneumonia in pregnancy 284
Pneumothorax 285
Poisoning 285
Poliomyelitis 286
Polyarteritis nodosa 286
Polycystic kidney disease 286
Polycystic ovary syndrome 287
Polycythaemia 287
Polymyalgia rheumatica 288
Polymyositis/dermatomyositis 288
Polyneuritis 289
Polyneuropathy 289
Porphyria 289
Post-transfusion purpura 292
Pre-eclampsia 292
Pregnancy 294
Priapism 297

Procalcitonin 297
Proctitis 297
Progressive multifocal leukoen-
  cephalopathy 298
Protein C 298
Protein S 299
Proteinuria 299
Prussian blue 300
Pseudogout 300
Pseudohyperkalaemia 300
Pseudohyponatraemia 300
Pseudohypoparathryoidism 301
Pseudomembranous colitis 301
Pseudo-obstruction of the colon 301
Pseudo primary aldosteronism 301
Psoriasis 301
Ptosis 302
Pulmonary alveolar proteinosis 302
Pulmonary hypertension 303
Pulmonary infiltrates 305
Pulmonary infiltration with eosinophilia 306
Pulmonary nodules 306
Pulmonary oedema 307
Pulmonary veno-occlusive disease 307
Purpura 307
Pyoderma gangrenosum 308
Pyrexia 308
Pyroglutamic acid 313

Q
Q Fever 313

R
Rabies 314
Radiation injury 314
Rat bites 315
Raynaud's phenomenon/disease 315
Reactive arthritis 316
Reiter's syndrome 316
Relapsing fever 317
Renal artery occlusion 317
Renal calculous disease 318
Renal cortical necrosis 318
Renal cystic disease 319
Renal tubular acidosis 320
Renal vein thrombosis 321
Renin–angiotensin–aldosterone 321
Respiratory burns 322

xi

Respiratory diseases 322
Restless legs 324
Reticulocytes 324
Retinal haemorrhage 325
Retrobulbar neuritis 325
Reye's syndrome 325
Rhabdomyolysis 326
Rheumatology 327
Rickettsial diseases 328

S
Salicylism 330
Salpingitis 330
Sarcoidosis 330
Scalded skin syndrome 333
Scarlet fever 333
Schistosomiasis 333
Schonlein–Henoch purpura 334
Scleroderma 334
Scombroid 335
Scorpion stings 336
Scurvy 336
Selenium 336
Serotonin syndrome 337
Serpins 337
Serum sickness 337
Sheehan's syndrome 337
Short bowel syndrome 337
Shy–Drager disease 337
Sickle cell anaemia 337
Sideroblastic anaemia 337
Situs inversus 337
Sjögren's syndrome 338
Skin necrosis 339
Skin signs of internal malignant disease 339
Sleep disorders of breathing 339
Smoke inhalation 341
Snake bites 341
Sodium nitroprusside 341
Somatomedin C 341
Somatostatin 341
Spider bites 341
Splenomegaly 341
Spondyloarthritis 342
Spotted fevers 342
Staphylococcal scalded skin syndrome 342
Stevens–Johnson syndrome 342
Stings 342

Stomatitis 342
Storage disorders 343
Stridor 343
Strychnine 343
Sturge–Weber syndrome 343
Sucralfate 344
Sweating 344
Sweet's syndrome 345
Swimming 345
Syndrome of inappropriate antidiuretic
    hormone 345
Syphilis 346
Syringomyelia 347
Systemic diseases and the lung 347
Systemic lupus erythematosus 348

T
Takayasu's disease 351
Tardive dyskinesia 351
Temporal arteritis 351
Tetanus 351
Tetrahydroaminoacridine (THA) 352
Tetralogy of Fallot 352
Tetrodotoxin 352
Thalassaemia 352
Thallium 353
Thermoregulation 353
Thiamine deficiency 353
Thrombasthenia 353
Thrombocythaemia 353
Thrombocytopenia 353
Thrombocytosis/thrombocythaemia 357
Thromboembolism 358
Thrombophilia 358
Thrombopoietin 359
Thrombotic thrombocytopenic purpura 359
Thyroid function 359
Thyroid storm 359
Ticks 359
Tinnitus 359
Tongue 359
Torulosis 359
Toxic epidermal necrolysis 359
Toxic erythemas 359
Toxic gases and fumes 359
Toxic-shock syndrome 359
Toxoplasmosis 361
Trace elements 361

Transverse myelitis 362
Trauma 362
Trauma in pregnancy 363
Trench fever 364
Trichlorethylene 364
Tropical eosinophilia 364
Tuberculosis 364
Tuberous sclerosis 365
Tubulointerstitial diseases 365
Tumour lysis syndrome 367
Typhoid fever 367
Typhus 367

U
Ulcerative colitis 368
Ulcers 368
Urticaria 368

V
Varicella 370
Vasculitis 370
Vasopressin 372
Vertigo 372
Vesiculobullous diseases 372
VIPoma 373
Viral haemorrhagic fever 373
Vitamin deficiency 373
Vitamin B_{12} deficiency 373

Vitamin K deficiency 374
Vitiligo 374
Von Recklinghausen's disease 374
Von Willebrand's disease 374

W
Waldenstrom's macroglobulinaemia 376
Warfare agents 376
Wasp stings 377
Water-related accidents 377
Waterhouse–Friderichsen syndrome 377
WDHA syndrome 377
Weil's disease 377
Wegener's granulomatosis 377
Wernicke–Korsakoff syndrome 379
Whipple's disease 379
Wilson's disease 379
Woolsorter's disease 379

Y
Yellow fever 380

Z
Zinc 381
Zollinger–Ellison syndrome 381
Zoonoses 381
Zoster 381

xiii

Preface

This book is intended to be different, though whether it is in fact so and more importantly how usefully so is a matter for the reader to judge. For though there are many Intensive Care books, their general theme regardless of their size is always one of coverage of the major topics, or groups of specialized topics, encountered most commonly in the field. Usually, and appropriately, emergency management is emphasized, sometimes even in the form of a didactic recipe.

Yet topics related to the care of the seriously ill, probably like those in most other areas, fall into three categories – the common, the uncommon and the incidental. Common problems should not need to be looked up in a textbook by those in the field, except perhaps by the most junior. Rather, the most useful references are journals and monographs reporting new information. Incidental problems are those not relevant to the current Intensive Care diagnosis and management of a particular patient. For the curious, suitable information can readily be sought as a rule in appropriate general or specialist texts. Uncommon problems are another matter. Even experienced clinicians cannot retain in their memory all the relevant details of so many varied topics, yet these problems may have a direct impact on acute patient care. Some, of course, do not carry any major or immediate therapeutic implication, though knowledge is always desirable, especially if readily obtainable. Some can be buried or overlooked in even a major Intensive Care textbook. Most can be found sooner or later in a major current textbook or journal for the relevant specialty, but then the impact on Intensive Care management is unlikely to be made apparent.

A solution for most clinicians and departments has generally been to collect or perhaps to have on-line, a bank of suitable references from the literature, but this can be a tedious task, may not be comprehensive and is often inefficient in data retrieval.

This book offers another approach. Uncommon problems relevant to Intensive Care have been gathered into a single volume, in which they have been described in sufficient detail to obviate much of the need to refer to specialized texts. Moreover, their implications for Intensive Care management have been highlighted. Although many of these problems can be reviewed in a more leisurely way than the more common and pressing disorders in Intensive Care, it could be convenient to have them collated in a single volume. The individual topics have been arranged alphabetically, as in an encyclopaedia and with ample cross-referencing, so that no index is required. The book is thus intended to provide an easy and practical reference for the clinician at any level faced with an uncommon clinical problem at the bedside.

There are many things this book is not intended to do. It does not replace major specialized Intensive Care texts, for it is not designed to cover the front-line disorders and emergencies which are the 'bread-and-butter' of the care of the seriously ill. Nor does it replace in-depth specialist reviews and more importantly consultant opinion of specialist colleagues – rather it is hoped to be a partner with these in the large and important boundary between

Intensive Care and many other medical and surgical specialties. Some may say that such a volume would need to be enormous to be truly useful and that a more modest-sized text may do justice to nothing. A few may believe that Intensive Care is primarily about managing the general principles of disordered physiology and that diagnosis except for the most obvious can be made by others if necessary. A greater difficulty lies in where to draw the line in breadth and in depth of coverage. In this, comments and suggestions would of course be welcome.

The following colleagues from the Royal Melbourne Hospital and the University of Melbourne have kindly made expert comments on the topics in their own areas of specialist knowledge – Dr David Baraclough (rheumatology), Prof. Graham Brown (infectious diseases), Dr Peter Colman (metabolism & nutrition, endocrinology), Prof. Stephen Davis (neurology), Dr David Hunt (cardiovascular diseases), Dr Benno Ihle (metabolism & nutrition, obstetrics & gynaecology, nephrology), Dr Tom Kay (immunology), Dr Peter Morley (drugs, environment, trauma), Prof. Rob Moulds (drugs, poisoning), Dr Jeff Presneill (respiratory diseases, miscellaneous diseases), Prof. Michael Quinn (obstetrics & gynaecology), Prof. James St John (gastroenterology, hepatic diseases) and Dr George Varigos (dermatology). Their assistance is gratefully acknowledged, though the entire content including any errors remains the responsibility of the author.

The author was fortunate to be able to persuade Mr Ron Tandberg, Australia's leading political cartoonist, to illustrate the book. His incisive wit is expected to enliven and illuminate an otherwise perhaps tedious text, but it is hoped that his contribution does not become the book's main attraction!

Finally, the author thanks the editorial staff at Greenwich Medical for their encouragement, patience and expertise.

J.F.C.
Melbourne, 2001

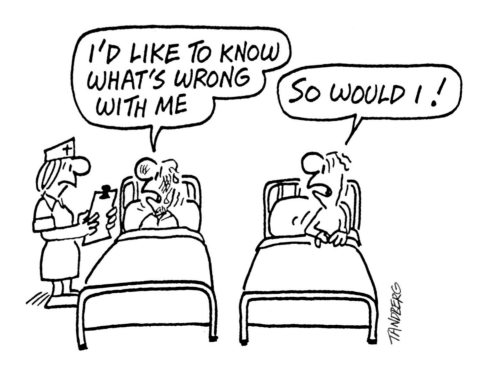

Abciximab

Abciximab (c7E3 Fab, ReoPro – Eli Lilly) is a novel antiplatelet agent. It is a chimeric monoclonal humanized murine IgG antibody to the platelet receptor, glycoprotein (GP) IIb/IIIc. GP IIb/IIIc is the receptor which, following platelet activation, binds fibrinogen and other adhesive molecules, so that platelet aggregation can proceed. Abciximab thus blocks this receptor and causes a temporary thrombasthenia-type platelet function defect.

Abciximab has a short half-life, with an initial phase of 10 min and a subsequent phase of 30 min. However, being platelet-bound it stays in the circulation for several days, though clinically adequate platelet function returns within 48 h.

It is used primarily in percutaneous transluminal coronary angioplasty (PTCA) as an adjunct to heparin and aspirin, where it has been shown to enhance significantly coronary patency rates. It has also been studied in a variety of other acute thrombotic situations where antiplatelet therapy could be of value.

It is given in a standard dose of 0.25 mg/kg by iv bolus followed by 0.125 μg/kg/h by continuous IV infusion for 12 h. It is very expensive. Its chief adverse effects are bleeding and sometimes thrombocytopenia.

Bibliography

Adgey AA 1998 An overview of the results of clinical trials with glycoprotein IIb/IIIa inhibitors. Am Heart J 135: S43.

Coller BS, Anderson KM, Weisman HE 1996 The anti-GPIIb/IIIa agents: fundamental and clinical aspects. Haemostasis 26: 285.

Hayes R, Chesebro JH, Fuster V et al 2000 Antithrombotic effects of abciximab. Am J Cardiol 85: 1167.

Kereiakes DJ, Berkowitz SD, Lincoff AM et al 2000 Clinical correlates and course of thrombocytopenia during percutaneous coronary intervention in the era of abciximab platelet glycoprotein IIb/IIIa blockade. Am Heart J 140: 74.

Sane DC, Damaraju LV, Topol EJ et al 2000 Occurrence and clinical significance of pseudothrombocytopenia during abciximab therapy. J Am Coll Cardiol 36: 75.

Topol EJ 1995 Novel antithrombotic approaches to coronary artery disease. Am J Cardiol 75: 27.

The EPIC investigation 1994 Use of a monoclonal antibody directed against the platelet glycoprotein IIb/IIIa receptor in high-risk coronary angioplasty. N Engl J Med 330: 956.

Abortion (see Pregnancy)

Acanthosis nigricans (see Pigmentation disorders)

Acetazolamide (see Carbonic anhydrase inhibitors)

Acetylsalicylic acid (see Aspirin)

Achlorhydria

Achlorhydria refers to the lack of secretion of gastric acid. The diagnosis of achlorhydria may be less than rigorous if it is based on the pH of spot samples of gastric contents rather than on formal testing of basal or stimulated gastric secretion.

The absence of gastric acid even after stimulation (i.e. absolute achlorhydria) has a number of associations, including

- gastric carcinoma;
- gastric polyps;
- pernicious anaemia;
- iron deficiency;
- hypogammaglobulinaemia;
- increased susceptibility to gastrointestinal infection.

Achlorhydria is, of course, also seen after:

- extensive gastric surgery or irradiation (permanently);
- potent ATPase inhibitors (temporarily).

Gastric acid is a prerequisite for peptic ulceration, and the demonstration of increased acid secretion may sometimes be helpful in the assessment of refractory or recurrent peptic ulceration (see Zollinger–Ellison syndrome).

Bibliography
Wolfe MM, Jensen RT 1987 Zollinger–Ellison syndrome: current concepts in diagnosis and management. N Engl J Med 317: 1200.

Acidosis, renal tubular (see Renal tubular acidosis)

Acquired immunodeficiency syndrome

Acquired immunodeficiency syndrome (AIDS) has become a well recognized entity throughout all of clinical medicine and beyond.

In Intensive Care, as in many other specialties, the most common presenting features of AIDS are **opportunistic infections**. Patients presenting with these, even if their HIV status is unknown and provided they have no other known immunodeficiency, are generally not difficult to recognize as likely to have AIDS.

These infections are often unusually chronic, recurrent or invasive. In many such patients presenting with fever and a presumptive diagnosis of infection, a specific microbiological cause is never identified. Although the patient may be a risk to others, particularly if tuberculosis is not promptly recognized, the patient is clearly also at risk of acquiring other, nosocomial infections while in hospital and especially while in Intensive Care.

Respiratory infections are the most common infections suffered by AIDS patients admitted for Intensive Care, but the clinical presentation is dependent on the patient's immune status, most simply assessed by the CD4 count.

- If the CD4 count is normal or nearly so, the infection is most likely to be bacterial or perhaps tuberculosis.
- If the CD4 count is < 200/μL, the infection is most likely to be caused by, in order,

  - *P. carinii*;
  - bacteria (especially pneumococci, but also legionella, listeria, nocardia, salmonella);
  - mycobacteria (either TB or MAC);
  - fungi (candida, aspergillus);
  - protozoa (toxoplasma);
  - viruses (CMV, HSV, VZV, E–B).

Bacillary angiomatosis and bacillary peliosis hepatis are serious infective complications of cat-scratch disease (q.v.), seen in immunocompromised patients such as those with AIDS.

The second most common group of presenting features comprises **neoplastic conditions**, especially Kaposi's sarcoma, but also non-Hodgkin's lymphoma and primary cerebral lymphoma.

Less common presenting features may be seen as the **direct effects** of HIV infection. A very broad collection of such features may be seen, including

- an acute infectious mononucleosis-like illness which commonly persists for several months;
- thrombocytopenia;
- wasting;
- neurological disease:

  - subacute encephalitis;
  - encephalopathy;
  - myelopathy;
  - peripheral neuropathy;
  - aseptic meningitis;

- abnormalities of:

  - myocardium;
  - kidneys;
  - gut;
  - thyroid;
  - joints.

Bibliography

Brookmeyer R 1991 Reconstruction and future trends of the AIDS epidemic in the United States. Science 253: 37.

Levine SJ, White DA 1988 *Pneumocystis carinii*. Clin Chest Med 9: 395.

Mann JM 1992 AIDS – the second decade: a global perspective. J Infect Dis 165: 245.

Miller R 1996 HIV-associated respiratory diseases. Lancet 348: 307.

1996 Update: provisional public health service recommendations for *chemoprophylaxis* after occupational exposure to HIV. MMWR 45: 468.

Acromegaly (see also Pituitary)

Acromegaly is a rare condition, produced in adults by excessive growth hormone which is usually derived from a pituitary adenoma. Its incidence is about 4 cases per million per year and its prevalence is about 50 cases per million of the population.

The pituitary adenoma usually arises from somatic mutation of the gene coding for part of a regulatory G protein, thus causing the production of growth hormone to become continuous instead of varying greatly during the day as it normally does in response to many stimuli, including exercise, stress, hypoglycaemia and adrenergic influences. Excessive growth hormone in children may produce **gigantism** as an occasional phenomenon.

Growth hormone (GH) is a 191 amino acid peptide, which is secreted by the anterior pituitary and which acts by stimulating the hepatic production of **somatomedin C** (or insulin-like growth factor 1, IGF-1), one of the body's many growth factors which circulate and bind to target cell receptors. IGF, which as an ultimate anabolic agent has been called the 'wonder drug of the late 20th century', is now described as a system and is the subject of an extensive literature.

The pituitary secretion of growth hormone is regulated by two neuropeptides secreted by the hypothalamus into the pituitary portal circulation, namely growth hormone releasing hormone (GHRH) which is stimulatory and somatostatin which is inhibitory. Acromegaly may thus also occur from excessive pituitary stimulation by GHRH either from the hypothalamus or ectopically from tumours, particularly benign foregut tumours such as bronchial carcinoid or pancreatic adenoma.

> The clinical features of acromegaly include both local (mechanical or parasellar) and distal (hormonal) changes, as for all pituitary tumours.
>
> - **Local** (mechanical or parasellar) features include headache and visual impairment (both of fields and of acuity).
> - **Distal** (hormonal) features include acral and soft tissue overgrowth (affecting especially the face, hands and feet), increased bodily hair, sweating and odour, sleep apnoea, husky voice, diabetes and skin tags (fibroma molluscum).
>
> Most patients have sleep apnoea (q.v.), and both the obstructive and central forms of this condition may occur. Since the hormonal changes of acromegaly which lead to clinical recognition tend to develop slowly, the adenoma is generally a macro-adenoma (i.e. >10 mm) and parasellar features are usual when the diagnosis is made.

Investigations show an elevated plasma growth hormone level which is not suppressed after a glucose load (i.e. > 3 µg/L, despite glucose 75 g 1–2 h previously in a standard oral glucose tolerance test). The plasma somatomedin C level which reflects average growth hormone activity is increased. The sella itself is best imaged by CT or perhaps MRI. If pituitary hyperplasia rather than a discrete adenoma is present, the source of GHRH should be sought either in the hypothalamus or an ectopic site.

*Treatment of a pituitary adenoma is usually by trans-sphenoidal **resection**.*

- *Postoperative **radiotherapy** is required if the GH and IGF-1 remain elevated, as is often the case.*

- *If GH levels still remain elevated, symptoms may be improved by medical treatment, using agents such as* **bromocriptine** *(a dopamine agonist, given in a dose of 2.5–10 mg orally twice daily) or* **octreotide** *(a synthetic analogue of somatostatin, given in a dose of 250 µg sc twice or thrice daily). Bromocriptine is particularly useful in patients with prolactin-secreting tumours.*

Pituitary apoplexy is an emergency complication which can complicate any pituitary tumour. It presents with headache, coma and abnormal eye signs.

It requires urgent treatment with **corticosteroids** *and* **surgery**.

Bibliography

Bach LA 1999 The insulin-like growth factor system: basic and clinical aspects. Aust NZ J Med 29: 355.

Bills DC, Meyer FB, Laws ER et al 1993 A retrospective analysis of pituitary apoplexy. Neurosurgery 33: 602.

Cardoso ER, Peterson EW 1984 Pituitary apoplexy: a review. Neurosurgery 14: 363.

Cheung NW, Taylor L, Boyages SC 1997 An audit of long-term octreotide therapy for acromegaly. Aust NZ J Med 27: 12.

Lamberts S, van der Lely AJ, de Herder WW et al 1996 Octreotide. N Engl J Med 334: 246.

Melmed S. Acromegaly 1990 N Engl J Med 322: 966.

Randeva H, Schoebel J Byrne J et al 1999 Classical pituitary apoplexy: clinical features, management and outcome. Clin Endo 51: 181.

ACTH (see Adrenocorticotropic hormone)

Actinomycosis

Actinomycosis is due to infection with a Gram-positive bacterium, *Actinomyces israelii*, previously thought to be a fungus because of its filamentous hyphae-like appearance. It is an obligate anaerobe, related to nocardia and often part of the normal oral flora.

Infection arises when there is injury to the mucosal barrier, especially in association with necrotic tissue or a foreign body. Most infections are facio-cervical, but occasionally the infection may involve the lungs or become disseminated. It is also an uncommon cause of pelvic inflammatory disease in women.

It is a chronic deep granulomatous infection with sinus formation. Inspection of exuded material may show the characteristic 'sulfur granules', tiny pale particles which on microscopy are masses of filaments.

Laboratory identification can sometimes be difficult, as the organisms on smear may fragment to give coccobacilli appearing like diphtheroids and on culture are slow growing under anaerobic conditions.

Treatment is with **penicillin** *7.2–14.4 g (12–24 million U) iv daily in divided doses for 2–4 weeks, then orally in reduced dose for 3–6 months. In penicillin-sensitive patients, tetracycline may be used.*

- *Surgical clearance may be required, and hyperbaric oxygen should be considered in severe infections.*

The prognosis is generally good.

Bibliography

Weese WC 1975 Smith IM. A study of 57 cases of actinomycosis over a 36-year period. Arch Intern Med 135: 1562.

Acute brain syndrome (see Delirium)

Acute fatty liver of pregnancy

Acute fatty liver of pregnancy is a rare and potentially fatal condition of the third trimester. It presents with nausea, vomiting, abdominal pain and jaundice.

Liver function tests are abnormal, and there is usually a coagulopathy. Hypoglycaemia can be severe and sustained. The liver biopsy shows diffuse panlobular fatty change (i.e. steatosis).

Treatment is with emergency **delivery** *and Intensive Care support.*

Acute pulmonary oedema

Acute lung irritation

Acute lung irritation can be produced by a large number of chemical pollutants in the form of noxious gases and fumes (see Occupational lung diseases). Irritation generally occurs in the upper respiratory tract (and often elsewhere), as well as in the lung.

Clinical features of acute lung irritation thus include;

- sneezing, rhinorrhoea, lacrimation;
- stridor;
- cough;
- wheeze;
- dyspnoea.

Systemic effects may also be seen on occasion, including

- fever;
- chills;
- leukocytosis.

Bronchiolitis, pulmonary oedema and subsequent bronchopneumonia are possible consequences of acute lung irritation.

Toxic gases and fumes include:

- ammonia;
- chlorine;
- sulfur dioxide;
- oxides of nitrogen;
- ozone;
- isocyanates, which may also cause occupational asthma (q.v.);
- osmium tetroxide,
- metal fumes

  - especially oxides of copper, magnesium and zinc;
  - also oxides of antimony, beryllium, cadmium, cobalt, iron, manganese, nickel, selenium, tin, tungsten and vanadium;

- mercury;
- platinum salts;

- polymer fumes (Teflon degradation products).

Systemic abnormalities are also produced following the inhalation of:

- carbon monoxide (q.v.);
- cyanide (q.v.).

Asphyxia may be caused by excess:

- carbon dioxide;
- nitrogen;
- methane.

Bibliography

Schwartz DA 1987 Acute inhalational injury. Occup Med 2: 297.

Acute pulmonary oedema

5

Pulmonary oedema is defined as an increased amount of extravascular fluid (water and solute) in the lung, where it may be interstitial or alveolar or both.

Pulmonary oedema is one of the commonest respiratory disorders and may follow a wide variety of local and systemic insults. Although pulmonary oedema due to left heart failure is the classical clinical picture, pulmonary oedema also occurs in a number of other common settings. In these, the left atrial pressure may be normal or even low.

These non-cardiac settings include:

- serious medical or surgical illness in the form of the acute (adult) respiratory distress syndrome (ARDS);
- an important component in:

  - viral pneumonia;
  - aspiration pneumonitis;
  - respiratory burns;
  - uraemia;
  - endotoxaemia (systemic inflammatory response syndrome);
  - drowning;
  - head injury;

– severe upper airway obstruction;
– altitude-related illness.

Pulmonary oedema may therefore present in diverse settings with different pathogenetic mechanisms and thus with different therapeutic implications.

The causes of pulmonary oedema are:

1. Increased capillary hydrostatic pressure

- cardiogenic (left heart failure);
- blood volume overload;
- pulmonary veno-occlusive disease.

2. Increased capillary permeability

- acute (adult) respiratory distress syndrome (ARDS);
- viral and other pneumonia;
- inhaled toxic substances (including oxygen);
- circulating toxic agents (including sepsis);
- disseminated intravascular coagulation;
- uraemia, radiation, burns, near-downing.

3. Decreased plasma oncotic pressure

- hypoalbuminaemia.

4. Decreased tissue hydrostatic pressure

- rapid lung re-expansion, after

   – drainage of a pneumothorax or large pleural effusion;
   – pneumonectomy;

- laryngospasm (and other causes of acute upper airway obstruction, when associated with strong inspiratory effort).

5. Decreased lymphatic drainage

- lymphangitis carcinomatosa;
- lymphangiomyomatosis;
- lung transplantation.

6. Uncertain mechanisms

- high altitude;
- neurogenic (raised intracranial pressure);
- drug overdose (especially IV heroin);
- pulmonary embolism.

In practice

- the first two groups of causes are by far the most commonly encountered;
- the third group is probably not a cause in its own right, but lowers the threshold for pulmonary oedema from other causes;
- groups four, five and six are less common.

Bibliography

Albertson TE, Walby WF, Derlet RW 1995 Stimulant-induced pulmonary toxicity. Chest 108: 1140.

Colice GL 1985 Neurogenic pulmonary edema. Clin Chest Med 6: 473.

Harms BA, Kramer GC, Bodai BI et al 1981 Effect of hypoproteinemia on pulmonary and soft tissue edema formation. Crit Care Med 9: 503.

Hasegawa N, Husari AW, Hart WT et al 1994 Role of coagulation system in ARDS. Chest 105: 268.

Kollef MH, Pluss J 1991 Noncardiogenic pulmonary edema following upper airway obstruction. Medicine 70: 91.

McConkey PP 2000 Postobstructive pulmonary oedema. Anaes Intens Care 28: 72.

McHugh LG, Milberg JA, Whitcomb ME et al 1994 Recovery of function in survivors of the acute respiratory distress syndrome. Am J Respir Crit Care Med 150: 90.

Milberg JA, Davis DR, Steinberg KP et al 1995 Improved survival of patients with acute respiratory distress syndrome (ARDS): 1983–1993. JAMA 273: 306.

Richalet JP 1995 High altitude pulmonary oedema: still a place for controversy? Thorax 50: 923.

Rossaint R, Falke KJ, Lopez F et al 1993 Inhaled nitric oxide for the adult respiratory distress syndrome. N Engl J Med 328: 399.

Scherrer U, Vollenweider L, Delabays A et al 1996 Inhaled nitric oxide for high-altitude pulmonary edema. N Engl J Med 334: 624.

Schoene RB 1985 Pulmonary edema at high altitude: review, pathophysiology, and update. Clin Chest Med 6: 491.

Sibbald WJ, Cunningham DR, Chin DN 1983 Non-cardiac or cardiac pulmonary edema? Chest 84: 452.

Simon RP 1993 Neurogenic pulmonary edema. Neurol Clin 11: 309.

Taylor JR, Ryu J, Colby TV et al 1990
Lymphangioleiomyomatosis. N Engl J Med 323:
1254.
Timby J, Reed C, Zeilender S et al 1990 Mechanical
causes of pulmonary edema. Chest 98: 973.

Acute respiratory distress syndrome (see Acute pulmonary oedema)

Acyclovir

Acyclovir is the most important of the available
antiviral drugs. It has replaced vidarabine (ara-
A), the first available antiviral agent for systemic
use in serious infections. It is a synthetic purine
nucleoside analogue, structurally related to
guanosine. Its unique mechanism of action
inhibits DNA synthesis and thus viral
replication. It therefore does not affect the
latent virus. There is a low incidence of
development of resistance, but unwarranted use
is unwise.

The antiviral effects of acyclovir are particularly
relevant for herpesviruses, as follows. It is

- especially effective against **herpes simplex virus** (HSV) types 1 and 2;
- less effective but still very useful for **varicella-zoster virus** (VZV);
- of intermediate efficacy against **Epstein–Barr virus** (EBV);
- ineffective against **cytomegalovirus** (CMV) (the related agent, **ganciclovir**, is however effective against CMV–q.v.).

> The greatest value of acyclovir is in **HSV encephalitis**, in which trial results have
> shown a survival rate of about 80% and
> complete neurological recovery in about
> 50%. It is also of value in oral-labial, genital,
> rectal and neonatal HSV infections.

In **VZV infections**, it is helpful in:

- the elderly, especially those with widespread lesions or trigeminal involvement;

- herpes zoster encephalitis;
- varicella pneumonia;
- immunocompromised patients (in whom interferon alpha and/or VZV immune globulin are also useful).

Acyclovir

- is not indicated in **infectious mononucleosis**, except perhaps in severe cases,
- is not indicated in **cytomegalovirus infections**, except for prophylaxis after bone marrow transplantation in seropositive patients, in whom it is effective when given in high-dose, i.e. 500 mg/m^2 tds iv for the 1st month),
- is not effective in the **chronic fatigue syndrome**.

Acyclovir is not protein-bound but is distributed
evenly throughout the total body water, except
in the CSF in which the level is 25–50% of that
in plasma. The urinary concentration is about 10
times the plasma concentration. It has a half-life
of about 3 h, which rises six-fold in severe renal
failure, since it is primarily excreted in the urine.
It is 60% removed by dialysis. It is probably not
mutagenic nor carcinogenic. Although fetal risk
has not been shown, it crosses the placenta and
should be used in pregnancy only if there is a
strong maternal indication. It is excreted into
breast milk.

It is available as a powder for iv administration,
as capsules for oral use and as an ointment for
mucocutaneous lesions or keratitis.
Intravenously, it is given as 5–10 mg/kg 8
hourly for 5–10 days. Typically, 500 mg are
reconstituted in 20 mL, diluted to 100 mL and
administered over 1 h, giving a mean steady-
state peak plasma concentration of 20 μg/mL.

Although the solution is widely compatible, it
undergoes irreversible crystallization if
refrigerated. Intravenous acyclovir is normally
well tolerated, but it is potentially phlebitic
because of its alkaline nature unless given
diluted and slowly, and it can sometimes give
rise to nausea or a rash. Rarely, reversible

encephalopathy or renal dysfunction may occur from very high concentrations.

Ganciclovir is structurally similar to acyclovir and is given in the same dosage. Its chief difference is that it is active against cytomegalovirus (q.v.). It is therefore used, often with immune globulin, in CMV retinitis or pneumonia, for example after bone marrow transplantation. Unlike acyclovir, it can produce bone marrow depression. It is teratogenic and mutagenic in animals. The usual dose is 5 mg/kg iv 12 hourly.

Bibliography

Ernest ME, Franey RJ 1998 Acyclovir and ganciclovir-induced neurotoxicity. Ann Pharmacother 32: 111.

Jackson JL, Gibbons R, Meyer G et al 1997 The effect of treating herpes zoster with oral acyclovir in preventing postherpetic neuralgia: a meta-analysis. Arch Intern Med 157: 909.

Laskin OL 1984 Acyclovir: pharmacology and clinical experience. Arch Intern Med 144: 1241.

Prentice HG, Gluckman E, Powles RL et al 1994 Impact of long-term acyclovir on cytomegalovirus infection and survival after allogenic bone marrow transplantation: European Acyclovir for CMV Prophylaxis Study Group. Lancet 343: 749.

Addison's disease (see Adrenal insufficiency)

Adenosine

Adenosine is an **autacoid**, one of a broad range of substances normally present in the body and functioning in humoral regulation at a local level (and thus separate from hormones, neurotransmitters and cytokines). Autacoids have short half-lives, since they act near to their site of synthesis and are not blood-borne. In addition to adenosine, other examples of autacoids include bradykinin, eicosanoids, histamine, PAF and serotonin.

Adenosine is an endogenous purine nucleoside of molecular weight 267 d, and it has receptors (A1 or A2) on most cell membranes. It is released when ATP is used and may thus help maintain the balance between oxygen availability and utilization. It is involved in many local regulatory processes and in particular is a vasodilator and an inhibitor of neuronal discharge.

Its cardiac effects were first recognized in 1929 and are extensive. They especially involve decreased conduction and ventricular automaticity, coronary vasodilatation and the blunting of the effects of catecholamines. On balance, it is thus 'cardioprotective'. Both A1 and A2 receptors are present in the heart, A1 in the cardiomyocytes and A2 in the endothelial cells and vascular smooth muscle cells.

> Clinically, its particular use is in the diagnosis and treatment of tachyarrhythmias.

- It is of most value in the treatment of supraventricular tachycardia, especially that associated with the WPW syndrome, with an average time to termination of arrhythmia of 30 s.
- It has no effect in atrial fibrillation or atrial flutter.
- It is not of value in ventricular tachycardia unless catecholamine-induced.

Its effects are antagonized by theophylline and potentiated by dipyridamole, but it may be administered without altered efficacy in the presence of other cardiac drugs or in liver or renal disease. It is of potential clinical use in electrophysiological studies, in cardiac stress testing and in the assessment of coronary blood flow reserve. It has no useful effect on coronary ischaemia. Since its half-life is only 10 s, it is given as a rapid iv bolus of 3–6 mg. A further bolus of 12 mg may be given 1–3 min later if necessary.

It can produce unpleasant and marked though transient side-effects, including flushing, sweating, tingling, headache, light-headedness, nausea and apprehension. Bronchospasm may be precipitated in asthmatics. It can also produce cardiac pain, which is angina-like but not in fact ischaemic.

Adrenal insufficiency

Acute adrenal insufficiency is an uncommon condition and is usually due to haemorrhage (especially from heparin), hypotension or shock (as in the Waterhouse–Friderichsen syndrome, q.v.).

> It thus occurs mostly in seriously ill patients, in whom it should remembered as an uncommon cause of hyperdynamic shock.

The clinical features include nausea, weakness and abdominal pain, as well as circulatory failure. Typically, there is hyponatraemia with hyperkalaemia, and the plasma urea may be elevated.

Relevant investigations include failure of the plasma cortisol level to increase after the injection of synthetic ACTH (see below) and direct imaging with CT.

Treatment is with physiological doses of **hydrocortisone** *iv.*

Chronic adrenal insufficiency (Addison's disease) is due to:

- autoimmune disease (sometimes polyglandular);
- a space-occupying lesion, typically a metastasis or granuloma (e.g. TB);
- pituitary deficiency, due either to
  - global hypopituitarism (when hypothyroidism is also typically present), or
  - previous administration of corticosteroids in pharmacological doses (when diabetes is commonly associated);
- HIV infection, with associated CMV adrenal infection,
- drugs, such as ketoconazole, rifampicin.

Clinical features comprise:

- weakness;
- weight loss;
- pigmentation especially in body creases;
- hypotension;
- hypovolaemia (except that blood volume remains normal in pituitary deficiency, since aldosterone secretion is primarily controlled by the renin–angiotensin system).

Investigations show mild hyperkalaemia and proneness to hyponatraemia from water overload. In patients who are sufficiently hypovolaemic to have pre-renal renal failure, there is more marked hyperkalaemia with hypoglycaemia, raised plasma urea and raised haematocrit. Specific testing shows a low plasma cortisol, which fails to rise after **synthetic ACTH** 250 μg iv (normal >150 nmol/L and a rise at 30 min by at least 300 nmol/L to a peak of >550 nmol/L). This short synthetic ACTH stimulation test is simple and safe.

If adrenal insufficiency is clinically overt and corticosteroids have been commenced, confirmatory testing is very difficult, unless dexamethasone can be temporarily substituted and then ceased pending a long (i.e. 3 day) synthetic ACTH stimulation test.

The plasma ACTH level is >20 pmol/L in primary adrenal failure, but in hypopituitarism it is low (as are the other pituitary hormones – q.v.). A rise in plasma cortisol still occurs in hypopituitarism following ACTH, though this may be subnormal due to chronic ACTH deficiency.

Treatment of adrenal insufficiency is urgent if there is circulatory failure (i.e. adrenal crisis), with **hydrocortisone** *100 mg iv then 10–15 mg/h, together with fluids, electrolytes and glucose. Chronic treatment requires maintenance therapy with cortisone (approximately 35 mg daily given about 2/3 in the morning and 1/3 in the evening), together with fludrocortisone 100 μg daily.*

> Patients with adrenal insufficiency exposed to stress require increased doses of corticosteroids. Typically, double the usual dose is used for minor stress and hydrocortisone 100 mg/8 h iv for severe stress, though recently it has become recognized that these doses are excessive. In fact, doses of 25–150mg of hydrocortisone per day for a maximum of 3 days are adequate.

Hypothalamic–pituitary–adrenal function is suppressed by previously administered corticosteroids in pharmacological doses.

- This may not recover for a year or more after such steroids are ceased.
- There is no simple and accurate prediction of hormonal reserve function, based on the previous dose or duration of steroid treatment.
- Prophylactic hydrocortisone (as above) is also routinely recommended in such patients exposed to stress. This cover is continued for two days, and then if the clinical situation is satisfactory it is tapered over the next few days.

If time permits, the cortisol response to ACTH may be assessed prior to anticipated stress, such as elective major surgery, but a normal value after ACTH does not necessarily imply a normal response to other stress. A more relevant adrenal assessment may be provided by the cortisol response to insulin-induced hypoglycaemia, but this test is probably unsafe.

Bibliography

Claussen MS, Landercasper J, Cogbill TH 1992 Acute adrenal insufficiency presenting as shock after trauma and surgery: three cases and review of the literature. J Trauma 32: 94.

Editorial 1980 Corticosteroids and hypothalamic–pituitary–adrenocortical function. Br Med J 280: 813.

Loriaux DL 1985 The polyendocrine deficiency syndromes. N Engl J Med 312: 1568.

Salem M, Tainsh RE, Bromberg J et al 1994 Perioperative glucocorticoid coverage: a reassessment 42 years after emergence of a problem. Ann Surg 219: 416.

Szalados JE, Vukmir RB 1994 Acute adrenal insufficiency resulting from adrenal hemorrhage as indicated by post-operative hypotension. Intens Care Med 20: 216.

Vance ML 1994 Hypopituitarism. N Engl J Med 330: 1651.

Vita JA, Silverberg SJ, Goland RS et al 1985 Clinical clues to the cause of Addison's disease. Am J Med 78: 461.

Adrenocorticotropic hormone (see also Adrenal insufficiency, Cushing's syndrome and Ectopic hormone production)

Adrenocorticotropic hormone (corticotropin, ACTH) is the main controlling factor for the adrenal production of cortisol and androgens. It is produced in the anterior pituitary by cleavage of a large and complex polypeptide (241 amino acids), called **propiomelanocortin** (POMC), which also includes melanocyte-stimulating hormone (MSH), beta-endorphin, met-enkephalin, beta-lipotropin, and a number of other peptides of presently unknown function.

The secretion of ACTH is controlled primarily by the hypothalamus-derived **corticotropin releasing hormone** (CRH) and secondarily by catecholamines and vasopressin. ACTH release is also stimulated by stress and by hypoglycaemia. CRH production and ACTH release is inhibited by both natural and synthetic corticosteroids, which suppress mRNA for POMC synthesis. ACTH is released in pulses, especially in the mornings, thus explaining the diurnal rhythm of cortisol secretion. The normal level of ACTH is 1.3–16.7 pmol/L.

Bibliography

Editorial 1980 Corticosteroids and hypothalamic–pituitary–adrenocortical function. Br Med J 280: 813.

Imura H 1987 Control of biosynthesis and secretion of ACTH: a review. Horm Metab Res 16 (suppl): 1.

Orth DN 1992 Corticotropin-releasing hormone in humans. Endocr Rev 13:164.

Adult respiratory distress syndrome (see Acute pulmonary oedema)

Agammaglobulinaemia

Agammaglobulinaemia was the first described immunodeficiency disorder. It is a congenital X-linked condition, caused by mutations in a gene on the long arm of the X-chromosome which encodes for a tyrosine kinase expressed in pre-B cells.

- There is a life-long susceptibility to infection:

  - particularly with encapsulated pyogenic micro-organisms;
  - less so to viruses, fungi and even most Gram-negative bacteria (except for *H. influenzae*).

- Infections, particularly of the respiratory tract, show an:

  - increased frequency;
  - increased severity;
  - increased recurrence rate;
  - decreased responsiveness to treatment.

Chronic meningoencephalitis, due to an echovirus, can be a particularly troublesome complication.

In about 30% of patients, agammaglobulinaemia is associated with a rheumatoid arthritis-like disease and sometimes with dermatomyositis, probably due to an enterovirus. On investigation, all the immunoglobulins are decreased (with IgA, IgM and IgD often undetectable and IgG < 1 g/L) and there are no B cells. There is no antibody response (e.g. to diphtheria–pertussis–tetanus immunization), but there is normal cell-mediated immunity.

*Treatment with intravenous **immunoglobulin** (30 mg/kg/month iv) significantly improves the prognosis. Screening of at-risk family members is recommended.*

Bibliography

Buckley RH, Schiff RI 1991 The use of intravenous immune globulin in immunodeficiency diseases. N Engl J Med 325: 110.

Van de Meer JWM 1994 Defects in host–defense mechanisms. In: Rubin RH, Young LS (eds) Clinical Approach to Infections in the Compromised Host. 3rd edition. New York: Plenum. p 33.

Agranulocytosis

Agranulocytosis for practical purposes is synonymous with **neutropenia** (q.v.). Theoretically, the term also includes deficiency of the other granulocytes, namely eosinophils and basophils.

Bibliography

Vincent PC 1986 Drug-induced aplastic anemia and agranulocytosis. Drugs 31: 52.

AIDS (see Acquired immunodeficiency syndrome)

Air embolism (see Diving)

Alcohol, methyl (see Methanol)

Aldosterone (see also Renin–angiotensin–aldosterone and Conn's syndrome)

Aldosterone is produced in the zona glomerulosa of the adrenal gland from cholesterol and acetate precursors. It is the chief mineralocorticoid and promotes the renal tubular reabsorption of sodium and water.

- It is stimulated chiefly by angiotensin but also by ACTH, hyperkalaemia, hyponatraemia and hypovolaemia.
- It is inhibited by dopamine in low doses which thus causes a natriuresis, an important phenomenon in Intensive Care patients, in whom secondary aldosteronism is common.

Aldosterone circulates in the free form and is metabolized in the liver, so that its level is increased in many liver disorders. Aldosterone causes an increased blood volume and cardiac output via sodium and water retention, and there may be associated increased blood pressure from the vasoconstrictor effects of angiotensin II. These volume and blood pressure signals cause the juxtaglomerular apparatus in the kidney to reduce renin release, a negative feedback effect.

Bibliography

Melby JC 1991 Diagnosis of hyperaldosteronism. Endocrinol Metab Clin North Am 20: 247.

Quinn SJ, Williams GH 1988 Regulation of aldosterone secretion. Ann Rev Physiol 50: 409.

White PC 1994 Disorders of aldosterone biosynthesis and action. N Engl J Med 331: 250.

Alkaloids

Alkaloids are a class of organic compounds containing carbon, hydrogen and nitrogen and often possessing powerful physiological effects. They are usually derived from flowering plants and are complex structures generally containing some type of ring. They are chemically basic (i.e. alkaline), hence their name. Their role in nature is unknown.

Alkaloids include substances such as:

- ephedrine;
- morphine;
- nicotine;
- quinine;
- strychnine.

Some plant alkaloids are common cancer chemotherapy agents (e.g. vincristine, vinblastine). They bind to structural proteins in the cytoplasm and thus prevent the formation of microtubules and the spindle apparatus in mitosis.

Alkaloids of the pyrrolizidine class are found in many plants and are sometimes ingested in herbal or bush teas, following which they may produce hepatic veno-occlusive disease (q.v.).

Allergic bronchopulmonary aspergillosis (see Aspergillosis and Eosinophilia and lung infiltration)

Allergic granulomatosis and angiitis (see Churg–Strauss syndrome)

Alopecia

Alopecia, which refers to loss of bodily hair, can have many causes and may vary in extent from the loss of an area of hair on the scalp to the loss of all bodily hair, even including eyebrows and eyelashes.

1. **Alopecia areata** is a localized condition of unknown cause, occurring in young people and with one or more areas of complete hair loss, usually on the scalp. There is minimal inflammation clinically (although histological examination shows lymphoid cells around the hair bulbs), and the process is usually reversible within three years.

As it is (like vitiligo) associated with several autoimmune diseases, especially Addison's disease, thyroiditis and pernicious anaemia, it is probably an autoimmune phenomenon itself.

It is treated with local steroids. Local irritants assist and phototherapy and/or minoxidil may help in some patients.

2. **Androgenetic alopecia** or male baldness has well known features, though an underlying endocrine disorder should be sought if it occurs in young women.

If the result is cosmetically unacceptable, it may be treated with oestrogens and antiandrogens if indicated for other reasons (e.g. hirsutism) or with minoxidil topically (1 mL of 2% in alcohol bd).

3. **Stress alopecia** (telogen effluvium) is a diffuse thinning of the hair following a severe physiological insult which has altered the growth cycle of hairs so as to convert the majority in the active phase to the resting phase.

- It is well known to follow severe clinical disease, such as fever, haemorrhage, surgery, trauma, starvation, childbirth or psychiatric illness.

- It may also accompany specific diseases, such as iron deficiency, thyroid disease and secondary syphilis.
- It may follow the use of a number of drugs, most notably cytotoxic agents (which interfere with mitosis in the hair follicles, rather than converting them to the resting phase) but also allopurinol, heparin, indomethacin, lithium, nitrofurantoin and propranolol. Oral contraceptives on the other hand can give an androgenetic alopecia.

4. **Cicatricial alopecia** is permanent loss of hair due to destruction of the hair follicles from severe viral, bacterial or fungal infection. It is associated with trauma, neoplasia, scleroderma, discoid lupus, atrophic lichen planus or occasionally severe acne.

5. **Traction alopecia** refers to local hair loss from mechanical trauma, sometimes from fingers (trichotillomania).

Bibliography
Munro DD, Darley CR 1979 Hair. In: Fitzpatrick TB, Eisen AZ, Wolff K et al (eds) Dermatology in General Medicine. New York: McGraw-Hill. p 395.

Shapiro J, Price VH 1998 Hair regrowth: therapeutic options. Dermatol Clin 16: 341.

Tosti A, Piraccini BM 1999 Androgenetic alopecia. Int J Dermatol 38 (suppl 1): 1.

Alpha-fetoprotein

Alpha-fetoprotein (AFP, tumour-associated antigen) is an oncofetal antigen, present in fetal tissue but not in the corresponding normal adult tissue. It is, however, elaborated in a number of adult malignant cells, because most of the antigen is carbohydrate-determined and post-translational modification is readily achieved by differential glycosylation (which becomes similar to that in fetal tissue). The normal level is <7.75 μg/L. Its half-life is 6 days.

Increased levels of alpha-fetoprotein are found in:

- hepatoma;
- liver metastases from gastrointestinal cancer;
- acute and chronic hepatitis;
- non-seminoma testicular cancer;
- extragonadal germ cell tumour (e.g. in the anterior mediastinum);
- fetal neural tube defects, when it may be demonstrated in both the maternal blood and in the embryonic fluid.

Bibliography
McIntire KR, Waldmann TA, Moertel CG et al 1975 Serum alpha-fetoprotein in patients with neoplasms of the gastrointestinal tract. Cancer Res 35: 991.

Alpha₁-antitrypsin deficiency

Alpha₁-antitrypsin deficiency was first described as a serum electrophoretic abnormality by Laurell and Eriksson in Scandinavia in 1963 and was soon recognized to be associated with chronic airway obstruction.

Alpha₁-antitrypsin (α_1 AT) is one of the major plasma antiproteases. It is thus a member of the serpin superfamily, inhibitors controlling coagulation, fibrinolysis and complement activation. It is also an acute phase reactact. It has 392 amino acid sequence, and its molecular weight is 52 kd. It is synthesized mainly in the liver and has a plasma concentration of about 1–2 g/L. In the alveolar wall, it is presumed to function to inactivate proteases, especially neutrophil elastase, and thus to prevent interstitial injury from the recurrent release of this enzyme from phagocytes.

Alpha₁-antitrypsin has a complex inheritance with over 30 autosomal codominant alleles at a single locus called Pi ('protease inhibitor') on chromosome 14 producing gene products which are separately identifiable by their different electrophoretic mobility, though most are associated with a normal concentration of the protein in plasma. The most frequent protein is Pi^M, i.e. of medium mobility, and is found in 90% or more of the population. However, homozygous Pi^{ZZ} occurs in 1:1000 or less of the population and is associated with only 10–15% of the normal plasma concentration. The Z variant has only a single amino acid difference from the normal M protein, but this difference impairs hepatic excretion of the molecule, so that there are granular cytoplasmic inclusion bodies in the liver associated with the plasma deficiency in affected subjects.

The clinical importance of alpha₁-antitrypsin deficiency (α_1-ATD) is its association with emphysema in most patients (80%). The incidence is 100% in those who also smoke. The emphysema occurs early, i.e. by 35–40 y in smokers and by 45–55 y in non-smokers. It is usually panacinar and especially affects the lower lobes. It is responsible for about 2% of cases of emphysema.

Hepatic cirrhosis also occurs in 10–20% of patients, mainly in those over 50 y.

In severe α_1-ATD, there may be an increased incidence of asthma.

The heterozygotes Pi^{MZ} have about 50% of the normal plasma concentration, which is now considered not to be associated with clinical disease, the threshold for which is probably about 40% of normal.

*Treatment consists of **replacement therapy**, either 60 mg/kg weekly or 250 mg/kg monthly, though trial evidence of its value is incomplete. However, even in the absence of randomized, placebo-controlled trials of mortality reduction, replacement therapy although expensive (about US$50 000 per year) has been calculated to be probably cost-effective.*

- *Clearly smoking should be avoided.*
- *Successful lung transplantation has been reported.*

Bibliography

Alkins SA, O'Malley P 2000 Should health-care systems pay for replacement therapy in patients with α_1-antitrypsin deficiency? Chest 117: 875.

Burdon JGW, Knight KR, Brenton S et al 1996 Antiproteinase deficiency, emphysema and replacement therapy. Aust NZ J Med 26: 769.

Carrell RW, Whisstock J, Lomas DA 1994 Conformational changes in serpins and the mechanism of alpha₁-antitrypsin deficiency. Am J Resp Crit Care Med 150: S171.

Eden E, Mitchell D, Mehlman B et al 1997 Atopy, asthma, and emphysema in patients with severe α-1-antitrypsin deficiency. Am J Repir Crit Care Med 156: 68.

Gadek JE (ed) 1997 Alpha₁-antitrypsin: A world view. Chest 110 (suppl).

Hutchison DCS, Hughes MD 1997 Alpha-1-antitrypsin replacement therapy: will its efficacy ever be proved? Eur Respir J 10: 2191.

Larsson C 1978 Natural history and life expectancy in severe α_1-antitrypsin PiZ. Acta Med Scand 204: 345.

Laurell C-B, Erikson S 1963 The electrophoretic α_1-globin pattern of serum in α_1-antitrypsin deficiency. Scand J Clin Lab Invest 15: 132.

Stoller JK 1997 Clinical features and natural history of severe α_1-antitrypsin deficiency. Chest 111: 123S.

Altitude (see High altitude)

Aluminium

Aluminium (A1, atomic number 13, atomic weight 27, first called **aluminum**) is a light metal of the boron group, first isolated in 1825. Although it is the most abundant metal in the earth's outer crust, comprising 8% by weight (and exceeded in abundance only by the elements oxygen and silicon), it is never found pure in nature because of its great reactivity, and it is usually obtained as hydrated oxides (bauxite). Following modern production in 1886, it progressively became the most used non-ferrous metal, and since 1960 it was exceeded only by iron in world metal production.

Aluminium is important in clinical medicine because of:

- its use in gastric medications, and
- its toxicity.

Aluminium-containing antacids are commonly prescribed but should be used with care, particularly in renal failure, because they are very constipating and because of the possibility of aluminium absorption.

Aluminium is also contained within multiple negatively charged sulfated groups in sucralfate, which is a basic aluminium salt of sulfated sucrose. Although aluminium can be released from sucralfate with the production of detectable levels in serum, clinical harm from this phenomenon is unlikely, except perhaps in patients with renal failure in whom toxic levels (i.e. >3.7 μmol/L) have been reported.

Aluminium toxicity is seen primarily in patients with renal failure, since it is normally excreted via the kidney. It occurs either because of intake from aluminium-contaminated dialysis solution or from oral aluminium-containing phosphate binders. The normal serum aluminium is usually <10 μg/L and toxicity is seen at levels >100 μg/L. However, serum levels are an indirect indication of body load and can be normal even if tissues such as bone and brain are loaded.

Toxicity is manifest by:

- encephalopathy;
- osteomalacia;
- anaemia.

The **encephalopathy** has been termed dialysis dementia and may be a progressive and eventually fatal process. Increased neurological difficulty occurs with confusion, aphasia, myoclonus and focal signs, which typically are worse after each dialysis. However, it should be remembered that an encephalopathy of non-specific nature is also seen in uraemia and following dialysis. This latter encephalopathy does not correlate with identifiable biochemical changes but is probably related to rapid dialysis-induced biochemical dysequilibrium, when the serum osmolality becomes less than the cerebral osmolality with resultant cerebral oedema causing stupor, fits and raised intracranial pressure.

The **osteomalacia** is vitamin D-resistant, typically with a slightly increased plasma calcium level, a low PTH level, weakness and proximal myopathy, and severe bone pain with pathological fractures. This arises because aluminium blocks the mineralization of osteoid. Since the process is vitamin D-resistant, the administration of vitamin D may result in marked hypercalcaemia. Osteomalacia of a similar nature has been reported with long-term total parenteral nutrition, also from aluminium deposition.

The **anaemia** is usually normochromic and normocytic and occurs because aluminium inhibits iron utilization and thus the erythroid precursors. The irons stores and serum ferritin levels are normal.

The diagnosis of aluminium toxicity is made by desferrioxamine (DFO) challenge and confirmed by bone biopsy. The DFO challenge consists of the administration of 40 mg/kg iv over 30 min and the demonstration of an increase in serum aluminium level of >200 μg/L at 48 h. Bone biopsy shows the typical changes of aluminium-induced osteomalacia, with decreased bone formation and aluminium deposits on the calcifying front on trabecular surfaces.

The treatment of aluminium toxicity is also with **desferrioxamine** *(DFO), in a dose 2 g iv over 30 min after dialysis. The DFO–aluminium complex is removed by the next dialysis, though aluminium itself is not normally removed by dialysis because it is protein-bound. Improvement can take six months or more, and in the meantime DFO treatment can cause hypotension, retinal and auditory toxicity, proneness to opportunistic infections (especially with Yersinia) and increased dialysis encephalopathy (see Chelating agents).*

Bibliography
Alfrey AC 1984 Aluminum intoxication. N Engl J Med 310: 1113.

Ciba Foundation 1992 Aluminium in Biology and Medicine. London.

Cooke K, Gould MH 1991 The health effects of aluminium – a review. J R Soc Health 111: 163.

Kaiser L, Schwartz KA 1985 Aluminum-induced anemia. Am J Kidney Dis 6: 348.

McCarthy DM 1991 Drug therapy (sucralfate) N Engl J Med 325: 1017.

Mulla H, Peek G, Upton D et al 2001 Plasma aluminum levels during sucralfate prophylaxis for stress ulceration in critically ill patients on continuous venovenous hemofiltration: a randomized controlled trial. Crit Care Med 29: 267.

Wills MR, Savory J 1983 Aluminium poisoning: dialysis encephalopathy, osteomalacia, and anaemia. Lancet 2: 29.

Alveolar hypoventilation (see Sleep disorders of breathing)

Alzheimer's disease (see Dementia)

Amanita (see Mushroom poisoning)

Amenorrhoea

Primary amenorrhoea (i.e. failure of periods to commence) is relatively rare.

Secondary amenorrhoea (i.e. the cessation of periods) is of much greater clinical importance. The commonest causes are pregnancy or the menopause, but otherwise the condition is probably due to anovulation.

Failure of ovulation can be due to a variety of disorders and can occur at several levels, namely:

- hypothalamus (this probably includes athlete's amenorrhoea, which appears to be a reversible neuro-endocrine disturbance, and amenorrhoea due to significant weight loss),
- pituitary (especially due to a microadenoma, which is associated with hyperprolactinaemia),
- ovary (associated with the polycystic ovary

syndrome or with systemic problems, such as autoimmune disease or cytotoxic therapy).

Bibliography

Nattiv A, Agostini R, Drinkwater B et al 1994 The female athlete triad: the inter-relatedness of disordered eating, amenorrhea, and osteoporosis. Clin sports Med 13: 405.

Tan SL, Jacobs HS 1985 Recent advances in the management of patients with amenorrhoea. Clin Obstet Gynaecol 12: 725.

Aminoaciduria

Aminoaciduria occurs in many forms of renal disease. These include some types of:

- glomerulonephritis (e.g. focal GN);
- tubulointerstitial disease (e.g. Fanconi syndrome).

It is often associated with normoglycaemic glycosuria.

Aminocaproic acid (see Angioedema, Fibrinolysis and Von Willebrand's disease)

Ammonia (see Acute lung irritation and Burns, respiratory complications)

Amnesia

Amnesia (memory impairment) may be due to a variety of disorders, which may grouped as follows:

- drugs

  - such as, classically, alcohol or sedatives (particularly benzodiazepines);
  - but also unexpectedly sometimes with ranitidine, simvastatin, selective serotonin reuptake inhibitors (SSRIs),

- metabolic disorders

  - such as hypoglycaemia or multi-organ failure;

- structural problems

  - such as cerebrovascular disease, head injury, organic psychosis;

- transient global amnesia

  - a brief and benign state with a good prognosis;

- miscellaneous conditions

  - such as narcolepsy, though this does not usually cause amnesia.

Amniotic fluid embolism

Amniotic fluid embolism (AFE) is an uncommon but serious complication of labour, delivery or the early postpartum state. Although it may accompany any obstetric procedure, it is most frequently seen following Caesarean section. It may also occur in prolonged labour, following fetal death in utero or with elective evacuation of a missed second trimester abortion. Its overall prevalence is 1 in 8000–80 000 live births. It presents acutely, and its severity may range from subclinical to fulminating.

Typically, the clinical features are of the sudden onset of:

- respiratory failure, with an ARDS-like picture;
- disseminated intravascular coagulation.

There may be shock, coma or fits.

Haemodynamic findings include pulmonary hypertension, elevated pulmonary artery wedge pressure and impaired left ventricular function (e.g. decreased LVSWI).

Diagnosis is clinical, as laboratory evidence of circulating fetal material in the mother is non-specific. Recently, the serological identification in maternal serum of sialyl TN (STN) antigen, derived from fetal mucin, has been reported to be a highly sensitive diagnostic test for AFE.

The differential diagnosis includes:

- placental abruption;
- septic shock;
- pulmonary embolism;
- tension pneumothorax;
- myocardial ischaemia.

Treatment is prompt **resuscitation**, *and cardiorespiratory and haematological support, since the condition is self-limited.*

The mortality in severe cases used to be about 80%, with up to half dying in the first hour. It is doubtful if the prognosis is currently as poor as this, but the condition is still the cause of about 10% of all maternal deaths.

Bibliography
Choi DMA, Duffy BL 1995 Amniotic fluid embolism. Anaes Intens Care 23: 741.
McDougall RJ, Duke GJ 1995 Amniotic fluid embolism syndrome: case report and review. Anaes Intens Care 23: 735.
Morgan M 1979 Amniotic fluid embolism. Anaesthesia 34: 20.
Oi H, Kobayashi H, Hirashima Y et al 1998 Serological and immunohistochemical diagnosis of amniotic fluid embolism. Semin Thromb Hemost 24: 479.

Amoebiasis

Amoebiasis is due to infection with *Entamoeba histolytica*, the main human pathogen in this class. Infection occurs following the ingestion of cysts from infected human faeces and is thus via water-borne or food-borne routes. There is a worldwide prevalence of up to 10%.

Clinical infection usually involves either the colon or the liver.

- Although most cases of colitis are asymptomatic, abdominal discomfort and diarrhoea, even to the extent of dysentery, may be seen. In these cases, there is extensive colonic invasion with necrosis and ulceration. Occasionally, an abdominal mass (amoeboma) may be felt.
- The liver is involved via haematogenous

spread. The right lobe is particularly involved, and there is often a solitary abscess which may be up to 20 cm in diameter. In most such cases, the colitis has been asymptomatic and instead there is abdominal pain, hepatomegaly and marked systemic symptoms if the abscess ruptures into the chest.

Investigations typically show anaemia, leukocytosis and raised alkaline phosphatase. The faeces are positive for occult blood and may show Charcot–Leyden crystals. Imaging confirms a liver mass. However, definitive diagnosis requires microscopic examination of faeces or biopsy material for cysts or trophozoites. Serology is sensitive and specific for invasive disease, though not for colitis alone.

The differential diagnosis of amoebic colitis includes:

- diverticulitis;
- ulcerative colitis;
- Crohn's disease;
- infection with campylobacter, salmonella or shigella;
- irritable bowel syndrome.

The differential diagnosis of an amoebic liver mass includes:

- pyogenic or hydatid abscess.

Treatment is with **metronidazole** *750 mg orally tds for 5–10 days. This is so effective even for liver abscess that drainage is not usually necessary. However, metronidazole may be associated with unpleasant side-effects, including nausea, headache, dizziness, a metallic taste, dark urine and a disulfiram-like effect following ingestion of alcohol.*

Bibliography
Adams EB, Macleod IN 1977 Invasive amebiasis. Medicine 56: 315, 325.

Amphetamines

Amphetamine (alpha-methylphenethylamine) has few medical indications approved nowadays (e.g. narcolepsy, childhood hyperactivity). Its main use is non-medical, as a CNS-stimulant. It is thus popular with long-distance truck drivers and students prior to examinations.

The amphetamines are racemic β-phenolisopropylamine, although the d-isomer (dexamphetamine) is the main therapeutic agent. A related drug is 3.4-methylenedioxyamphetamine (MDMA or Ectasy), a derivative synthesized in 1914 as an appetite suppressant but never marketed.

CNS stimulation gives psychic effects of alertness, euphoria, increased concentration, increased mental performance (but only for simple tasks), increased physical performance (but not aerobic power), but also anorexia, headache and confusion. MDMA (Ecstasy) prompts abnormal behaviour, such as marathon dancing, especially when taken by a group (aggregation toxicology) as at 'rave' parties.

The toxic effects of amphetamine are numerous and can be life-threatening. They include the following.

- **Central effects**

  - Those described above are accompanied by an acute psychosis.
  - This consists of aggression, hallucinations, paranoia and enhanced libido, followed later by depression and fatigue.
  - Fatal coma, seizures or cerebral haemorrhage may occur.
  - Hyponatraemia may result from vasopressin stimulation.

- **Cardiovascular features**

  - These are usually prominent due to the drug's sympathomimetic effects.
  - Hypertension, arrhythmias, angina and vasculitis are seen.

- **Hyperthermia and rhabdomyolysis**

  - These are followed by coagulopathy and acute renal failure.

– These features are seen especially with MDMA and resemble the 'serotonin syndrome' (see below).

- **Dry mouth, metallic taste and abdominal pain**
- **Acute liver failure, with damage resembling hepatitis**

The toxic effects of amphetamine are not simply related to excess dosage, as they can be either

- severe following a dose as low as 30 mg (which is only a maximum daily therapeutic dose), or
- not fatal at doses as high as 300 mg.

Acute treatment consists of **urinary acidification** *(e.g. with ammonium chloride, which increases excretion), sedation and blood pressure control (e.g. with sodium nitroprusside). Dantrolene and serotonin antagonists may be useful in the management of MDMA-induced hyperthermia.*

Chronic use can result in considerable tolerance. Thus, despite increasingly high doses, euphoria disappears and fatigue, depression, irritability and even paranoia appear. Headache, nausea, tremor, dilated pupils and hypertension are common.

Abrupt withdrawal leads to profound psychological though not physical consequences, in particular with depression which may be severe and prolonged.

The related anorectic drugs, **fenfluramine**, **dexfenfluramine** and **phentermine**, were recently withdrawn from the market worldwide, because of the discovery of an increased incidence of pulmonary hypertension (20-fold risk above baseline) and a potentially important association with acquired heart valve abnormalities. The valvulopathy typically causes mitral and/or aortic regurgitation and sometimes requires valve replacement. The pathogenesis of this latter unexpected effect is unknown, but it has been postulated to be similar to the cardiac impact of the carcinoid

syndrome or ergot derivatives. Neither its progression nor its reversibility is presently known.

The **'serotonin syndrome'** comprises:

- altered mental state (agitation, confusion);
- autonomic dysfunction (sweating, shivering, fever, diarrhoea);
- increased neuromuscular activity (hyperreflexia, tremor, myoclonus).

It is due to a drug reaction involving one or more serotonergic agents, including:

- amphetamine and related compounds;
- selective serotonin reuptake inhibitors (SSRIs, e.g. fluoxetine, paroxetine, sertraline);
- tricyclic antidepressants;
- monoamine oxidase inhibitors;
- pethidine;
- pseudoephedrine.

It usually responds to drug cessation and supportive care. Occasionally, it may be fulminating and require serotonin antagonist therapy, such as with cyproheptadine, methysergide, chlorpromazine or benzodiazepines.

Bibliography

Chan BSH, Graudins A, Whyte IM et al 1998 Serotonin syndrome resulting from drug interactions. Med J Aust 169: 523.

Connolly HM, Crary JL, McGoon MD et al 1997 Valvular heart disease associated with fenfluramine-phentermine. N Engl J Med 337: 581.

Fishman AP 1999 Aminorex to fen/phen: an epidemic foretold. Circulation 99: 156.

Henry JA, Jeffreys KJ, Dawling S 1992 Toxicity and deaths from 3.4-methylenedioxy-methamphetamine ('ecstasy'). Lancet 340: 384.

Milroy CM 1999 Ten years of 'ecstasy'. J R Soc Med 92: 68.

Parrott AC (ed) 2000 MDMA (Methylenedioxy-methamphetamine). Basel: Karger.

Screaton GR, Cairns HS, Sarner M et al 1992

Hyperpyrexia and rhabdomyolysis after MDMA ('ecstasy') abuse. Lancet 339: 677.

Sternbach H 1991 The serotonin syndrome. Am J Psych 148:705.

Amyloid (see Multiple myeloma)

Amyotrophic lateral sclerosis

Amyotrophic lateral sclerosis (motor neurone disease) is a condition of degeneration of the pyramidal motor neurones from the cortex as far as the anterior horn cells of the spinal cord. It is an uncommon condition of unknown aetiology, most commonly affecting middle-aged men.

Clinical features comprise a slowly progressive weakness and wasting, associated with fasciculation, hyper-reflexia and muscle cramps. The process can be distal or proximal early, but progressive proximal involvement then occurs.

There are no sensory or autonomic features and no eye involvement, but there may be bulbar or pseudobulbar palsy.

The EMG shows denervation. The differential diagnosis includes:

- cervical cord compression;
- polymyositis;
- **multifocal motor neuropathy** (MMN). This recently described condition is similar to motor neurone disease, but it is due to a slowly progressive nerve conduction defect of asymmetric distribution, particularly involving the upper limbs. It responds to immune globulin.

There is no treatment for amyotrophic lateral sclerosis. Survival is about 3 y from diagnosis.

Bibliography
Pestronk A 1991 Motor neuropathies, motor neuron disorders, and antiglycolipid antibodies. Muscle Nerve 14: 927.

Anaemia

Anaemia refers to decreased circulating haemoglobin, but as for many biological parameters any definition based on a single number is of limited value. Thus, acute blood loss is not initially associated with a decreased haemoglobin concentration, while haemodilution (e.g. in pregnancy) can cause a decreased haemoglobin concentration while being associated with an increased red blood cell mass.

Nevertheless, anaemia is defined as a haemoglobin level below the lower limit of normal for the sex and age of the patient, which in turn depends on the range determined in a specific clinical laboratory (the typical normal range being 130–170 g/L for men and 115–150 g/L for women). For practical purposes, anaemia may be considered present if the Hb is <100 g/L in men and <90 g/L in women.

Anaemia is traditionally classified on the basis of red blood cell kinetics and morphology into three main aetiological groups, namely those due to:

- blood loss;
- haemolysis;
- impaired production.

---

1. Anaemia due to blood loss

Although blood loss is usually readily apparent, sometimes it may be occult, especially from the gastrointestinal tract. Blood loss whether overt or occult is most commonly from the gastrointestinal tract or in women from obstetric or gynaecological causes. In Intensive Care patients, it may be iatrogenic.

Rarer causes of a similar anaemia include:

- long-distance athletic performance;
- paroxysmal nocturnal haemoglobinuria.

In acute blood loss, the haemoglobin concentration may take up to three days to reach its new (lower) plateau.

After acute blood loss, the bone marrow reserve is less than 2-fold (unlike in haemolysis when it is up to 8-fold), because iron is mobilized less easily from the tissues than from the destroyed red blood cells. Moreover, the maximum amount of iron that can be mobilized from stores is insufficient to replace even normally senescent red blood cells.

The clinical features of blood loss or iron deficiency anaemia are those of any form of hypoxia. In addition, there is:

- increased susceptibility to infections in general

    – but paradoxically a possibly increased resistance to *E. coli* and malaria,

- cold intolerance;
- gastro-oesophageal mucosal atrophy

    – with dysphagia (Plummer–Vinson syndrome) and achlorhydria;

- koilonychia;
- blue sclerae;
- abnormal fetal and childhood development;
- sometimes pica

    – especially compulsive eating of abnormal material, such as ice.

The differential diagnosis of anaemia due to blood loss includes:

- the anaemia of chronic disease;
- haemoglobinopathy (especially thalassaemia);
- sideroblastic anaemia.

Unless the condition is mild, when diagnosis may be difficult, there is:

- hypochromia and microcytosis on the peripheral blood film;
- low serum iron;
- low iron-binding saturation (ratio of serum iron to serum transferrin or iron-binding capacity is <20%) – a more important finding;

- low serum ferritin (which reflects iron stores) – also a more important finding.

However, the serum iron, transferrin and iron binding saturation are also low in anaemia of chronic disease, and the serum ferritin may be elevated by concomitant disease, such as infection or malignancy.

Treatment with iron supplementation is straightforward, but failure of response suggests:
- *persistent bleeding;*
- *concurrent inflammation;*
- *associated folic acid deficiency;*
- *failure of iron absorption (malabsorption or iron-binding foods);*
- *an alternative diagnosis.*

2. Anaemia due to haemolysis

Haemolytic anaemia occurs when the rate of red blood cell destruction exceeds the bone marrow's productive capacity. Thus, although the normal life-span of red blood cells in the circulation is about 115 days (with thus about 1% or the equivalent of 50 mL of blood being destroyed and replaced daily), the marrow reserve is such that it can compensate for a red blood cell life-span of 30 days or less. The marrow reserve is thus considerable, being normally about 5-fold and rising to perhaps 8-fold with severe and prolonged stimulation, provided there is an adequate haematinic supply.

The hallmarks of haemolysis are:

- anaemia;
- jaundice;
- a marked reticulocytosis on peripheral blood film;
- pigment gallstones in longstanding cases.

Haemolysis is due to either **intracorpuscular** or **extracorpuscular** defects. The sites of destruction are usually **extravascular** (i.e. the reticuloendothelial system), except in severe cases when it can be **intravascular** (with resultant haemoglobinaemia, haemoglobinuria and disseminated intravascular coagulation).

Intracorpuscular defects indicate an abnormal red blood cell. All such conditions are hereditary, except for paroxysmal nocturnal haemoglobinuria. Intracorpuscular defects may be of haemoglobin, cell membrane or cell metabolism.

- **Haemoglobin defects** are numerous (see Haemoglobin disorders) and particularly include sickle cell anaemia and thalassaemia.
- **Red blood cell membrane defects** include:

  – hereditary spherocytosis,
  – paroxysmal nocturnal haemoglobinuria (PNH), which in addition to anaemia is also associated with neutropenia, thrombocytopenia, thromboembolism, and occasionally aplastic anaemia or even leukaemia.

- **Red blood cell metabolic defects** particularly include glucose 6-phosphate dehydrogenase (G6PD) deficiency (q.v.).

Extracorpuscular defects include the following.

- **Autoimmune haemolytic anaemia** (AHA). This may be either idiopathic or secondary to conditions such as lymphoma, multiple myeloma, SLE, ulcerative colitis. The direct Coombs test is positive, and there may be jaundice, hepatosplenomegaly and lymphadenopathy in severe cases. In addition to spherocytosis, there is macrocytosis and sometimes leukopenia or thrombocytopenia.

*The condition usually responds to **corticosteroids**, but sometimes splenectomy or immunosuppressive therapy may be needed.*

Blood cross-matching is difficult.

- **Microangiopathic haemolysis**

q.v.

- **Cold agglutinin disease**

q.v.

- **Drug-induced haemolysis**

Methyldopa in particular, but also laevodopa and procainamide, can cause an acquired haemolytic anaemia.

Aspirin, beta-lactam antibiotics, isoniazid, quinidine, rifampicin and sulfonamides can contribute to immune haemolysis.

Nitroglycerin, 'recreational' nitrites and dapsone can occupy the oxygen-binding cleft of haemoglobin and generate free radicals with the consequent production of methaemoglobin (q.v.) and possibly haemolysis due to membrane damage. A similar picture has been reported after paraquat ingestion.

Haemolysis similar to that induced by drugs may also be found with:

  – exposure to toxins (e.g. snake venom);
  – physical agents (e.g. cardiopulmonary bypass, fresh-water drowning, burns, intravenous water);
  – liver disease;
  – renal disease;
  – lead poisoning (q.v.);
  – infections (clostridial, infectious mononucleosis, *H. influenzae* type b, malaria);
  – hypophosphataemia (<0.3 mmol/L).

A similar picture has also been reported following Intralipid overdose.

- **Incompatible blood transfusion**
- **March haemoglobinuria**. This is similar to microangiopathic haemolysis (q.v.), except that it occurs after prolonged running, especially on a hard surface. It is presumed to be due to destruction of red blood cells in the vessels in the soles of the feet. There is haemoglobinaemia and haemoglobinuria, which may be clinically apparent for up to 24 h.

- **Hypersplenism**

q.v.

3. **Anaemia due to impaired production**

Anaemia due to impaired production may be associated with a bone marrow which is:

- hypoplastic;
- normal;
- hyperplastic.

Marrow hypoplasia usually results in concomitant neutropenia and/or thrombocytopenia (and thus infection and/or haemorrhage) as well as anaemia. Compensatory extramedullary haemopoiesis is evident from the leukoerythroblastic peripheral blood film. There may be immunological damage to pluripotential haematopoietic stem cells in the marrow, regardless of the causative trigger. The condition is referred to as **aplastic anaemia**. It is caused by:

- drugs
    - cytotoxics, sometimes chloramphenicol, gold and previously phenylbutazone;
- toxic inhalants
    - e.g. organic solvents, such as benzene;
- irradiation;
- infections
    - especially hepatitis C;
- immune diseases
    - SLE, graft-versus-host disease;
- pre-leukaemia or paroxysmal nocturnal haemoglobinuria;
- thymoma
    - which is typically associated with a pure red cell aplasia.

Pure red cell aplasia (PRCA) is a separate condition on cytogenetic testing and appears to be a prodrome to acute myeloid leukaemia or a myelodysplastic disorder.

Normal-appearing bone marrow may be associated with defective red cell production and thus anaemia in systemic disease and in renal disease.

Systemic diseases, such as inflammation, neoplasia and trauma, cause **anaemia of chronic disease**. This is normochromic and normocytic, with both the serum iron and iron binding capacity low and ferritin normal. The serum erythropoietin level is often low. The anaemia is generally mild and may be multifactorial, with IL-1 causing the trapping in macrophages of the iron from senescent red blood cells.

In chronic renal disease, especially during haemodialysis programmes, the anaemia is generally moderate (5–8 g/L) and is erythropoietin-responsive.

Marrow hyperplasia may paradoxically be associated with anaemia if there is ineffective erythropoiesis. An erythroid defect causes premature cell death in the bone marrow and thus some of the features of haemolysis. This condition is seen in some cases of:

- megaloblastic anaemia (q.v.),
- sideroblastic anaemia (q.v.),
- thalassaemia (q.v.),
- myelofibrosis (agnogenic myeloid metaplasia).

Bibliography

Anderson KC, Weinstein HJ 1990 Transfusion-associated graft-versus-host disease. N Engl J Med 323: 315.

Barrett-Connor E 1972 Anemia and infection. Am J Med 52: 242.

Editorial 1992 Paroxysmal nocturnal haemoglobinuria. Lancet 339: 395.

Engelfriet CP, Overbeeke MAM, von dem Borne AEGK 1992 Autoimmune hemolytic anemia. Semin Hematol 29: 3.

Finch CA 1982 Erythropoiesis, erythropoietin, and iron. Blood 60: 1241.

Henry DH, Spivak JL 1995 Clinical use of erythropoietin. Curr Opin Hematol 2: 118.

Krantz SB 1991 Erythropoietin. Blood 77: 419.

Marmont AM 1991 Therapy of pure red cell aplasia. Semin Hematol 28: 285.

Marsh JCW, Socie G, Schrezenmeier H et al 1994 Haemopoietic growth factors in aplastic anaemia: a cautionary note. Lancet 344: 172.

Means RT 1999 Advances in the anemia of chronic disease. Int J Hematol 70: 7.

Means RT, Krantz SB 1992 Progress in understanding the pathogenesis of the anemia of chronic disease. Blood 80: 1639.

Vincent PC 1986 Drug-induced aplastic anemia and agranulocytosis. Drugs 31: 52.

Young NS 1992 The problem of clonality in aplastic anaemia: Dr. Damashek's riddle, restated. Blood 79: 1385.

Anaphylaxis (see Drug allergy)

ANCA (see Wegener's granulomatosis)

Aneurysms, mycotic (see Mycotic aneurysms)

Angiodysplasia

Angiodysplasia comprises multiple degenerative vascular lesions. They can occur anywhere in the bowel, though they are most frequently found in the caecum and ascending colon. They are an uncommon but important cause of acute or chronic gastrointestinal blood loss.

Diagnosis is by colonoscopy, angiography or nuclear scan.

Although acute bleeding generally stops spontaneously, surgical resection or colonoscopic electrocoagulation is required for continued haemorrhage.

Angioedema

Hereditary angioedema (HAE) is due to a deficiency of C_1 inhibitor (C_1 INH), a serine protease like many activated coagulation factors. HAE is an autosomal dominant condition, with affected heterozygotes having 5–30% of the normal concentration of C_1 INH.

- Clinically, there are recurrent attacks of non-pitting oedema, lasting 48–72 h and affecting skin, respiratory tract and gut.
- The most dramatic feature is laryngeal oedema, causing potentially fatal upper airway obstruction.
- The oedema is not associated with erythema, pruritus or local discomfort (except sometimes for intestinal colic, due to associated visceral angioedema).
- The attacks are classically initiated by trauma, though more commonly no obvious precipitant is identified.

- Recently, cases have been reported to have been caused by ACE inhibitors and occasionally by the complementary medicine, echinacea. Drug-induced angioedema is of course well known as one of the major features of anaphylaxis, the most dramatic manifestation of drug allergy (q.v.).

Investigations show elevated C_1 and decreased C_4 and C_2 during the attack. Since C_1 INH also inhibits factor XIIa and kallikrein, the coagulation, fibrinolytic and kinin systems are also activated. The formation of the peptide, bradykinin, may be the main pathogenetic mechanism for the increased vascular permeability.

Prophylactic treatment is not generally used, but **epsilon aminocaproic acid (EACA)** *may be helpful. Its mechanism of action in this setting is unknown, though it is a well-recognized inhibitor of fibrinolysis. Anabolic steroids (e.g. danazol) may also be used for prophylaxis.*

There is no specific treatment for acute episodes, but fresh frozen plasma has been reported to be helpful. **Purified C_1 inhibitor** *is available, but it is extremely expensive. There are case reports of this inhibitor also helping ameliorate graft failure after lung transplantation and streptococcal toxic shock syndrome.*

Bibliography

Agah R, Bandi V, Guntupalli KK 1997 Angioedema: the role of ACE inhibitors and factors associated with poor clinical outcome. Intens Care Med 23: 793.

Colten HR 1987 Hereditary angioneurotic edema, 1887 to 1987. N Engl J Med 317: 43.

Fronhoffs S, Luyken J, Steuer K et al 2000 The effect of C1-esterase inhibitor in definite and suspected streptococcal toxic shock syndrome. Intens Care Med 26: 1566.

Gabb GM, Ryan P, Wing LMH et al 1996 Epidemiological study of angioedema and ACE inhibitors. Aust NZ J Med 26: 777.

Waytes AT, Rosen FS, Frank MM 1996 Treatment of hereditary angioedema with a vapor-heated C1 inhibitor concentrate. N Engl J Med 334: 1630.

Angiotensin (see

Renin–angiotensin–aldosterone)

Angiotensin-converting enzyme

(see also angiotensin II receptor antagonists in Renin–angiotensin–aldosterone)

Angiotensin-converting enzyme (ACE) is a membrane-bound enzyme in the pulmonary vessels which converts angiotensin I to angiotensin II in a single passage through the lungs (see Renin–angiotensin–aldosterone). Interestingly, an identical enzyme degrades bradykinin, the vasodilator peptide of the kallikrein-kinin system.

The plasma ACE level is characteristically increased in active sarcoidosis, and also sometimes in biliary cirrhosis, leprosy, pneumoconiosis and tuberculosis.

The **ACE inhibitors** (captopril, enalapril and the several more recent agents) have become major therapeutic agents in cardiovascular disease, especially hypertension and cardiac failure. In hypertension, they have become the most commonly prescribed drugs. In cardiac failure, deterioration and mortality are reduced by ACE inhibitors, not just because of vasodilatation but perhaps also because of remodelling and normalized cell growth. This could occur because angiotensin II is a growth factor, contributing to the maladaptation and thus changed molecular composition rather than just hypertrophy seen in cardiomyopathic processes (see Renin–angiotensin–aldosterone). Cough and angioedema are two interesting side-effects of ACE inhibition, perhaps caused by decreased kinin catabolism.

In addition, there is recent evidence that ACE inhibitors reduce proteinuria in diabetic patients, independent of their effect of blood pressure, and slow the progression of renal failure in nondiabetics.

Bibliography

Curry SC, Arnold-Capell P 1991 Nitroprusside, nitroglycerin, and angiotensin-converting enzyme inhibitors. Crit Care Clin 7: 555.

Franzosi MG, Santoro E, Zuanetti G et al 1998 Indications for ACE inhibitors in the early treatment of acute myocardial infarction: systematic overview of individual data from 100,000 patients in randomized trials. Circulation 97: 2202.

ISIS-4 (Fourth International Study of Infarct Survival) Collaborative Group 1995 ISIS-4: A randomised factorial trial assessing early oral captopril, oral mononitrate, and intravenous magnesium sulphate in 58 050 patients with suspected acute myocardial infarction. Lancet 345: 669.

Lewis EJ, Hunsicker LG, Bain RP et al 1993; The effect of angiotensin-converting-enzyme inhibition on diabetic nephropathy. N Engl J Med 329: 1456.

Luiz W, Wiemer G, Gohlke P et al 1995 Contributions of kinins to the cardiovascular actions of angiotensin-converting enzyme inhibitors. Pharmacol Rev 47: 25.

Pfeffer MA, Lamas GA, Vaughan DE et al 1988 Effect of captopril on progressive ventricular dilatation after anterior myocardial infarction. N Engl J Med 319: 80.

Pitt B, Segal R, Martinez FA et al 1997 Randomised trial of losartan versus captopril in patients over 65 with heart failure (Evaluation of Losartan in the Elderly Study, ELITE). Lancet 349: 747.

Quinn SJ, Williams GH 1988 Regulation of aldosterone secretion. Ann Rev Physiol 50: 409.

Sharpe N, Smith H, Murphy J et al 1991 Early prevention of left ventricular dysfunction after myocardial infarction with angiotensin-converting-enzyme inhibition. Lancet 337: 872.

Vaughn DE, Pfeffer MA 1994 Angiotensin converting enzyme inhibitors and cardiovascular remodelling. Cardiovasc Res 28: 159.

Animal bites (see Bites and stings)

Ankylosing spondylitis

Ankylosing spondylitis is a subgroup of the **spondyloarthropathies** (q.v.), conditions characterized by the combination of sacroiliitis and seronegative peripheral arthropathy.

Although the aetiology is unknown, it may possibly be precipitated by a number of bacterial antigens. There is also a presumed immunogenetic susceptibility, as evidenced by clustering in families and some ethnic groups.

There is a strong correlation with the HLA antigen B27. Thus, 95% of patients with ankylosing spondylitis are B27-positive and ankylosing spondylitis occurs in 10–20% of B27-positive individuals. B27-positive adults comprise about 10% of Caucasian populations and from <1% to about 50% of different ethnic groups around the world.

There is a predominance in men (70%), especially younger men. The clinical presentation usually is of chronic back discomfort. Typically, there is night pain, morning stiffness and improvement after exercise. Early in its course, the condition is often misdiagnosed as mechanical back disease. If it progresses, there is obvious limitation of lumbar spinal mobility and chest expansion. Peripheral arthropathy occurs in 20–30% of cases, usually in large, lower limb joints. Amyloidosis or IgA nephropathy may occur late in the disease.

More severe disease may be associated with:

- systemic symptoms;
- multi-organ changes.

Systemic symptoms include:

- mild fever;
- fatigue;
- weight loss.

Multi-organ changes, especially involve the:

- eye
  - uveitis;
- cardiovascular system
  - aortic valve incompetence;
  - conduction defects;
- lung
  - cystic changes, sometimes with aspergillus superinfection;
  - pulmonary fibrosis.

The X-ray shows sacroiliitis and sometimes involvement higher in the spine. Laboratory results may be normal, though usually there is a raised ESR or increased IgA. Synovial biopsy shows non-specific changes similar to those of rheumatoid arthritis, with inflammatory cell infiltrate, lymphoid follicles and intimal cell hyperplasia.

The diagnosis can sometimes be difficult. Radiological evidence of sacroiliitis remains the strongest evidence, when combined with the clinical features of back pain and stiffness, decreased spinal flexion and decreased chest expansion. HLA–B27 gene testing is not diagnostically helpful.

Treatment is primarily with physical measures and **NSAIDs***.*

- *Sometimes, sulfasalazine, methotrexate and/or corticosteroids are indicated.*
- *Radiotherapy was used successfully in the past, but this led to an increased incidence of leukaemia.*

The prognosis is generally favourable, as the course of the disease is usually very long and mild involvement of the sacroiliac joints only is seen for periods of up to 30 y. However, the natural history is variable, and in some patients the condition progresses to involve the entire spine and there are extra–articular manifestations. If permanent spinal stiffness occurs, the spine is more 'brittle' and fractures can occur with relatively minor trauma.

Bibliography

Callin A, Ellswood J, Riggs S et al 1988 Ankylosing spondylitis – an analytical review of 1500 patients: the changing pattern of disease. J Rheumatol 15: 1234.

Davies D 1972 Ankylosing spondylitis and lung fibrosis. Q J Med 41: 395.

Kahn MA (ed) 1994 Spondyloarthropathies. Curr Opin Rheumatol 6: 351.

Kapasi K, Chui B, Inman RD 1992 HLA-B27/microbial mimicry: an in vivo analysis. Immunology 77: 456.

McEwen C, DiTata D, Lingg C et al 1971 Ankylosing spondylitis and spondylitis accompanying ulcerative colitis, regional enteritis, psoriasis and Reiter's disease. Arthritis Rheum 14: 291.

Anorectal infections

Anorectal infections are most commonly seen in homosexual men. Such infections are, therefore, often sexually transmitted diseases. They include:

- chancroid;
- chlamydial infection;
- condylomata accuminata;
- gonorrhoea;
- granuloma inguinale;
- herpes (HSV);
- syphilis;
- HIV infection.

Rectal inflammation, **proctitis**, may be associated with:

- the anorectal infections described above;
- campylobacter-like organisms;
- meningococci;
- more proximal inflammatory bowel disease;
- radiation.

Anorectic agents (see Amphetamines and Pulmonary hypertension)

Anorexia nervosa

Anorexia nervosa is an uncommon but potentially severe eating disorder, associated with a major decrease in food intake and with resultant weight loss, perhaps up to 30% or more of the ideal body weight.

Its aetiology is unknown, but it is thought that it could be related to a distortion of the modern perception of an ideal body image. This view would be consistent with its increased incidence in recent decades, especially in the more affluent. Its greatest incidence is in adolescent women.

The clinical features are those of starvation, with associated secondary changes, such as endocrine disturbances (including hypothalamic dysfunction and amenorrhoea), lanugo and depression. Clinical features also include coldness, bradycardia, hypotension and cognitive impairment.

Investigations typically show anaemia, leukopenia, hypokalaemia, possibly cardiomyopathy with failure and/or arrhythmias, and occasionally fatty liver, pancreatitis, seizures and parotitis.

Treatment derived from clinical trials is not available, but the usual therapeutic principles include motivation, decreased physical activity and restoration of nutrition. If the process is severe, the daily intake may need to be high (e.g. over 3000 kcal or 12 500 kJ) to ensure progress. Nasogastric tube feeding is rarely required, but drugs such as cyproheptadine or currently fluoxetine may assist.

The prognosis is often disappointing, with only about half the patients being normal after 5 y and about 25% having a continuing poor outlook. The mortality is up to 10%, with half the deaths from suicide. Interestingly, in about 5% of the patients, the outcome is obesity.

Bibliography
Gilchrist PN, Ben-Tovim DI, Hay PJ et al 1998 Eating disorders revisited. 1: anorexia nervosa. Med J Aust 169: 438.

Anthrax

Anthrax is chiefly a disease of animals which is sometimes transmitted to humans from contact with animal products, particularly hides and wool. It is caused by the large, aerobic and highly pathogenic Gram-positive rod, *Bacillus anthracis*, first identified by Koch in 1877. The organism also produces long-lived and resistant spores in the external environment though not in its host. Anthrax is a disease of documented antiquity and may have been the cause of the plagues of Egypt recorded in the Bible 3500 years ago.

The particular current interest in anthrax relates to its potential role in germ warfare and especially in bioterrorist attack. For example, about 100 000 people could be killed by a single strategically dispersed bomb containing only 50 kg of spores.

The clinical manifestations can be several.

1. Cutaneous

The classical presentation is with a necrotic and oedematous but painless ulcer at the site of an infected abrasion.

2. Pulmonary

More rarely, inhalational anthrax causes a serious flu-like pulmonary infection, but with characteristic haemorrhagic mediastinitis, respiratory distress, pleural effusions, meningitis and shock. This form of anthrax was previously called 'woolsorter's disease' and is the form which would be seen in modern germ warfare. It can be produced by the inhalation of as few as 10 000 spores and results in intense bacteraemia.

3. Intestinal

Occasionally, intestinal anthrax may occur due to the ingestion of infected meat. The diagnosis may be late because its clinical features are initially non-specific and it may be unsuspected. The organism is readily identified from blood cultures and serology is positive.

*Treatment is with **antibiotics** (high-dose penicillin) and intensive care with isolation. The organism is also sensitive to tetracycline, amoxycillin, erythromycin and ciprofloxacin but not third-generation cephalosporins.*

Vaccination is available for people at risk. Animal vaccination was introduced by Pasteur in 1881. Without prompt antibiotic therapy, inhalational anthrax is generally fatal and cutaneous anthrax has a mortality of 20%.

Bibliography
LaForce FM 1994 Anthrax. Clin Infect Dis 19: 1009.
Penn CC, Klotz SA 1997 Anthrax pneumonia. Semin Respir Infect 12: 28.
Pile JC, Malone JD, Eitzen EM et al 1998 Anthrax as a potential biological warfare agent. Arch Intern Med 158: 429.
Shafazand S, Doyle R, Ruoss S et al 1999 Inhalational anthrax: epidemiology, diagnosis, and management. Chest 116: 1369.

Antibiotic-associated colitis (see Colitis)

Anticardiolipin antibody (see Antiphospholipid syndrome)

Anticholinergic (cholinolytic) agents

Anticholinergic effects are produced by the following agents:

- atropine and related compounds, including

  - the belladonna alkaloids, such as scopolamine;
  - the synthetic quaternary ammonium compounds with anti-muscarinic action, such as homatropine, ipratropium and propantheline;

- antidepressants (tricyclics);
- antipsychotics (phenothiazines);
- antiparkinsonian drugs (especially benztropine);
- disopyramide;
- mushroom poisons (q.v.);
- nerve agent antidotes.

Anticholinergic effects comprise three actions, namely:

- **anti-muscarinic**;
- **ganglion-blocking**;
- **neuromuscular blocking**.

Clinically, anticholinergic effects are manifest as:

- dry mouth;
- tachycardia;
- constipation;
- urinary retention;

- delirium, particularly in the elderly;
- predisposition to heat stroke.

They are picturesquely described by the mnemonic:

'blind as a bat, dry as a bone, hot as a hare, mad as a hatter and red as a beet'.

These effects are particularly likely to occur in the presence of polypharmacy, including antispasmodics, antidiarrhoeals, antihistamines and some sedatives.

Overdoses of anticholinergic drugs are treated with the anticholinesterases, **physostigmine** (a tertiary amine which penetrates the blood–brain barrier) and **pyridostigmine** (a quaternary amine which has poor cerebral penetration). Both reversibly inhibit acetylcholinesterase and thus protect it. Physostigmine reverses the CNS effects of anticholinergic drugs, though other effects of such poisoning (e.g. cardiac) are not reversed. It is given in a dose of 1–2 mg iv over 5 min and repeated if necessary each 20 min. Since pyridostigmine does not penetrate the blood–brain barrier, it does not impair CNS performance like physostigmine and is therefore useful as prophylaxis.

Since the entire cholinergic spectrum is particularly seen with nerve agents (q.v.), they are antagonized by atropine (in doses up to 6 mg), though newer antagonists with greater CNS effects have been developed. These antagonists particularly include the oximes, e.g. **pralidoxime**, organic compounds which complex with anticholinesterase agents and thus free the enzyme, acetylcholinesterase, so that cholinergic function is restored.

Bibliography

Goldfrank L, Flomenbaum N Levin N et al 1982 Anticholinergic poisoning. J Toxicol Clin Toxicol 19: 17.

Anticholinesterases

Anticholinesterases comprise:

- neostigmine and pyridostigmine;
- edrophonium;
- tetrahydroaminoacridine (THA, tacrine);
- nerve agents (e.g. insecticides, chemical warfare agents).

Acetylcholinesterase (AChE) terminates the action of acetylcholine at cholinergic nerve endings. Therefore, anticholinesterases allow acetylcholine to accumulate at its extensive central and peripheral sites.

Neostigmine and **pyridostigmine** are the main therapeutic anticholinesterases. They permit the accumulation of acetylcholine at neuromuscular junctions and autonomic synapses. They also give rise to muscarinic effects of salivation, sweating, abdominal cramps, diarrhoea, bradycardia and even asystole. Their use and that of **edrophonium** is discussed in the section on myasthenia gravis (q.v.).

THA acts at the neuromuscular junction without a muscarinic effect. THA is also a mild analeptic, prolongs the paralysis induced by suxamethonium and can be used with neostigmine to reverse curarization.

Because of its central actions, it was considered to provide modest therapeutic benefit in Alzheimer's disease, but this benefit has not been confirmed in subsequent studies. A newer anticholinesterase, donepezil, has however been confirmed in large studies to provide symptomatic benefit, though there has been no evidence of decreased disease progression.

Bibliography

Cladwell JE 1995 Reversal of residual neuromuscular block with neostigmine at one to four hours after a single intubating dose of vecuronium. Anesth Analg 80: 1168.

Davis KL, Powchik P 1995 Tacrine. Lancet 345: 625.

Mayeux R, Sano M 1999 Drug therapy: treatment of Alzheimer's disease. N Engl J Med 341: 1670.

Peter JV, Cherian AM 2000 Organic insecticides. Anaes Intens Care 28: 11.

Antidiuretic hormone (see

Desmopressin)

Antinuclear antibodies

Antinuclear antibodies (ANA) are most characteristically associated with SLE, but in fact they are also diagnostically useful in other autoimmune diseases, including Sjögren's syndrome, scleroderma and mixed connective tissue disease.

Several nuclear antigens are recognized by autoantibodies in SLE, with the resultant circulating immune complexes able to injure a number of organs and structures, especially renal glomeruli. Antibodies to native double-strand DNA and soluble (extractable) nuclear antigen called Sm are specific for SLE. Other antibodies include those to denatured single-strand DNA, RNA, nucleoprotein, histones and nucleoli.

While the presence of antinuclear antibodies is diagnostically useful, their pathogenetic role is doubtful, except in congenital heart block which is strongly associated with placental passage of maternal autoantibodies to Ro(SS-A) and La(SS-B).

Antiphospholipid syndrome

The antiphospholipid syndrome (APS) is a hypercoagulable state associated with the presence of anticardiolipin antibody, lupus anticoagulant and possibly other antibodies.

In the 1950s, some patients with SLE were observed to have a long clotting time but a paradoxical thrombotic tendency. In the 1970s, the responsible substance became referred to as the lupus anticoagulant (LA). Subsequently, LA was observed in other (especially autoimmune) diseases and even in some healthy people, so that it was then referred to as the 'lupus-like anticoagulant' (LLA). This 'anticoagulant' was later found to be closely related to antibodies to negatively charged phospholipids such as cardiolipin, so that the syndrome was then referred to as the anticardiolipin syndrome. In 1983, the broader name antiphospholipid syndrome was given to describe the clinical propensity to arterial and venous thrombosis in association with such antibodies. More recently, the name 'Hughes' syndrome' has been proposed.

Although the anticardiolipin antibody (which is responsible for a false positive syphilis test) and the lupus anticoagulant are both antiphospholipids, the immune response appears to be directed to modified proteins rather than to lipids, since a cofactor (most commonly, beta-2 glycoprotein I (β2-GPI), an activator of lipoprotein lipase) is required for anionic phospholipid binding prior to antibody formation. The lipid-binding peptide of β2-GPI is similar to those found in some bacteria and viruses, implying the potential for an infection to stimulate anticardiolipin antibody formation. The antibodies themselves are heterogenerous and usually polyclonal IgG or IgM. Although many different mechanisms have been postulated to explain their in vitro anticoagulant but in vivo thrombotic effects, it is likely that the antibodies themselves are directly responsible for the clinical effects and that the clotting test results are artifacts of non-flowing blood.

Clinical features of APS comprise:

- thromboses

  - including recurrent DVT and other forms of venous thrombosis;

- pulmonary hypertension;
- cerebral artery occlusion

  - with TIA, stroke, ischaemic dementia, ocular ischaemia;

- livedo reticularis

  - i.e. necrotizing purpura;

- heart valve disease

  - including valvular degeneration and verrucous endocarditis;

- resembling culture-negative bacterial endocarditis;
- spontaneous abortion and fetal death;
- miscellaneous problems
  - such as labile hypertension, epilepsy, migraine, transverse myelopathy, thrombocytopenia and depression.

The condition may also be:

- drug-related, especially to chlorpromazine or hydralazine;
- associated with opportunistic infections, as in AIDS.

There is an increased incidence of anticardiolipin antibodies in Behçet's disease.

In Intensive Care patients, '**catastrophic APS**' may be associated with:

- ARDS;
- multi-organ failure;
- thrombocytopenia;
- Budd–Chiari syndrome.

These are all probably related to a widespread thrombotic tendency.

Investigations typically show a prolonged APTT, although this is an in vitro phenomenon only and due to the antibody effect on cephalin which is the phospholipid source in the APTT test. Although not associated with a bleeding tendency, the prolonged APTT is of clinical significance in patients requiring heparin therapy, since it makes control difficult. The presence of a lupus anticoagulant is confirmed by mixing studies, because the APTT becomes normal in this way if its prolongation is due to a circulating inhibitor. The anticardiolipin antibody (aCL) may be directly assayed, usually by ELISA.

Treatment issues have as much uncertainty as do those related to pathogenesis and investigation.

- *Anticoagulation with even full doses of heparin is often insufficient and warfarin is probably best.*

The optimal dose of warfarin appears to be high, with a required INR of at least 3.

- *Low-dose aspirin may be ineffective, and corticosteroids are contraindicated in some settings (e.g. in pregnancy they are associated with an increased incidence of pre-eclampsia).*
- *Gamma globulin iv has been reported to be helpful.*

Bibliography

Bick RL (ed) 1994 Antiphospholipid syndromes. Semin Thromb Hemost 20: 1.

Bick RL 1997 The antiphospholipid thrombosis syndromes: a common multidisciplinary medical problem. Clin Appl Thromb Hemost 3: 270.

Brighton TA, Chesterman CN 2000 The clinical significance of antiphospholipid antibodies in patients without autoimmune disease. Aust NZ J Med 30: 693.

Briley DP, Coull BM, Goodnight SH 1989 Neurological disease associated with antiphospholipid antibodies. Ann Neurol 25: 221.

Copeman PW 1975 Livedo reticularis: signs in the skin of disturbance of blood viscosity and blood flow. Br J Dermatol 93: 519.

Cowchock FS, Reece EA, Balaban D et al 1992 Repeated fetal losses associated with antiphospholipid antibodies: a collaborative randomised trial comparing prednisolone with low dose heparin treatment. Am J Obstet Gynecol 166: 1318.

de Groot PG, Derksen RHWM 1995 Specificity and clinical relevance of lupus anticoagulant. Vessels 1: 22.

Galve E, Ordi J, Barquinero J et al 1992 Valvular heart disease in the primary antiphospholipid syndrome. Ann Intern Med 116: 293.

Ginsberg JS, Brill-Edwards P, Johnston M et al 1992 Relationship of antiphospholipid antibodies to pregnancy loss in patients with systemic lupus erythematosus. Blood 80: 975.

Hughes GR 1993 The antiphospholipid syndrome: ten years on. Lancet 342: 341.

Khamashta MA, Cuadrado MJ, Mujic F et al 1995 The management of thrombosis in the antiphospholipid-antibody syndrome. N Engl J Med 332: 993.

Laskin CA, Bombardier C, Hannah ME 1997
   Prednisolone and aspirin in women with
   autoantibodies and unexplained recurrent fetal loss.
   N Engl J Med 337: 148.
Lockshin MD 1992 Antiphospholipid antibody
   syndrome. JAMA 268: 1451.
Morgan M, Downs K, Chesterman CN, Biggs JC
   1993 Clinical analysis of 125 patients with the
   lupus anticoagulant. Aust NZ J Med 23: 151.
Roubey RAS 1994 Autoantibodies to phospholipid-
   binding plasma proteins: a new view of lupus
   anticoagulants and other "antiphospholipid"
   autoantibodies. Blood 84: 2864.
Ryan P, Street A 1993 Thrombosis and
   antiphospholipid antibodies – an evolving story.
   Aust NZ J Med 23: 148.

Antiprotease (see Alpha$_1$-antitrypsin deficiency and Antithrombin III)

Antithrombin III

Antithrombin III (AT-III) is a circulating plasma protein of molecular weight 58 kd. It is the most important natural inhibitor of the serine proteases (activated coagulation factors II, X, IX, XI and XII). This antiprotease activity is slow, except in the presence of heparin, which binds to a lys residue and produces an allosteric effect, which in turn results in greater accessibility of the active site for stoichiometric protease binding. Antiprotease activity is thereby enhanced 1000-fold.

Antithrombin III is normally present in a plasma concentration of about 300 mg/L (5 μM), corresponding to 100% activity, and is sufficient to neutralize all the thrombin that can be generated from the same volume of blood. Its half-life is about 48 h.

Antithrombin III deficiency may be hereditary or acquired.

Hereditary AT III deficiency is an autosomal dominant condition with several different genotypes. There is a positive family history and the onset of a thrombotic tendency from early adult life, especially following stimuli such as surgery or pregnancy. Although heterozygotes are generally asymptomatic carriers, the disease is manifest even at levels of circulating AT-III up to 60% of normal. By middle age, there is a 90% incidence of thrombosis.

Acquired AT III deficiency occurs:

- in disseminated intravascular coagulation (or other major consumptive disorders, such as extensive thromboembolism or trauma);
- in the postoperative state;
- in liver disease;
- in the nephrotic syndrome;
- in vasculitis;
- after asparaginase (which is better known for causing hypofibrinogenaemia).

Treatment of an acute thrombosis in AT-III deficiency requires **heparin***, plus* **AT-III replacement** *if there is heparin resistance (i.e. the APTT does not increase as expected with the usual doses of heparin). AT-III may be given as specific concentrate (20–50 U/kg is required to raise the level to 100%) or fresh frozen plasma.*

For prevention of thrombosis, life-long warfarin is required. Since warfarin is contraindicated in pregnancy, heparin and AT-III concentrate are given at labour. Asymptomatic patients are usually not given prophylaxis, though oral anabolic steroids may be helpful in some.

Antithrombin III concentrates have been studied in the treatment of sepsis, since plasma AT-III levels have been found to be low in that condition and to correlate with outcome. Variable results have been reported to date, and the initial results of current larger studies appear disappointing. Antithrombin III concentrates have perhaps more usefully been used in the treatment of disseminated intravascular coagulation.

Bibliography
Levi M, ten Cate H 1999 Disseminated intravascular
   coagulation. N Engl J Med 341:586.
Wheeler AP, Bernard GR 1999 Treating patients
   with severe sepsis. N Engl J Med 340: 207.

Aortic coarctation

Aortic coarctation refers to narrowing of the aorta, usually distal to the origin of the left subclavian artery. It is usually congenital, but rarely it can follow aortitis or blunt trauma.

- Congenital aortic coarctation may be associated with a bicuspid aortic valve, ventricular septal defect or Turner's syndrome.
- Coarctation due to aortitis occurs most commonly in young women with idiopathic Takayasu's disease, though occasionally it may be associated with a collagen-vascular disease and involve the abdominal and lower thoracic aorta.
- Coarctation following trauma is usually mild and is referred to pseudocoarctation.

Clinical features comprise hypertension, sometimes associated with headache, and coldness and fatigue of the lower extremities. The femoral pulses are reduced and delayed compared with the radial pulses. A bruit may be heard over the back.

The hypertension is detectable only in the arms, in which the systolic pressure is at least 20 mmHg higher than in the legs. The blood pressure rises markedly on exertion, much more so than for essential hypertension of similar degree. The hypertension may be irreversible, if surgical correction is late or if there is residual or recurrent coarctation. Clearly, examination for aortic coarctation should be included in the assessment of patients with hypertension.

The complications of coarctation include:

- cardiac failure;
- intracranial haemorrhage;
- aortic dissection;
- bacterial endocarditis.

Chest X-ray shows:

- cardiomegaly;
- rib notching from dilated collateral intercostal vessels;

- an abnormal silhouette of the aortic knob (the so-called figure-of-three).

Diagnosis is confirmed by angiography and/or CT scanning.

The obstruction is usually moderate, though it can occasionally be complete. Sometimes it is mild, as in pseudocoarctation.

Significant obstruction has traditionally been treated by surgical **resection**, *which is usually very successful, though aneurysm formation, recurrent coarctation and persistent hypertension may occur postoperatively.* **Angioplasty** *with or without stenting is currently the preferred treatment. It is especially appropriate for narrowing after aortitis or for recurrence after surgery.*

Bibliography

Arend WP, Michel BA, Bloch DA et al 1990 The American College of Rheumatology 1990 criteria for the classification of Takayasu arteritis. Arthritis Rheum 33: 1129.

Calhoun DA, Oparil S 1990 Treatment of hypertensive crisis. N Engl J Med 323: 1177.

Hijazi ZM, Geggel R 1995 Balloon angioplasty for postoperative recurrent coarctation of the aorta. J Interv Cardiol 8: 509.

Kerr GS, Hallahan CW, Giordano J et al 1994 Takayasu arteritis. Ann Intern Med 120: 919.

Rothman A 1998 Coarctation of the aorta: an update. Curr Probl Pediatr 28: 33.

Aortic dissection

Aortic dissection, sometimes erroneously referred to as a dissecting aneurysm, is a spontaneous tear in the aortic intima, giving rise to a false channel within the aortic wall. The blood in this channel dissects along the aorta, including its branches, and eventually ruptures either back into the lumen or out through the adventitia.

The most common sites of the initial tear are in the ascending aorta (type A dissection) and in the descending aorta immediately distal to the origin of the left subclavian artery (type B dissection).

Type A dissection

- is caused by medial degeneration, or cystic medionecrosis, of the aortic wall;
- usually occurs in middle age;
- is not associated with hypertension;
- may be associated with Marfan's syndrome;
- may dissect retrograde to the sinuses of Valsalva, then possibly either causing aortic regurgitation or rupturing into the pericardium causing tamponade;
- may dissect antegrade to any of the major aortic branches.

Type B dissection

- occurs primarily in elderly hypertensive and/or atherosclerotic patients;
- typically presents with chest pain radiating to the back;
- usually dissects antegrade and extends as far as the abdomen.

The clinical features of aortic dissection include:

- sudden chest pain mimicking acute myocardial infarction but without ECG changes;
- unequal pulses;
- aortic regurgitation;
- neurological signs;
- a widened mediastinum on chest X-ray.

The diagnosis is confirmed by transoesophageal echocardiography, CT scanning and/or angiography, or possibly MRI.

Treatment is either medical or surgical.

- ***Medical treatment*** *may be in preparation for surgery or may be the primary therapy especially for type B dissection. Treatment emphasis is to decrease the physical stress on the aortic wall by potent antihypertensive agents, usually sodium nitroprusside and beta-blockers.*
- ***Surgery*** *is indicated for type A dissection as an emergency and for chronic dissection electively. Surgery for type B dissection generally carries a higher mortality than nonoperative treatment.*

In patients who survive, the incidence of recurrence of dissection is considerable, ranging from 15–40%. Aneurysmal dilatation may become a late problem.

Bibliography

Calhoun DA, Oparil S 1990 Treatment of hypertensive crisis. N Engl J Med 323: 1177.

Crawford ES 1990 The diagnosis and management of aortic dissection. JAMA 264: 2537.

DeSanctis RW, Doroghazi RM, Austen WG et al 1987 Aortic dissection. N Engl J Med 317: 1060.

Treasure T, Raphael MJ 1991 Investigation of suspected dissection of the thoracic aorta. Lancet 338: 490.

Aplastic anaemia (see Anaemia)

ARDS (see Acute pulmonary oedema)

Arnold–Chiari malformation

The Arnold–Chiari malformation is one of the congenital neural tube defects. These also include meningomyelocele, syringomyelia, and stenosis of the aqueduct of Sylvius. The most severe form is of course anencephaly.

There is an increased incidence of neural tube defects in babies of mothers who are folic acid deficient or who fail to take folic acid supplementation during pregnancy.

The Arnold–Chiari malformation comprises downward displacement of the lower medulla and cerebellar tonsils through the foramen magnum. Half of the cases are associated with syringomyelia (q.v.).

Although developmental, it commonly presents initially in adults, with pain in the back of the head, extending down over the shoulders and arms and exacerbated by coughing. Sometimes, there may be associated:

- bulbar symptoms;
- blurred vision;

- nystagmus;
- vertigo;
- ataxia;
- respiratory failure (occasionally);
- sleep apnoea (occasionally).

*Treatment is with surgical **decompression**.*

Bibliography

Lemire RJ 1988 Neural tube defects. JAMA 259: 558.

Paul KS, Lye RH, Strang FA et al 1983 Arnold–Chiari malformation. J Neurosurg 58: 183.

Arsenic

Arsenic (As, atomic number 33, atomic weight 75) is a non-metallic element in the nitrogen family. Although arsenic-containing compounds have been known since antiquity and arsenic is widely distributed in nature in various forms, the element was not identified until 1649. Arsenicals are used in herbicides, pesticides and various manufacturing processes.

> Arsenic poisoning may be occupational, accidental or deliberate (either as a classical criminal agent or as a military poison).

Toxicity from arsenic arises from inactivation of cellular enzymes, though there is great individual variation in susceptibility and many famous cases of tolerance. Most such preparations are arsenates.

- Arsenious oxide (As_4O_6) is a colourless, odourless and tasteless compound, much beloved in detective fiction and presumably as commonly in reality.
- Arsine (arsenic hydride, $AsH3$) is a colourless gas, used as a doping agent for semi-conductors and also as a military poison.
- Potassium arsenate was known pharmaceutically as Fowler's solution, though arsenicals are no longer used clinically.

- Arsenic may also be contained in tobacco, from which it is oxidized like other heavy metals as the tobacco is burned.

Arsenate is isostructural with orthophosphate and thus can become misincorporated into DNA. Various international standards recommend the limitation of exposure to inorganic arsenic to not >10 $\mu g/m^3$/8 h or 2 $\mu g/m^3$/15 min, beyond which dermatitis and cancer of the lung and of the lymphoid tissues may occur.

> Arsenic poisoning may be either acute or chronic.

Acute poisoning is manifest by:

- nausea;
- burning of the mouth;
- abdominal pain;
- acute haemolytic anaemia;
- shock and death within an hour.

Chronic poisoning is manifest by:

- weakness;
- paralysis;
- confusion;
- toxic neuropathy;
- skin pigmentation, keratoses and cancer;
- streaking of the nails;
- anaemia;
- hepatic cirrhosis;
- renal failure.

The neuropathy is similar to that produced by many toxic agents and indeed drugs.

The skin pigmentation is bronze in colour and is the characteristic skin lesion, with 'rain drop' areas of hypopigmentation due to hypomelanotic macules.

In addition to keratoses, there may be skin cancer, either basal cell carcinoma or squamous cell carcinoma. Although Bowen's disease, which resembles superficial basal cell carcinoma, usually arises from solar exposure, when it follows arsenic ingestion it can occur in covered areas of the skin.

The anaemia of chronic poisoning is due to decreased red blood cell production.

The hepatic cirrhosis is similar to that produced by excess vitamin A and methotrexate.

The renal failure is due initially to tubular damage and later to residual tubulointerstitial scarring giving rise to a chronic nephropathy, similar to that produced by mercury.

The treatment of arsenic poisoning is with **gastric lavage** *if recently ingested. Both acute and chronic poisoning are treated with* **dimercaprol** *(BAL)(q.v.).*

Bibliography
Kyle RA, Pease GL 1965 Hematologic aspects of arsenic intoxication. N Engl J Med 273: 18.

Arteriovenous malformations

Arteriovenous malformations (AVMs) may occur either as a widespread phenomenon (the Osler–Weber–Rendu disease) or as isolated lesions (usually affecting either the cerebral or pulmonary circulation).

Osler–Weber–Rendu disease (hereditary haemorrhagic telangiectasia, HHT) is an autosomal dominant condition causing ectasia of small blood vessels. There is multisystem vascular dysplasia and haemorrhage.

Genetically, the condition is heterogeneous with a variety of responsible mutations reported. The end-result appears to be impairment of the function of endoglin, a membrane glycoprotein which assists the binding to various cells, particularly endothelial cells, of transforming growth factor β (TGF-β).

The condition becomes manifest after puberty, with a penetrance of almost 100% by the age of 40 y. It presents particularly as spider naevi on the skin of the face and fingers and on the mucous membranes of the mouth and nose. Ectatic vessels may also develop in the gut, urinary tract, liver and brain. The lung is involved in about 20% of cases (see below). There may be associated platelet dysfunction, but coagulation is normal.

Patients commonly present with bleeding, either acute and local or chronic with anaemia.

Cerebral AVMs are congenital but usually do not present until early adult life (average age 35 years).

Most become manifest as intracerebral and/or intraventricular or subarachnoid haemorrhage. The annual rate of recurrent bleeding from such lesions is about 4%.

The AVM should be obliterated by **surgery** *or* **embolization** *or if these are not successful or feasible by stereotactic* **irradiation***.*

Pulmonary AVMs or arteriovenous fistulae are one of the causes of single lung nodules either small or large. However, in about one third of the cases, the lesions are multiple and often bilateral. As with cerebral AVMs, the condition is congenital but becomes apparent only in adult life. About half the cases with multiple lesions in fact have Osler–Weber–Rendu disease (see above) with multiple AVMs elsewhere throughout the body.

Clinical features include hypoxaemia (from right-to-left shunt), haemoptysis, paradoxical systemic embolization, and exertional dyspnoea if the condition is severe and especially if there is associated anaemia. Cyanosis and clubbing may be seen and also polycythaemia if there is no systemic bleeding. Pulmonary hypertension, cardiac failure and AVM rupture with haemoptysis or haemothorax are uncommon.

The condition should be suspected if the lesion on chest X-ray is seen to have a leash (containing the feeding artery and draining vein). Pulmonary angiography is required for definitive diagnosis.

Surgical **resection** *may be considered if the lesion is single and large, but resection is usually unsatisfactory because other small lesions may subsequently enlarge. Radiological* **embolization** *provides a more satisfactory solution.*

Bibliography

Gossage JR, Kanj G 1998 Pulmonary arteriovenous malformations. Am J Respir Crit Care Med 158: 643.

Guttmacher AE, Marchuk DA, White RI 1995 Hereditary hemorrhagic telangiectasia. New Engl J Med 333: 918.

Ondra SL, Troupp H, George ED et al 1990 The natural history of symptomatic arteriovenous malformations of the brain. J Neurosurg 73: 387.

Terry PB, Barth KH, Kaufman SL et al 1980 Balloon embolization for the treatment of pulmonary arteriovenous fistulas. N Engl J Med 302: 1189.

White RJ, Lynch-Nyhan A, Terry P et al 1988 Pulmonary arteriovenous malformation: techniques and long-term outcome of embolotherapy. Radiology 169: 663.

Arteritis

Most type of arteritis are more appropriately discussed in the more general section on vasculitis (q.v.).

However, three conditions may be considered as specifically arteritic, namely:

- cerebral arteritis;
- giant cell arteritis;
- endarteritis.

Cerebral arteritis is a diffuse inflammation of the intracranial arteries which may be either primary or secondary.

- **Primary arteritis** is an isolated condition causing a fluctuating encephalopathy over weeks or months, with headache, confusion and focal neurological signs. The diagnosis is made angiographically and treatment is with corticosteroids and immunosuppression.
- **Secondary arteritis** occurs in giant cell arteritis, AIDS, HZV infection, TB, sarcoidosis, collagen-vascular diseases and Hodgkin's disease.

Giant cell arteritis (temporal arteritis) is the most common and important form of arteritis, because it may have serious complications if untreated.

It usually presents in patients older than 50 years and is associated with both

- systemic features of fever, anorexia and weight loss;
- local features of headache and scalp tenderness with palpable nodules.

There may be associated polymyalgia rheumatica (q.v.).

Clinical features may be present for many weeks, and blindness, neuropathy, cerebral ischaemia, vertigo or depression may occur before the diagnosis is made. In particular, the blindness which is due to ischaemic neuritis is sudden and irreversible and may sometimes be bilateral.

Diagnosis is assisted by the finding of mild anaemia and raised ESR and is confirmed by temporal artery biopsy.

*Treatment with **corticosteroids** provides a rapid response.*

Endarteritis is an infective lesion of the endothelium analogous with endocarditis (q.v.). It usually affects the abdominal aorta or iliofemoral arteries and may involve atherosclerotic plaques and aneurysms, as well as the normal vessel wall.

- Endarteritis is usually bacterial (especially from salmonella), but it can be due to fungi, rickettsiae or chlamydiae.
- Endarteritis may also be produced by irradiation, which causes inflammation and eventually fibrosis of the vaso vasorum, though initially the condition may be steroid-responsive.

Bibliography

Bahlas S, Ramos-Remus C, Davis P 1998 Clinical outcome of 149 patients with polymyalgia rheumatica and giant cell arteritis. J Rheumatol 25: 99.

Calabrese L, Dune G, Lie J 1997 Vasculitis in the central nervous system. Arthritis Rheum 40: 1189.

Hamilton CR, Shelley WM, Tumulty PA 1971 Giant cell arteritis: including temporal arteritis and polymyalgia rheumatica. Medicine 50: 1.

Hunder GG, Bloch DA, Michel BA et al 1990 The American College of Rheumatology 1990 criteria for the classification of giant cell arteritis. Arthritis Rheum 33: 1122.

Moore PM 1989 Diagnosis and management of isolated angiitis of the central nervous system. Neurology 39: 167.

Oz MC, Brener BJ, Buda JA et al 1989 A ten-year experience with bacterial aortitis. J Vasc Surg 10: 439.

Zilko PJ 1996 Polymyalgia rheumatica and giant cell arteritis. Med J Aust 165: 438.

Arthritis

Arthritis (and arthropathies) describe conditions affecting joints. They are traditionally classified as:

- **degenerative**

  – primary or secondary;

- **infective** (or septic)

  – usually direct viral, bacterial, fungal or parasitic infection in joints;

  – polymicrobial in about 10% of cases;

  – sometimes indirect (i.e. **'reactive'** arthritis), with an infection at some other site precipitating with arthritis by a presumed immunological mechanism (see Reiter's syndrome).

- **metabolic disorders**

  – including crystal-induced arthritis (e.g. gout and pseudogout);

- **connective tissue diseases**

  – including rheumatoid arthritis, SLE, scleroderma, polyarteritis nodosa, Sjögren's syndrome, Behçet's syndrome, overlap syndromes;

- **neuropathic**;
- **spondyloarthritis**

  – q.v.;

- **miscellaneous** conditions

  – such as drug-induced joint manifestations (e.g. in SLE, serum sickness).

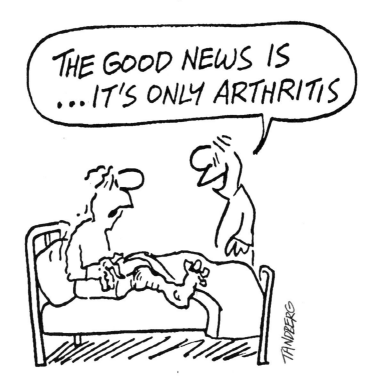

THE GOOD NEWS IS ...IT'S ONLY ARTHRITIS

Acute **monoarthritis** is typically infective, though it may often be associated with systemic disease, especially if there are other concomitant clinical features. Thus, the additional presence of:

- erythema nodosum suggests inflammatory bowel disease, sarcoidosis, SLE;
- mouth ulcers suggest Behçet's syndrome, Reiter's syndrome, SLE;
- splinter haemorrhages suggest bacterial endocarditis.

Bibliography
Editorial 1980 Reactive arthritis. Br Med J 281: 311.

Gibofsky A, Zabriskie JB 1995 Rheumatic fever and poststreptococcal reactive arthritis. Curr Opin Rheumatol 7: 299.

Hamerman D 1989 The biology of osteoarthritis. N Engl J Med 320: 1322.

Smith JW 1990 Infectious arthritis. Infect Dis Clin North Am 4: 523.

Weston VC, Jones AC, Bradbury N et al 1999 Clinical features and outcome of septic arthritis in a single UK health district 1982–1991. Ann Rheum Dis 58: 214.

Winblad S 1975 Arthritis associated with *Yersinia enterocolitica* infections. Scand J Infect Dis 7: 191.

Arthropathies (see Arthritis)

Arthus reaction (see Immune complex disease)

Asbestos (see also Occupational lung diseases)

Asbestos is a natural mineral fibre freed from crushed rock, usually chrysotile, and composed of magnesium silicate. It is resistant to fire, acid and alkali. Because it is virtually indestructible, its smooth brittle fibres have been widely used commercially since the 19th century both for building and for thermal insulation. In the body, the silicate groups gradually dissociate and then substitute for phosphates, thus deranging

DNA. Safe exposure limits of <100–$200\,000$ fibres of $>5\ \mu m/m^3/8$ h have been set.

Calculations of the worldwide health burden from occupational and environmental exposure to asbestos suggest a projected 5–10 million cancers, with 30 000 in Australia alone (two thirds lung cancer, one third mesothelioma). Because of this and because there are now safe and economic alternatives, an international ban on all mining and use of asbestos has been recommended.

The risks from asbestos exposure include:

- lung cancer;
- mesothelioma;
- pneumoconiosis (asbestosis);
- pleural plaques.

Lung cancer follows heavy exposure and the risk is enhanced 8-fold by concomitant cigarette smoking.

Mesothelioma (usually pleural but sometimes peritoneal) on the other hand can occur even after a single exposure and may have a latent period of up to 30 or more years.

Pneumoconiosis (asbestosis) consists of a diffuse pulmonary infiltrate. The risk is dose-related, with a long latent period of 20 years or more, followed by a slowly progressive fibrosis, with cough and dyspnoea. The characteristic findings include particularly decreased gas transfer, also decreased lung volumes and impaired gas exchange, but normal lung mechanics. The lung function abnormalities precede both symptoms and radiographic changes. Asbestos bodies can be recovered in bronchoalveolar lavage fluid.

Pleural plaques are discrete connective tissue collections on the parietal pleura and follow heavy exposure to asbestos or sometimes other inorganic fibres. They are usually seen on the lateral posterior or basal pleural surfaces and not in the costophrenic angle nor in the upper third of the thorax. They vary greatly in diameter and have an average thickness of 5 mm. If not calcified, they may be seen only in tangential views. They develop slowly with a latent period of 20 years or more. They are a marker only of asbestos exposure and do not predispose to symptoms, functional changes or malignancy. If non-calcified, they should be distinguished from other causes of local pleural thickening, such as inflammation, trauma or malignancy.

Sometimes there may be more diffuse pleural fibrosis rather than discrete collections.

Bibliography

Berry G 1995 Environmental mesothelioma incidence, time since exposure to asbestos and level of exposure. Environmetrics 6: 221.

Mossman BT, Bignon J, Corn M et al 1990 Asbestos: scientific developments and implications for public policy. Science 247: 294.

Peto J, Decarli A, La Vecchia C et al 1999 The European mesothelioma epidemic. Br J Cancer 79: 566.

Sterman DH, Kaiser LR, Albelda SM 1999 Advances in the treatment of malignant pleural mesothelioma. Chest 116: 504.

Teirstein AS 1998 Diagnosing malignant pleural mesothelioma. Chest 114: 666.

Aspergillosis (see Eosinophilia and lung infiltration (asthmatic pulmonary eosinophilia))

Aspergillosis is caused by the fungus aspergillus, most commonly *A. fumigatus* but occasionally others, e.g. *A. flavus*. Aspergillus is a ubiquitous saprophyte in nature, and infection arises only when it is aerosolized into a normally sterile site (thus, it is usually a pulmonary infection). Moreover, its isolation from normal subjects may not be significant, whereas its presence in an immunocompromised patient should be taken very seriously.

It may produce one of three pulmonary conditions, namely:

- mycetoma;
- allergic disease;
- invasive disease.

Mycetoma is a fungus ball which occupies an existing cavity. Aspergillus is the most common cause of a fungus ball (then often called an aspergilloma), though sometimes other fungi may produce a similar condition. Haemorrhage occurs in more than half the patients and can be fatal. There is an overall mortality of 5–10%. The sputum is usually negative for the organism.

*Treatment is with **surgery**.*

Allergic bronchopulmonary aspergillosis is associated with wheeze, eosinophilia and brown plugs of sputum. The sputum is usually positive for the organism, and skin tests and serum precipitins are also usually positive.

*Treatment is with **corticosteroids**.*

*The oral antifungal agent, **itraconazole** (200 mg twice daily), has recently been shown to add further improvement without toxicity in patients with this condition who were steroid-dependent.*

Invasive disease usually occurs only in immunocompromised hosts. There is a necrotizing pneumonia with haemorrhagic infarction and cavitation, and sometimes systemic metastases. Sputum cultures are only sometimes positive for the organism (about 30%), blood cultures are always negative and serology is unhelpful.

*Treatment is with **amphotericin** in high doses, though the response may be poor.*

Bibliography

Chatzimichalis A, Massard G, Kessler R et al 1998 Bronchopulmonary aspergilloma: a reappraisal. Ann Thorac Surg 65: 927.

Janssen JJWM, Strack van Schijndel RJM, van der Poest Clement EH et al 1996 Outcome of ICU treatment in invasive aspergillosis. Intens Care Med 22: 1315.

Levitz SM 1989 Aspergillosis. Infect Dis Clin North Am 3: 1.

Oakley EJ, Petrou M, Goldstraw P 1997 Indications and outcome of surgery for pulmonary aspergilloma. Thorax 52: 813.

Stevens DA, Schwartz HJ, Lee JY et al 2000 A randomized trial of itraconazole in allergic bronchopulmonary aspergillosis. N Engl J Med 342: 756.

Aspiration

Aspiration pneumonitis (chemical pneumonia, Mendelson's syndrome) refers to the inhalation of gastric contents. The original description of this condition was in obstetric patients in whom it is still a significant problem.

Aspiration of gastric contents is a serious complication in the patient whose airway is unprotected because of impaired consciousness and/or disturbance of gastro-oesophageal function. Many of the procedures in caring for the unconscious patient, particularly in Anaesthesia and in Intensive Care, relate to airway protection and thus prevention of aspiration.

The pathogenesis of aspiration is related to the acidity of the gastric contents and is especially significant when the pH is less than 2.5. Acid inhalation causes immediate chemical damage to the bronchial mucosal cells or alveolar epithelial cells, with resulting inflammatory exudate and cellular infiltrate.

The clinical features start with the aspiration event itself, which may be witnessed.

- Immediate asphyxia may occasionally result, especially if the aspiration is large and particulate.
- More typically, cough, frothy sputum, dyspnoea and wheeze occur, usually within an hour or so.
- Hypoxaemia occurs and is sometimes severe.
- There may be circulatory failure due to hypovolaemia or reflex responses.
- The features of bronchopneumonia become apparent within 24 to 48 h. Secondary aerobic or anaerobic infection may occur in the next few days.
- Specific problems occur if the aspiration is infected or if large food particles are retained.
- If the aspirate includes mineral oil, formerly a popular night-time laxative, chronic lipoid

pneumonia can be produced by repeated aspiration.

> Diagnosis of aspiration is often straightforward. However, it may be difficult if:
>
> - the aspiration has not been witnessed,
> - if the patient is already ill for other reasons,
> - no food particles or patchy inflammation are found in the tracheobronchial tree at fibreoptic bronchoscopy.
>
> Conversely, if food particles are found in the oropharynx, a mistaken diagnosis of aspiration may be made.

*The treatment of aspiration is **supportive**.*

- *Since the chemical reaction is immediate, measures such as instillation of bicarbonate or saline lavage are not helpful.*
- *Corticosteroids have been shown to be ineffective, and prophylactic antibiotics are not generally indicated.*
- *Treatment thus consists of oxygenation, cardiovascular resuscitation if necessary, intubation and mechanical ventilation in seriously affected patients, and bronchodilators when bronchospasm is prominent.*

Bibliography
Wright BA, Jeffrey PH 1990 Lipoid pneumonia. Semin Respir Infect 5: 314.

Aspirin

Aspirin (acetylsalicylic acid) was first prepared by Hoffman at Bayer and introduced into clinical medicine in 1899 as an anti-inflammatory agent. It had been preceded by sodium salicylate, which had been used since 1875 for its antipyretic and uricosuric as well as anti-inflammatory properties. This in turn had been preceded in previous centuries by the use of willowbark (salicylate-containing) as an antipyretic for ague. Aspirin consists of benzoic acid with an acetyl group at the ortho position, i.e. it is the salicylate ester of acetic acid.

Its use as an analgesic (for integumental but not visceral pain), anti-inflammatory drug, antipyretic and antiplatelet agent are well known.

In the Intensive Care Unit, common but important issues include:

- drug interactions;
- toxic effects;
- side-effects;
- Reye's syndrome (q.v.).

Drug interactions (q.v.) are common, because the acetyl group of aspirin acetylates proteins and thus displaces protein-bound drugs.

Toxic effects of aspirin in high doses are widespread, since the drug is distributed in most tissues and fluids. These effects may include:

- circulatory depression and peripheral vasodilatation;
- respiratory stimulation initially but depression with very high doses, the initial hyperventilation comprising some increase in tidal volume but a much greater increase in respiratory rate;
- tinnitus and confusion, with coma after very high dose;
- impaired haemostasis;
- increased renal loss of sodium, potassium and water;
- increased metabolic rate and metabolic acidosis, due to uncoupling of phosphorylation and the accumulation of metabolic products.

Treatment of salicylate toxicity includes:

- *gastric lavage;*
- *correction of fluid, electrolyte, acid–base, haemostasis and temperature disturbances;*
- *forced alkaline diuresis;*
- *dialysis or charcoal haemoperfusion in severe cases.*

Side-effects of aspirin are associated with therapeutic rather than excessive doses and include:

- gastric irritability;
- salicylism (nausea and tinnitus);
- exacerbation of asthma (and also of rhinitis and the rare systemic mastocytosis);
- an enhanced bleeding tendency;
- more rarely, hepatotoxicity, with a reversible and asymptomatic 'transaminitis', especially in the presence of collagen-vascular diseases, though it has also occasionally been implicated in chronic drug-induced hepatitis;
- contribution to analgesic nephropathy (chronic interstitial nephritis);
- decreased mucociliary clearance, though the clinical significance of this phenomenon is unknown.

Bibliography

Gabow P, Anderson RJ, Potts DE et al 1978 Acid-base disturbances in the salicylate-intoxicated adult. Arch Intern Med 138: 1481.

Leatherman JW, Schmitz PG 1991 Fever, hyperdynamic shock, and multiple-system organ failure: a pseudo-sepsis syndrome associated with chronic salicylate intoxication. Chest 100: 1391.

Asthma (see also Occupational lung diseases)

Asthma-like symptoms can develop in any subject given a severe enough stimulus, such as a toxic gas. The presence of a viral infection heightens the susceptibility of normal subjects as well as of asthmatics to such stimuli.

Since anyone can develop asthma-like symptoms given a sufficient stimulus, it is clearly important that the definition of clinical asthma includes the concept of abnormally increased bronchial reactivity.

The differential diagnosis of asthma includes conditions producing dyspnoea with wheeze, i.e. airways obstruction, namely:

- chronic bronchitis and emphysema;
- acute pulmonary oedema

  – 'cardiac asthma';

- pulmonary embolism;

- aspiration;
- drugs (see Drugs and the lung)

  - hypersensitivity;
  - irritation;
  - smooth muscle cell contraction;
  - prostaglandin inhibition;

- acute lung irritation;
- cystic fibrosis;
- pulmonary infiltration with eosinophilia

  - specifically, allergic bronchopulmonary aspergillosis;

- some restrictive lung diseases

  - with bronchial involvement, e.g. sarcoidosis, rheumatoid lung,

- polyarteritis nodosa

  - including Churg–Strauss syndrome;

- carcinoid tumour

  - especially with liver metastases;

- local obstruction

  - giving local wheeze.

- laryngeal oedema

  - e.g. anaphylaxis;

- laryngospasm;
- neoplasia;
- neurological disease

  - laryngospasm, vocal cord paralysis;

- vocal cord dysfunction.

The clinical features of upper airway obstruction include a history of local disease and findings of hoarse voice and abnormal cough as well as stridor. Gas exchange is normal, but there is an abnormal flow–volume loop. Specific investigations include inspection by bronchoscopy and CT imaging. Of course, in patients with symptoms severe enough to warrant endotracheal intubation, there is immediate relief of the features of airway obstruction following this procedure. Moreover, the patient is able to be ventilated at normal pressures and flows and with normal gas exchange.

Stridor (i.e. upper airway obstruction) needs to be excluded. Upper airway obstruction can sometimes be variable and may even be exacerbated by exercise and improved with corticosteroids, thus mimicking asthma.

The most common causes of stridor are:

- extrinsic compression

  - e.g. goitre;

- foreign body;
- infection

  - croup, epiglottitis, diphtheria;

- inflammation

  - tonsils, granulations, cricoarytenoid arthritis, tracheomalacia, stenosis, relapsing polychondritis, sarcoidosis, amyloid;

Bibliography

Barrett GE, Koopman CF, Coulthard SW 1984 Retropharyngeal abscess. Laryngoscope 94: 455.

Editorial 1990 Cardiac asthma. Lancet 335: 693.

Kryger M, Bode F, Antic R et al 1976 Diagnosis of obstruction of the upper and central airways. Am J Med 61: 85.

Mayo-Smith M, Hirsch PJ, Wodzinski SF et al 1986 Acute epiglottitis in adults. N Engl J Med 314: 1133.

McCaughan BC, Martini N, Bains MS 1985 Bronchial carcinoids. J Thorac Cardiovsc Surg 89: 8.

Murray DM, Lawler PG 1998 All that wheezes is not asthma: paradoxical vocal cord movement presenting as severe acute asthma requiring ventilatory support. Anaesthesia 53: 1006.

Ricketti AJ, Greenberger PA, Mintzer RA et al 1983 Allergic bronchopulmonary aspergillosis. Arch Intern Med 143: 1553.

Schuyler MR 1983 Allergic bronchopulmonary aspergillosis. Clin Chest Med 4: 15.

Shapiro J, Eavey RD, Baker AS 1988 Adult supraglottitis: a prospective analysis. JAMA 259: 563.

Asthmatic pulmonary eosinophilia (see Eosinophilia and lung infiltration)

Atrial natriuretic factor

Atrial natriuretic factor (ANF) is a peptide which is stored in the atrial myocardial cells and released during atrial dilatation. It is one of a family of five structurally related natriuretic peptides of 22–53 amino acids, each peptide being secreted by different tissues. ANP is a natural antagonist to the renin–angiotensin–aldosterone system and promotes renal excretion of sodium and water. It is also a potent vasodilator and may thus play a homeostatic role in vascular control.

Excess release of ANF may contribute to hypotension in right ventricular infarction and like inappropriate ADH contribute to hyponatraemia. Experimentally, ANP helps to prevent and may even reverse postischaemic acute tubular necrosis, though this benefit has not been confirmed in humans. Theoretically, circulating natriuretic peptides and their degradation products may be useful biological markers of tissue injury, though such a role has yet to be confirmed by major clinical trial.

Bibliography

Davidson NC, Naas AA, Hanson JK et al 1996 Comparison of atrial natriuretic peptide, B-type natriuretic peptide, and N-terminal proatrial natriuretic peptide as indicators of left ventricular dysfunction. Am J Cardiol 77: 828.

Diringer M, Ladenson PW, Stern BJ et al 1988 Plasma atrial natriuretic factor and subarachnoid hemorrhage. Stroke 19: 1119.

Needleman P, Greenwald JE 1986 Atriopeptin: a cardiac hormone intimately involved in fluid, electrolyte, and blood-pressure homeostasis. N Engl J Med 314: 828.

Stein BC, Levin RI 1998 Natriuretic peptides: physiology, therapeutic potential, and risk stratification in ischemic heart disease. Am Heart J 135: 914.

Wei C-M, Heublein DM, Perrella MA et al 1993 Natriuretic peptide system in human heart failure. Circulation 88: 1004.

Autacoids (see Adenosine)

Auto-erythrocyte purpura (see Purpura)

Autoimmune disorders

Autoimmune disorders comprise a large group of diseases caused by an immune reaction to a self (or auto) antigen. Self-reactive lymphocytes, both T cells and B cells, are largely eliminated during development, but some appear to persist in a mature state in peripheral lymphoid tissue, where they can be activated to cause autoimmunity.

Mechanisms of activation of autoimmunity include:

- exposure of a normally sequestered self-antigen;
- structural alteration of a self-antigen (e.g. by drugs or viruses);
- molecular mimicry in which an appropriate immune response occurs to bacterial or viral proteins which are closely related to host antigens.

Genetic predisposition to autoimmunity is also important, and the MHC (HLA) locus is the best defined risk factor for most such diseases.

In general, the mechanism of antibody production requires both a genetic predisposition and then a trigger, presumably of environmental origin, since concordance for autoimmune disease is only about 30–50% in identical twins.

Pathology may be caused by:

- cell damage from the binding of antibodies to cell surface antigens;
- agonist or antagonist actions of autoantibodies binding to cell surface receptors;
- immune complex disease (especially with nuclear antigens);
- cell-mediated immunity.

Autoimmune disorders may be either:

- organ-specific, or
- systemic.

The antigens recognized are usually correspondingly organ-specific or widespread.

Organ-specific disorders include most commonly:

- insulin-dependent diabetes mellitus (IDDM);
- Graves' disease;
- Hashimoto's thyroiditis;
- pernicious anaemia;
- vitiligo.

Other organ-specific conditions include:

- Addison's disease;
- autoimmune haemolytic anaemia;
- chronic active hepatitis;
- hypoparathyroidism;
- idiopathic thrombocytopenic purpura;
- lymphocytic hypophysitis;
- multiple sclerosis;
- myasthenia gravis;
- pemphigus;
- primary biliary cirrhosis.

Many organ-specific disorders are thus endocrine, with auto-antigens often being enzymes or receptors. Polyglandular syndromes may occur in some families.

- In IDDM, antibodies recognize islet cells (ICA), and the specific proteins recognized include insulin (IAA), glutamic acid decarboxylase (anti-GAD) or the recently described tyrosine phosphatase, IA-2.
- In Graves' disease, the antibody is to TSH receptors (TRAb).
- In Hashimoto's thyroiditis, the main antibody specificity is to thyroid peroxidase

(anti-TPO, formerly called microsomal antibody).

Non-organ-specific disorders, i.e. multi-system or systemic disorders, include:

- systemic lupus erythematosus;
- Sjögren's disease;
- scleroderma;
- rheumatoid arthritis;
- rheumatic fever;
- polymyositis;
- Goodpasture's syndrome.

Therapeutic opportunities for immunomodulation include:

- *non-specific immune suppression (e.g. corticosteroids, cyclosporin, intravenous gammaglobulin, plasmapheresis, thalidomide);*
- *semispecific therapy (e.g. anti-TNF antibodies);*
- *specific manipulation (e.g. antigen-based therapies, some of which are now in clinical trials).*

Bibliography

Austen KF, Burakoff SJ, Rosen FS et al (eds) 1996 Therapeutic Immunology. Cambridge: Blackwell.

Dwyer JM 1992 Manipulating the immune system with immune globulin. N Engl J Med 326:107.

Loriaux DL 1985 The polyendocrine deficiency syndromes. N Engl J Med 312: 1568.

Naparstek Y, Plotz PH 1993 The role of autoantibodies in autoimmune disease. Annu Rev Immunol 11: 79.

Nossal GJV 1989 Immunologic tolerance: collaboration between antigen and lymphokines. Science 245: 147.

Peter JB, Shoenfeld Y 1996 Autoantibodies. Amsterdam: Elsevier.

Reimann PM, Mason PD 1990 Plasmapheresis: technique and complications. Intens Care Med 16: 3.

Tan EM 1991 Autoantibodies in pathology and cell biology. Cell 67: 841.

Yu Z, Lennon VA 1999 Mechanism of intravenous immune globulin therapy in antibody-mediated autoimmune diseases. N Engl J Med 340: 227.

Bacillary angiomatosis (see Cat-scratch disease)

Bacillary peliosis hepatis (see Cat-scratch disease)

Bacitracin

Bacitracin is a polypeptide antibiotic produced from the micro-organism, *B. subtilis*, and is active against Gram-positive bacteria. It is however nephrotoxic, so that it is no longer used parenterally.

Its local administration remains useful, either

- orally for *Clostridium difficile* diarrhoea, or
- as an ointment for a variety of infected dermatological conditions, when it is usually combined with other antibacterial agents, such as neomycin and/or polymyxin and often also with corticosteroids.

BAL (see Chelating agents and Warfare agents)

Barotrauma (see also Diving)

Barotrauma refers to air forced outside the normal air spaces. It thus comprises:

- pneumothorax;
- interstitial emphysema;
- pneumomediastinum;
- pneumopericardium;
- pneumoperitoneum;
- subcutaneous emphysema;
- gas embolism (via pulmonary veins).

More subtle abnormalities may be seen histologically or on CT scan and include:

- alveolar rupture;
- emphysema;
- pseudocysts (pneumatoceles).

Barotrauma is a potential complication of mechanical ventilation, especially if inspired pressures or volumes are high or excessive PEEP is used. An alveolar distending pressure of 30–35 mmHg is the injury threshold in most animal studies, so that the end-inspiratory plateau pressure in ventilated patients should be kept below this level if possible. However, there is no direct correlation of clinical injury with the level of pressure used, and indeed it has recently become popular to use the term **volutrauma** rather than barotrauma when discussing pneumothorax etc. in ventilated patients to indicate that the problem is considered to be an overdistended volume rather than an overdistending pressure.

Bibliography

Abolnik I, Lossos IS, Breuer R 1991 Spontaneous pneumomediastinum. Chest 100: 93.

Maunder RJ, Pierson DJ, Hudson LD 1984 Subcutaneous and mediastinal emphysema: pathophysiology, diagnosis, and management. Arch Intern Med 144: 1447.

Basophilia

Basophilia refers to an increased number of circulating basophils ($>0.1 \times 10^9$/L). These cells originate from the pluripotent stem cell via the myeloblast. They have prominent granules containing heparin, histamine and leukotrienes. Like the closely related tissue mast cells, they mediate hypersensitivity reactions.

Basophilia is seen in:

- myeloproliferative disorders (most commonly);
- iron deficiency;
- lung cancer;
- varicella infection.

Bibliography

Denburg JA 1992 Basophil and mast cell lineage in vitro and in vivo. Blood 79: 846.

Echtenacher B, Mannel DN, Hultner L 1996 Critical protective role of mast cells in a model of acute septic peritonitis. Nature 381: 75.

Bat bites (see Bites and stings)

Bathing

Bathing or swimming may be associated with folliculitis from contaminated water or with swimmer's ear.

Exposure to hot tubs or saunas may cause hyperthermia (q.v.). This is particularly important in patients with cardiac disease, who may suffer failure or arrhythmias, and in pregnancy, when a raised core temperature during the first trimester may give rise to neural tube defect in the fetus.

Bibliography
Allison TG, Miller TD, Squires RW et al 1993 Cardiovascular responses to immersion in a hot tub in comparison with exercise in male subjects with coronary artery disease. Mayo Clin Proc 68: 19.
Castle SP 1985 Public health implications regarding the epidemiology and microbiology of public whirlpools. Infect Control 6: 418.
Kosatsky T, Kleeman J 1985 Superficial and systemic illness related to a hot tub. Am J Med 79: 10.
Lemire RJ 1988 Neural tube defects. JAMA 259: 558.
Milunsky A, Ulcickas M, Rothman K et al 1992 Maternal heat exposure and neural tube defects. JAMA 268: 882.
Ridge BR, Budd GM 1990 How long is too long in a spa pool. N Engl J Med 323: 835.

Bed rest

Bed rest is an important therapeutic measure for a number of disorders (particularly cardiac failure and pre-eclampsia), but it is more often nowadays a consequence of illness rather than a prescribed therapy.

Bed rest may be regarded as the opposite of exercise training and may thus result in a number of physiological derangements. These may be seen in the elderly within 48 h and in other patients by 1–3 weeks.

The adverse changes of bed rest include the following.

- **Circulatory**, with
  - decreased cardiac output,
  - decreased blood volume (by an average of 750 mL),
  - orthostatic hypotension,
  - decreased red blood cell mass,
  - increased blood viscosity,
  - increased venous stasis with thromboembolism.

- **Respiratory**, with
  - decreased lung volumes, especially vital capacity and functional residual capacity,
  - decreased arterial saturation.

- **Muscular**, with
  - decrease in muscle mass and contractility.

- **Metabolic**, with
  - loss of bone mineralization,
  - impaired glucose tolerance,
  - increased blood cholesterol.

- **Neurological**, with
  - blunted sensation and motor activity, due to sensory deprivation and especially in Intensive Care,
  - emotional lability.

Clearly, these changes are undesirable but equally clearly they are inevitable, particularly in Intensive Care patients, when the changes are often compounded by a septic or catabolic state.

Bee stings (see Bites and stings)

Behçet's syndrome

Behçet's syndrome (Behçet's disease) is a multisystem disease of unknown cause, affecting primarily young adults of Eastern Mediterranean or Japanese origin.

Clinical features comprise most commonly:

- painful mouth ulcers (similar to aphthous stomatitis) and genital ulcers;
- eye signs (iritis, episcleritis, retinal vasculitis, optic neuritis).

Less commonly, there may be:

- seronegative, non-destructive arthritis;
- colitis;
- vasculitis and/or thrombophlebitis, sometimes associated with anticardiolipin antibodies and arterial or venous thrombosis (and possibly infarction);
- neurological involvement, with cranial nerve palsy, brainstem dysfunction or meningoencephalitis.

The diagnosis is based on the clinical features.

In Intensive Care practice, it should be considered in the differential diagnosis of multisystem dysfunction, if the cause is not otherwise apparent and the clinical setting is appropriate.

Treatment consists of **corticosteroids**, *with added cytotoxic therapy in cases of recurrence or relapse.*

Colchicine, thalidomide and more recently cyclosporin have been reported to be of benefit in some patients.

The prognosis is mostly favourable over several years.

Bibliography

James DG 1979 Behçet's syndrome. N Engl J Med 301: 431.
Lee S, Bang D, Lee E et al 2000 Behçet's Disease. Berlin: Springer-Verlag.
Shimizu T, Ehrlich GE, Inaba G et al 1979 Behçet's disease (Behçet's syndrome). Semin Arthritis Rheum 8: 223.

Bell's palsy

Bell's palsy refers to paralysis of the facial (VII) nerve. It is produced by inflammation in the facial canal within the temporal bone, but the cause of this process is uncertain. Recently, herpes simplex virus type 1 has been implicated.

There is the rapid onset of paralysis, which is sometimes complete. There is no sensory change, though there may be impaired lacrimation, salivation and taste.

The differential diagnosis includes:

- 7th nerve herpes zoster (Ramsay Hunt syndrome);
- diabetic 7th nerve palsy;
- neoplastic or vascular lesions of the pons or cerebellopontine angle;
- Guillain–Barré syndrome;
- Lyme disease;
- sarcoidosis;
- carcinomatous meningitis.

Treatment with **corticosteroids** *is commonly given, but significant benefit has been difficult to confirm in controlled trials.*

- *Recently,* **acyclovir** *has been shown to be helpful.*
- *The eye should be covered if the cornea is exposed.*

Most cases recover, at least sufficiently to give a good cosmetic result, though 5–10% have some permanent weakness.

Bibliography

Adour KK 1982 Diagnosis and management of facial paralysis. N Engl J Med 307: 348.
Devriese PP, Schumacher T, Scheide A et al 1990 Incidence, prognosis and recovery of Bell's palsy. Clin Otolaryngol 15: 15.
Halperin J, Luft BJ, Volkman DJ et al 1990 Lyme neuroborreliosis: peripheral nervous system manifestations. Brain 113: 1207.
Murakami S, Mizobuchi M, Nakashiro Y et al 1996 Bell palsy and herpes simplex virus identification of viral DNA in endoneurial fluid and muscle. Ann Intern Med 124: 27.

Bence Jones protein (see also Multiple myeloma)

Bence Jones protein is a low molecular weight protein originally described in the urine of patients with multiple myeloma. It was noted to coagulate on gentle heating of the urine but to redissolve on boiling, only to precipitate again on cooling below 60°C.

Its presence is virtually pathognomonic of multiple myeloma, though it is present in only 50% of such cases. The urine shows a positive dipstick test for protein, and there is a single band on urine electrophoresis. The protein is also present in serum but in low concentration.

The protein is the kappa or lambda light chain of IgG. Its presence is regarded as mild if the daily urinary excretion is <4 g and severe if it is >12 g.

Bence Jones protein can cause renal tubular damage either directly or associated with cast production. Casts occur from the aggregation of the Bence Jones protein with the locally produced 14 kd glycoprotein, nephrocalcin. Distal tubular obstruction and inflammation may result.

Benign intracranial hypertension

Benign intracranial hypertension (idiopathic intracranial hypertension, pseudotumour cerebri) refers to chronically increased intracranial pressure without hydrocephalus.

> It usually occurs in obese young women and without known cause. It can also be related to:
>
> - some drugs;
>   - including indomethacin, isotretinoin, nitrofurantoin, oral contraceptives, tetracycline (especially minocycline, the most lipid-soluble member of the group);
> - cerebral venous thrombosis;
> - endocrine disorders (sometimes).

Clinical features include:

- headache;
- visual impairment, with
  - visual loss (sometimes permanent);
  - peripheral field defects;
  - diplopia;
  - papilloedema.

Treatment is with **CSF drainage***,* **diuretics** *or, if refractory,* **corticosteroids** *(in moderate doses for about 3 months).*

- *CSF drainage may be by repeated lumbar puncture (e.g. 20–40 mL taken several times weekly) or a shunt (e.g. lumboperitoneal).*
- *Suitable diuretics include frusemide or acetazolamide. Glycerol orally can be effective.*
- *Weight reduction is recommended.*
- *Surgical decompression is sometimes required, e.g. optic nerve sheath decompression if vision is threatened.*

Bibliography

Giuseffi V, Wall M, Siegel PZ et al 1991 Symptoms and disease associations in idiopathic intracranial hypertension (pseudotumor cerebri). Neurology 41: 239.

Lyons MK, Meyer FB 1990 Cerebrospinal fluid physiology and the management of increased intracranial pressure. Mayo Clin Proc 65: 684.

Wall M, George D 1991 Idiopathic intracranial hypertension. Brain 114: 155.

Beriberi

Beriberi is vitamin B1 (thiamine) deficiency, and the name is derived from the Sinhalese meaning extreme weakness. In developed countries, it is sometimes seen as part of the nutritional deficiency associated with alcoholism. It is thus usually accompanied by other stigmata of alcoholism, especially Wernicke's encephalopathy (q.v.).

So-called 'wet' beriberi is manifested by a dilated cardiomyopathy with hyperdynamic circulatory failure.

In Intensive Care, beriberi should thus be remembered as one of the uncommon causes of the hyperdynamic state. Its importance lies in its rapid response to thiamine (100 mg iv).

Beryllium

Beryllium (Be, atomic number 4, atomic weight 9) is a brittle, alkaline-earth metal and was discovered in 1798. It is not free in nature and there are no large deposits, beryllium most frequently appearing as beryllium aluminium silicate in gem stones (including emeralds). It has a very high melting point (1278°C) and is a good conductor of both heat and electricity. Its particular use has been as a hardening agent in metallurgy. Exposure levels of not $>0.5–3$ $\mu g/m^3/8$ h are recommended.

Soluble beryllium compounds are toxic

- **Acute toxicity** occurs in mining or metallurgy and consists of a burning rash, nose and eye irritation, cough and chest tightness. Fatal respiratory failure within 72 h may occasionally occur, but more commonly there is recovery over a few months.
- **Chronic toxicity** is seen in scientific or industrial workers and follows a latent period of up to 15 years. Permanent, though often mild, respiratory disability occurs with cough and dyspnoea. The diffuse pulmonary changes are referred to as **berylliosis**, in which granulomas histologically identical to sarcoidosis are seen and even bilateral hilar lymphadenopathy. Chronic beryllium exposure can also predispose to lung cancer.

Bibliography

Rossman MD, Kern JA, Elias JA et al 1988 Proliferative responses of bronchoalveolar lymphocytes to beryllium: a test for chronic beryllium disease. Ann Intern Med 108: 687.

Beta$_2$-microglobulin

Beta$_2$-microglobulin is the beta or light-chain of the HLA-Class I molecule required for cell-cell recognition. It is a small protein of 11.5 kd and is present on most cell membranes though not on mature red blood cells. There is considerable amino acid sequence homology between beta$_2$-microglobulin, the heavy chain of the MHC Class I antigen and the constant region of the heavy chain of IgG.

Beta$_2$-microglobulin is released during cell breakdown and is then metabolized and cleared by the kidney. Its plasma level is thus increased with renal impairment. It is also increased following complement activation and IL-1 generation, due to increased synthesis.

The proteinuria in tubulointerstitial disease is predominantly low molecular weight material, such as beta$_2$-microglobulin, rather than albumin as in glomerular diseases.

Beta$_2$-microglobulin provides the protein subunit for dialysis-related amyloid.

Biliary cirrhosis (see also Cholangitis and Cholestasis)

Biliary cirrhosis may be either primary or secondary.

Primary biliary cirrhosis is an autoimmune disease. It is thus also associated with other autoimmune diseases, particularly scleroderma, CREST syndrome, Sjögren's syndrome and renal tubular acidosis. There is a genetic predisposition because of the association with the HLA-DR8 haplotype.

Clinical features of primary biliary cirrhosis typically are manifest in women aged 30–50 y. There is the gradual onset of pruritus, fatigue and increased skin pigmentation. Late features include jaundice, hepatosplenomegaly, multiple xanthomas, osteoporosis (with bone pain and pathological fractures). Eventually, ascites and oedema occur.

Investigations show liver function disturbance with chiefly an increased alkaline phosphatase. Anti-mitochondrial antibody is typically present, and the serum cholesterol is raised. Liver biopsy shows a specific histological picture in only a few patients, as in most the findings are similar to those seen in chronic active hepatitis.

The differential diagnosis includes:

- secondary biliary cirrhosis;
- cholangitis;
- chronic biliary obstruction.

Treatment modalities including corticosteroids, cytotoxic agents, colchicine, penicillamine and cyclosporin are all at best poorly effective and are associated with significant side-effects.

- *Cholestyramine may alleviate pruritus, for which antihistamines are usually ineffective.*
- *The bile acid **ursodiol** (ursodeoxycholic acid, 12–15 mg/kg per day orally) diminishes the potentially toxic endogenous bile acid pool and is moderately effective as well as safe, though it is expensive.*
- *Vitamin supplementation is required.*

The course of the disease is slow, with a median survival of 10 years.

Secondary biliary cirrhosis arises from chronic biliary tract disease due to obstruction or prolonged inflammation. This leads to the irreversible histological changes of cirrhosis.

Bibliography
James SP, Hoofnagle JH, Strober W et al 1983 Primary biliary cirrhosis: a model autoimmune disease. Ann Intern Med 99: 500.
Poupon RE, Poupon R, Balkau B 1994 Ursodiol for the long-term treatment of primary biliary cirrhosis. N Engl J Med 330: 1342.

Bioterrorism (see Anthrax)

Bird fancier's lung (see Hypersensitivity pneumonitis)

Bismuth

Bismuth (Bi, atomic number 83, atomic weight 209, melting point 271°C) is the most metallic of the elements in the nitrogen family. It was first described in 1450 and is a hard, brittle, greyish substance, which does not tarnish in air and which is difficult to magnetize. In addition to its widespread use in manufacturing, its salts in a variety of colloidal forms have long been in common use in medicine as a gastrointestinal soothing agent, in ointments, and as a radio-opaque medium. It is also commonly used as an antibacterial in the prevention or treatment of diarrhoea, e.g. in travellers.

More recently, it has been used for peptic ulceration, despite its lack of antacid effect. In this setting, it inhibits pepsin, increases mucus and most importantly detaches *Helicobacter pylori* from the gastric epithelium thus permitting its lysis.

Non-absorbable preparations are used, because systemic levels can cause encephalopathy and osteodystrophy. It should not be used in renal failure, as any small amounts that may be absorbed are normally excreted in the urine. The oral administration of bismuth compounds can produce a dark mouth, a phenomenon which is reversible.

The most common compound is bismuth subcitrate (tripotassium dicitratobismuthate), but subnitrate, subgallate and subsalicylate compounds are also prepared.

Bites and stings

Bites and stings may be inflicted by many creatures. Their clinical effects depend on:

- the site and severity of the bite or sting itself;
- the injection of potentially pathogenic organisms. Infecting organisms may come

from the biting mouth or stinging part of the attacking creature or from the recipient's skin;

- the injection of toxin (venom).

Venom refers to a poisonous secretion from specialized glands, often associated with the teeth, spines, stings or other piercing parts of the attacking creature. Venoms are a mixture of toxic enzymes and other proteins. In nature, venoms are used for attacking prey or for defence. When injected into man, they produce the syndrome of **envenomation**.

Venomous creatures may be found worldwide and are represented in most major animal phyla, although they are especially found in the rural tropics. The best known such creatures are snakes, spiders, scorpions, insects and marine vertebrates and invertebrates. The most venomous creatures reside in Australia, which has some 2000 such species.

Nevertheless, death from envenomation is rare in a developed country (e.g. about two deaths per year in Australia, all without appropriate first-aid), though it has been estimated that over 100000 people die each year from envenomation worldwide. In developed countries, anaphylaxis from bee or wasp venom is a more common cause of death. In Australia, there are about 10 hospital admissions per day from bites and stings, with 38% from spiders, 28% from bees and wasps, and 16% from snakes.

> The clinical features of envenomation may be:
>
> - neurotoxic;
> - haemotoxic;
> - allergic.
>
> These features may vary greatly in severity from asymptomatic to serious or even fatal.

The general principles of treatment of bites and stings relate to local trauma (if any) and to the risks of infection or of envenomation.

- ***Potentially infected bites***, *especially on the hand, should be treated with prophylactic oral antibiotics (e.g. amoxycillin/clavulanic acid),*

though these may safely be omitted if the bite is minor. If infection actually occurs or if the patient presents late, intravenous antibiotics are preferable. Since the Gram-stain from the wound usually provides inadequate information, microbiological culture is important. Appropriate tetanus prophylaxis is required, as is basic wound care.

- ***Potentially venomous bites*** *should be treated with bodily rest and immobilization of the affected part by the bandage and splint technique (except after fish, red-back spider or Crotalid envenomation because local pressure increases pain and possibly local tissue damage). Transport should be arranged to a hospital, and unless the injury is minor, the patient should be admitted to Intensive Care for circulatory, respiratory, renal and coagulation support. Treatment of circulatory failure (due especially to hypovolaemia), respiratory failure (due primarily to paralysis), coagulopathy, haemolysis and rhabdomyolysis are the chief priorities.*

> If there are clinical or investigational features of systemic envenomation, specific antivenom (antivenene) should be urgently given, following species identification (if necessary using a venom detection kit. If the responsible species cannot be identified with confidence, polyvalent antivenom should be given. The antivenom is given diluted and iv and the dose is based on the amount of venom injected and not on the patient's body size. The dose in one container is designed to neutralize the amount of venom in a standard or milked bite; this dose needs to be increased or repeated if there have been multiple bites, delay in treatment or relapse.
>
> **Adrenaline** is required either for anaphylaxis or prior to antivenom in patients with a previous reaction.
>
> **Corticosteroids** and **antihistamine** should be given iv if the patient is hypersensitive to horse serum or has had a previous exposure.
>
> Tetanus prophylaxis is required, but antibiotics are not indicated.

The bites and/or stings from a number of creatures may present specific problems.

Bats from all continents except Australia have been recorded to harbour rabies. In Australia, some fruit bats have been found to carry a related organism, lyssavirus. This can cause encephalitis in humans, *which should be treated as for rabies.*

Bees and wasps may give acute allergic reactions and even anaphylaxis in some patients. This is because hymenopteran venom contains enzymes (proteins), as well as vasoactive amines and small peptides. Even a large local reaction is generally allergic, as infectious cellulitis is rare after insect stings. If very numerous, such stings may produce severe systemic toxicity with hypotension.

*Acute treatment of a clinically significant reaction is with an anti-H1 **antihistamine** and if severe with **corticosteroids**, as well as symptomatic measures such as ice and analgesia. Either desensitization or self-administered adrenaline should be offered to those who have had a previous severe reaction.*

Cats can give an infective bite, the risk being higher than for a dog bite because of the cat's sharper teeth (and thus the bite and anaerobic inoculum is generally deeper). The usual pathogen in domestic cats is *P. multocida*, though organisms similar to those in the human mouth (see below) may also be present, as may be *C. canimorsus* found in dogs (see below). Similar flora ('fang flora') exist in the mouths of large cats, though clearly the bites from these animals are also associated with much more severe injuries, including particularly spinal damage from a crushing bite to the neck. A cat bite can also lead to cat-scratch disease (q.v.).

Dog bites are usually from a known animal and are on an extremity, except in children when the face is commonly bitten. Although the dog mouth contains many aerobic and anaerobic bacteria, the main pathogens are *P. multocida* and *Capnocytophaga canimorsus* (formerly called DF-2), a slowly-growing Gram-negative rod. The latter can cause death even in normal hosts and is especially prone to cause septicaemia in alcoholics or in patients with significant underlying disease. The septicaemia is indistinguishable clinically from other forms of severe sepsis, except for the presence of a wound usually with painful cellulitis. Systemic symptoms occur 1–8 days after the bite, and the reported mortality is about 30%. Despite this potential, most dogs' bites are in fact not infectious and prophylaxis is often unnecessary.

Wild animal bites should be considered a risk for rabies, unless in a rabies-free country (see Rabies).

Human bites may occur anywhere on the body but most commonly on the fingers. Similar lesions may also occur on the knuckles of a clenched fist or may be self-inflicted on the hands or lips. The organism most commonly involved is *S. viridans*. Other organisms are also commonly involved, including *S. aureus, H. influenzae, E. corrodens*, and a variety of anaerobes, including bacteroides, fusobacteria and peptostreptococci.

*Prophylaxis with **penicillin** (or flucloxacillin or amoxycillin/clavulanic acid) is usually required.*

Insects, including mosquitoes, ticks, lice and mites, are the vectors for the transmission to humans of a wide variety of infectious diseases (q.v.). In particular, **ticks** may inject a neurotoxin, which can produce diplopia, weakness and ataxia, sometimes with associated rhabdomyolysis, myocarditis or lymphadenopathy (see also Lyme disease).

Antitoxin treatment is available.

Marine invertebrates which can cause envenomation in man particularly include members of the Coelenterata phylum, such as **jellyfish** (the best known being the Portuguese Man of War and the most toxic being the Box Jellyfish). Their sting can cause local pain (which may be extreme) and cutaneous eruption (which may be followed by skin necrosis), and systemic features of vomiting, sweating, dyspnoea, hypotension and even anaphylaxis. Following contact with Box

Jellyfish tentacles, hypotension, paralysis and cardiorespiratory failure may develop within minutes.

Emergency treatment of jellyfish stings is with local vinegar and immobilization. Analgesia, volume expanders, inotopes and ventilatory support may be required until antivenom becomes available.

The blue-ringed **octopus** may inject tetrodotoxin (a neuromuscular blocking neurotoxin). The bite itself may be painless, but paralysis may result.

Treatment of an octopus bite is supportive, as no antivenom is currently available, though anticholinesterase therapy (q.v.) has been reported to be possibly helpful.

Marine vertebrates can also produce venom, particularly in fish spines. The **puffer fish** contains tetrodotoxin (see blue-ringed octopus above). **Stone fish** spines are typically a risk to humans from being trodden on. There is severe local pain (and possibly skin necrosis subsequently) and sometimes major systemic symptoms, such as paralysis and circulatory collapse.

Antivenom *should be given, except in mild cases, and local anaesthesia is symptomatically effective.*

Monkey bites can potentially cause infection with herpesvirus simiae (monkey B virus), which is a fatal neurotropic viral infection.

Rat saliva may contain the organisms, *Spirillum minus* or *Streptobacillus moniliformis*.

Scorpion stings are common in tropical and subtropical countries. The sting causes considerable local pain and often general intoxication, but the mortality is generally less than 1%. The general intoxication comprises neurological, respiratory and especially cardiovascular responses. The latter is due to intense adrenergic stimulation, which causes arrhythmias, cardiac failure and even shock.

Antivenom *treatment is available.*

Snake bite is a potential emergency, although the mortality is in fact low. In untreated cases,

up to 10% of deaths occur within 3 h, though over 80% occur after 7 h (and thus usually well after medical assistance can be obtained) and nearly half occur after 24 h. The fang marks themselves may be difficult to identify, but there is usually local pain and inflammation. Local tissue damage is most evident following cobra or rattlesnake bites. Following a suspected snake bite, the patient should be observed for at least 12 h for signs of envenomation. Snake venoms are complex products, generally with neurotoxins, but also commonly with haemotoxins, myotoxins, nephrotoxins, cardiotoxins and proteolytic enzymes which cause local tissue damage.

Systemic symptoms generally appear within 4 h and sometimes much earlier. They include:

- neurological features

  – paraesthesiae, weakness, strange taste, drowsiness, bulbar signs, fits;

- nausea;
- bleeding;
- dyspnoea;
- shock.

Anaphylaxis may occur in patients who have been similarly envenomated previously (e.g. snake handlers).

Investigations include full blood examination (especially for haematocrit and platelet count), coagulation screen, electrolytes, renal function, and urinalysis. These should be carried out initially and then 8 hourly until any major acute changes have resolved.

Treatment principles are outlined above.

Spider bites mostly are harmless, though there are some major exceptions. The **Sydney funnel-web spider** is the world's most deadly spider and may cause potentially lethal envenomation, with a dramatic clinical picture of tachycardia, hypertension, salivation, muscle spasm, pulmonary oedema, raised intracranial pressure and acidosis. This is sometimes referred to as an autonomic storm.

Treatment of a funnel-web spider bite consists of immobilization, support of respiratory and circulatory failure, and the administration of **antivenom***, the beneficial effects of which are rapid.*

Red-back spider bites cause severe and prompt local pain, followed by sweating, nausea, vomiting, headache, and sometimes tachycardia, hypertension and paralysis. This spider is a member of the Lactodectus genus, which includes the American black widow spider.

Treatment of a red-back spider bite is with local ice packs, diazepam and specific **antivenom***.*

Extensive local tissue damage (**necrotic arachnidism**) may sometimes be produced by the bites of some spiders (e.g. recluse, white-tailed, wolf).

Treatment of this injury is primarily on its local merits, but associated vasculitis may be helped with heparin and/or corticosteroids. Useful measures for necrosis probably include hyperbaric oxygen but not debridement, grafting or antibiotics.

Brown recluse and **black widow** spiders are important causes of envenomation in the USA. **Tarantulas** have become common household 'pets', and the bites of these large hairy creatures are correspondingly frequent. Local pain, erythema and swelling are accompanied by systemic features of anaphylaxis in those allergic to the venom. Eye injuries from released barbs can occur.

Toad bites may occasionally cause envenomation.

There has been a recent report of its successful treatment with **digoxin-specific antibody** *(q.v.).*

Bibliography

Aghababian RV, Conte JE 1980 Mammalian bite wounds. Ann Emerg Med 9: 79.

Auerbach PS 1991 Marine envenomation. N Engl J Med 325: 486.

Brubacher JR, Ravikumar PR, Bania T et al 1996 Treatment of toad venom poisoning with digoxin-specific Fab fragments. Chest 110: 1282.

Burnett JW, Calton GJ 1987 Jellyfish envenomation syndromes updated. Ann Emerg Med 16: 1000.

Callahan M 1980 Dog bite wounds. JAMA 244: 2327.

CSL Ltd 1992 Treatment of Snake Bite in Australia and Papua New Guinea using Antivenom. Melbourne: Commonwealth Serum Laboratories.

Cummings P 1994 Antibiotics to prevent infection in patients with dog bite wounds: a meta-analysis of randomized trials. Ann Emerg Med 23: 535.

Cuthbertson BH, Fisher M 1998 Envenomation. Int J Intens Care 5: 64.

Dire DJ 1991 Cat bite wounds: risk factors for infection. Ann Emerg Med 20: 973.

Fenner PJ, Williamson JA 1996 Worldwide deaths and severe envenomation from jellyfish stings. Med J Aust 165: 658.

Fisher MM, Carr GA, McGuinness R, Warden JC 1980 Atrax robustus envenomation. Anaesth Intens Care 8: 410.

Goldstein EJC 1992 Bite wounds and infection. Clin Infect Dis 14: 633.

Griego RD, Rosen T, Orengo IF et al 1995 Dog, cat, and human bites. J Am Acad Dermatol 33: 1019.

Hovenga S, Tulleken JE, Moller LVM et al 1997 Dog-bite induced sepsis: a report of four cases. Intens Care Med 23: 1179.

Hunt GR 1981 Bites and stings of uncommon arthropods. Postgrad Med 70: 91, 107.

Janda DH, Ringler DH, Hilliard JK et al 1990 Nonhuman primate bites. J Orthop Res 8: 146.

Javaid M, Feldberg L, Gipson M 1998 Primary repair of dog bites to the face. J R Soc Med 91: 414.

Klein M 1985 Nondomestic mammalian bites. Am Fam Physician 32: 137.

McHugh TP, Bartlett RL, Raymond JI 1985 Rat bite fever. Ann Emerg Med 14: 1116.

O'Hehir RE, Douglass JA 1999 Stinging insect allergy. Med J Aust 171: 649.

Pennell TC, Babu S-S, Meredith JW 1987 The management of snake and spider bites in the southeastern United States. Ann Surg 53: 198.

Pers C, Gahrm-Hansen B, Frederiksen W. 1996 *Capnocytophaga canimorsus* septicaemia in Denmark, 1982–1995: review of 39 cases. Clin Infect Dis 23: 71.

Reisman RE 1994 Insect stings. N Engl J Med 331: 523.

Sofer S 1995 Scorpion envenomation. Intens Care Med 21: 626.

Sutherland SK 1983 Australian Animal Toxins. Melbourne: Oxford University Press.

Sutherland SK, Leonard RL 1995 Snakebite deaths in Australia 1992–1994 and a management update. Med J Aust 163: 616.

Sutherland S, Nolch G 2000 Dangerous Australian Animals. Sydney: Hyland House.

Sutherland SK, Coulter AR, Harris RD 1979 Rationalisation of first-aid measures for elapid snakebite. Lancet 1: 183.

Tibballs J 1992 Diagnosis and treatment of confirmed and suspected snake bite. Med J Aust 156: 270.

Underhill D 1990 Australia's Dangerous Creatures. Sydney: Reader's Digest.

Warrell DA, Fenner PJ 1993 Venomous bites and stings. Br Med Bull 49: 423.

Weiner S. 1961 Redback spider bites in Australia. Med J Aust 2: 44.

White J 1995 CSL Antivenom Handbook. Melbourne: CSL.

White J 1999 Necrotising arachnidism. Med J Aust 171: 98.

Williamson JA, Le Ray LE, Wohlfahrt M et al 1984 Acute management of serious envenomation by box-jellyfish (*Chironex fleckeri*). Med J Aust 141: 851.

Bleomycin

Bleomycin is a mixture of related glycopeptides used in cancer chemotherapy, especially for squamous cell carcinomas, as well as for lymphoma and testicular cancer. It produces little bone marrow or immune suppression. Its unique action is to fragment DNA, and it is commonly used in multidrug combinations.

Its side-effects include fever, stomatitis, alopecia, and rash with pruritus and vesiculation.

In the Intensive Care Unit, two uncommon but important side-effects may be relevant.

A **fulminant reaction** may be seen in about 1% of patients overall and in 5% of patients with lymphomas. This reaction occurs within a few hours of the first or second dose and is characterized by confusion, fever, wheeze and hypotension. It does not appear to be anaphylactic and may be related to the release of endogenous pyrogens.

Pulmonary toxicity which can be severe and even fatal may be a late complication. It occurs 4–10 weeks after the start of treatment in 5–10% of patients. The risk is increased with higher doses, in the elderly, with oxygen and with irradiation. It is characterized by cough, crackles on auscultation, and a diffuse basal infiltrate on chest X-ray. The value of corticosteroids is unknown, but they are probably helpful. If recovery occurs, pulmonary function returns to normal. Nevertheless, the risk of post-anaesthetic ARDS persists for 6–12 months after treatment, and it is important in such patients to avoid excessive fluid administration and to keep the inspired oxygen concentration below 30% (though the added pulmonary risk from 'hyperoxia' is controversial).

Bibliography
Mathes DD 1995 Bleomycin and hyperoxia exposure in the operating room. Anesth Analg 81: 624.

Blisters (see Vesiculobullous diseases)

Boerhaave's syndrome (see Mallory–Weiss syndrome)

Botulism (see also Food poisoning)

Botulism is produced by the neurotoxin from the anaerobic Gram-positive bacillus, *Clostridium botulinum*, which blocks acetylcholine release at peripheral nerve endings.

The use of **botulinum toxin** in hemifacial spasm and related disorders is an interesting and valuable clinical application of this otherwise undesirable toxin.

Although the toxin is labile, the spores are heat-stable and may thus produce new toxin if cooked food is left at room temperature for more than 16 h. Most commonly, botulism arises from the ingestion of poorly processed home foods, though it occasionally occurs as a wound infection. Recently, cases have been reported following the ingestion of fish gut. The incubation period ranges from 6 h to 8 days, though it usually 18–36 h.

The patient experiences diplopia, ptosis, dysphagia, dysarthria and descending paralysis. The mouth is dry and there are usually gastrointestinal symptoms. There is no fever.

The differential diagnosis includes:

- Guillain–Barré syndrome;
- brainstem stroke;
- poisoning;
- diphtheria.

Treatment is with **antitoxin**, *administered as soon as the diagnosis is established, and with mechanical ventilation.*

The mortality is still about 20%.

Bibliography

Jankovic J, Brin MF 1991 Therapeutic uses of botulinum toxin. N Engl J Med 324: 1186.

Lecour H, Ramos H, Almeida B et al 1988 Food-borne botulism: a review of 13 outbreaks. Arch Intern Med 148: 578.

Merson MH, Dowell VR 1973 Epidemiologic, clinical and laboratory aspects of wound botulism. N Engl J Med 289: 1005.

Bovine spongiform encephalopathy (see Creutzfeldt–Jakob disease)

Bromocriptine (see Acromegaly and Neuroleptic malignant syndrome)

Bronchiectasis

Bronchiectasis is defined on anatomical grounds as chronic abnormal dilatation of larger bronchi. This process comprises airway obstruction and damage following chronic inflammation, because the pooling of bronchial secretions rich in inflammatory products and in released intracellular proteases weakens the bronchial wall. In addition to severe, necrotizing lung infections, the aetiology probably also includes congenital factors.

The association of bronchiectasis with congenital dextrocardia and sinusitis is referred to as **Kartagener's syndrome** (see Situs inversus). Bronchiectasis may also complicate:

- cystic fibrosis;
- hypogammaglobulinaemia;
- rheumatoid lung;
- asthmatic pulmonary eosinophilia.

The clinical features are cough, purulent sputum and proneness to recurrent or persistent lower respiratory tract infection. The sputum can be copious and particularly offensive. Haemoptysis, dyspnoea and wheeze may occur, and there are crackles on auscultation and clubbing of the fingers.

The diagnosis was made formerly by bronchography (or autopsy) but is made nowadays by CT scanning. The bronchographic distinction of cylindrical, varicose (fusiform) and cystic (saccular) changes probably has little clinical significance.

Treatment is primarily with physiotherapy and antibiotics, the latter in most patients preferably only for exacerbations. Surgical resection is only occasionally indicated nowadays.

Prevention is of major importance and includes particularly the prompt and effective treatment of respiratory infections and of airway obstruction by foreign bodies.

Bibliography

Afzelius BA 1976 A human syndrome caused by immotile cilia. Science 193: 317.

Agasthian T, Deschamps C, Trastek VF et al 1996 Surgical management of bronchiectasis. Ann Thorac Surg 62: 976.

Mygind N, Nielsen MH, Pedersen M 1983 Kartagener's syndrome and abnormal cilia. Eur J Respir Dis 64 (suppl 127): 1.

Bronchiolitis obliterans

Bronchiolitis obliterans (BO) (obliterative bronchiolitis, bronchiolitis fibrosa obliterans) is a rare condition and probably a very severe form of chronic obstructive bronchitis with pathological changes implied by its name, namely chronic organizing inflammation of small airways. Its pathogenesis is presumably bronchiolar epithelial injury followed by an excessively proliferative repair process.

It is most usually due to the inhalation a few weeks previously of a toxic gas, for example an industrial chemical (such as nitrogen dioxide, as in silo-filler's disease) or a military poison.

It has occasionally followed severe infections, usually viral pneumonia, when it may sometimes take the form of **bronchiolitis obliterans organizing pneumonia** (BOOP). In this situation, there are prominent nodules of granulation tissue within the small airways. The relationship between BO and BOOP is not always clear.

It has more recently been appreciated that a similar end-result can also follow collagen-vascular disease, graft-versus-host disease and lung transplantation in which it is a common form of chronic rejection.

The chest X-ray typically shows diffuse fine nodules with subsequent hyperinflation.

Treatment is generally ineffective.

The prognosis is often poor.

Bibliography
Boehler A, Kesten S, Weder W et al 1998 Bronchiolitis obliterans after lung transplantation: a review. Chest 114: 1411.
Epler GR, Colby TV, McLoud TC et al 1985 Bronchiolitis obliterans organizing pneumonia. N Engl J Med 312: 152.
Ramirez J, Dowell AR 1971 Silo-filler's disease: nitrogen dioxide-induced lung injury: long-term follow-up and review of the literature. Ann Intern Med 74: 569.
Schwartz DA 1987 Acute inhalational injury. Occup Med 2: 297.
Theodore J, Starnes VA, Lewiston NJ 1990 Obliterative bronchiolitis. Clin Chest Med 11: 309.
Wohl MEB, Chernick V 1978 Bronchiolitis. Am Rev Respir Dis 118: 759.

Bronchocentric granulomatosis

(see Wegener's granulomatosis)

Brucellosis

Brucellosis is due to infection with a small slowly growing Gram-negative aerobic bacillus, discovered by Bruce in 1887, which is normally seen in animals – *B. abortus* in cattle, *B. suis* in pigs, *B. melitensis* in goats and *B. canis* in dogs, as well as other more recently identified strains in other animals, including marine mammals. Infection thus usually arises following exposure to animals and so particularly affects meat workers. Dairy products are not nowadays a source of infection in most countries.

Following a variable incubation period of days to months, there is an insidious onset of fever and variable local findings, e.g. endocarditis, meningitis, osteomyelitis.

Investigations may show a normal white cell count and ESR. The microbiological diagnosis is made from blood cultures or from an increased titre of serum agglutinins. Specimens must be handled with special care in the laboratory, so as to avoid accidental infection of the staff.

*Treatment is with **tetracycline** (e.g. doxycycline 100 mg twice daily) and/or rifampicin (600–900 mg daily) for 3–6 weeks. If there is severe local disease, such as endocarditis or meningitis, combination therapy of tetracycline with added cotrimoxazole and/or rifampicin and/or an aminoglycoside is used for several months.*

The prognosis is now good, with a mortality of <1%. There is no presently available vaccine.

Bibliography
Corbell MJ 1997 Brucellosis: an overview. Emerg Infect Dis 3: 2.

Radolf J 1994 Brucellosis: don't let it get your goat! Am J Med Sci 307: 64.

Budd–Chiari syndrome

The Budd–Chiari syndrome arises from hepatic vein thrombosis.

It is seen

- in thrombophilias

  – such as antithrombin III deficiency,

- in myelodysplastic disorders

  – such as polycythaemia vera,

- in veno-occlusive disease

  – such as in poisoning from plant alkaloids, as are found in herbal or bush teas,

- following high-dose chemotherapy

  – in association with bone marrow transplantation.

The clinical features comprise acute tender hepatomegaly, with jaundice, ascites and peripheral oedema.

*Treatment is traditionally with **anticoagulation** (heparin followed by warfarin), but there have been case reports of successful thrombolytic therapy given either locally or systemically.*

Even if acute recovery occurs, cardiac cirrhosis may result and may then become a longer-term problem.

Bibliography
Bach N, Thung SN, Schaffner F 1989 Comfrey herb tea-induced hepatic veno-occlusive disease. Am J Med 87: 97.
Broughton BJ 1991 Hepatic and portal vein thrombosis closely associated with myeloproliferative disorders. Br Med J 302: 192.
Klein AS, Sitzmann JV, Coleman J et al 1990 Current management of the Budd–Chiari syndrome. Ann Surg 212: 144.
Mitchell MC, Boitnott JK, Kaufman S et al 1982 Budd–Chiari syndrome: etiology, diagnosis and management. Medicine 61: 199.
Shulman HM, Hinterberger W 1992 Hepatic veno-occlusive disease – liver toxicity syndrome after bone marrow transplantation. Bone Marrow Transpl 10: 197.
Valla D, Casadevall N, Lacombe C et al 1985 Primary myeloproliferative disorder and hepatic vein thrombosis. Ann Intern Med 103: 329.
Vassal G, Hartmann O, Benhamou E 1990 Busulfan and veno-occlusive disease of the liver. Ann Intern Med 112: 881.

Bullae (see Vesiculobullous diseases)

Burns, respiratory complications

The respiratory complications of burns (inhalation injury) can result in significant morbidity and mortality in those initially surviving a fire. Respiratory tract injury results from the inhalation of products of combustion, which may be numerous, and has an even greater impact on mortality than the two important factors in burn injury of patient age and surface area involved.

Smoke, the most obvious such product, is a suspension of carbon particles in air and other gases. The particles are often coated with chemicals, such as organic acids and aldehydes. The other gases may include carbon monoxide and toxic fumes, such as sulfur dioxide, nitrogen oxides, ammonia, hydrogen cyanide and hydrochloric acid, these being vaporized chemicals often released from the burning of modern synthetic materials, such as PVC.

Smoke may be hot, but usually it has only a low thermal capacity, so that any burns involve only the upper respiratory tract, in contrast to steam which has a high thermal capacity (4000 times that of dry air) and can burn as far as the bronchioles. Fortunately, burns due to steam are uncommon.

Respiratory burns may comprise:

- direct thermal injury;
- smoke inhalation;

- inhalation of toxic products of combustion;
- later respiratory complications.

Direct thermal injury, particularly of the upper respiratory tract, is common and is usually associated with facial burns. Severe acute upper airways obstruction may result.

As indicated above, thermal injury of the lower respiratory tract and lung parenchyma is difficult to produce except by superheated steam.

Smoke inhalation is also a common thermal injury. It gives rise to irritation, sometimes severe, of the tracheobronchial tree and usually causes immediate respiratory distress, though this may be delayed for up to 48 h. There is a chemical bronchitis, with mucosal injury, cilial dysfunction, mucous plugging, atelectasis and bronchorrhoea. There may also be mucosal oedema and increased vascular permeability.

The upper respiratory tract injury may appear minor at first, but its progress over the next 48 h needs to be carefully monitored. The patient may develop clinical features of stridor, cough, charcoal-containing sputum, dyspnoea, wheeze, hypoxia and respiratory distress. Bronchial casts may subsequently be coughed.

Inhalation of toxic products of combustion results from fires in confined spaces, e.g. buildings or aircraft. These products give rise to a severe form of acute lung irritation (q.v.) and are a major cause of fatality.

If the serum lactate level is markedly elevated (e.g. 10 mmol/L or more), carbon monoxide (q.v.) or cyanide (q.v.) toxicity should be considered. Death can occur from tissue hypoxia produced by either of these two gases.

Later respiratory complications are common, such as pulmonary oedema (especially volume overload), acute (adult) respiratory distress syndrome (ARDS) and secondary bacterial infection. Of burns patients requiring intubation, about 50% develop ARDS, but inhalation injury does not appear to be a major

risk factor for this complication. In contrast to other critical care settings, ARDS occurs much later after burns (average time to onset of about 7 days) and confers little added mortality (perhaps since the average underlying mortality is about 40%).

Hospitalization is required for any person exposed to smoke or fumes or with a singed face, with careful observation for at least the first two days. Early fibreoptic bronchoscopy provides the best way to assess the extent and severity of respiratory tract injury.

Treatment of respiratory burns is with **respiratory support** *and with management of any complications on their individual merits.*

- *Early endotracheal intubation is wise, because of its great technical difficulty if delayed.*
- *Bronchodilators are helpful if there is wheeze.*
- *Recently, inhaled heparin with acetylcysteine has been reported to reduce cast formation, atelectasis, reintubation and mortality compared with historical controls.*

Long-term lung function abnormalities and sometimes significant respiratory complications, such as tracheal or bronchial stenosis and obliterative bronchiolitis, have been reported in survivors of respiratory burns.

Bibliography

Baud FJ, Barriot P, Toffis V et al 1991 Elevated blood cyanide concentrations in victims of smoke inhalation. N Engl J Med 325: 1761.

Crapo RO 1981 Smoke-inhalation injuries. JAMA 246: 1694.

Dancey DR, Hayes J, Gomez M et al 1999 ARDS in patients with thermal injury. Intens Care Med 25: 1231.

Dietch E 1990 The management of burns. N Engl J Med 323: 1249.

Dyer RF, Esch VH 1976 Polyvinyl chloride toxicity in fires: hydrogen chloride toxicity in firefighters. JAMA 235: 393.

Fogarty PW, George PJM, Solomon M et al 1991 Long term effects of smoke inhalation in survivors of the King's Cross underground station fire. Thorax 46: 914.

Gueugniaud P-Y, Carsin H, Bertin-Maghit M et al 2000 Current advances in the initial management of major thermal burns. Intens Care Med 26: 848.

Haponik E, Munster A (eds) 1990 Respiratory Injury: Smoke Inhalation and Burns. New York: McGraw-Hill.

Large AA, Owens GR, Hoffman LA 1990 The short-term effects of smoke exposure on the pulmonary function of firefighters. Chest 97: 806.

Schulz JT, Ryan CM 2000 The frustrating problem of smoke inhalation injury. Crit Care Med 28: 1677.

Byssinosis (see Occupational lung diseases)

Cadmium

Cadmium (Cd, atomic number 48, atomic weight 112) is a soft, highly polishable metal of the zinc group with a low melting point (321°C). It was discovered in 1817 and is associated in nature with zinc. It is widely used in metallurgy, the most common compounds being cadmium oxide and cadmium sulfide (artist's yellow). Its vapour and dust are toxic with recommended levels not $>0/1 mg/m^3/8$ h for fumes and $0.2 mg/m^3/8$ h for dust.

The clinical features of toxicity depend upon the route and duration of exposure.

- **Acute toxicity** from ingestion produces prompt but transient nausea, diarrhoea and prostration (onset within 15 min and offset by 24 h).
- **Acute toxicity** from inhalation can produce a potentially fatal pneumonitis.
- **Chronic inhalation** at a lower level gives rise to anosmia, cough, dyspnoea, weight loss, renal damage (tubulointerstitial damage like that from other heavy metals, especially lead), liver damage and increased risk of cancer of the lung, kidney and prostate.

Treatment of cadmium toxicity is with **calcium edetate** *(q.v.).*

Bibliography

Ellis KJ, Yuen N, Yasumura S et al 1984 Dose–response analysis of cadmium in man: body-burden vs. kidney dysfunction. Environ Res 33: 216.

Calcitonin

Calcitonin is a polypeptide hormone secreted by the parafollicular cells of the thyroid gland and is one of the three regulators of calcium balance, together with parathyroid hormone and vitamin D. Calcitonin blocks the release of calcium and phosphorus from bone by inhibiting osteoclastic bone reabsorption, so that it opposes the effects of parathyroid hormone and vitamin D.

However, neither abnormally increased plasma levels of calcitonin (e.g. with tumours) or abnormally decreased levels (e.g. following thyroidectomy) result in detectable changes in serum calcium level nor in any apparent clinical effect, so that the physiological role of calcitonin and of its controls remain unknown. In fact, its synthesis is closely related to that of several other peptides with probable neurotransmitter rather than hormonal roles, including calcitonin gene-related peptide, the most potent natural vasodilator.

Nevertheless, the clinical significance of calcitonin is two-fold.

- Its level is increased in **medullary thyroid carcinoma**, for which it is a marker. It is also produced ectopically from a number of other tumours, particularly phaeochromocytoma and thus especially in patients with MEN type II (q.v.).
- It has considerable pharmacological value in **Paget's disease** (q.v.), in which it produces an immediate response of falling serum and urine hydroxyproline levels.

Side-effects include local discomfort, as well as flushing, nausea and abnormal taste. The synthetic salmon polypeptide preparation, unlike the synthetic human form, may induce antibodies.

Procalcitonin (PCT), the precursor of calcitonin, has recently been found to be a new and unexpected marker of severe infection. Procalcitonin is a 116 amino acid glycoprotein with a molecular weight of 13 kd, derived from the larger preprocalcitonin (141 AA). Cleavage by a specific protease produces calcitonin (32 AA from the mid region) and other fragments of unknown function. The half-life of procalcitonin is 25–30 h (compared with 10 min for calcitonin), but plasma levels are undetectable in normal subjects (i.e. <0.1 ng/mL). However, PCT may rise to 100 ng/mL or more in severe sepsis and septic shock, in which its rise is similar to that of the cytokines, except for a slower onset and greater duration. In these circumstances, it is probably produced by extra-thyroid cells, perhaps leukocytes or neuroendocrine cells of the lung or intestine, and is not degraded to calcitonin.

Bibliography

Assicot M, Gendrel D, Carsin H et al 1993 High serum procalcitonin concentrations in patients with sepsis and infection. Lancet 341: 515.

de Werra I, Jaccard C, Corradin SB et al 1997 Cytokines, nitrite/nitrate, soluble tumor necrosis factor receptors, and procalcitonin concentrations: comparison in patients with septic shock, cardiogenic shock, and bacterial pneumonia. Crit Care Med 25: 607.

McDermott MT 1992 Calcitonin and its clinical applications. Endocrinologist 2: 366.

Stevenson JC, Hillyard CJ, MacIntyre I et al 1979 A physiological role for calcitonin: protection of the maternal skeleton. Lancet 2: 769.

Calcium (see Hypercalcaemia and Hypocalcaemia)

Calcium disodium edetate (see Chelating agents)

Cancer

Patients with the common cancers are frequently seen in Intensive Care, either because of concomitant disease or because of specific cancer complications, procedures or treatments. Less common tumours or complications are considered in this book, including:

- amyloid;
- Bence Jones protein;
- cancer complications;
- carcinoid syndrome;
- glucagonoma;
- haemangioma;
- islet cell tumour;
- multiple myeloma;
- paraneoplastic syndromes;
- phaeochromocytoma;
- skin signs of internal malignant disease;
- Waldenstrom's macroglobulinaemia.

63

Bibliography

Aaronson SA 1991 Growth factors and cancer. Science 254: 1146.

Angell M 1982 The quality of mercy. N Engl J Med 306: 98.

Holzman D 1995 New cancer genes crowd the

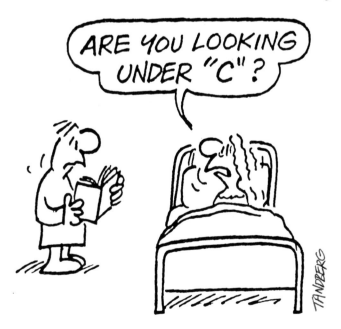

ARE YOU LOOKING UNDER "C"?

horizon, create possibilities. J Natl Cancer Inst 87: 1108.

Kerr JFR, Winterford CM, Harmon BV 1994 Apoptosis: its significance to cancer and cancer therapy. Cancer 73: 2013.

Krontiris TG 1995 Oncogenes. N Engl J Med 333: 303.

Lowe S, Bodis S, McClatchey A et al 1994 Status and efficacy of cancer therapy in vivo. Science 266: 807.

Pardoll DM 1994 Tumour antigens: a new look for the 1990s. Nature 1369: 357.

Rosenberg SA 1992 The immunotherapy and gene therapy of cancer. J Clin Oncol 10: 180.

Seleznick MJ 1992 Tumor markers. Prim Care 19: 715.

Solomon E, Borrow J, Goddard AD 1991 Chromosome aberrations and cancer. Science 254: 1153.

Weinberg RA 1991 Tumor suppressor genes. Science 254: 1138.

zur Hausen H 1991 Viruses in human cancers. Science 254: 1167.

Cancer complications

By far the majority of patients with cancer seen in an Intensive Care Unit present with concomitant or incidental problems. The most frequently encountered concomitant problems are opportunistic infections and postoperative complications.

Uncommonly, more specific problems of Intensive Care relevance are encountered. These may be classified as follows.

- **cardiac**
  - non-bacterial endocarditis, pericardial tamponade;

- **cutaneous**
  - various dermatoses (see Paraneoplastic syndromes);

- **endocrine/metabolic**
  - adrenal insufficiency, diabetes insipidus, ectopic hormone production, hypercalcaemia, hyperuricaemia;

- **general**
  - fever, metastases, weight loss;

- **haematological**
  - anaemia, disseminated intravascular coagulation, neutropenia, thrombocytopenia, thromboembolism;

- **neurological**
  - myopathy, neuropathy;

- **renal**
  - tumour-lysis syndrome.

The **tumour-lysis syndrome** results from the massive release of cellular components, especially purines (but also potassium and phosphate), following extensive acute lysis of tumour cells. The syndrome is particularly seen following induction chemotherapy in haematological malignancies.

Purine metabolism gives rise to uric acid and phosphate release.

- The former may give rise to oliguric renal failure due to acute uric acid nephropathy.
- The latter leads to hypocalcaemia and thus cardiac arrhythmias and fits.

Prevention is with:

- fluid loading, e.g. saline to give a urine output of at least 100 mL/h;
- bicarbonate (to give a urinary pH of at least 6.5, since uric acid is then converted to the more soluble urate);
- allopurinol.

Treatment is with:

- *fluid administration (titrated against cardiac filling pressures);*
- *loop diuretics;*
- *dialysis if necessary.*

Bibliography

Adelstein DJ, Hines SG, Carter SF et al 1988 Thromboembolic events in patients with malignant superior vena cava syndrome and the role of anticoagulation. Cancer 62: 2258.

Arrambide K, Toto RD 1993 Tumor lysis syndrome. Semin Nephrol 13: 273.

Barton JC 1989 Tumor lysis syndrome in nonhematopoietic neoplasms. Cancer 64: 738.

Bell DR, Woods, RL, Levi JA 1986 Superior vena cava obstruction. Med J Aust 145: 566.

Bick RL 1992 Coagulation abnormalities in malignancy: a review. Semin Thromb Hemost 18: 353.

Cascino TL 1993 Neurologic complications of systemic cancer. Med Clin North Am 77: 265.

Chan A, Woodruff RK 1992 Complications and failure of anticoagulation therapy in the treatment of venous thromboembolism in patients with disseminated malignancy. Aust NZ J Med 22: 119.

Colman RW, Rubin RN 1990 Disseminated intravascular coagulation due to malignancy. Semin Oncol 17: 172.

Langstein HN, Norton JA 1991 Mechanisms of cancer cachexia. Hematol Oncol Clin North Am 5: 103.

Lazarus HM, Creger RJ, Gerson SL 1989 Infectious emergencies in oncology patients. Semin Oncol 16: 543.

Pizzo PA 1993 Management of fever in patients with cancer and treatment-induced neutropenia. N Engl J Med 328: 1323.

Rosen PJ 1992 Bleeding problems in the cancer patient. Hematol Oncol Clin North Am 6: 1315.

Silverman P, Distelhorst CW 1989 Metabolic emergencies in clinical oncology. Semin Oncol 16: 504.

Silverstein RL, Nachman RL 1992 Cancer and clotting – Trousseau's warning. N Engl J Med 327: 1163.

Weiss HW, Walker MD, Wiernik PH 1974 Neurotoxicity of commonly used antineoplastic agents. N Engl J Med 291: 75, 127.

Zacharski LR, Wojtukiewicz MZ, Costantini V et al 1992 Pathways of coagulation/fibrinolysis activation in malignancy. Semin Thromb Hemost 18: 104.

Carbon monoxide

Carbon monoxide is a colourless, odourless, non-irritant and flammable gas with physical properties similar to nitrogen. It is produced from the incomplete combustion of carbon-containing fuels and is thus a common product in motor vehicle exhausts, faulty domestic heating and cooking devices, and in industry. In most countries, its predominant source is motor vehicle exhaust fumes, from which death can occur within 15 min if inside a confined space.

Carbon monoxide is the most common lethal poison in all societies.

- It has an estimated incidence of about one in 25 000 of the population per year.
- Nearly one third of cases are fatal.
- Most cases nowadays are suicidal, though some can be accidental.

Although carbon monoxide poisoning carries significant mortality and substantial late morbidity and has been known since last century, understanding of its pathogenetic consequence of tissue hypoxia remains surprisingly incomplete. Thus, although carbon monoxide displaces oxygen from haemoglobin, having a 200-fold greater affinity than oxygen for haemoglobin, anaemic hypoxia does not explain carbon monoxide's toxicity, because oxygen transport and even oxygen consumption are increased due to a compensatory rise in cardiac output. Direct tissue toxicity is also an unsatisfactory explanation, and it is more likely that carbon monoxide alters a number of intracellular enzymes.

Nevertheless, the level of carboxyhaemoglobin is a guide to severity, in that levels up to 20% represent mild poisoning and 30–50% severe poisoning, with >50% often associated with fatality, especially in the presence of metabolic acidosis. These levels should be seen in the context of 5–10% in heavy smokers and up to 6% in some industries and in some cities. Levels below 5% are considered safe. However, a low level does not exclude the possibility of a previously high level, so that (as for any drug) the time from the initial exposure should be taken into account when interpreting a blood level (T½ of COHb is ≈ 2 h). Moreover, even levels of 3–6% may impair exercise tolerance and increase arrhythmias in cardiac patients, and levels of 5–8% reduce vigilance in healthy subjects.

Several clinical patterns of poisoning may be seen

- If the onset of poisoning is gradual, the patient may present with a flu-like illness, comprising headache, dizziness, weakness, nausea and finally coma. If a number of people are so affected, a mistaken diagnosis of food poisoning may be made.
- If the onset is sudden, rapid coma occurs with fitting and then death.
- The classical cherry-red appearance of the skin is in fact uncommon, though the presence of retinal haemorrhages is a useful diagnostic clue.
- Cardiac arrhythmias are common, especially in patients with associated heart disease.
- Exposure during pregnancy may cause fetal damage.

> The clinical course is variable and unpredictable.
>
> A biphasic response is common, with up to 20% of severely affected patients having a late recovery on the one hand and on the other hand about 10% of patients suffering a late deterioration which may be severe. This delayed relapse may occur up to one month after hospital discharge and after seemingly full recovery. It is primarily neurological with a fluctuating mental state and tremor, dysphasia, ataxia and incontinence, though most of these features disappear again within the next year.
>
> In patients who survive, permanent neurological damage may result, especially disorders of personality and cognition. Infarction of skin, heart, peripheral nerve and bowel may be seen.

Treatment modalities are as follows.

- **100% oxygen** *should be administered and possibly mechanical ventilation. 100% oxygen*

increases the elimination of carbon monoxide 5-fold compared with room air.
- **Hyperbaric oxygen**, *though not formally confirmed as effective in controlled studies, is commonly recommended in severe cases; one or two treatments are given within the first 12 h; this form of treatment may be useful up to 16 h after the initial event, but beyond 24 h it does not appear to influence outcome.*
- *Other measures, such as exchange transfusion, hypothermia and barbiturate or other sedation have been found to be ineffective.*

Bibliography

Caravanti EM, Adams CJ, Joyce SM et al 1988 Fetal toxicity associated with maternal carbon monoxide poisoning. Ann Emerg Med 17: 714.

Choi IS 1983 Delayed neurologic sequelae in carbon monoxide intoxication. Arch Neurol 40: 433.

Cobb N, Etzel RA 1991 Unintentional carbon monoxide-related deaths in the United States, 1979 through 1988. JAMA 266: 659.

Hardy KR, Thom DR 1994 Pathophysiology and treatment of carbon monoxide poisoning. Clin Toxicol 32: 613.

Runciman WW, Gorman DF 1993 Carbon monoxide poisoning: from old dogma to new uncertainties. Med J Aust 158: 439.

Scheinkestel CD, Bailey M, Myles PS et al 1999 Hyperbaric or normobaric oxygen for acute carbon monoxide poisoning: a randomised controlled clinical trial. Med J Aust 170: 203.

Smith SJ, Brandon S 1973 Morbidity from acute carbon monoxide poisoning at three-year follow-up. Br Med J 1:318.

Walden SM, Gottlieb SO 1990 Urban angina, urban arrhythmias: carbon monoxide and the heart. Ann Intern Med 113: 337.

Winter PM, Miller JN 1976 Carbon monoxide poisoning. JAMA 236: 1502.

Ziser A, Shupak A, Halpern P et al 1984 Delayed hyperbaric oxygen treatment for acute carbon monoxide poisoning. Br Med J 289: 960

Carbon tetrachloride

Carbon tetrachloride (tetrachormethane) is a heavy, colourless, volatile (boiling point 77°C), non-flammable, water-insoluble, toxic liquid with a characteristic odour. It is an organic halogen compound (a chlorinated hydrocarbon), first prepared in 1839 from combining chloroform with chlorine. It has been used as a refrigerant, a solvent, a dry cleaning agent until replaced by **tetrachloroethylene** (a more stable and less toxic agent), and even as an anaesthetic (although the industrial solvent, **trichloroethylene**, became much more commonly used than carbon tetrachloride for this latter purpose, until recognized to be a potential carcinogen).

Carbon tetrachloride is well absorbed from the lungs and the gut. Poisoning may thus result from

- inhalation as a result of either industrial exposure or sniffing (solvent abuse),
- accidental or deliberate ingestion.

Clinical features include local irritation, gastrointestinal symptoms which may be severe, neurological features of headache, convulsions and coma, cardiovascular findings of hypotension and arrhythmias, and most importantly hepatorenal damage which is often delayed for at least two days after exposure. In particular, hepatic necrosis with later fatty infiltration may be produced. Other organ damage may involve the lungs, adrenal, pancreas, bone marrow, cerebellum and optic nerve.

Treatment is with removal from further exposure, gastric lavage if there has been recent ingestion, and symptomatic support. Subsequent exposure must be avoided, as even low concentrations may then produce fever, fatigue and depression.

Bibliography
Wartenberg D, Reyner D, Scott CS 2000 Trichlorethylene and cancer: epidemiological evidence. Environ Health Perspect 108: 161.

Carbonic anhydrase inhibitors

The prototype carbonic anhydrase inhibitor is **acetazolamide**, a non-bacteriostatic sulfonamide with a molecular weight of 222 d. It is a potent reversible inhibitor of the enzyme, carbonic anhydrase. Its potential therapeutic uses are:

- as a diuretic, though not nowadays since its diuretic effect is mild and comparable only with that of thiazides;
- to alkalinize the urine in glaucoma;
- in acute mountain sickness;
- in some convulsive disorders;
- in periodic paralysis (even in the presence of hypokalaemia).

In Intensive Care, acetazolamide is sometimes used in the management of severe metabolic alkalosis, since it enhances the urinary excretion of bicarbonate 5-fold and thus produces metabolic acidosis. However, if carbon dioxide excretion is limited, as in some patients with chronic lung disease, increased hypercapnia may result.

It is given in a dose of 500 mg 8 hourly, but only short-term use is recommended as tolerance rapidly develops. Among many occasional adverse reactions, hypokalaemia can be important. Toxic effects include:

- drowsiness;
- paraesthesiae;
- rare hypersensitivity, including erythema multiforme;
- teratogenicity.

It is contraindicated in:

- hyponatraemia;
- hypokalaemia;
- hyperchloraemia;
- metabolic acidosis;
- severe liver or renal disease;
- hypersensitivity to sulfonamides.

Bibliography
Preisig PA, Toto RD, Alpern RJ 1987 Carbonic anhydrase inhibitors. Renal Physiol 10: 136.

Carboxyhaemoglobin (see Carbon monoxide)

Carcinoembryonic antigen

Carcinoembryonic antigen (CEA), like alpha-fetoprotein, is a glycoprotein which behaves an oncofetal antigen. The normal level is <3 μg/L and its half-life is about 2 weeks.

It is a useful maker in a number of conditions, namely:

- gastrointestinal cancers;
- some non-gastrointestinal cancers;
- some non-malignant gastrointestinal diseases.

In **gastrointestinal cancers** (originally colorectal cancer), CEA is increased only when the bowel wall has become penetrated, so that it is not a useful screening test. Although not quantitatively related to tumour bulk, it becomes particularly increased with liver metastases, even if they are small. On the other hand, it can be normal if the cancer is poorly differentiated. It may provide some preoperative guide to operability and more usefully a postoperative indication of the completeness of resection, the presence of recurrence or the response of metastatic disease to treatment.

Non-gastrointestinal cancers include particularly lung cancer. This is especially so if there has been extrathoracic spread and more particularly if there are liver metastases from squamous cell carcinoma.

Non-malignant gastrointestinal diseases comprise conditions such as inflammatory bowel disease.

Bibliography
Fletcher RH 1986 Carcinoembryonic antigen. Ann Intern Med 104: 66.

Carcinoid syndrome

Carcinoid tumours are the most common endocrine-secreting tumours of the gut, though most such tumours do not secrete sufficient quantities of mediators to produce the overt clinical features referred to as the **carcinoid syndrome**.

The tumours may arise anywhere in the gut and occasionally in the bronchial tree. The appendix is the commonest site (40%), followed by the small intestine (24%, half in the ileum), rectum (14%) and lung (10%). Gut tumours metastasize to the liver, but lung tumours tend to metastasize to bone. Carcinoid tumours can be associated with the multiple endocrine neoplasia (type I) condition (q.v.).

Most silent carcinoid tumours occur in the appendix and most secretory tumours occur in the ileum. To provide enough tumour mass to produce symptoms, most clinically apparent tumours are associated with hepatic metastases.

The tumours contain argentaffin cells, which secrete a number of biologically active substances, characteristically serotonin but also histamine, bradykinin, catecholamines, prostaglandins, growth hormone releasing factor, adrenocorticotrophic hormone and pancreatic polypeptide.

Symptoms are mostly, though not solely, attributable to serotonin. The typical clinical feature is of paroxysmal vasomotor disturbance, seen in 90% of patients as red-purple cyanotic flushing of the face and neck, which is triggered by alcohol, food, emotion or exertion. The episode lasts for a few minutes and is associated with tachycardia and hypotension. Eventually, many patients (40%) develop large purple telangiectases.

Since bronchial carcinoids secrete directly into the systemic circulation, they can produce much more severe and prolonged flushing episodes (up to two weeks), which spread to the trunk and are associated with lacrimation, rhinorrhoea, salivation and even facial oedema.

Sometimes, a full **carcinoid storm** may occur with:

- tachycardia;
- hypotension;

- oliguria;
- tremor;
- coma;
- even death.

Many other clinical features may also be seen in the carcinoid syndrome, namely

- **cardiac**
  - endocardial fibrosis may occur with a resultant murmur;
  - oedema is frequent;
  - tricuspid valve regurgitation may be seen.

- **cutaneous**
  - the rash of pellagra is seen in 10% of patients, being caused by the diversion of tryptophan to 5-hydroxytryptamine (serotonin);
  - hyperpigmentation may also occur.

- **endocrine**
  - occasionally Zollinger–Ellison, Cushing's or MEN syndromes may be seen.

- **gastrointestinal**
  - diarrhoea from increased peristalsis occurs in most patients (90%);
  - abdominal cramps are frequent (40%);
  - there is an increased incidence of peptic ulceration (14%);
  - hepatomegaly, ascites and an abdominal mass are common.

- **general**
  - fever, night sweats, mental changes and bone pain are sometimes seen.

- **respiratory**
  - dyspnoea due to bronchoconstriction occurs in up to 50% of patients.

The diagnosis is made from the measurement of increased 5-hydroxyindoleacetic acid (5-HIAA) in urine to >125 μmol/day and usually to >250–500 μmol/day. False-positive results may occur from many foods, including avocados, bananas, mushrooms, pineapples, plums and walnuts and from guaiacolate in cough medicines. False-negative may occur from phenothiazines.

Treatment is surgical if possible. **Resection** *is performed if the tumour can be identified and there are no metastases. Otherwise, surgical debulking is performed if feasible, and liver transplantation has even been reported.*

- *Diarrhoea is improved with* **cyproheptadine** *or with an H_1–H_2 combination, e.g. diphenhydramine and ranitidine, if histamine is a major contributor.*
- *Somatostatin (and especially the synthetic analogue,* **octreotide***, 50–100 μg sc bd) blocks the release of mediators, although refractoriness commonly eventuates.*
- *Interferon is probably helpful in some patients.*

In carcinoid storm, fluids and inotropes are required, though adrenaline should be used with care as it may aggravate hypotension.

The prognosis is good in the short term, since the tumours are very slowly growing. The average 5-year survival is 50%, though it is greater for tumours in the appendix, rectum and lung.

Bibliography

Coupe M, Levi S, Ellis M et al 1989 Therapy for symptoms in the carcinoid syndrome. Q J Med 73: 1021.

Godwin JD 1975 Carcinoid tumors: an analysis of 2837 cases. Cancer 36: 560.

McCaughan BC, Martini N, Bains MS 1985 Bronchial carcinoids. J Thorac Cardiovsc Surg 89: 8.

Cardiac tumours

Cardiac tumours are relatively common, though most are asymptomatic and the diagnosis is often difficult. Cardiac tumours may be primary or secondary.

- **Primary tumours** are generally histologically benign and are **myxomas** (see below), but occasionally a fibroma, lipoma or hamartoma (as in tuberous sclerosis) may occur. Rarely, primary tumours may be malignant, in which case they are usually sarcomas.

- **Secondary tumours** comprise at least 95% of cardiac neoplasms at autopsy and are found in about 10% of patients with terminal malignant disease. They usually arise from haematogenous spread and derive primarily from cancers of the lung or breast, from melanoma and from lymphoma.

Cardiac tumour should be suspected if there is otherwise unexplained:

- arrhythmia;
- failure;
- murmur;
- syncope;
- systemic embolization;
- pericardial effusion;
- abnormal cardiac silhouette.

Diagnosis is confirmed by non-invasive imaging with echocardiography, CT scanning or, perhaps, preferably MRI.

Cardiac myxoma arises from the endothelium, usually in the left atrium on the fossa ovalis. Clinical features are due to local obstruction, systemic symptoms or systemic embolization.

- **Local obstruction** of the mitral valve or pulmonary veins may give rise to dyspnoea, cardiac failure and fatigue. Syncope may occur and is typically positional. There may be a varying murmur.
- **Systemic symptoms** are due to the release of 'toxic' products and include fever, weight loss, malaise and even myalgia and Raynaud's phenomenon.
- **Systemic embolization** occurs in one third of cases and although the tumours are histologically benign, they can occasionally continue to grow in sites of distal implantation.

A **'myxoma complex'** may sometimes be seen, in which there are multicentric tumours,

which are prone to recurrence and which are associated with skin pigmentation, endocrine hypersecretion (especially Cushing's syndrome), and testicular tumour in men or breast fibroadenoma in women.

Laboratory investigations typically show anaemia, leukocytosis, thrombocytopenia, raised ESR, increased IgG and often increased IL-6.

The chief differential diagnosis is mitral valve disease and bacterial endocarditis.

*Treatment is with **surgical removal**, but recurrence is sometimes seen.*

Bibliography

Goodwin JF 1963 Diagnosis of left atrial myxoma. Lancet 1: 464.

Klatt EL, Heitz DR 1990 Cardiac metastases. Cancer 65: 1456.

Hancock EW 1990 Malignant pericardial disease. Cardiol Clin 8: 673.

McGregor GA, Cullen RA 1959 The syndrome of fever, anaemia and high sedimentation rate with an atrial myxoma. Br Med J 2: 991.

Reynan K 1995; Cardiac myxomas. N Engl J Med 333: 1610.

Salcedo EE, Cohen GI, White RD et al 1992 Cardiac tumors: diagnosis and management. Curr Probl Cardiol 17: 73.

Tazelaar HD, Locke TJ, McGregor CGA 1992 Pathology of surgically excised primary cardiac tumors. Mayo Clin Proc 67: 957.

Cardiomyopathies

Cardiomyopathies are a heterogeneous group of myocardial diseases, specifically separate from hypertensive, valvular or ischaemic cardiac disease.

Cardiomyopathies are traditionally classified into four (or three) types, namely:

- dilated;
- hypertrophic;
- restrictive;
- obliterative (this being regarded by some as a variant of restrictive).

Dilated cardiomyopathy is nowadays usually idiopathic. Many of these cases are familial and are associated with a variety of recently described mutations, involving actin, dystrophin or nuclear envelope proteins. Asymptomatic relatives commonly have echocardiographic abnormalities. Dilated cardiomyopathy may also be seen:

- in alcoholism;
- in malnutrition (beriberi, selenium deficiency);
- post-partum;
- in post-infective states (viral, diphtheritic, parasitic, systemic septic);
- with toxic agents (cocaine, anti-cancer drugs of the anthracycline group, and zidovudine);
- in a variety of diseases (collagen-vascular diseases, sarcoidosis, thyrotoxicosis, myxoedema, phaeochromocytoma, acromegaly and muscular dystrophy).

The most common virus involved is probably coxsachie B, and the main parasitic form is Chagas' disease seen in South America.

There is dilatation of both the left and right ventricles with cardiac failure, arrhythmias, dyspnoea, fatigue and embolization. Acute pulmonary oedema may be much less than otherwise expected because of concomitant right ventricular failure. The failure is of the hyperdynamic type in beriberi and thyrotoxicosis. Clinical examination shows heart failure, gallop rhythm and mitral regurgitation.

The chest X-ray shows marked cardiomegaly and pulmonary congestion. The ECG shows a variety of changes, including LVH, often LBBB, abnormal P waves, first degree heart block, a variety of arrhythmias, and ST-T abnormalities which may mimic acute myocardial infarction. Cardiac catheterization is not commonly performed nowadays but shows a decreased cardiac output with reduced ejection fraction and increased LVEDP. The diagnosis is confirmed by echocardiography and/or radionuclide studies.

> The differential diagnosis of dilated cardiomyopathy is:
>
> - myocarditis, or
> - advanced hypertensive, valvular or ischaemic disease.

Treatment is of the underlying disorder if identified.

- *Cardiac therapy includes digitalis, diuretics, vasodilators, salt restriction and rest. Digoxin has now been confirmed to be both symptomatically and functionally helpful, even in patients in sinus rhythm.*
- *Hypokalaemia and hypomagnesaemia should be avoided.*
- *Warfarin is indicated for systemic or pulmonary embolism.*
- *Sometimes, parenteral inotropes (dobutamine or milrinone) may be used for a few days to stabilize a difficult situation.*
- *Cardiac transplantation may be indicated in advanced cases.*

Hypertrophic cardiomyopathy is mostly (60%) hereditary, being inherited as an autosomal dominant. It has recently been considered a genetic disease of the cardiac muscle sarcomere. About one third of such cases have an abnormality on chromosome 14 of the gene which codes for the beta heavy chain of cardiac myosin, transcripts of which may be detectable in peripheral blood lymphocytes, thus providing a convenient screening test. Other cases have a variety of mutations (over 100 having now been described), involving chromosomes 1, 2, 11, 15, 16 or 18, giving single amino acid substitutions. The same defect occurs in all affected members of the same family.

There are variable patterns of ventricular hypertrophy, mostly involving the septum, which may be massive and cause a pressure gradient from the apex of left ventricle to the aorta, with frank obstruction in about 25% of cases. Histologically, the individual myofibrils are hypertrophied and disordered.

Hypertrophic cardiomyopathy is commonly associated with obstruction and is then referred to as hypertrophic obstructive cardiomyopathy (HOCM) or its variants, asymmetrical septal hypertrophy (ASM) or systolic anterior movement of the mitral valve (SAM). It used to be referred to as idiopathic hypertrophic subaortic stenosis (IHSS).

Clinical features include angina, syncope, arrhythmias, left heart failure and systemic embolization. On examination, there is an abnormal carotid pulse in obstructed cases, raised jugular venous pressure, gallop rhythm, and systolic murmur either from left ventricular outflow obstruction or mitral regurgitation.

The abnormal clinical findings are exacerbated by agents which cause

- tachycardia or increased myocardial contractility, e.g. beta agonists, digitalis;
- decreased preload or afterload, e.g. vasodilators, hypovolaemia, tachycardia, standing, Valsalva manoeuvre.

The chest X-ray is non-specific. The ECG shows LVH, sometimes with extensive Q waves due to the massive septal hypertrophy (and thus resembling AMI).

Definitive diagnosis is made by echocardiography and occasionally by cardiac catheterization, which typically shows normal systolic performance, with normal cardiac output and LVEDP, increased contractility with increased ejection fraction, but markedly decreased left ventricular compliance. The haemodynamic problem is thus obstruction and/or abnormal diastolic performance, so that the failure occurs even when the ejection fraction is as high as 80%.

The differential diagnosis of hypertrophic cardiomyopathy is:

- aortic stenosis, or
- subvalvular membranous stenosis.

Treatment is medical with beta blockers (and sometimes calcium-channel blockers) in moderate to high doses.

- *Digitalis, nitrates and diuretics are contraindicated.*
- *Arrhythmias can be difficult to treat.*
- *Strenuous sport should be avoided.*
- *Atrioventricular pacing with a dual chamber sequential device may favourably alter the pattern of ventricular depolarization and decrease obstruction.*
- *Surgery is indicated in about 10% of cases in due course, with myotomy or myectomy usually achieving a satisfactory symptomatic result, though the incidence of sudden death is not changed.*
- *More recently, successful chemical septal ablation has been described.*

The prognosis is very variable, with a mortality of 2–3% per year due to sudden death, though the condition often becomes more stable in older patients. It is the commonest cause of sudden cardiac death in patients under 35 years of age, including athletes, in whom the condition may have previously been entirely silent. Some of the variability in prognosis relates to the different mutations that may give rise to the condition. Family screening is recommended.

Restrictive cardiomyopathy

- may occasionally be familial,
- may sometimes be idiopathic,
- is usually due to myocardial infiltration in malignancy, amyloidosis, haemochromatosis or glycogen storage diseases.

The clinical features include cardiac failure, especially right heart failure, gallop rhythm and Kussmaul's sign (i.e. paradoxical increase in JVP on inspiration).

The chest X-ray only sometimes shows cardiomegaly. The ECG typically shows low voltages. Echocardiography (or cardiac catheterization) shows the findings of a rigid and incompliant ventricle, with impaired diastolic filling and a picture somewhat resembling constrictive pericarditis. The LVEDP is increased, and the cardiac output and ejection fraction may be deceased. However, unlike constrictive pericarditis in which the pressures tend to be equalized from the LVEDP to the right atrium, the LVEDP is much higher than the RVEDP and there is often pulmonary hypertension.

There is no satisfactory treatment, except sometimes that of the primary disease.

Obliterative cardiomyopathy is sometimes regarded as a variant of restrictive cardiomyopathy. It is due to massive endocardial fibrosis, and it is usually seen only in Third World countries, especially in Africa where it is common. It is probably hypereosinophilic in origin. There is associated intracardiac thrombosis, as well as endocardial hypertrophy.

Clinical features include cardiac failure, arrhythmias and embolization. Mitral and tricuspid regurgitation are usual.

Treatment is not effective, except for surgery in some cases.

The mortality is 25% within a year and two thirds within five years.

Bibliography

Cannon RO, Tripodi D, Dilsizian V et al 1994 Results of permanent dual-chamber pacing in symptomatic nonobstructive hypertrophic cardiomyopathy. Am J Cardiol 73: 571.

Cherian KM, John TA, Abraham KA 1983 Endomyocardial fibrosis. Am Heart J 105: 706.

Fatkin D, MacRae C, Sasaki T et al 1999 Missense mutations in the rod domain of the lamin A/C gene as causes of dilated cardiomyopathy and conduction-system disease. N Engl J Med 341: 1715.

Gheorghiade M, Zarowitz BJ 1992 Review of randomized trials of digoxin therapy in patients with chronic heart failure. Am J Cardiol 69: 48G.

Gupta PN, Valiathan MS, Balakrishnan KG et al 1989 Clinical course of endomyocardial fibrosis. Br Heart J 62: 450.

Katritsis D, Wilmshurst PT, Wendon JA et al 1991 Primary restrictive cardiomyopathy: clinical and pathologic characteristics. J Am Coll Cardiol 18: 1230.

Kelly DP, Strauss AW 1994 Inherited cardiomyopathies. N Engl J Med 330: 913.

Maron BJ, Bonow RO, Cannon RO 1987 Hypertrophic cardiomyopathy. N Engl J Med 316: 780, 844.

Maron BJ, Shirani J, Poliac LC et al 1996 Sudden death in young competitive athletes – clinical, demographic and pathological profiles. JAMA 276: 199.

Nishimura R, Trusty JM, Hayes DL et al 1997 Dual-chamber pacing for hypertrophic cardiomyopathy. A randomized double-blind crossover trial. J Am Coll Cardiol 29: 435.

Seggewiss H, Geichmann U, Faber L et al 1998; Percutaneous transluminal septal myocardial ablation in hypertrophic cardiomyopathy. J Am Coll Cardiol 1: 252.

Spirito P, Seidman CE, McKenna WJ et al 1997 The management of hypertrophic cardiomyopathy. N Engl J Med 336: 775.

Sugrue DD, Rodeheffer RJ, Codd MB et al 1992 The clinical course of idiopathic dilated cardiomyopathy. Ann Intern Med 117: 117.

Cardiovascular diseases

Many cardiovascular disorders are encountered so commonly in Intensive Care that they are regarded as 'core' to the specialty. These conditions include myocardial ischaemia and infarction, heart failure, arrhythmias, shock and hypertension.

However, numerous other cardiovascular disorders are sometimes seen, and it is these which are considered in this book. They include:

- aortic coarctation;
- aortic dissection;
- arteriovenous malformations;
- arteritis;
- atrial natriuretic factor;
- cardiac tumours;
- cardiomyopathies;
- Eisenmenger syndrome;
- endocarditis;
- Marfan's syndrome;
- mycotic aneurysms;
- tetralogy of Fallot;

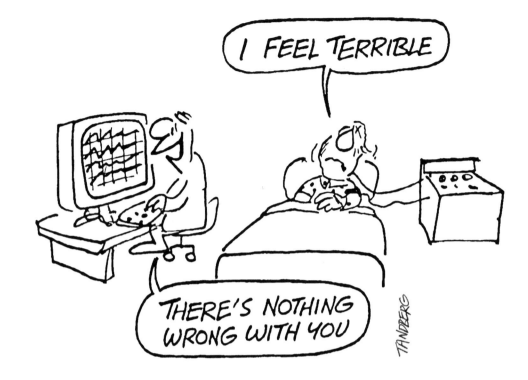

- toxic–shock syndrome;
- vasculitis.

Bibliography

Braunwald E 1992 Heart Disease. A Textbook of Cardiovascular Medicine. Philadelphia: WB Saunders.

Calhoun DA, Oparil S 1990 Treatment of hypertensive crisis. N Engl J Med 323: 1177.

Gheorghiade M, Zarowitz BJ 1992 Review of randomized trials of digoxin therapy in patients with chronic heart failure. Am J Cardiol 69: 48G.

Guyton AC 1991 Blood pressure control: special role of the kidney and body fluids. Science 252: 1813.

Heusch G, Schulz R 1997 Characterization of hibernating and stunned myocardium. Eur Heart J 18 (Suppl. D): 102.

ISIS-4 (Fourth International Study of Infarct Survival) Collaborative Group 1995 ISIS-4: A randomised factorial trial assessing early oral captopril, oral mononitrate, and intravenous magnesium sulphate in 58050 patients with suspected acute myocardial infarction. Lancet 345: 669.

Levin HJ, Paulker SG, Salzman EW et al 1992 Antithrombotic therapy in valvular heart disease. Chest 102: S434.

Loscalzo J, Creager MA, Dzau VJ (eds) 1992 Vascular Medicine. A Textbook of Vascular Biology and Diseases. Boston: Little, Brown.

Marik P, Varon J 1998 The obese patient in the ICU. Chest 113: 492.

Muller DWM 1994 Gene therapy for cardiovascular disease. Br Heart J 72: 309.

Nora JJ 1993 Causes of congenital heart disease: old and new modes, mechanisms, and models. Am Heart J 125: 1409.

Stein PD, Alpert JS, Copeland J et al 1992 Antithrombotic therapy in patients with mechanical and biological prosthetic heart valves. Chest 102: S445.

Wilson NJ, Neutze JM 1993 Adult congenital heart disease: principles and management guidelines. Aust NZ J Med 23: 498, 697.

Cat bites (see Bites and stings)

Cat-scratch disease

Cat-scratch disease (CSD) is still a disease of incompletely defined cause.

The first organism to be clearly associated with this disease was a small pleomorphic Gram-negative bacillus initially identified in 1988 and designated *Afipia felis* in 1992. Subsequently, the novel α-proteobacterium, *Rochalimaea henselae*, was identified by PCR in bacillary angiomatosis, particularly in immunocompromised patients, and it is now thought to be the actual causative agent of cat-scratch disease. This organism is related to rickettsiae and to bartonella and brucella. Indeed, the genus designation bartonella has replaced the former name rochalimaea, so that the aetiological agent of CSD is now referred to as *B. henselae*.

The apparent reservoir for these organisms is the domestic cat, in which they reside asymptomatically, but they can cause a variety of lesions in humans (and in armadillos!). The cat flea is the likely vector for transmission of the organism between animals.

Usually the scratch from an infected cat gives rise to a self-limited local lymphadenitis, which in up to 10% may suppurate. At the site of the scratch, an inflammatory lesion appears within 3–14 days and is followed in 1–3 weeks by the lymphadenopathy, which can last a very variable time from 2 weeks to 8 months. Mild systemic symptoms are common. The illness lasts 6–12 weeks.

In immunocompromised patients, disseminated disease may sometimes occur. This may comprise pneumonitis with hilar lymphadenopathy, encephalitis, retinitis, hepatitis, splenomegaly, thrombocytopenia or metastatic abscess.

Bacillary angiomatosis (BA) is an angioproliferative response, in which atypical endothelial cells form numerous poorly structured capillary channels. BA and the related **bacillary peliosis hepatis** arise in the skin and viscera in response to the presence of *B. henselae* (and probably other similar organisms, such as *B. quintana* in louse-infested or homeless environments). These complications occur particularly in immunocompromised patients, such as those with AIDS. In the skin, small angiomatous nodules are seen. The viscera affected include the liver, spleen, lymph nodes, bone marrow, lungs and brain.

Laboratory tests are generally unhelpful, and the diagnosis is traditionally made clinically and by exclusion. A positive skin test has been reported but is non-specific. Serology has a low sensitivity and moreover does not distinguish between past exposure and current disease. Culture of the organism is difficult because bacteraemia is infrequent and the organism is fastidious and slowly growing. Recently, PCR testing of biopsy tissue has been reported to have a sensitivity of up to 100%, though the test so far has limited availability. BA is diagnosed histologically.

The differential diagnosis includes:

- other infections

    - infectious mononucleosis;
    - pyogenic bacteria;
    - brucellosis;
    - toxoplasmosis;
    - fungal disease;
    - tuberculosis;
    - lymphogranuloma venereum;

- sarcoidosis;
- Hodgkin's disease.

Treatment is symptomatic only, as antibiotics are not helpful, though gentamicin or ciprofloxacin often with corticosteroids may be helpful in immunocompromised patients. BA is treated with erythromycin or doxycycline for four weeks.

The course is benign and self-limited, though it may run for several months. Disseminated BA may be fatal. A single episode of cat-scratch disease gives rise to immunity.

Bibliography

Anderson B, Sims K, Regnery R et al 1994 Detection of *Rochalimaea henselae* DNA in cat scratch disease patients by PCR. J Clin Microbiol 32: 942.

Bergmans AM, Peeters MF, Schellkens JF et al 1997

Pitfalls and fallacies of cat scratch disease serology. J Clin Microbiol 35: 1931.

Karim AA, Cockerell CJ, Petri WA 1994 Cat scratch disease, bacillary angiomatosis, and other infections due to Rochalimaea. N Engl J Med 330: 1509.

Regnery R, Tappero J 1995 Unraveling mysteries associated with cat-scratch disease, bacillary angiomatosis, and related syndromes. Emerg Infect Dis 1: 1.

Regnery RL, Martin M, Olson J 1992 Naturally occurring "Rochalimaea henselae" infection in domestic cat. Lancet 340: 557.

Relman DA, Falkow S, LeBoit PE et al 1991 The organism causing bacillary angiomatosis, peliosis hepatis, and fever and bacteremia in immunocompromised patients. N Engl J Med 324: 1514.

Slater LN, Welch DF, Hensel D et al 1990 A newly recognized fastidious gram-negative pathogen as a cause of fever and bacteremia. N Engl J Med 323: 1587.

Zangwill KM, Hamilton DH, Perkins BA et al 1993 Cat scratch disease in Connecticut – epidemiology, risk factors, and evaluation of a new diagnostic test. N Engl J Med 329: 8.

Cavitation

The chief causes of one or more **lung cavities** are:

- necrotizing pneumonia

    – often leading to lung abscess and/or empyema;

- cancer

    – bronchogenic carcinoma, metastases;

- tuberculosis

    – or fungal or parasitic infection;

- septic infarct;
- infected cysts or bullae;
- vasculitis

    – rheumatoid, Wegener's;

- lymphomatoid granulomatosis;
- angiocentric lymphoma.

Necrotizing pneumonia, **lung abscess** and **empyema** represent the extreme of pyogenic infections in the lung. Empyema is one of the causes of failure of resolution of chest infection.

The responsible organisms are usually klebsiella, staphylococci, pseudomonas or mixed anaerobic organisms, and they may follow aspiration.

The clinical features of empyema are those of:

- persistent infection (fever, cough, dyspnoea, chest pain);
- signs of pleural effusion (either a single loculus or multiloculated);
- finger clubbing (if the diagnosis is delayed).

Rupture through the skin (empyema necessitans) or into the bronchial tree (bronchopleural fistula) may occur.

Diagnosis is established by chest X-ray and aspiration of pleural fluid.

Treatment of necrotizing pneumonia, lung abscess and/or empyema consists of prolonged antibiotic therapy. An empyema should be drained, either by traditional chest tube or by image-guided catheter. Intrapleural fibrinolytic therapy (e.g. streptokinase 250 000 U in 20 mL of saline) may be of value if the empyema is loculated. If loculation still causes difficulty in drainage, video-assisted thoracoscopic surgery (VATS) is indicated for this task. Surgical resection, including decortication of organized, thickened pleura, is rarely required nowadays.

The prognosis nowadays is generally good, since the responsible infection is likely to respond well to antibiotics.

Bibliography

Angelillo Mackinlay TA, Lyons GA, Chimondeguy DJ et al 1996 VATS debridement versus thoracotomy in the treatment of loculated postpneumonia empyema. Ann Thorac Surg 61: 1626.

Bryant RE, Salmon CJ 1996 Pleural empyema. Clin Infect Dis 22: 747.

Davies RJO, Traill ZC, Gleeson FV 1997 Randomised controlled trial of intrapleural streptokinase in community acquired pleural infection. Thorax 52: 416.

Jerjes-Sanchez C, Ramirez-Rivera A, Elizalde JJ et al 1996 Intrapleural fibrinolysis with streptokinase as an adjunctive treatment in hemothorax and empyema: a multicenter trial. Chest 109: 1514.

Landreneau RJ, Keenan RJ, Hazelrigg SR et al 1995 Thoracoscopy for empyema and hemothorax. Chest 109: 18.

Leatherman JW, Mcdonald FM, Niewohner DE 1985 Fluid-containing bullae in the lung. South Med J 78: 708.

Muers MF 1997 Streptokinase for empyema. Lancet 349: 1491.

Sahn SA 1993 Management of complicated parapneumonic effusions. Am Rev Respir Dis 148: 813.

Silverman SC, Mueller PR, Saini S et al 1988 Thoracic empyema: management with image-guided catheter drainage. Radiology 169: 5.

Temes RT, Follis F, Kessler et al 1996 Intrapleural fibrinolysis in management of empyema thoracis. Chest 110: 102.

Walt MA, Sharma S, Hohn J et al 1997 A randomized trial of empyema therapy. Chest 111: 1548.

Weissberg D, Refaelyb Y 1996 Pleural empyema: 24-year experience. Ann Thorac Surg 62: 1026.

Cellulitis (see Gangrene)

Central pontine myelinolysis

Central pontine myelinolysis refers to demyelination primarily in the pons, though this process is also apparent in the basal ganglia and cerebellum on sensitive MRI examination.

Central pontine myelinolysis was originally described in alcoholism and malnutrition. Nowadays it is most commonly seen in patients who have been hyponatraemic, in whom it is thought to have been produced by osmotic injury from over-zealous correction of the hyponatraemia (especially correction which is too rapid).

Clinical features include:

- quadriparesis or paraparesis;
- dysarthria and dysphagia;
- mutism and possibly the locked-in state.

The process may be irreversible and may sometimes be fatal.

*Treatment is **preventative**.*

*Repair of **hyponatraemia** should be not >0.5 mmol/L per h, unless the hyponatraemia is associated with encephalopathy, in which case the sodium should be corrected by up to 2 mmol/L per h.*

In general, a plasma concentration of about 120 mmol/L is a symptomatically safe goal. Above this, further normalization can be leisurely.

Thus, if for example the plasma sodium concentration is 105 mmol/L, the amount of sodium required for acute repair in a 70 kg person is (120 − 105) × 60% × 70 kg = 630 mmol, which should be given as 4 L of N saline (or preferably 1.2 L of 3% saline) over 8–30 h.

However, if the originating process has been acute, symptoms of hyponatraemia may seen at higher levels, sometimes up to 130 mmol/L. In this case, the treatment goals need to be shifted up accordingly.

Bibliography

Arieff AI, Guisado R 1976 Effects on the central nervous system of hypernatremic and hyponatremic states. Kidney Int 10: 104.

Ayus JC, Krothapalli RK, Arieff AI 1987 Treatment of symptomatic hyponatremia and its relation to brain damage: a prospective study. N Engl J Med 317: 1190.

Berl T 1990 Treating hyponatremia: damned if we do and damned if we don't. Kidney Int 37: 1006.

Brunner JE, Redmond JM, Haggar AM et al 1990 Central pontine myelinolysis and pontine lesions after rapid correction of hyponatremia: a prospective magnetic resonance imaging study. Ann Neurol 27: 61.

Laureno R, Karp BI 1988 Pontine and extrapontine myelinolysis following rapid correction of hyponatraemia. Lancet 1: 1439.

Soupart A, Decaux G 1996 Therapeutic recommendations for management of severe hyponatremia: Current concepts on pathogenesis and prevention of neurologic complications. Clin Nephrol 46: 149.

Sterns RH, Riggs JE, Schochet SS 1986 Osmotic demyelination syndrome following correction of hyponatremia. N Engl J Med 314: 1535.

Sterns RH, Cappuccio JD, Silver SM et al 1994 Neurologic sequelae after treatment of severe hyponatremia: a multicenter perspective. J Am Soc Nephrol 4: 1522.

Strange K 1992 Regulation of solute and water balance and cell volume in the central nervous system. J Am Soc Nephrol 3: 12.

Tien R, Arieff AI, Kucharczyk W et al 1992 Hyponatremic encephalopathy: is central pontine myelinolysis a component? Am J Med 92: 513.

Cerebellar degeneration

Cerebellar degeneration occurs in a number of forms.

1. **Hereditary, spinocerebellar degenerative disorders**

These are unrelated conditions, except for the marked clinical feature of ataxia. A number of different mutational mechanisms and inheritance patterns have recently been identified.

The best known of these conditions is **Friedreich's ataxia**, which is manifest by areflexia and loss of proprioception as well as ataxia. There is associated cardiomyopathy and skeletal abnormality, particularly of the chest wall.

2. **Subacute cerebellar degeneration**

This is a paraneoplastic condition (q.v.), especially in carcinoma of the lung or ovary. In addition to ataxia, there may be sensory symptoms and mental changes.

Plasmapheresis is ineffective, even though circulating antibodies to cerebellar Purkinje cells have been found.

3. **Cerebellar degeneration due to alcoholism or nutritional deficiency**

Cerebellar degeneration is most commonly caused by alcohol. Myxoedema may sometimes be implicated. Deficiency of vitamin E, which arises from fat malabsorption (q.v.), has also been reported as a rare cause.

Bibliography

Campuzano V, Montermini L, Molto MD et al 1996 Friedreich's ataxia: autosomal recessive disease caused by intronic GAA triplet repeat expansion. Science 271: 1423.

Durr A, Cossee M, Agid Y et al 1996 Clinical and genetic abnormalities in patients with Friedreich's ataxia. N Engl J Med 335: 1169.

Gotoda T, Arita M, Arai H et al 1995 Adult-onset spinocerebellar dysfunction caused by a mutation in the gene for the α-tocopherol-transfer protein. N Engl J Med 333: 1313.

Cerebral arterial gas embolism
(see Diving)

Cerebral arteritis (see Arteritis)

Charcot–Marie–Tooth disease (see also Neuropathy)

Charcot–Marie–Tooth disease (CMT, peroneal muscular atrophy) is the most common hereditary polyneuropathy. It is usually an autosomal dominant condition, though several separate gene loci have been identified.

There is segmental demyelination (with local nerve hypertrophy) and consequent distal weakness and atrophy of the legs, often with pes cavus. Sensory as well as motor impairment occurs, and the hands may eventually be involved.

It is a benign condition with no major morbidity and no mortality.

Chelating agents

A chelate is a complex compound with a central metal atom attached to a larger molecule (a ligand) in a ring structure. A chelating agent refers to the ligand which can attach to the metal ion at two or more points, thus forming a ring.

Chelates are more stable than non-chelated compounds of comparable composition. Haemoglobin and chlorophyll are examples of chelate compounds in nature. Chelates are widely used in industrial and laboratory processes.

In clinical medicine, chelating agents are used in the treatment of metal poisoning, because they bind the metal more strongly than do the vulnerable components of the living organism.

Although man has always had environmental exposure to heavy metals in food, water and cooking utensils, this exposure increased markedly after industrialization. These metals cannot be metabolized but persist in the body, where they produce prolonged toxic effects by combining with a reactive group (a ligand) thereby affecting chemical function.

Chelating agents are heavy metal antagonists, since they compete with these reactive groups in the body for the metal and therefore they can prevent or treat toxic effects by permitting excretion. Clearly, a selective chelator is required so as not to bind the body's own essential metals, though it must distribute in the same body spaces. It must also have a greater affinity than the body's own ligands, it must produce non-toxic complexes pending excretion and it must be able to mobilize the metal after binding so as to permit excretion.

The heavy metals of most relevance in this setting are:

- arsenic (q.v.);
- cadmium (q.v.);
- iron (q.v.);
- lead (q.v.);
- mercury (q.v.).

There are four important chelating agents for clinical use, namely:

- calcium disodium edetate;
- dimercaprol;
- penicillamine;
- desferrioxamine.

Calcium disodium edetate (sodium calciumedetate, ethylene-diaminetetra-acetate, EDTA) is chiefly used in lead poisoning, though it is also of value in enhancing the clearance of cadmium (and also chromium, cobalt, copper, magnesium, nickel, selenium, uranium, vanadium, zinc) and (in double dosage) of the radioactive products from nuclear accidents (e.g. plutonium). The toxic metal displaces calcium from the chelator. It has also been used in atherosclerosis but without evidence to support this indication.

Since it is poorly absorbed from the gut, it is given intravenously; 2 g (two 5 mL ampoules of 200 mg/mL each) are diluted to 500–1000 mL in isotonic dextrose or saline and are administered daily for 5 days in two divided doses each over 1 h. If combined with BAL for lead poisoning, there should be a four h delay between the administration of the two agents, with BAL given first.

EDTA has a half-life of about 40 min, distributes in the extracellular fluid and is excreted in the urine (50% in the first hour), so that it is contraindicated in anuria.

The side-effects of EDTA include:

- fever;
- thirst;
- nausea;
- myalgia;
- hypotension;
- reversible renal tubular damage;
- T-wave inversion on ECG;
- increased intracranial pressure;
- increased prothrombin time;
- dermatitis;
- phlebitis.

Dimercaprol (2,3-dimercaptopropanol, British anti-Lewisite, BAL) was designed to combat arsenic-containing military gas in the Second World War. Later, its use was extended to other heavy metal poisoning, particularly from lead and mercury. It is an oily pungent liquid, which is given intramuscularly and metabolized and excreted within 4–6 h.

The individual doses are 3–5 mg/kg (3 mg/kg for arsenic, 4 mg/kg for lead and 5 mg/kg for mercury). The urine should be alkalinized concomitantly to decrease the breakdown of chelate complex.

- In arsenic poisoning, it is given 4 hourly until abdominal symptoms subside.
- In lead poisoning, it is given 4 hourly for 48 h, 6 hourly for 48 h and then 12 hourly for 5–7 days, usually in combination with EDTA.
- It may also be of use in gold, bismuth, antimony and thallium poisoning.
- It is not of use in cadmium poisoning.

The side-effects of BAL can be dramatic, though they are reversible and not usually serious. They reach their peak within 20 min of injection and disappear by 2 h. They include:

- tachycardia;
- hypertension;
- nausea;
- sweating;
- lacrimation;
- anxiety;
- generalized burning and tingling, particularly of the mouth and penis;
- chest and abdominal pain.

They are probably reduced by the administration of ephedrine, 30–60 mg orally, 30 min beforehand.

Pencillamine, a characteristic product of penicillins, was first found in 1953 in the urine of patients with liver disease given penicillin. It is the D-isomer of β, β-dimethylcysteine (D-3 mercaptovaline).

It is used in poisoning from antimony, copper, gold, lead, mercury and zinc (and also arsenic,

cadmium, cobalt, nickel), but it is a second choice after BAL. It is also commonly used in Wilson's disease (q.v.), cystinuria and rheumatoid arthritis. It may possibly be of value in scleroderma (q.v.) and in primary biliary cirrhosis (q.v.).

It is well absorbed from the gut and is given orally in a dose of 0.5–2 g/day in four divided doses. The usual course of therapy for heavy metal poisoning is five days.

Although there is a theoretical risk of penicillin anaphylaxis, there are no traces of penicillin in the preparations nowadays available, but care should be taken in patients who are allergic to penicillin. Elective surgery is contraindicated for six weeks after administration because of poor collagen cross-linking.

The side-effects of penicillamine are common.

- About 30% of patients get fever and itch, perhaps because of cross-reactivity with penicillin.
- Skin lesions are common during long-term administration and consist of

  – friability;
  – maculopapular rash;
  – pemphigoid;
  – even SLE.

- Anorexia, nausea, abdominal discomfort and diarrhoea are also common.
- Rarer reactions include:

  – marrow aplasia, which can occasionally be fatal;
  – haemolytic anaemia;
  – nephrotic syndrome;
  – bronchoalveolitis;
  – myasthenia gravis.

Desferrioxamine (deferoxamine, DFO) is isolated initially as an iron chelate from *Streptomyces pilosus* from which the iron is then removed chemically to produce a ligand with a high affinity for ferric iron. DFO is able to remove iron from haemosiderin and ferritin and to a lesser extent from transferrin, but not from haemoglobin, myoglobin, cytochromes and other iron-containing enzymes. The chelate complex produced is excreted in the urine and is also dialysable.

DFO is used:

- in the treatment of acute iron poisoning;
- in transfusion haemosiderosis, e.g. in the chronic treatment of thalassaemia;
- in the diagnosis and treatment of iron storage disease;
- sometimes in the treatment of aluminium toxicity in dialysis patients;
- not in haemochromatosis.

Since iron overload conditions probably predispose to infection, sometimes with exotic micro-organisms (e.g. *Yersinia*), careful microbiological surveillance is recommended.

It is given parenterally, preferably intravenously if the patient has circulatory impairment, in which case a dose of up to 1 g/h or 4 g over 12 h and up to 16 g/day may be given. In acute iron poisoning, the need for further doses depends on the serum iron level. During iron elimination in this way, the urine becomes orange-red in colour.

Bibliography

Burns CB, Currie B 1995 The efficacy of chelation therapy and factors influencing mortality in intoxicated petrol sniffers. Aust NZ J Med 25: 197.

Jackson TW, Ling LJ, Washington V 1995 The effect of oral deferoxamine in iron absorption in humans. J Toxicol Clin Toxicol 33: 325.

Mathieu D, Mathieu-Nolf M, Germain-Alonso M et al 1992 Massive arsenic poisoning: effect of haemodialysis and dimercaprol on arsenic kinetics. Intens Care Med 18: 47.

Mills KC, Curry SC 1994 Acute iron poisoning. Emerg Clin North Am 12: 397.

Proper R, Shurn S, Nathan D 1976 Reassessment of the use of deferoxamine B in iron overload. N Engl J Med 294: 1421.

Proudfoot AT, Simpson D, Dyson EH 1986 Management of acute iron poisoning. Med Toxicol 1: 83.

Chemical poisoning

Chemical poisoning due to drug overdosage is a very commonly encountered problem in Intensive Care and its management principles are well known. However, many other chemical agents, generally of a non-therapeutic nature, may cause uncommon forms of poisoning following ingestion or other exposure. In particular, chemical exposure is a common environmental hazard in many parts of the world and in many industrial or accidental situations.

Important poisonings or exposures described in this book are those involving:

- aluminium;
- arsenic;
- asbestos;
- beryllium;
- cadmium;
- carbon monoxide;
- carbon tetrachloride;
- chlorine;
- cocaine;
- cyanide;
- dioxins;
- ergot;
- ethylene glycol;
- formaldehyde;
- gamma-hydroxybutyric acid;
- hydrogen sulfide;
- lead;
- mercury;
- methanol;
- paraquat;
- strychnine;
- thallium;
- warfare agents.

Some uncommon drug poisonings (e.g. amphetamines) are also considered under the headings of the individual drugs themselves (see Drugs).

Bibliography

American College of Physicians 1990 Occupational and environmental medicine: the internist's role. Ann Intern Med 113: 974.

Bascom R, Bromberg PA, Costa DL et al 1996;
Health effects of outdoor pollution. Am J Resp
Crit Care Med 153: 3, 477.

Cugell DW 1992 The hard metal diseases. Clin
Chest Med 13: 269.

Haddad LM, Shannon MW, Winchester JF (eds)
1997 Clinical Management of Poisoning and Drug
Overdose. 3rd edition. Philadelphia: WB
Saunders.

Nriagu JO, Pacyna JM 1988 Quantitative assessment
of worldwide contamination of air, water and soils
by trace metals. Nature 333: 134.

Olson KR (ed) 1998 Poisoning and Drug Overdose.
3rd edition. Norwalk: Appleton & Lange

Redlich CA, Sparer JS, Cullen MR 1997 Sick
building syndrome. Lancet 349: 1013.

Rosenstock L, Cullen M (eds) 1994 Textbook of
Clinical Occupational and Environmental
Medicine. Philadelphia: Saunders.

Roxe DM, Krumlovsky FA 1988 Toxic interstitial
nephropathy from metals, metabolites, and
radiation. Semin Nephrol 8: 72.

Trujillo MH, Guerrero J, Fragachan C et al 1998
Pharmacologic antidotes in critical care medicine:
a practical guide for drug administration. Crit Care
Med 26: 377.

Chest wall disorders

Chest wall disorders include:

- congenital conditions

  – pectus carinatum or excavatum;

- kyphoscoliosis (q.v.);
- ankylosing spondylitis (q.v.);
- old thoracoplasty;
- obesity;
- neuromuscular disorders;
- inflammation

  – costochondritis (Tietze's syndrome);

- trauma;
- tumour

  – primary (usually benign);
  – secondary (more common).

Bibliography
Bergofsky EH 1979 Respiratory failure in disorders
of the thoracic cage. Am Rev Respir Dis 119: 643.

Davies D 1972 Ankylosing spondylitis and lung
fibrosis. Q J Med 41: 395.

Libby DM, Briscoe WA, Boyce B et al 1982 Acute
respiratory failure in scoliosis or kyphosis:
prolonged survival and treatment. Am J Med 73:
532.

Ray CS, Sue DY, Bray G et al 1983 Effects of
obesity on respiratory function. Am Rev Respir
Dis 128: 501.

Chinese-restaurant syndrome (see also Food poisoning)

The Chinese-restaurant syndrome is probably
due to the ingestion of monosodium glutamate
(MSG). Symptoms appear within 20 min and
last up to 2 h. These comprise a generalized
burning feeling, with pressure sensations,
sweating and occasionally headache,
palpitations and even syncope. The syndrome is
self-limited and harmless, though it can
produce consternation, particularly in cardiac
patients.

Bibliography
Schaumburg HH, Byck R, Gerstl R et al 1969
Monosodium L-glutamate: its pharmacology and
role in the Chinese restaurant syndrome. Science
163: 826.

Chlorine (see also Acute lung irritation)

Chlorine (Cl, atomic number 17, atomic
weight 35) is the second lightest halogen after
fluorine. It is a corrosive, pungent, greenish-
yellowish gas, 2½ times heavier than air and
with a boiling point of −34°C. It was first
isolated in 1774 and is the main anion in salt
water. The chlorine molecule, which consists
of two atoms of chlorine (i.e. Cl_2), is a very
reactive substance, readily giving rise to
chlorides and various oxidative species,
including ions and oxides.

Chlorine is widely used as an industrial bleach,
and because of its toxicity it has been used as a
military poison. The maximum recommended
exposure levels are not >3 mg/m^3 (1 ppm).

Levels above this cause eye and respiratory irritation (see Acute lung irritation), with higher levels causing suffocation and pulmonary oedema. Levels 1000-fold higher cause death within minutes.

*Treatment of chlorine poisoning is **symptomatic** and supportive.*

Bibliography

Centres for Disease Control 1991 Chlorine gas toxicity from mixture of bleach with other cleaning products. JAMA 256: 2529.

Schonhofer B, Voshaar T, Kohler D 1996 Long-term lung sequelae following accidental chlorine gas exposure. Respiration 63: 155.

Cholangitis

Acute cholangitis is usually associated with biliary obstruction, and this in turn is usually due to choledocholithiasis. **Acute cholecystitis** is due to cystic duct obstruction, and this in turn is virtually always due to cholelithiasis. However, most gallstones remain silent.

The clinical features are dominated by biliary colic, i.e. severe pain in the right upper quadrant, rapid in onset, constant in nature (and thus not true colic), lasting up to one hour and associated with nausea, vomiting and often a high fever.

The differential diagnosis includes:

- pancreatitis;
- ureteric colic;
- acute myocardial infarction;
- hepatitis;
- other causes of biliary obstruction at the porta hepatis;
- acute intermittent porphyria.

The diagnosis is made most conveniently on ultrasonography.

---

*Treatment is with **antibiotics** and endoscopic or surgical **removal** of the obstructing stone.*

Chronic cholangitis is also usually due to biliary duct obstruction, but the causes include stricture or carcinoma as well as stones. **Recurrent pyogenic cholangitis** may also occur. This is occasionally secondary to intestinal parasites. **Sclerosing cholangitis** may sometimes be seen, involving both intrahepatic and extrahepatic bile ducts. This is a condition of unknown aetiology, but it is mostly associated with ulcerative colitis. It carries a 30% mortality over 5 years.

The clinical features of chronic cholangitis include jaundice, fever, anorexia, weight loss and fatigue.

Liver function tests, particularly the alkaline phosphatase and gamma GT, are abnormal. The causative lesion is best defined by ERCP.

*The obstruction should be dealt with on its surgical merits, because without **mechanical relief** chronic cholangitis may lead to biliary cirrhosis. Endoscopic stricture dilatation may be helpful in selected patients. **Ursodiol** (see Biliary cirrhosis) provides symptomatic and biochemical benefit but no survival advantage.*

Bibliography

Angulo P, Lindor KD 1999 Primary sclerosing cholangitis. Hepatology 30: 325.

Berger MY, van der Velden JJ, Lijmer JG et al 2000 Abdominal symptoms: do they predict gallstones? A systematic review. Scand J Gastroenterol 35: 70.

Johnston DE, Kaplan MM 1993 Pathogenesis and treatment of gallstones. N Engl J Med 328: 412.

LaRusso NF, Wiesner RH, Ludwig J et al 1984 Primary sclerosing cholangitis. N Engl J Med 310: 899.

Vennes JA, Bond JH 1983 Approach to the jaundiced patient. Gastroenterology 84: 1615.

Cholera

Cholera is an acute diarrhoeal disease caused by the Gram-negative bacillus, *Vibrio cholerae*. The usual pathogen was the 01 strain, mostly confined until 1961 to Asia. Subsequently, the 7th world pandemic was caused by the El Tor biotype. More recently, the 8th world pandemic which started in Southern and Eastern India in 1992 was caused by a new serogroup, 0139-Bengal.

As humans are the only natural host, infection arises from faecal contamination of water or food. The organisms multiply in the proximal small bowel, where they secrete enterotoxin but do not invade the bowel wall. The molecular mechanisms of the pathogenesis of cholera have been particularly well studied.

Clinically, there is painless, acute, severe, watery diarrhoea after an incubation period of a few days. Up to a litre per hour of isotonic fluid is lost in this way, with resultant hypovolaemia. The illness lasts from 1–7 days.

The diagnosis is made clinically and from microscopic examination of the stool, in which the organism is readily seen and from which it can be readily grown.

Treatment is with **fluid resuscitation**, *including rapid restoration of the circulation and continuing maintenance. The latter may require up to 10 L in the first 24 h, preferably of half-normal saline, with 50 mmol/L of NaHCO₃ and 12.5 mmol/L of KCl.*

Tetracycline, *2 g/day for two days, eradicates the organism and reduces the severity and duration of illness.*

The mortality is 50%, if hypovolaemia is severe and simple resuscitative measures are not available. Natural infection gives long-lasting immunity, but available vaccines are only of limited and temporary efficacy.

Other tetracycline-sensitive vibrio species can also give clinical disease, including:

- diarrhoea;
- cellulitis;
- septicaemia.

Bibliography
Popovic T, Fields PL, Olsvik O et al 1995 Molecular subtyping of toxigenic *Vibrio cholerae* O139 causing epidemic cholera in India and Bangladesh, 1992–1993. J Infect Dis 171: 122.

Cholestasis

Cholestasis occurs in a number of settings. These include:

- biliary tract obstruction;
- benign postoperative intrahepatic cholestasis;
- pregnancy;
- drugs.

1. **Biliary tract obstruction** (see Cholangitis)

2. **Benign postoperative intrahepatic cholestasis**

This is usually seen after major surgery, in which there have been operative difficulties entailing undue prolongation, hypotension or massive transfusion.

The liver function tests are normal, apart from increased conjugated bilirubin.

The process appears within 1–2 days of surgery and lasts 2–4 weeks.

3. **Pregnancy**

Cholestasis is sometimes seen in late pregnancy, but it disappears after delivery, though it may recur with oral contraceptives.

4. **Drugs**

These include particularly phenothiazines, erythromycin estolate, oral contraceptives, and the anti-staphyococcal antibiotics, flucloxacillin and dicloxacillin (especially the former drug).

Bibliography
Johnston DE, Kaplan MM 1993 Pathogenesis and treatment of gallstones. N Engl J Med 328: 412.
LaMont JT, Isselbacher KJ 1973 Postoperative jaundice. N Engl J Med 288: 305.
Vennes JA, Bond JH 1983 Approach to the jaundiced patient. Gastroenterology 84: 1615.

Cholinergic agonists

Cholinergic agonists include:

- acetylcholine;
- methacholine;
- bethanechol, carbachol;
- choline esters;

- cholinomimetic alkaloids (pilocarpine, muscarine);
- mushroom poisons (mycetism) (q.v.).

The traditional pharmacology of cholinergic agonists is well known, comprising both muscarinic and nicotinic effects. The **muscarinic effects** occur in autonomic ganglia, CNS, heart, secretory glands and smooth muscle (and are antagonized by atropine). The **nicotinic effects** are exerted at the neuromuscular junction (and antagonized by curare) and in the autonomic ganglia, adrenal gland and CNS (all antagonized by trimethaphan). However, cholinergic pharmacology has become complex over the last decade, because of new data derived from the molecular cloning of receptors and from the pharmacology of pirenzepine.

Cholinergic crisis

A cholinergic crisis may occur:

- during the treatment of myasthenia gravis (q.v.),
- from exposure to nerve agents in chemical warfare (q.v.).

In myasthenia gravis, it arises from the excess dosage of anticholinesterase drugs which increase weakness because of depolarization of muscle. Although the differentiation of overtreatment from undertreatment with such drugs can be difficult, cholinergic excess typically occurs at the time of the peak effect of the drug, and is associated with muscarinic side-effects of salivation, sweating, gastrointestinal distress, bradycardia and constricted pupils.

If necessary, the diagnosis can be confirmed by giving edrophonium 1–2 mg/iv, though in this case muscle weakness will be temporarily worsened and brief respiratory support may be required.

Atropine should thus not be given routinely to such patients, as it could mask these important (muscarinic) markers of cholinergic overdose.

Christmas disease (see Haemophilia)

Chromium

Chromium (Cr, atomic number 24, atomic weight 52) is a hard grey metal, discovered in 1797 and so named because of its multi-coloured compounds (e.g. in gem stones), because while abundant in nature it is always present as a compound. Its main industrial use is to increase the strength and corrosion resistance of alloys. Chromium is present in meat, eggs and dairy foods and is an essential trace element.

Its clinical deficiency is uncommon. It is seen in the presence of prolonged poor oral intake and especially in prolonged total parenteral nutrition administration, unless replacement is given.

The clinical manifestations of chromium deficiency have been reported to include glucose intolerance (with a syndrome indistinguishable from non-insulin-dependent diabetes mellitus) and neuropathy.

The average daily requirement is 10–50 μg orally and the recommended iv dose is 0.2–0.4 μmol/day.

Chronic fatigue syndrome (see Acyclovir and Ciguatera)

Churg–Strauss syndrome

Churg–Strauss syndrome comprises:

- asthma;
- eosinophilia;
- systemic vasculitis.

It may be a subtype of polyarteritis nodosa (q.v.), with extravascular granulomas and eosinophilic vasculitis affecting both small arteries and venules. It may be related to Wegener's granulomatosis (q.v.), i.e. it is one of the ANCA-associated systemic vasculitides.

Recently, several cases have been reported following the use of the new leukotriene antagonists, zafirlukast and later montelukast, in patients with asthma. The probable mechanism is the unmasking of an underlying but hitherto unrecognized vasculitis.

> Clinical features include fever, anorexia, weight loss, arthralgia, polyneuropathy, and lung and renal involvement.

Investigations often show an increased anti-neutrophil cytoplasmic antibody (ANCA), an autoantibody found especially in Wegener's granulomatosis but also in polyarteritis nodosa and in idiopathic crescentic glomerulonephritis. The class of ANCA found is usually p-ANCA, unlike the c-ANCA typically found in Wegener's granulomatosis.

Diagnosis is confirmed by biopsy.

Treatment is with **corticosteroids** *and possibly with cyclophosphamide.*

The outlook is limited.

A variant is **allergic granulomatosis and angiitis**, which is seen in patients with prior asthma and allergy for many years.

> Clinical features include fever, dyspnoea, purpura, skin nodules, polyneuropathy and sometimes acute myocardial infarction. Pulmonary involvement occurs in 25% of cases and includes peripheral infiltrate, non-cavitating nodules and pleural effusion. It may sometimes be fulminating.

There is anaemia and leukocytosis with marked eosinophilia. The diagnosis is made clinically and histologically.

Treatment is with **corticosteroids** *and added cyclophosphamide if refractory.*

Bibliography
Choi YH, Im J-G, Han, BK et al 2000 Thoracic manifestations of Churg–Strauss syndrome. Chest 117: 117.
Chumbley LC, Harrison EG, DeRemee RA 1977 Allergic granulomatosis and angiitis (Churg–Strauss syndrome). Mayo Clin Proc 52: 477.
Churg J, Strauss L 1951 Allergic granulomatosis, allergic angiitis, and periarteritis nodosa. Am J Pathol 27: 277.
Guillevin L, Cohen P, Gayraud M et al 1999 Churg–Strauss syndrome: clinical study and long-term follow-up of 96 patients. Medicine 78: 26.
Lanham JG, Elkon KB, Pusey CD et al 1984 Systemic vasculitis with asthma and eosinophilia: a clinical approach to the Churg–Strauss syndrome. Medicine 63: 65.
Salama AD 1999 Pathogenesis and treatment of ANCA-associated systemic vasculitis. J R Soc Med 92: 456.
Wechsler ME, Finn D, Gunawardena D et al 2000 Churg–Strauss syndrome in patients receiving montelukast as treatment for asthma. Chest 117: 708.
Wechsler ME, Garpestad E, Kocher O et al 1998 Pulmonary infiltrates, eosinophilia, and cardiomyopathy following corticosteroid withdrawal in patients with asthma receiving zafirlukast. JAMA 279: 455.

Chylothorax (see Pleural cavity)

Ciguatera (see also Food poisoning)

Ciguatera arises from a toxin produced by algae, which are ingested by small fish, which in turn are consumed by larger bottom-dwelling fish which concentrate the toxin. Such fish are most common around coral reefs. The toxin is lipid-soluble and heat-stable, but there is no practical laboratory test for it in human samples. Its half-life is unknown.

The onset of symptoms is usually within a few hours and consists of gastrointestinal symptoms, sweating, itching and abnormal sensory perception. There is occasional circulatory failure. It generally lasts for only a few days and is rarely fatal.

Uncommonly, there is prolonged convalescence, referred to as chronic ciguatera poisoning. This condition is one of the differential diagnoses of chronic fatigue syndrome (myalgic encephalomyelitis).

*Treatment is with **emesis** and resuscitation if necessary. **Atropine** may improve some symptoms, and **mannitol** 25–50 g iv has been reported to be very helpful.*

Bibliography

Gillespie NC, Lewis RJ, Pearn JH et al 1986 Ciguatera in Australia: occurrence, clinical features, pathophysiology and management. Med J Aust 145: 584.

Lehane L 2000 Ciguatera update. Med J Aust 172: 176.

Morris JG 1980 Ciguatera fish poisoning. JAMA 244: 273.

Pearn JH 1997 Chronic fatigue syndrome: chronic ciguatera poisoning as a differential diagnosis. Med J Aust 166: 309.

Clostridial infections

These are caused by anaerobic spore-forming Gram-positive bacilli which secrete potent exotoxins. There are three major disease groups, namely:

- histotoxic (chiefly *C. perfringens*);
- enterotoxigenic (*C. perfringens* and *C. difficile*);
- neurotoxic (*C. tetani* and *C. botulinum*).

1. Histotoxic

C. perfringens is found in the lower gut and in the soil, and it enters a new site such as a wound, uterus or burn following appropriate trauma. The disease so produced is **gas gangrene**, an uncommon condition which requires in addition to the presence of the organism, associated necrosis, avascularity and/or a foreign body. The alpha toxin produced gives rise to haemolysis, necrosis and myocardial depression.

There is an incubation period of 8–72 h, followed by:

- local symptoms
  - pain, swelling, skin discolouration, crepitus, and foul-smelling, brown discharge;

- systemic features
  - fever, hypotension, oliguria, haemolysis, myonecrosis.

Uterine infection is usually post-abortal. Sometimes, a benign and localized gas abscess, i.e. a Welch abscess, only is formed.

The differential diagnosis of a gas-forming or crepitant cellulitis includes:

- Gram-negative infection
  - especially in diabetics;
- mixed anaerobic infection
  - e.g. perineal phlegmon from a peri-rectal abscess;
- trapped air
  - see Gas in soft tissues.

Treatment is with:

- *resuscitation;*
- *extensive surgical clearance;*
- *penicillin (7.2–14.4 g or 12–24 million U iv daily for two weeks);*
- *antitoxin (though this has never been proven to be useful);*
- *hyperbaric oxygenation as an adjunct.*

The average mortality is 15–30% and up to 50% if the abdominal wall or uterine cavity is severely infected.

2. Enterotoxigenic

Food poisoning caused by *C. perfringens* is second only to staphylococcal in incidence. The organisms are usually ingested from rewarmed meat and multiply in the small intestine, where they produce enterotoxin and thus diarrhoea.

There is an incubation period of about 12 h. There are no systemic symptoms, and the condition subsides within 24 h.

Pig-bel (necrotic jejunitis) seen in New Guinea is probably caused by the same organism.

Colitis is produced by *C. difficile*, which is found in soil and in normal faecal flora and which may overgrow when the normal flora are altered by antibiotic therapy (see Colitis).

3. Neurotoxic

The neurotoxic organisms gives rise to the specific diseases of:

- tetanus (q.v.);
- botulism (q.v.).

Bibliography

Loewenstein MS 1972 Epidemiology of *Clostridium perfringens* food poisoning. N Engl J Med 286: 1026.
Murrell TGC, Roth L, Egerton J et al 1966 Pig-bel: enteritis necroticans, a study in diagnosis and management. Lancet 1: 217.
Unsworth IP, Sharp PA 1984 Gas gangrene: an 11-year review of 73 cases managed with hyperbaric oxygen. Med J Aust 140: 256.
Weinstein L, Barza MA 1973 Gas gangrene. N Engl J Med 289: 1129.

Clostridium difficile (see Colitis)

Coagulation disorders

Coagulation disorders comprise a group of conditions, which together with

- thrombocytopenia,
- platelet function disorders,
- abnormally enhanced fibrinolysis,
- vascular fragility

comprise the broader group of **disorders of haemostasis**.

Coagulation disorders may be hereditary or acquired.

Hereditary coagulation disorders can comprise a deficiency of any of the individual coagulation factors. Each deficiency (except for factor XII deficiency which is asymptomatic) gives rise to a specific coagulopathy. The better known and most common hereditary coagulation disorders are:

- von Willebrand's disease (q.v.),
- haemophilia (q.v.).

Acquired coagulation disorders on the other hand usually demonstrate deficiency of multiple coagulation factors. These disorders include:

- disseminated intravascular coagulation (q.v.);
- liver disease;
- vitamin K deficiency (q.v.).

Occasional cases are iatrogenic.

Coagulation factors are of course plasma proteins, and the characteristics of the individual coagulation factors are shown in the table below.

Coagulation factors

Coagulation factor	Molecular weight	Plasma concentration (μcg/mL)	Plasma concentration (μM)
Fibrinogen (I)	330 000	3000	9.1
Prothrombin (II)	72 000	100	1.39
Factor V	330 000	10	0.03
Factor VII	50 000	0.5	0.01
Factor VIII	330 000	0.1	0.0003
Factor IX	56 000	5	0.089
Factor X	58 800	8	0.136
Factor XI	160 000	5	0.031
Factor XII	80 000	30	0.375
Factor XIII	320 000	10	0.031

Bibliography

Flier JS, Underhill LH 1992 Molecular and cellular biology of blood coagulation. N Engl J Med 326: 800.

Greenberg CS, Sane DC 1990 Coagulation problems in critical care medicine. In: Lumb PD, Shoemaker WC (eds). Critical Care: State of the Art, Chapter 9. Fullerton: Society of Critical Care Medicine. p 187.

Levi M, ten Cate H 1999 Disseminated intravascular coagulation. N Engl J Med 341:586.

Peyvandi F, Mannucci PM 1999 Rare coagulation disorders. Thromb Haemost 82: 1207.

Rapaport SI 1983 Preoperative hemostatic evaluation: which tests, if any? Blood 61: 229.

Cocaine

Cocaine is a white, crystalline alkaloid derived from the leaves of the South American coca plant. It has the composition of $C_{17}H_{21}NO_4$. The usual form is cocaine hydrochloride, a powder which may be inhaled or sniffed but is poorly absorbed and cannot be smoked. It is irritant and gives chronic rhinitis or even nasal ulceration. It is a mucous membrane anaesthetic, hence its application in clinical medicine. It produces rapid euphoria and alertness, which last for up to 90 min, and is addictive.

The freebase form (crack) which appeared in the 1980s is well absorbed and may be smoked or injected. It produces even more intense euphoria, but its action is brief and it is more addictive.

Clinical features of toxicity are numerous.

- **Acute toxicity** is manifest neurologically by headache, dizziness, dysphoria, formication, focal signs, fits and coma. Prolonged use may give rise to depression, irritability, disordered sleep, confusion, paranoia and fits. These neurological effects are due to excess dopaminergic neurotransmission.
- **Cardiovascular effects** of arrhythmias (including cardiac arrest), myocardial infarction, hypertension or stroke may be seen, even in the absence of high doses or concomitant cardiac disease. These effects are due to excess noradrenaline action. Long-term use may produce premature atherosclerosis.
- **Respiratory effects** include upper respiratory tract damage, pulmonary oedema and spontaneous barotrauma. When inhaled with smoke, it may cause permanent lung damage.
- **Systemic effects** such as hyperthermia, rhabdomyolysis, renal failure, liver failure, disseminated intravascular coagulation and bowel ischaemia may be seen.
- **Fetal damage** can occur.

Acute treatment is with **benzodiazepines** *and if necessary a calcium antagonist and/or antiarrhythmic agent. Vigabatrin (γ-vinyl-GABA, GVG) has shown promise in early studies in treating cocaine addiction. However, medical care attends clearly to only a small part of a much wider societal problem.*

Bibliography

Benowitz NL 1993 Clinical Pharmacology and toxicology of cocaine. Pharmacol Toxicol 72:3.

Cregler LL, Mark H 1986 Medical complications of cocaine abuse. N Engl J Med 315: 1495.

Dellinger RP, Zimmerman JL 1990 Management of the critically ill cocaine abuser. In: Lumb PD, Shoemaker WC (eds). Critical Care: State of the Art, Chapter 6. Fullerton: Society of Critical Care Medicine. p 115.

Dewey SL, Morgan AE, Ashby CR et al 1998 A novel strategy for the treatment of cocaine addiction. Synapse 30: 119.

Forrester JM, Steele AW, Waldron JA et al 1990 Crack lung: an acute pulmonary syndrome with a spectrum of clinical and histopathologic findings. Am Rev Respir Dis 142: 462.

Gawin FH 1991 Cocaine addiction: psychology and neurophysiology. Science 251: 1580.

Hollander JE 1995 The management of cocaine-associated myocardial ischaemia. N Engl J Med 333: 1267.

Karch SB 1999 Cocaine: history, use, abuse. J R Soc Med 92: 393.

Levine SR, Brust JCM, Futrell N et al 1990 Cerebrovascular complications of the use of the "crack" form of alkaloidal cocaine. N Engl J Med 323: 699.

Cold

Cold is one of the important Physical exposures (q.v.) and is represented by:

- frostbite (q.v.);
- hypothermia (q.v.).

Other cold-induced injuries occur following prolonged exposure to temperatures which are low but greater than freezing. These injuries include:

- chilblains;
- trench foot;
- immersion injury;
- cold urticaria (see Urticaria).

Cold intolerance is seen in iron deficiency and in hypothyroidism.

Cold agglutinin disease

Cold agglutinin disease is produced by a temperature-sensitive complement-fixing antibody which occurs in a number of infections. The highest titres occur during *Mycoplasma pneumoniae* infections, in which an IgM antibody is produced to the red blood cell membrane protein, IAg. Presumably the antigen is altered by the micro-organism so as to become immunogenic. The cold agglutinin titre for type O red blood cells shows either a 4-fold rise or a titre >1:128. The thermal amplitude of the antibody is usually 30–34°C.

The antibody production is related to the severity of illness and is seen in about 60% of patients with pneumonia due to *M. pneumoniae*. Although antibiotics decrease the duration and severity of infection, they do not clear the micro-organism which usually persists for 3–8 weeks. Though the production of antibody is a self-limited process, it usually last therefore for a few weeks.

The clinical consequence of cold agglutinin production is **haemolysis**. Although there is a very high incidence (80%) of reticulocytosis and a positive direct Coombs test, overt haemolysis is much less common. Clinical haemolysis typically occurs in the second and third week of illness and is associated with jaundice and even haemoglobinuria. Its extent is related to the height of titre. If clinical haemolysis occurs, the environmental temperature should be kept above the thermal amplitude of the antibody.

Bibliography

Dowd PM 1987 Cold-related disorders. Prog Dermatol 21: 1.

Frank M, Atkinson JP, Gadek J 1977 Cold agglutinins and cold agglutinin disease. Annu Rev Med 28: 291.

Colitis

Colitis or enterocolitis occurs in a number of forms.

1. **Ulcerative colitis** and **Crohn's disease** (granulomatous colitis) (see Inflammatory bowel disease.

2. **Ischaemic colitis**

This most commonly affects the distal colon in elderly patients, in whom it presents as blood-stained diarrhoea without mucus. The process may resolve within 48 h (though subsequent stricture may occur), or it may progress very rapidly to a fatal outcome, often despite surgery.

3. **Antibiotic-associated colitis** (pseudomembranous colitis)

This was originally described after the use of clindamycin, though it is now recognized to follow the use of many different antibiotics. It is due to the overgrowth of the toxin-producing *C. difficile* following the suppression by antibiotics of the normal bowel flora. At least two toxins, A (enterotoxic) and B (cytotoxic) are produced. The 'incubation period' is usually 4–9 days after the commencement of the culprit antibiotic regimen, but it can be as short as 2 days or as long as 6 weeks.

The condition is most frequent in seriously ill patients and is commonly nosocomial (when it is not necessarily antibiotic-related). Because of this, enteric precautions are required in affected hospital patients.

About 50% of cases have the characteristic pseudomembranous changes evident on endoscopy, though only 20% get diarrhoea (often of a variable nature) and only 10% have severe symptoms of blood-stained diarrhoea with abdominal pain, fever and leukocytosis.

Toxic megacolon is a rare complication.

Diagnosis requires the demonstration of toxin by assay in the faeces, since culture though sensitive is non-specific, as up to 25% of hospital patients have been reported to have positive cultures anyway.

Treatment consists of removing the potentially offending antibiotics and giving oral metronidazole, vancomycin or bacitracin for 7–10 days.

Relapse is common and is not prevented by more prolonged therapy. A fatal outcome is sometimes seen.

4. **Infective enterocolitis** (see also Diarrhoea)

This may be due to:

- campylobacter;
- staphylococci;
- *E. coli* (0157:H7 strain which can cause haemorrhagic diarrhoea).

5. **Irritable bowel syndrome**

This has sometimes been referred to as mucous colitis or spastic colitis.

Bibliography

Blaser MJ, Smith PD, Ravdin JL et al (eds) 1995 Infections of the gastrointestinal tract. New York: Raven Press.

Field M, Rao MC, Chang EB 1989 Intestinal electrolyte transport and diarrheal disease. N Engl J Med 321: 800, 879.

Johnson S, Clabots CR, Linn FV et al 1990 Nosocomial *Clostridium difficile* colonization and disease. Lancet 336: 97.

Kelly CP, Pothoulakis C, La Mont JT 1994 *Clostridium difficile* colitis. N Engl J Med 330: 257.

Lyerly DM, Krivan HC, Wilkins TD 1988 *Clostridium difficile*: its disease and toxins. Clin Microbiol Rev 1: 1.

Schlager TA, Guerrant RL 1988 Seven possible mechanisms for *Escherichia coli* diarrhea. Infect Dis Clin North Am 2: 607.

Young GP, Bayley N, Ward P et al 1986 Antibiotic-associated colitis caused by *Clostridium difficile*: relapse and risk factors. Med J Aust 144: 303.

Complement deficiency

The complement system is one of the four plasma enzyme cascades and together with the coagulation, fibrinolysis and kinin systems, it is involved in the bodily responses to injury. In particular, the complement system provides the major link between the process of inflammation and the immune system. It is thus involved not only in host resistance to infection, both immunological and nonspecific, but also in the mechanisms of tissue injury.

The 18 plasma proteins of the complement system produce components which kill viruses and bacteria and which regulate white cell chemotaxis and phagocytosis, mediator release, solubilization of immune complexes, smooth muscle contraction and cell lysis. There is a complex nomenclature.

Activation occurs via either the **classical** or the **alternative** pathway, each resulting in the cleavage of C3 and the initiation of a common terminal sequence which results in the lytic complex (C5b67 with C8 and C9, i.e. C5b–9).

- The **classical pathway** is activated by immune complexes (containing IgG or IgM antibody). Deficiencies of this pathway thus predispose to immune complex disease.
- The **alternative pathway** (or properdin) is activated directly by bacteria or other cells. Deficiencies of this pathway thus predispose to bacterial infection.

As with coagulation, the components of the two pathways undergo a controlled but amplified cascade of limited proteolysis leading to the production of active fragments, many of which have biological activity in their own right, most notably C5a. C5a produces neutrophil chemotaxis, activation and aggregation, a process which can occur to excess in some conditions and give rise to cell damage, e.g. pulmonary endothelial cell damage and ARDS.

Like other immune processes both humoral and cellular and indeed other biological responses to injury, complement is a classical double-edged sword which, while geared to provide defence against infection, can cause host damage under certain circumstances of excessive local or systemic activation.

Complement deficiency may be inherited or acquired.

Inherited deficiencies in general predispose to either immune complex disease (the classical pathway) or bacterial infection (the alternative pathway) There are 15 described abnormalities of complement, 14 associated with disease.

- C_1 INH with HAE, i.e. hereditary angioedema,
- C_1, C_4, C_2 with autoimmune disease, especially SLE,
- C_3, factor D, control proteins I and H with bacterial infections,
- properdin, C5–9 with neisseria infections.

Acquired complement deficiency is secondary to overt activation. This form of hypocomplementaemia is associated with, and perhaps related to, some cases of:

- adult respiratory distress syndrome;
- septic shock;
- cellular damage from extracorporeal circuits;
- haemolysis;
- vasculitis.

Bibliography
Colten HR, Rosen FS 1992 Complement deficiencies. Annu Rev Immunol 10: 809.

Schifferli JA, Ng YC, Peters DK 1986 The role of complement and its receptors in the elimination of immune complexes. N Engl J Med 315: 488.

Tomlinson S 1993 Complement defense mechanisms. Curr Opinion Immunol 5: 83.

Van de Meer JWM 1994 Defects in host-defense mechanisms. In: Rubin RH, Young LS (eds). Clinical Approach to Infections in the Compromised Host. 3rd edition. New York: Plenum, p 33.

Conjunctivitis

Conjunctivitis and keratoconjunctivitis may be:

- allergic;
- infective;
- associated with specific diseases.

Allergic conjunctivitis is a common condition and is the eye equivalent of allergic rhinitis. It is thus a seasonal, IgE-mediated condition, with bilateral redness, swelling and itch.

The differential diagnosis from herpetic conjunctivitis is important, because corticosteroids are contraindicated in the latter condition. The other differential diagnoses include infective or contact-induced inflammation.

Infective conjunctivitis may be caused by viruses, bacteria or *Chlamydia trachomatis*.

- The common viruses are adenovirus or herpes simplex virus; enterovirus 70, the Newcastle disease virus of poultry, can give a haemorrhagic conjunctivitis in humans.

- The common bacteria are gonococci, haemophilus, meningococci and staphylococci.
- Infective conjunctivitis may also occur in systemic infectious diseases, such as measles and typhus.

Specific diseases associated with conjunctivitis include several systemic disorders, including:

- Behçet's syndrome;
- exophthalmos;
- Reiter's syndrome;
- Stevens–Johnson syndrome;
- toxic-shock syndrome.

In addition, keratoconjunctivitis is a major local feature of the sicca syndrome (Sjögren's syndrome, q.v.).

Conn's syndrome

Conn's syndrome comprises hypertension and hypokalaemia due to excess adrenal production of aldosterone. It is caused by:

- **benign unilateral adrenal adenoma** (most commonly);
- **bilateral adrenal hyperplasia**, which is probably pituitary in origin (less commonly);
- **adrenal carcinoma** (rarely);
- **genetic variant** (rarely). This is inherited as an autosomal dominant, in which an abnormal gene product presumably has combined synthetic enzyme activities, so that excess aldosterone is dependent on ACTH and not on angiotensin. This variant responds paradoxically to corticosteroids;
- **liquorice** ingestion in excess (>0.5 kg per week), since glycyrrhizic acid inhibits the renal inactivation of aldosterone and is thus salt-retaining (see Liquorice). This condition is sometimes called (**pseudo primary aldosteronism**).

Conn's syndrome is thus an uncommon cause of secondary hypertension, but while aldosterone causes salt and water retention and thus acute hypervolaemic hypertension, the mechanism for sustained hypertension in this

setting is unknown. Nevertheless, Conn's syndrome is usually discovered from screening hypertensive patients who have a borderline or low serum potassium level.

The hypokalaemia may be asymptomatic, though it may be associated with cardiac arrhythmias, muscle weakness, insulin-resistant glucose intolerance and polyuria due to a renal tubular defect. There is also an excessive proneness to hypokalaemia following diuretic therapy.

Investigations should be performed with the patient off any medication containing diuretics, beta blockers, calcium channel blockers and ACE inhibitors.

- There is a high 24-h urinary potassium excretion (at least 30 mmol despite hypokalaemia).
- Provided the patient is not hypokalaemic at the time of testing (since hypokalaemia can suppress aldosterone biosynthesis), there is a high plasma aldosterone level (>450 pmol/L) and a suppressed plasma renin activity (<1 μg/L). Autonomous aldosterone secretion is demonstrated by failure of it suppression by sodium loading (2 L os isotonic saline over 4 h), fludrrocortisone (0.4 mg daily for 3 days) or captopril (25 mg).
- The specific lesion should be localized with CT scanning, adrenal vein sampling if necessary and occasionally adrenal scintigraphy.

*Treatment is with **adrenalectomy**. Spironolactone should be used preoperatively and also for continuing medical treatment of bilateral hyperplasia.*

Bibliography
Blumenfeld JD, Sealey JE, Schlussel Y et al 1994 Diagnosis and treatment of primary hyperaldosteronism. Ann Intern Med 121: 877.
Editorial 1980 Corticosteroids and hypothalamic-pituitary-adrenocortical function. Br Med J 280: 813.
Gittler RD, Fajans SS 1995 Primary aldosteronism (Conn's syndrome). J Clin Endocrinol Metab 80: 3438.

Melby JC 1991 Diagnosis of hyperaldosteronism. Endocrinol Metab Clin North Am 20: 247.

Quinn SJ, Williams GH 1988 Regulation of aldosterone secretion. Ann Rev Physiol 50: 409.

Copper

Copper (Cu, atomic number 29, atomic weight 64) is a red ductile metal. Since it is found free in nature, it was used as the first metal substitute for stone implements from about 8000 BC and was subsequently combined with tin to form bronze. It may also be combined with zinc to form brass and with zinc and nickel to form nickel silver. Since it is a very good conductor of heat and electricity, its greatest use is in the electrical industry and in alloys.

Copper is chiefly ingested from shellfish or animal organs. Most of the body's copper (100–150 mg) is found in the liver, where it is attached to copper-binding proteins or present in metalloenzymes. These play a key role in mitochondrial function, collagen and elastin cross-linking, and melatonin production. It is thus an essential trace element.

In plasma, copper is mostly bound to caeruloplasmin, and the normal serum copper is 11–24 μmol/L. The normal daily requirements are 300–1000 μg/day orally and the recommended iv dose is 5–20 μmol/day. These doses should be increased if there are excessive gastrointestinal losses and decreased if there is hepatobiliary disease.

The serum copper level is increased by oestrogens, since they increase caeruloplasmin. Increased serum copper is also seen in lymphoma and Wilson's disease (see below).

Copper deficiency is uncommon. It occurs primarily with prolonged gastrointestinal losses, since it is normally excreted via the bile. Copper deficiency gives rise to anaemia and leukopenia.

Wilson's disease is a rare autosomal recessive disorder due to a defect on chromosome 13, resulting in impaired excretion of copper into

the bile. Copper thus accumulates in the tissues, especially in the liver and brain, giving rise to 'hepatolenticular degeneration'.

Clinical manifestations are usually apparent by early adulthood with:

- hepatosplenomegaly;
- abnormal liver function tests;
- haemolysis;
- neurological deterioration (clumsiness, tremor, rigidity, dysarthria and personality changes);
- pathognomonic Kayser–Fleischer corneal rings, which are thin, brown and peripheral.

Investigations show a low or absent serum caeruloplasmin, increased urinary copper and increased hepatic copper.

*Treatment is with **penicillamine** (see Chelating agents). This binds copper and enhances its urinary excretion up to 3-fold. The usual dose is 1 g daily.*

- *Concomitant pyridoxine 50 mg/week is required.*
- *If penicillamine is not tolerated, oral zinc or tetrathiomolybdate may be used.*

Bibliography

Chelly J, Monaco AP 1993. Cloning the Wilson disease gene. Nature Genetics 5: 317.

Ferenci P. Wilson's disease. Clin Liver Dis 1998; 2: 31.

Scheinberg IH, Sternlieb I 1965 Wilson's disease. Annu Rev Med 16: 119.

Schilsky ML 1996 Wilson disease: genetic basis of copper toxicity and natural history. Semin Liver Dis 16: 83.

Sternlieb I 1990 Perspectives on Wilson's disease. Hepatology 12: 1234.

Strickland GT, Leu M 1975 Wilson's disease – clinical and laboratory manifestations in 40 patients. Medicine 54: 113.

Wilson SAK 1912 Progressive lenticular degeneration. A familial nervous disease associated with cirrhosis of the liver. Brain 34: 295.

Yarze JC, Martin P, Munoz SJ et al 1992 Wilson's disease: current status. Am J Med 92: 643.

Costochondritis (see Chest wall disorders)

CREST syndrome (see Scleroderma)

Creutzfeldt–Jakob disease

Creutzfeldt–Jakob disease (CJ disease, CJD) is an encephalopathy due to infection with a small transmissible proteinaceous particle called a prion. It is the human form of transmissible dementia, generally transmitted in nature by ingestion of infected animal tissues. It is related to the human disease, kuru, and to the animal diseases, scrapie and bovine spongiform encephalopathy (BSE, 'mad cow disease').

It is still a mystery how a variant of a normal cell membrane protein without RNA or DNA can be an infectious agent. Moreover, there is no detectable serological response. At all events, insoluble aggregates of prion protein (PrP) appear responsible for the plaques and fibrils seen in the brains of infected subjects. Presumably, there has been a mutation in the PrP gene on chromosome 20 in non-iatrogenic cases.

A few cases are familial (about 10%) but most are sporadic. Some are iatrogenic (perhaps 200 cases worldwide) and have occurred particularly in middle-aged patients who have had surgery (especially neurosurgery) or trauma. It has also been reported in patients formerly given the human pituitary-derived hormones, growth hormone for short stature or gonadotrophin for infertility, between 1960 and 1985. It may possibly occur after ingestion of animal brains (and perhaps other tissues of infected animals), since ritualistic cannibalism of human brains was the practice which used to lead to kuru.

A variant form (nvCJD) was recently reported in a cluster of cases among young patients in the UK. It followed the epidemic of BSE which commenced in 1986 in that country and has been shown to be caused by the same strain of transmissible agent as BSE. There is new concern about its potential transmission from apparently healthy persons incubating the disease to others via blood, blood products, organ donation or instrumentation, though there is no epidemiological evidence that this has so far occurred.

The incubation period has been reported to be 1–3 years in patients with a single definable culprit event, but it is perhaps much longer in some patients. The patient is infectious during this time.

Clinical features comprise dementia, together with myoclonus and pyramidal, extrapyramidal and cerebellar signs. Cerebellar signs are dominant in the familial variant referred to as Gerstmann–Straussler syndrome.

The CSF is normal and the CT scan shows cerebral atrophy. The diagnosis can only be made histologically, with the demonstration of spongiform changes (neuronal vacuolation), astrocyte proliferation, neuronal loss and amyloid plaques, but no inflammatory response. Genetic screening for PrP gene variants (and thus susceptibility to exogenous prion infection) is now possible.

There is no effective treatment.

The outcome is always fatal, after a clinical illness of about 6 months.

The following points are of importance in Intensive Care practice.

- Special care needs to be taken in handling potentially infectious material.

  - The infectious agent may be present widely throughout the body.
  - Importantly, it is not inactivated by routine techniques used to destroy nucleic acids, viz. boiling, irradiation, ethylene oxide, glutaraldehyde, formalin, alcohol or iodine.
  - It is however inactivated by prolonged autoclaving or by sodium hydroxide or hypochlorite.

- Due to difficulties in diagnosis, the human prion diseases may be more common than previously thought.

  - Moreover, most body tissues and fluids may be infectious for prolonged periods.

Creutzfeldt–Jakob disease

– This has adverse implications for blood, tissue and organ donation and transplantation.

Bibliography

Andrews NJ, Farrington CP, Cousens SN et al 2000 Incidence of variant Creutzfeldt–Jakob disease in the UK. Lancet 356: 481.

Brown P, Cervenakova L, Goldfarb LG et al 1994 Iatrogenic Creutzfeldt–Jakob disease: an example of the interplay between ancient genes and modern medicine. Neurology 44: 291.

Brown P, Will RG, Bradley R et al 2001 Bovine spongiform encephalopathy and variant Creutzfeldt–Jakob disease: background, evolution and current concerns. Emerg Infect Dis 7: 1.

Bruce ME, Will RG, Ironside JW et al 1997 Transmissions of mice indicate that 'new variant' CJD is caused by the BSE agent. Nature 389: 448.

Collins S, Masters CL 1996 Iatrogenic and zoonotic Creutzfeldt–Jakob disease. Med J Aust 164: 598.

DeArmond SJ 1993 Overview of the transmissible spongiform encephalopathies: prion protein disorders. Br Med Bull 49: 725.

Edney ATB 1996 Spongiform encephalopathies: still many unanswered questions. J Roy Soc Med 89: 423.

Holman RC, Khan AS, Belay ED et al 1996 Creutzfeldt–Jakob disease in the United States, 1979–1994: using national mortality data to assess the possible occurrence of variant cases. Emerg Infect Dis 2: 4.

Masters CL 2001 The emerging European epidemic of variant Creutzfeldt–Jakob disease and bovine spongiform encephalopathy. Med J Aust 174: 160.

Mitchell AR 1996 Creutzfeldt–Jakob disease. Lancet 347: 1704.

Parchi P, Castellani R, Capellari S et al 1996 Molecular basis of phenotypic variability in sporadic Creutzfeldt–Jakob disease. Ann Neurol 39: 767.

Pattison J 1998 The emergence of bovine spongiform encephalopathy and related diseases. Emerg Infect Dis 4: 3.

Prusiner SB 1991 Molecular biology of prion disease. Science 252: 1515.

Prusiner SB, Hsiao KK 1994 Human prion diseases. Ann Neurol 35: 385.

Will RG 1994 Gene influence on Creutzfeldt–Jakob disease. Lancet 344: 1310.

Will RG, Ironside JW, Zeidler M et al 1996 A new variant of Creutzfeldt–Jakob disease in the UK. Lancet 347: 921.

Wilson K, Code C, Ricketts MN 2000 Risk of acquiring Creutzfeldt–Jakob disease from blood transfusions. Br Med J 321: 17.

Cricoarytenoid arthritis

The cricoarytenoid joints may be affected in rheumatoid arthritis, as may the temporomandibular joints. The condition is often mild and asymptomatic.

Cricoarytenoid arthritis, if severe, is one of the causes of upper airway obstruction and can thus be especially relevant in Intensive Care.

- Acutely,

    – there is stridor, hoarseness and dysphagia,
    – sometimes, there is pain radiating to the ear,
    – the larynx is tender, and the arytenoids are red and swollen at laryngoscopy.

- Chronically,

    – there may also be stridor or hoarseness due to ankylosis of these joints.

Bibliography

Montgomery WW 1963 Cricoarytenoid arthritis. Laryngoscope 73: 801.

Critical illness myopathy (see Myopathy)

Critical illness polyneuropathy (see Neuropathy)

Crohn's disease (see Inflammatory bowel disease)

Cryoglobulinaemia (see Multiple myeloma)

Cryptococcosis

Cryptococcosis (torulosis) is a systemic disease caused by the yeast-like organism, *C. neoformans*. The organism is found worldwide, usually in avian excreta, especially from pigeons. Exposure to inhaled particles, and thus asymptomatic infection, is probably very common, with clinical infection occurring mostly from either massive exposure or in compromised hosts, especially those with impaired cell-mediated immunity. The pathogenesis is probably similar to that of tuberculosis or other mycoses, and the pulmonary effects are chiefly due to a mass rather than to the virulence of the micro-organism.

Perhaps up to a third of documented cases and presumably a higher proportion of total cases are asymptomatic, despite even extensive X-ray changes. In the others, there are chest symptoms which are chronic and rarely progressive. Occasionally, there may be dissemination to the meninges in compromised hosts. Chronic meningitis or the symptoms of a space-occupying lesion then become apparent. Dissemination elsewhere in the body may also occur, particularly to the skin where ulcerated papules may occur.

The diagnosis is made by demonstrating the presence of the organism or its antigen in blood or CSF. The demonstration of the organism in sputum is non-specific. The CSF in cases of meningitis additionally shows a positive India ink stain in 50% of cases and increased pressure, lymphocytes and protein, and decreased glucose. Biopsy of appropriate material is also diagnostic. Chest X-ray typically shows a mass with or without cavitation, sometimes multiple and occasionally diffuse. Hilar lymphadenopathy is sometimes seen, as is pleural effusion.

Treatment is required for extrapulmonary disease in all cases. For pulmonary disease, treatment is required only if the involvement is extensive or the patient is immunocompromised.

- *Treatment is with **amphotericin B** to a total of 2–3 g over 6 weeks. If renal function and bone marrow function are normal, the addition of flucytosine 10 g daily in divided doses permits a lower dose of amphotericin and results in fewer failures.*
- *If pulmonary resection is to be performed, fluconazole should be used to prevent associated meningitis, for which there is a 5% risk.*

The mortality of cryptococcal meningitis is always 100% without treatment, but it is reduced to about 40% with treatment.

Cushing's syndrome

Cushing's syndrome refers to adrenal cortical hyperactivity.

> Cushing's syndrome is caused by:
> - excess adrenal stimulation;
> - intrinsic adrenal overactivity;
> - iatrogenic administration of corticosteroids in pharmacological doses.

1. **Excess adrenal stimulation** arises from excess ACTH, which may be secreted either by the pituitary (Cushing's disease) or ectopically.

- Excess pituitary secretion of ACTH causes bilateral adrenal hyperplasia and is responsible for two thirds of the cases of Cushing's syndrome. The original pituitary cause is often unclear because, although there is sometimes an adenoma, some cases are postulated to be due to excess hypothalamic secretion of CRH, causing in turn a hyperplastic response in the pituitary.

- Ectopic production of ACTH is either from a carcinoma (lung, pancreas, kidney, thymus) or a carcinoid tumour (which can also secrete CRH).

2. **Intrinsic adrenal overactivity** may be due to neoplasia or hyperplasia.

- Adrenal adenomas usually secrete cortisol only, whereas the uncommon carcinomas if secretory usually release androgens as well.
- Bilateral non-ACTH-dependent hyperplasia is an unusual entity with several forms, namely macronodular (probably originally pituitary in origin but with nodular autonomy later developing), micronodular (occasionally familial, thought by some to be due to autoantibodies to ACTH receptors) and a food-dependent form (in which adrenal cells inappropriately express gastric inhibitory peptide, GIP, which stimulates cortisol release).

3. The **iatrogenic causes** of Cushing's syndrome are well recognized, but these overt changes are much less common than the subclinical effects of the invariable hypothalamic–pituitary–adrenal suppression which is seen in all patients receiving such doses of corticosteroids. This is clearly an important phenomenon in the seriously ill (see Adrenal insufficiency).

The clinical features of Cushing's syndrome include facial plethora, skin fragility with easy bruising and poor wound healing, and susceptibility to infections. Diabetes, hypertension, obesity, osteoporosis, depression, amenorrhoea, hirsutism, cataracts, glaucoma, pancreatitis, oedema, renal calculi, benign intracranial hypertension and hypokalaemia may also occur. Proximal myopathy is also seen and together with osteoporosis and skin fragility represent catabolic changes.

As is well known, many of the clinical features of Cushing's syndrome, such as diabetes, hypertension, obesity and hirsutism, are common in a variety of other settings (e.g. alcoholism).

> An explosive onset of hypokalaemic alkalosis, pigmentation and severe weakness may result from ectopic ACTH produced by a small cell lung carcinoma.

The most usual screening test is the dexamethasone suppression test, in which following dexamethasone 1 mg orally at midnight, the serum cortisol level at 9 am is >140 nmol/L. Apart from Cushing's syndrome, the level may also be increased (i.e. fail to be suppressed to the normal level by dexamethasone 1 mg) in association with stress, alcohol, oestrogens, depression or Intensive Care. A 24 h basal urinary free cortisol should also be measured (normal <200 nmol). If both tests are normal, no further testing is required.

Abnormal screening tests have traditionally been confirmed with a two-day low-dose dexamethasone suppression test, which if normal excludes Cushing's syndrome but if still abnormal should be followed by a two-day high-dose dexamethasone suppression test. More recently, abnormal screening tests have been followed by a high-dose dexamethasone (8 mg) suppression test, with the ACTH level measured before and after.

- If the ACTH level is low (<2 pmol/L), the Cushing's syndrome is of adrenal origin.
- If the ACTH level is normal or more usually high–normal (10–20 pmol/L) and suppressed, the Cushing's syndrome is of pituitary origin.
- If the ACTH level is high (>20 pmol/L) and not suppressed, the Cushing's syndrome is of ectopic origin. However, the plasma ACTH level may be normal even if there is ACTH dependence, since ACTH precursor or fragments may be responsible, especially in ectopic production.

Following biochemical confirmation of Cushing's syndrome, the primary site should be localized by CT scanning or MRI.

*Treatment is primarily **surgical**.*

- *Pituitary tumours are removed by trans-sphenoidal adenomectomy, which for small tumours has a 90% cure rate, though there is a small risk of postoperative diabetes insipidus or meningitis.*
- *Primary adrenal disorders require unilateral or bilateral adrenalectomy, depending on the nature*

of the pathology. In the presence of excess pituitary ACTH, bilateral adrenalectomy carries a 10–40% postoperative risk of Nelson's syndrome (markedly increased skin pigmentation and pituitary chromophobe tumour with visual defects), though this complication can be prevented by postoperative pituitary irradiation.

- *After even limited pituitary or adrenal surgery, endocrine function may take up to two years to recover, during which time replacement therapy is required.*

Bibliography

Aron DC, Findling JW, Tyrrell JB 1987 Cushing's disease. Endocrinol Metab Clin North Am 16: 705.

Bertagna X 1992 New causes of Cushing's syndrome. N Engl J Med 327: 1024.

Editorial 1980 Corticosteroids and hypothalamic–pituitary–adrenocortical function. Br Med J 280: 813.

Jeffcoate WJ 1988 Treating Cushing's disease. Br Med J 296: 227.

Kaye TB, Crapo L 1990 The Cushing syndrome: an update on diagnostic tests. Ann Intern Med 112: 434.

Odell WD 1991 Ectopic ACTH secretion: a misnomer. Endocrinol Metab Clin North Am 20: 371.

Cyanide

A cyanide is a compound containing the monovalent group, CN. Inorganic salts derived from hydrocyanic acid (such as sodium cyanide) are very toxic. Hydrogen cyanide (HCN) itself is a very volatile liquid. Organic cyanides are called nitriles and include acrylonitrile, which is used in the manufacture of plastics. In nature, cyanide is found in the pit of the wild cherry.

> Cyanide poisoning occurs traditionally from suicidal, accidental or homicidal ingestion, or from occupational exposure, though it may also occur from smoke inhalation (see Burns, respiratory complications) and more recently it has been observed after prolonged use of sodium nitroprusside.

Concentrations as low as 200 parts per million for 30 min or ingestion of 300 mg of salt or 100 mg of HCN are usually fatal.

The onset of poisoning is very rapid and requires prompt treatment. In non-fatal cases, complete recovery is the rule even without treatment, because of natural detoxification by hepatic rhodanase with the production of non-toxic sulfocyanides.

Since the circumstances of potential exposure are usually apparent, acute poisoning can generally be clinically suspected well before its biochemical confirmation. Clinical features include neurological dysfunction with impaired consciousness, headache, dizziness, agitation, confusion and fits, and systemic signs with tachycardia and tachypnoea.

Treatment is with 100% oxygen, mechanical ventilation and an appropriate antidote.

- ***Antidotes*** *include nitrites (amyl nitrite by inhalation, sodium nitrite by iv injection of 5 mg/kg over 3 min), sodium thiosulfate (50 mL of 25% solution iv) or a cobalt-containing compound, such as cobalt edetate (Kelocyanor) or hydroxycobalamin. These latter agents are the antidotes of choice and are given in a dose of 10.5 mg/kg and 70 mg/kg, respectively. The usual pharmaceutical preparation, cobalt edetate, can cause vomiting and hypotension.*

> In Intensive Care practice, the potential cyanide toxicity of **sodium nitroprusside** (SNP) is not widely appreciated. This toxicity occurs because SNP contains 44% cyanide which is degraded to thiocyanate in the liver, from where it is excreted in the urine. Toxicity is related to both the total dose and the rate of administration. Neurological damage, including neuropathy, encephalopathy, coma and focal signs may occur and can be irreversible. Unexplained cardiac arrest or death may occur.
>
> The greatest incidence is after open-heart surgery, where it has been estimated that perhaps 1000 deaths per year may occur

from SNP in the USA, though this number should be put in context of the large total usage of SNP of about 500 000 patient-days per year in that country.

This is a difficult subject to clarify, as most cases are probably unrecognized because of difficulties in measurement. Thus, increased levels of thiocyanate and even cyanide usually occur as late phenomena, as does metabolic (lactic) acidosis.

Bibliography

Curry SC, Arnold-Capell P 1991 Nitroprusside, nitroglycerin, and angiotensin-converting enzyme inhibitors. Crit Care Clin 7: 555.

Freeman AG 1988 Optic neuropathy and chronic cyanide intoxication: a review. J R Soc Med 81: 103.

Kulig K 1991 Cyanide antidotes and fire toxicology. N Engl J Med 325: 1801.

Robin ED, McCauley R 1992 Nitroprusside-related cyanide poisoning. Chest 102: 1842.

Vick JA, Froehlich H 1991 Treatment of cyanide poisoning. Milit Med 156: 330.

Zerbe NF, Wagner BK 1993 Use of vitamin B12 in the treatment and prevention of nitroprusside-induced cyanide toxicity. Crit Care Med 21: 465.

Cystic fibrosis

Cystic fibrosis is a common genetic disorder transmitted as an autosomal recessive trait. The abnormal gene is on the long arm of chromosome 7, a region which codes for a 1480 amino acid protein ('CF transmembrane regulator', CFTR). Over 700 CFTR mutations have now been described. In about 70% of patients with cystic fibrosis, amino acid no. 508 on this protein is missing. The resultant protein is abnormal in that it cannot glycosylated, so that it is retained in the Golgi apparatus rather than being transferred to the cell membrane.

The cell membrane then has an increased sodium absorption and decreased chloride transfer, with the result that exocrine gland secretions are abnormally viscid. Consequently, there is impaired clearance of respiratory secretions, with mucus plugging and secondary infection, especially due to *S. aureus* and *P. aeruginosa*. Although bronchiectasis, atelectasis and fibrosis are produced, the lesions rarely cavitate.

Clinical features of cystic fibrosis are usually present from childhood, though some variants first appear in adult life.

- There is progressive, chronic airways obstruction,

    – with cough, sputum, dyspnoea and wheeze.

- Physical examination shows cyanosis, clubbing and hyperinflation.
- Haemoptysis and pneumothorax are common early complications.
- Cor pulmonale frequently occurs subsequently.
- Extrapulmonary manifestations include:

    – pancreatic insufficiency;
    – recurrent bowel obstruction;
    – hepatic cirrhosis;
    – aspermia.

The diagnosis is made on the basis of increased sodium and chloride levels in sweat, as follows:

- chloride >60 mmol/L is found in all patients and is diagnostic if the patient is <20 y,
- chloride >80 mmol/L is not seen in any other condition and is diagnostic if the patient is >20 y.

Treatment is with physiotherapy (postural drainage and breathing exercises), nebulized mist therapy, bronchodilators and intensive antibiotic therapy.

- *Pancreatic enzyme replacement is required, as is adequate salt and water balance and protection from proneness to heat exhaustion.*
- *Inhaled amiloride has been reported to be helpful, as it blocks membrane sodium channels.*
- *DNase (dornase alpha) has recently been found to reduce the incidence of chest infections in cystic fibrosis but at great cost and thus uncertain cost-effectiveness.*

- *Lung transplantation has been available in some centres since the 1980s for advanced cases.*
- *Future prospects clearly include gene therapy.*

With recent improvements in treatment, patients with cystic fibrosis generally now survive into adulthood, the median life expectancy at birth now being about 40 y.

Bibliography

Brock DJH 1996 Prenatal screening for cystic fibrosis. Lancet 347: 148.

Davidson DJ, Porteous DJ 1998 The genetics of cystic fibrosis lung disease. Thorax 53: 389.

Elborn JS, Shale DJ, Britton JR 1991 Cystic fibrosis: current survival and population estimates to the year 2000. Thorax 46: 881.

Frizzell RA 1995 Functions of the cystic fibrosis transmembrane conductance regulator protein. Am J Respir Crit Care Med 151: S54.

Fuchs HJ, Borowitz DS, Christiansen DH et al 1994 Effect of recombinant human DNase on exacerbations of respiratory symptoms and on pulmonary function in patients with cystic fibrosis. N Engl J Med 331: 637.

Hilman BC 1997 Genetic and immunologic aspects of cystic fibrosis. Ann Allergy Asthma Immunol 79: 379.

Knowles MR, Church NL, Waltner WE et al 1990 A pilot study of aerosolized amiloride for the treatment of lung disease in cystic fibrosis. N Engl J Med 322: 1189.

Orenstein DM 1985 Diagnosis of cystic fibrosis. Semin Respir Med 6: 252.

Robinson M, Regnis JA, Bailey DL et al 1996 Effect of hypertonic saline, amiloride, and cough on mucociliary clearance in patients with cystic fibrosis. Am J Resp Crit Care Med 153: 1503.

Rosenstein BJ, Zeitlin PL 1998 Cystic fibrosis. Lancet 351: 277.

Rubin BK 1999 Emerging therapies for cystic fibrosis lung disease. Chest 115: 1120.

Sawyer SM, Robertson CF, Bowes G 1997 Cystic fibrosis: a changing clinical perspective. Aust NZ J Med 27: 6.

The Cystic Fibrosis Genotype-Phenotype Consortium 1993 Correlation between genotype and phenotype in patients with cystic fibrosis. N Engl J Med 329: 1308.

Tsui L-C 1995 The cystic fibrosis transmembrane conductance regulator gene. Am J Respir Crit Care Med 151: S47.

Wallis G 1997 Diagnosing cystic fibrosis: blood, sweat, and tears. Arch Dis Child 76: 85.

Welsh MJ, Smith AE 1995 Cystic fibrosis. Sci Amer 273: 36.

Yankaskas JR, Mallory GB 1998 Lung transplantation in cystic fibrosis: consensus conference statement. Chest 113: 217.

Cytomegalovirus

Cytomegalovirus (CMV) is a ubiquitous DNA virus and one of the 7 human herpesviruses. It is present in many bodily fluids and is transmitted from person to person across the placenta, in breast milk, in child care centres, from communal living, from close personal contact, in blood transfusion and in transplanted organs.

Following initial infection, the virus is carried for life in many different cells in many different organs. It remains dormant until reactivation and replication during periods of immunocompromise, especially during T cell dysfunction.

CMV causes the following disease states.

- Mononucleosis may be produced at any age but especially in young adults. It is similar to that produced by EBV infection, except that there is no heterophile antibody.
- It is the most common viral pathogen in patients after organ transplantation, especially bone marrow transplantation. After 1–4 months, there is fever, neutropenia, pneumonitis and occasionally disseminated disease.
- It is the most frequent and important pathogen in patients with AIDS. CMV and HIV potentiate each other's replication. Disseminated disease may include pneumonitis, gastrointestinal ulceration, encephalitis, polyradiculopathy and retinitis.

Diagnosis requires viral identification by isolation or PCR.

*Treatment is with **ganciclovir** iv (q.v.) or more recently with foscarnet. Oral ganciclovir may be used*

Cytomegalovirus

for prophylaxis or suppression in seropositive transplant recipients.

The mortality is up to 90% in CMV pneumonitis.

Bibliography

Goodgame, RW 1993 Gastrointestinal cytomegalovirus disease. Ann Intern Med 119: 924.

Jacobson MA, Mills J 1988 Serious cytomegalovirus disease in acquired immunodeficiency syndrome (AIDS): clinical findings, diagnosis, and treatment. Ann Intern Med 108: 585.

Merigan TC, Renlund DG, Keay S et al 1992 A controlled trial of ganciclovir to prevent cytomegalovirus disease after heart transplantation. N Engl J Med 326: 1182.

Dantrolene (see Amphetamines, Heat stroke, Malignant hyperthermia, Neuroleptic malignant syndrome and Rhabdomyolysis)

Decompression sickness (see Diving)

Delirium

Delirium describes acute cerebral dysfunction ('acute brain syndrome') and is manifest by disordered

- consciousness,
- orientation,
- expression,
- perception,
- attention span,
- memory,
- motor activity.

It has a rapid onset. It usually lasts only hours to days, during which time it may fluctuate in severity, being typically worse at night and improving even as far as lucidity during the day.

> Delirium is due to a specific organic problem. Most typically, this is a systemic infection.
>
> The cause can also be:
>
> - cardiac failure;
> - liver disease;
> - metabolic disorders;
> - renal disease;
> - CNS disease
>
>   – cerebrovascular, infection, trauma;
>
> - the postoperative state.
>
> It is also commonly seen
>
> - after drug withdrawal
>
>   – especially alcohol but also other sedatives,
>
> - in adverse environmental conditions
>   – especially those associated with sleep deprivation, and conflicting, overloaded or deprived sensory input.

Dementia

Dementia describes chronic cerebral dysfunction and is manifest by disturbed

- orientation,
- expression,
- memory.

There is usually no disturbance of consciousness, perception, attention span or motor activity, and no associated organic illness. Dementia may of course occur in association with delirium or with psychiatric illness.

> Most such patients have either Alzheimer's disease or multi-infarct dementia.
>
> Many other conditions (some treatable) may also cause dementia, including:
>
> - myxoedema;
> - thiamine deficiency;
> - syphilis;
> - aluminium toxicity;
> - quinidine;
> - Whipple's disease;
> - occult hydrocephalus;
> - cerebral tumour.

Ten per cent of the population over the age of 65 y and 20% over 80 y develop some degree of dementia. Genetic testing for Alzheimer's disease, especially for the apolipoprotein E gene (APOE) as a risk factor, is clinically and ethically controversial.

The centrally acting anticholinesterase, THA, was thought to provide therapeutic benefit in Alzheimer's disease, but this benefit was not confirmed in subsequent studies. However, more recently another cholinesterase inhibitor, donezepil, has been licensed for the symptomatic relief of Alzheimer's dementia on the basis of more convincing trial evidence.

Bibliography

Arie T 1983 Pseudodementia. Br Med J 286: 1301.

Bryson HM, Benfield P 1997 Donepezil. Drugs & Aging 10: 234.

Guttman R, Seleski M (eds) 1999 Diagnosis, Management and Treatment of Dementia. Chicago: American Medical Association.

Katzman R 1986 Alzheimer's disease. N Engl J Med 314: 964.

Mayeux, Saunders AM, Shea S et al 1998 Utility of the apolipoprotein E genotype in the diagnosis of Alzheimer's disease. N Engl J Med 338: 506.

Morantz RA, Walsh JW (eds) 1994 Brain Tumors. New York: Marcel Dekker.

Panegyres PK, Goldblatt J, Walpole I et al 2000 Genetic testing for Alzheimer's disease. Med J Aust 172: 339.

Saunders AM, Hulette C, Welsh-Bohmer KA et al 1996 Specificity, sensitivity, and predictive value of apolipoprotein-E genotyping for sporadic Alzheimer's disease. Lancet 348: 90.

Shah A, Royston MC 1997 Donezepil for dementia. J R Soc Med 90: 531.

Smith JS, Kiloh LG 1981 The investigation of dementia. Lancet 1: 824.

Wells CE (ed) 1977 Dementia. Philadelphia: Davis.

Demyelinating diseases

Demyelinating diseases are seen in several forms.

1. **Multiple sclerosis** (q.v.)

2. **Post-infectious disseminated encephalomyelitis**

This is a serious though fortunately rare complication of acute exanthematous viral infection (especially measles) or vaccination. It is associated with:

- stupor;
- fits;
- focal neurological signs.

3. **Progressive multifocal leukoencephalopathy (PML)**

This is an uncommon opportunistic infection of oligodendroglia due to a polyoma virus of the papovavirus family, called JC virus after the first

identified patient, though originally it was thought to be due to the monkey virus SV40.

> It is usually associated with systemic immunological disorders, such as:
>
> - AIDS;
> - chronic granulomatous disease;
> - lymphoma;
> - myeloproliferative disorders.

Clinical features include mental, visual and motor dysfunction.

The virus may be detected in peripheral blood lymphocytes, though its identification in brain biopsy is diagnostic. Viral identification in CSF by PCR may obviate the need for biopsy. The most useful imaging is with MRI.

There is no effective therapy.

The mortality is 80% within 1 y, with an average survival of only 4 months in patients with AIDS.

4. **Transverse myelitis**

This refers to the acute onset of motor and sensory impairment of the legs with hyporeflexia. There is associated bladder dysfunction, and the process may extend up to the chest or even neck.

The aetiology is unknown, though some cases are post-viral. If associated with bilateral optic neuritis, the condition is called Devic's disease. Usually, the condition is an initial manifestation of multiple sclerosis, but occasionally it occurs in patients with already known multiple sclerosis. It is sometimes associated with SLE.

> The differential diagnosis includes:
>
> - Guillain–Barré syndrome;
> - spinal cord infarction or compression.

The CSF typically contains lymphocytes. MRI of the brain and spinal cord is useful in diagnosis. The outlook is usually one of permanent neurological damage.

Bibliography
Brooks BR, Walker DL 1984 Progressive multifocal
   leukoencephalopathy. Neurol Clin 2: 299.
Tippett DS, Fishman PS, Panitch HS 1991 Relapsing
   transverse myelitis. Neurology 41: 703.

Dengue

Dengue is produced by a group B arborvirus, indistinguishable in appearance from the Yellow Fever virus. It is caused by one of four related but antigenically distinct serotypes within the genus flavovirus. It is transmitted by *Aedes aegypti* mosquitoes and is endemic in many tropical regions of Asia, the Pacific, Central America and West Africa, with epidemics after severe rainy seasons. The first epidemics were reported in 1779, and a global pandemic began after World War II, particularly in South East Asia. In temperate countries, it is seen only in travellers. Nowadays, it is primarily an urban disease of the tropics, with humans as the primary reservoir. It is the second most important tropical infection after malaria. Two forms of illness are seen.

- **Dengue fever** (DF) is a mild to moderate non-fatal illness which follows an incubation period of 5–7 days. There is fever, severe headache, myalgia, backache, bone pain, facial flush and profound weakness. A morbilliform rash involves the trunk and extremities and may desquamate. Neutropenia is typical. The illness subsides in 5–7 days, but it may be followed by prolonged asthenia.
- **Dengue haemorrhagic fever** (DHF) is a much more serious condition, usually confined to South East Asia and only 1/200th as common as DF. It is additionally associated with thrombocytopenia, petechiae, multiple haemorrhages and shock. The platelet count is $<100\times10^9$/L and there is haemoconcentration. It is possible that this form of illness may arise from a more virulent strain of organism.

The diagnosis is made from serology or viral isolation. The differential diagnosis, particularly in the returned traveller with shock, includes:

- various other infections, such as
  - viral haemorrhagic fever;
  - severe malaria;
  - yellow fever;
  - rickettsial disease;
  - toxic shock syndrome;
- non-infectious conditions, such as
  - drug-induced Stevens–Johnson syndrome.

*Treatment is **symptomatic** with analgesics, fluids and electrolytes. Clearly, avoidance of mosquito exposure is an important prophylactic measure. There is as yet no publically available vaccine.*

Bibliography
Gubler DJ, Clark GG 1995 Dengue/dengue
   hemorrhagic fever: the emergence of a global
   health problem. Emerg Infect Dis 1: 2.

Dermatitis

Dermatitis is a very general term encompassing a number of more specific entities.

1. **Atopic dermatitis** (atopic eczema) is well known.

It may have a complication called Kaposi's varicelliform eruption due to dissemination of HSV or VZV infection.

Treatment of severe refractory disease includes several options. Both immunosuppression with a variety of agents and traditional Chinese medicinal herbs have been reported to be helpful.

2. **Contact dermatitis** may be due to allergy, irritation or photosensitization.

The allergic form may be striking and is referred to as **acute**, **allergic**, **eczematous**, **contact dermatitis** (AECD). It encompasses the entity, **dermatitis medicamentosa**, which is produced by a variety of drugs, including transdermal patches, as well as preservatives and cosmetics. Photosensitization is also often drug-induced, especially with tetracyclines and thiazides.

3. **Exfoliative dermatitis** (q.v.).

4. **Dermatitis herpetiformis**.

5. **Seborrhoeic dermatitis**.

6. **Stasis dermatitis**, associated with pigmentation and due to venous hypertension and varicose veins.

Bibliography

Fisher AA 1986 Contact dermatitis. 3rd edition. Philadelphia: Lea & Febiger.

Hanifin JM 1991 Atopic dermatitis: new therapeutic considerations. J Am Acad Dermatol 24: 1097.

Katz SI, Hall RP, Lawley TJ et al 1980 Dermatitis herpetiformis: the skin and the gut. Ann Intern Med 93: 857.

LeBrec H, Bachot N, Gaspard I et al 1999 Mechanisms of drug-induced allergic contact dermatitis. Cell Biol Toxicol 15: 57.

Nicolis GD, Helwig EB 1973 Exfoliative dermatitis: a clinicopathologic study of 135 cases. Arch Dermatol 108: 788.

Dermatology

The care of skin disorders is mostly undertaken in the ambulatory setting, and it is rare for a dermatological condition to be the cause of an admission to an Intensive Care Unit. However, their frequency in the population means that many seriously ill patients have a concomitant skin disorder. Moreover, the skin is an important target organ for a variety of complications of serious illnesses, especially drug reactions. Yet dermatological problems retain perhaps a greater air of mystery for the non-specialist than almost any other organ–system disorder. In Intensive Care, the most important differential diagnoses are probably exfoliative dermatitis, skin necrosis and urticaria. Many other less common dermatological conditions may sometimes be encountered and those considered in this book include:

- alopecia;
- blisters;
- cellulitis;
- conjunctivitis;
- dermatitis;
- ecthyma;
- epidermolysis bullosa;
- erysipelas;
- erythema marginatum;
- erythema multiforme;
- erythema nodosum;
- flushing;

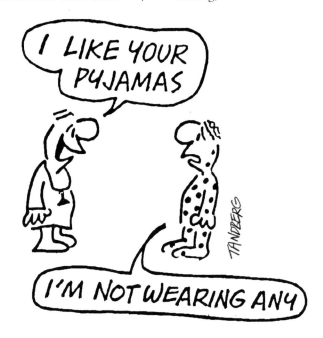

I LIKE YOUR PYJAMAS

I'M NOT WEARING ANY

- folliculitis;
- furunculosis;
- leukocytoclastic vasculitis;
- livedo reticularis;
- nail abnormalities;
- palmar erythema;
- pemphigus;
- pigmentation disorders;
- psoriasis;
- pyoderma gangrenosum;
- Raynaud's phenomenon/disease;
- scalded skin syndrome;
- skin signs of internal malignant disease;
- toxic erythemas;
- vesiculobullous diseases.

Bibliography

Badia M, Trujillano J, Gasco E et al 1999 Skin lesions in the ICU. Intens Care Med 25: 1271.

Champion RH 1984 Generalised pruritus. Br Med J 289: 751.

Denman ST 1986 A review of pruritus. J Am Acad Dermatol 14: 375.

Dowd PM 1987 Cold-related disorders. Prog Dermatol 21: 1.

Fitzpatrick TB, Eisen AZ, Wolff K et al (eds) 1979 Dermatology in General Medicine. New York: McGraw-Hill.

Fitzpatrick TB, Johnson RA, Wolff K et al 1997 Color Atlas and Synopsis of Clinical Dermatology. New York: McGraw-Hill.

Fox BJ, Odom RB 1985 Papulosquamous diseases: a review. J Am Acad Dermatol 12: 597.

Kvedar JC, Gibson M, Krusinski PA 1985 Hirsutism: evaluation and treatment. J Am Acad Dermatol 12: 215.

Peter RU 1998 Cutaneous manifestations in intensive care patients. Intens Care Med 24: 997.

Roujeau JC, Stern RS 1994 Severe adverse cutaneous reactions to drugs. N Engl J Med 10: 1272.

Sehgal VN, Gangwani OP 1987 Fixed drug eruption: current concepts. Int J Dermatol 26: 67.

Dermatomyositis (see Polymyositis)

Desferrioxamine (see Chelating agents)

Desmopressin

Antidiuretic hormone (ADH) is important in controlling water conservation in terrestrial species. However, it also acts at sites other than the kidney, and it is thus additionally a vasopressor (hence the name, vasopressin), a neurotransmitter and an oxytocic, and it can release clotting factors from endothelial cells. Natural vasopressin is a nonapeptide, 8-arginine vasopressin in humans. Vasopressin is also referred to as oxytocin.

Desmopressin (1–desamino-8-D-arginine vasopressin, DDAVP) is a synthetic analogue of vasopressin. It has an antidiuretic to pressor ratio of about 3000:1, compared with the usual 1:1 ratio for vasopressin. It has only minor oxytocic effects.

Desmopressin is the agent of choice for therapeutic use in this group. It has three main uses.

- **Antidiuretic agent**

This effect is exerted in the kidney by decreasing water reabsorption in the collecting tubule. The chief such use is in diabetes insipidus. This antidiuretic effect is inhibited by glibenclamide.

- **Haemostatic agent**

In bleeding disorders associated with a platelet function defect (including von Willebrand's disease, haemophilia, renal disease, aspirin use), desmopressin increases factor VIII levels and decreases bleeding time. It has been shown to decrease blood loss after cardiac surgery.

- **Splanchnic vasoconstrictor**

In portal hypertension with bleeding varices, it decreases portal blood pressure and so assists in controlling haemorrhage.

Desmopressin has a half-life of 8–80 min. It is given either intravenously or intranasally. As an antidiuretic in diabetes insipidus, it is given in a dose of 1–4 μg iv. In bleeding, it is given in a dose of 20 μg (i.e. 0.3 μg/kg) diluted in 50 mL and given over 30 min. This dose may be repeated in 6–12 h if necessary. If used prophylactically for anticipated bleeding, it should be given 30 min before the planned procedure.

Overhydration, with water intoxication and hyponatraemia, may occur with excess use.

Bibliography

Cattaneo M, Harris AS, Stromberg U, Mannucci PM 1995 The effect of desmopressin on reducing blood loss in cardiac surgery – a meta-analysis of double-blind placebo-controlled trials. Thromb Haemost 74: 1064.
Fogel MR, Knauer CM, Andres LL et al 1982 Continuous intravenous vasopressin in active upper gastrointestinal bleeding: a placebo-controlled trial. Ann Intern Med 96: 565.
Mannucci PM 1988 Desmopressin: a nontransfusional form of treatment for congenital and acquired bleeding disorders. Blood 72: 1449.
Richardson DW, Robinson AG 1985 Desmopressin. Ann Intern Med 103: 228.

Diaphragm

Diaphragmatic disorders include:

- congenital conditions

  - hernia, eventration (commonly congenital and usually left-sided);

- inflammation

  - subdiaphragmatic abscess, trichiniasis;

- paralysis;
- neuromuscular disorders

  - bilateral phrenic nerve injury (neuropathy, surgery, trauma);
  - unilateral paralysis (commonly asymptomatic, due to damage to a phrenic nerve from aneurysm, cardioplegia, lymphadenopathy, malignancy, neuropathy, surgery or trauma, or to direct damage to a hemidiaphragm);

- postoperative

  - irritation;

- spasmodic disorders

  - hiccup, tonic spasm, flutter;

- trauma;
- tumour.

Bibliography

Markand ON, Moorthy SS, Mahomed Y et al 1985 Postoperative phrenic nerve palsy in patients with open-heart surgery. Ann Thorac Surg 39: 68.
Riley EA 1962 Idiopathic diaphragmatic paralysis. Am J Med 32: 404.

Diarrhoea

Diarrhoea is a common condition, but it is worth having a classification, as it includes some uncommon causes. It should be remembered, however, that in about 50% of cases of chronic diarrhoea, no diagnosis is made. Acute diarrhoeal illnesses are even more elusive, as they are usually brief (up to 1–2 days), self-limited, caused by agents not detected by routine laboratory tests and not amenable in any event to specific therapy.

The presence of diarrhoea may be diagnosed on several different criteria related to the frequency, volume or fluidity of stools, but is commonly quantified as a stool output >200 g per day.

A practical subdivision of diarrhoea is into:

- large stools, which are usually of small bowel origin;
- small stools, which are usually of large bowel origin and associated with inflammation (and thus blood, mucus and tenesmus).

Diarrhoea is commonly classified on an aetiological basis into 5 groups, namely:
- osmotic;
- secretory;
- exudative;
- due to rapid transit time;
- due to drugs.

1. **Osmotic diarrhoea**

This is caused by:

- magnesium-, phosphate- or sulfate-containing medications

  - i.e. antacids or laxatives;

- carbohydrate malabsorption

  - e.g. lactose and sucrose in disaccharidase or lactase deficiency (q.v.);

- mannitol or sorbitol

  - i.e. sugar alcohols;

- lactulose

  - an indigestible disaccharide;

- excess legumes

  - these contain raffinose or stachyose.

2. **Secretory diarrhoea**

This occurs with:

- some bacterial infections

  - A number of bacteria, such as enteropathogenic *E. coli* (see below), *V. cholerae*, *C. botulinum*, *S. aureus*, may produce an enterotoxin which stimulates excess intestinal excretion. Toxigenic gastroenteritis thus results.
  - Enteropathogenic (enterotoxigenic, enterohaemorrhagic) *E. coli*, especially serotype O157:H7, was recognized as a human pathogen only 15 years ago. It is the commonest cause of traveller's diarrhoea and is spread from either contaminated food (especially from undercooked beef) or via the oral–faecal route. The infection is usually mild, though it can occasionally be severe and haemorrhagic and even cause haemolytic–uraemic syndrome (usually in children) (q.v.). A recent outbreak in South Australia is estimated to have cost about A$20 million and has prompted reassessment of surveillance programmes.

- irritative fatty acids

  - e.g. non-absorbable fatty acid laxatives such as castor oil or in malabsorption or bacterial overgrowth;

- bile acids

  - following ileal resection;

- hormone-producing tumours

  - These include carcinoid, gastrinoma, and vasoactive intestinal peptide tumour (VIPoma) of pancreas. VIPoma may give 'pancreatic cholera', i.e. watery diarrhoea, hypokalaemia and alkalosis (the WDHA or Verner–Morrison syndrome).
  - Hormonally produced secretory diarrhoea may respond to octreotide.

3. **Exudative diarrhoea**

This is usually seen following

- invasive bacterial infection with direct damage to the bowel wall.

In specific infections, the bacteria involved are typically campylobacter, salmonella, shigella and yersinia.

A variety of non-bacterial organisms are also commonly seen, including

  - viruses (Norwalk virus, rotavirus, enterovirus, adenovirus);
  - protozoa (giardia, entamoeba);
  - parasites (helminths);
  - fungi (candida).

These conditions thus give rise to a form of gastroenteritis, manifest particularly by bacterial dysentery.

- A similar condition is seen in

  - inflammatory bowel disease (q.v.);

  - antibiotic-associated (pseudomembranous) colitis (see Colitis).

4. **Rapid transit time**

A rapid transit time in the bowel may cause diarrhoea. This is seen following bowel resection and with entero-enteral fistulae. It may also be the basis of the irritable bowel syndrome.

5. Drugs

These are common causes of diarrhoea.

- Some may cause osmotic diarrhoea (see above).
- Some may cause pseudomembranous colitis (see Colitis).
- Many, such as colchicine, cytotoxics and ethanol, may have more direct effects.

Bibliography

Beers M, Cameron S 1995 Hemolytic uremic syndrome. Emerg Infect Dis 1: 4.

Blaser MJ, Smith PD, Ravdin JL et al (eds) 1995 Infections of the Gastrointestinal Tract. New York: Raven Press.

Fairchild PG, Blacklow NR 1988 Viral diarrhea. Infect Dis Clin North Am 2: 677.

Field M, Rao MC, Chang EB 1989 Intestinal electrolyte transport and diarrheal disease. N Engl J Med 321: 800, 879.

Hellard ME, Fairley CK 1997 Gastroenteritis in Australia: who, what, where, and how much? Aust NZ J Med 27: 147.

Kelly CP, Pothoulakis C, La Mont JT 1994 *Clostridium difficile* colitis. N Engl J Med 330: 257.

Krejs GJ 1987 VIPoma syndrome. Am J Med 82: 37.

Lyerly DM, Krivan HC, Wilkins TD 1988 *Clostridium difficile*: its disease and toxins. Clin Microbiol Rev 1: 1.

Phillips SF 1972 Diarrhea: a current view of the pathophysiology. Gastroenterology 63: 495.

Schlager TA, Guerrant RL 1988 Seven possible mechanisms for *Escherichia coli* diarrhea. Infect Dis Clin North Am 2: 607.

Slutsker L, Ries AA, Greene KD et al 1997 *Escherichia coli* 0157:H7 diarrhea in the United States: clinical and epidemiologic features. Ann Intern Med 126: 505.

Wanke CA, Guerrant RL 1987 Viral hepatitis and gastroenteritis transmitted by shellfish and water. Infect Dis Clin North Am 1: 649.

Young GP, Bayley N, Ward P et al 1986 Antibiotic-associated colitis caused by *Clostridium difficile*: relapse and risk factors. Med J Aust 144: 303.

Diffuse fibrosing alveolitis

Diffuse fibrosing alveolitis (idiopathic pulmonary fibrosis, interstitial pneumonitis, cryptogenic fibrosing alveolitis, Hamman–Rich syndrome) is a form of progressive diffuse inflammation distal to the terminal bronchiole.

Although its aetiology is uncertain and no single pathogenetic mechanism has yet been defined, there are common histological, radiological and clinical features exhibited by most patients with this condition, justifying its consideration as a separate entity. However, it may well represent a group of disorders, and in any event it is not easy to distinguish from similar processes associated with systemic disease (especially collagen-vascular diseases) or certain drugs (see Drugs and the lung).

Aetiological factors are probably immunological, because although no specific antigen has been identifiable, both cell-mediated and humoral changes can be shown and circulating immune complexes demonstrated in the cellular, pre-fibrotic stage of disease. An association with other autoimmune diseases has sometimes been found, and there appears to be some genetic predisposition. No infective agent has been identified, but some association with prior occupational exposure to wood and metal dusts has recently been reported.

The pathological changes consist of either

- thickening of alveolar walls due to a round cell infiltrate, leading to fibrosis, or
- no fibrosis and normal alveolar septa but alveolar filling with large mononuclear cells, mainly desquamated type II pneumocytes but also macrophages.

The former process, the more common, has a patchy distribution and is referred to as 'usual interstitial pneumonitis' (UIP).

The latter process is more evenly distributed and is referred to as 'desquamative interstitial pneumonitis' (DIP). Recently, this has been considered possibly a separate and more benign disease.

The two processes may or may not represent the same disease, with a better corticosteroid response likely to occur when the latter (presumably earlier) changes are more prominent. Eventually, cellularity decreases and fibrosis increases, so that there is diffuse though not uniform disorganization of the alveolar architecture, with fibrosis and with the appearance of cystic spaces (honeycombing). These processes are in fact common for many lung responses to injury.

> The clinical features of diffuse fibrosing alveolitis are usually dominated by progressive dyspnoea. The first presentation is sometimes as an apparent acute respiratory infection. A dry cough is common, as is fever and weight loss.
>
> On physical examination, there is frequently cyanosis, clubbing and tachypnoea. Diffuse crackles are heard, particularly at the lung bases. A late finding is cor pulmonale. Extrapulmonary manifestations suggest a systemic disorder.

The chest X-ray may initially be normal, even in the presence of dyspnoea. The radiological abnormalities predominantly affect the lower zones and tend to be diffuse, homogeneous or nodular opacities at first, reticulonodular later and eventually reticular, often with honeycombing. There is no hilar lymphadenopathy and no pleural effusion. High-resolution CT scanning (HRCT) is the imaging modality of current choice. Lung function tests show changes similar to those described for sarcoidosis (q.v.).

Although a presumptive diagnosis may be made on the basis of the clinical and radiological features together with the absence of systemic disease, or culprit exposures or drugs, lung biopsy is required for definitive diagnosis. However, a clinical diagnosis may sometimes be acceptable if the patient is particularly unwell and/or the features are unequivocal.

The chief differential diagnosis includes:

- late sarcoidosis;
- diffuse bronchiolitis obliterans (organizing pneumonia);
- lymphangitis carcinomatosa;
- lymphangiomyomatosis;
- histiocytosis X.

Biopsy is required to distinguish these diseases.

*Treatment comprises chiefly **corticosteroids**. In a few patients, there may be a dramatic response, but in most there is continued progression despite a modest symptomatic steroid response. Treatment is long-term and dosage should be titrated not only against symptoms but also appropriate lung function tests, particularly those of gas exchange, if these respond. There may be an adverse steroid response in those cases with patchy fibrosis and honeycombing.*

- *The place of immunosuppressive and anti-inflammatory therapy is unresolved, though cytotoxic therapy (cyclophosphamide) is indicated if corticosteroids are not effective. Colchicine and penicillamine have been shown to be ineffective.*
- *Long-term oxygen therapy may be symptomatically helpful.*
- *Successful lung transplantation has been reported.*

The course of the disease is very variable. The mean time from onset of symptoms to death is about four years, though reported survival has ranged from one month to over 20 years. The duration of survival appears to correlate with the severity of disease at the time of diagnosis, and the prognosis is better in patients with the acute desquamative form of the disease. Occasionally, spontaneous or corticosteroid-induced remissions occur.

Bibliography

Agusti C, Xaubet A, Roca J et al 1992 Interstitial pulmonary fibrosis with and without associated collagen vascular disease. Thorax 47: 1035.

Carrington CB, Gaensler EA, Coutu RE et al 1978 Natural history and treated course of usual and desquamative interstitial pneumonia. N Engl J Med 298: 801.

Cherniack RM, Colby TV, Flint A et al 1995 Correlation of structure and function in idiopathic pulmonary fibrosis. Am J Respir Crit Care Med 151: 1180.

Crystal RG, Bitterman PB, Rennard SI et al 1984

Interstitial lung diseases of unknown cause. N Engl J Med 310: 154, 235.

Homma Y, Ohtsuka Y, Tanimura K et al 1995 Can interstitial pneumonia as the sole presentation of collagen vascular disease be differentiated from idiopathic interstitial pneumonia. Respiration 62: 248.

Hubbard R, Lewis S, Richards K et al 1996 Occupational exposure to metal or wood dust and aetiology of cryptogenic fibrosing alveolitis. Lancet 347: 284.

International Consensus Statement 2000 Idiopathic pulmonary fibrosis: diagnosis and treatment. Am J Respir Crit Care Med 161:646.

Johnston IDA, Prescott RJ, Chalmers JC et al 1997 British Thoracic Society study of cryptogenic fibrosing alveolitis: current presentation and initial management. Thorax 52: 38.

Marinelli WA 1995 Idiopathic pulmonary fibrosis: progress and challenge. Chest 108: 297.

Michaelson JE, Aguayo SM, Roman J 2000 Idiopathic pulmonary fibrosis. Chest 118: 788.

Turner-Warwick M, Burrows B, Johnson A 1980 Cryptogenic fibrosing alveolitis. Thorax 35: 171.

Digoxin-specific antibody

Digoxin-specific immune antigen-binding Fab fragment (digoxin FAB antibodies, Digibind) is derived from antibodies made in sheep to digoxin conjugated with human albumin. It has a molecular weight of 50 kd. It binds to and thus decreases the concentration of free digoxin (and digitoxin) in plasma, and the complex thus formed is excreted in the urine. Since digoxin has greater affinity for the exogenous antibody than for tissue receptors, not only is less free drug available to interact with cardiac and other cell membranes but the drug is progressively removed from tissue receptors.

Its chief indication is life-threatening digoxin overdosage, usually associated with ventricular arrhythmias. Typically, more than 10 mg has been taken orally and plasma levels are greater than 10 ng/mL.

The dose is calculated as follows.

- Firstly, the body's digoxin load (in mg) is calculated as plasma level (ng/mL), multiplied by volume of distribution (5.6 L/kg), multiplied by body weight (kg), divided by 1000. Alternatively, the body load may be estimated based on the numbers of tablets taken, if known, as mg ingested divided by 0.8.

- Secondly, the number of vials required equals load (in mg) divided by 0.6 (the no. of mg of digoxin able to be bound per vial).

An average dose is 10 vials, though 20 vials should be given if the clinical situation is life-threatening and no levels or dosage are known. A vial containing 40 mg of powder is reconstituted to 4 mL and binds 0.6 mg of digoxin (or digitoxin). The drug is administered iv over 30 min using a 0.22 μm millipore filter.

Clinical improvement should be seen within 30 min. The plasma level of digoxin will increase markedly after administration of the antibody but almost all is bound. A new steady state plasma level is not achieved for 5–6 h.

The antibody may be used in renal failure, although excretion is delayed in that setting. Since digoxin overdose can cause hyperkalaemia, the serum potassium level must be monitored. Anaphylaxis associated with the antibody's use has not so far been reported, perhaps partly because no cases of re-challenge have yet been described. Re-emergence of digoxin toxicity has not been reported. As might be expected, any redigitalization needs to be deferred for several days.

Recently, the successful use of digoxin-specific immune antigen-binding Fab fragment has been reported in **toad venom poisoning**, since this venom may contain a digitalis-like substance (see Bites and stings).

Bibliography

Antman EM, Wenger TL, Butler VP et al 1990 Treatment of 150 cases of life-threatening digitalis intoxication with digoxin-specific Fab antibody fragments. Circulation 81: 1744.

Brubacher JR, Ravikumar PR, Bania T et al 1996 Treatment of toad venom poisoning with digoxin-specific Fab fragments. Chest 110: 1282.

Kelly RA, Smith TW 1992 Recognition and management of digitalis toxicity. Am J Cardiol 69: 1186.

Taboulet P, Baud FJ, Bismuth C 1993 Clinical features and management of digitalis poisoning – rationale for immunotherapy. J Toxicol Clin Toxicol 31: 247.

Dimercaprol (see Chelating agents)

Dioxins

A dioxin is a chemical compound consisting of two benzene rings connected by a pair of oxygen atoms. Since each ring contains 8 carbon atoms which can each bind to a hydrogen or other atom (the most concerning to health being chlorine), up to 75 isomers are possible. Dioxins are usually formed as a by-product of the manufacture of herbicides based on 2,4,5-trichlorophenol and are the most toxic of artificial substances.

The term dioxin particularly refers to one specific dioxin (2,3,7,8-tetrachlorodibenzo-p-dioxin, TCDD), a very stable substance which is insoluble in water but soluble in oils, so that it is not diluted environmentally but accumulates in animal tissues. It is not a useful substance but a by-product in the manufacture both of 2,4,5-trichlorophenoxyacetic acid (2,4,5-T), a major ingredient in the defoliant, Agent Orange, and of the antiseptic, hexachlorophene.

There is no safe level of 2,3,7,8-TCDD, which is lethal for some animal species at five parts per billion, i.e. as little as 60 μg can kill a mouse. It is a potential carcinogen. Agent Orange itself may increase the incidence of non-Hodgkin's lymphoma and soft tissue sarcoma. Other toxic effects include chloracne, neurological disorders, muscle dysfunction, impotence, birth defects and mutations. Industrial accidents since the 1970s have been associated with extensive loss of nearby animal life and the forced evacuation sometimes permanently of whole communities.

Related compounds include the PCBs (polychlorinated biphenols) and PCDFs (polychlorinated dibenzofurans).

- PCBs in particular are produced by electrical fires, which can cause widespread contamination of buildings. These substances give skin, liver and reproductive effects and are potential carcinogens.
- PCDFs have caused outbreaks of disease following contamination of cooking oil. The reproductive consequences of a generalized ectodermal disorder in offspring have been well documented.

Diphtheria

Diphtheria is caused by the dumbell-shaped Gram-positive bacillus, *Corynebacterium diphtheriae*, which produces a potent exotoxin. It is spread by droplets and thus primarily affects the pharynx, though sometimes primary sites elsewhere are seen. Bacterial multiplication occurs locally, and the exotoxin but not the bacteria become disseminated.

A characteristic grey, leathery and adherent local membrane is also produced by the toxin. The size of the membrane correlates with the extent of toxin produced.

The illness follows an incubation period of 2–4 days. Although the pharyngitis is generally mild, cervical lymphadenopathy can be marked, and there may be purpura and shock.

Cutaneous diphtheria is seen:

- in the tropics (jungle sore);
- after trauma (wound diphtheria);
- in association with poor hygiene (e.g. in poor alcoholics).

There are three important complications of diphtheria.

1. Upper airway obstruction

Obstruction from the pharyngeal membrane may give rise to a medical emergency.

2. **Myocarditis**

This occurs in 10–25% and is the usual cause of death. Cardiac involvement becomes apparent in the second week of illness, with ST abnormalities and then arrhythmias, complete heart block, bundle branch block, cardiac failure and shock. An AV conduction defect may persist after recovery.

3. **Peripheral neuritis**

This occurs in 10% of patients 2–6 weeks after the initial illness. It particularly involves the cranial nerves (III, VI, VII, IX and X) and peripheral motor nerves, including the phrenic nerve.

Sometimes, a Guillain–Barré syndrome-like condition may be seen.

The diagnosis is made clinically and confirmed by culture or fluorescent antibody detection of swab material.

A 'diphtheria-membrane' may also be seen in pharyngitis due to:

- Group A streptococci;
- infectious mononucleosis;
- viruses;
- candida.

However, generally the membrane in these conditions is less adherent.

*Treatment is with horse **antiserum**, if diagnosed within 48 h, in a dose of 20 000–100 000 U (50% im and 50% iv 1 h later).*

- *Antibiotics are not helpful in the acute illness, though erythromycin, penicillin or clindamycin may help eradicate a carrier state.*
- *Rest, isolation and treatment of complications are required.*

Prevention is with immunization, and the disease occurs only in the unimmunized. A 75% herd immunity is required to prevent community outbreaks, which are now seen in adults as well as in children in circumstances where there has been waning community immunity. Immunization does not prevent the carrier state. The Schick test is used for assessment of immunity and not for diagnosis.

Bibliography

Boyer NH, Weinstein L 1948 Diphtheritic myocarditis. N Engl J Med 239: 913.

Dobie RA, Tobey DN 1979 Clinical features of diphtheria in the respiratory tract. JAMA 242: 2197.

Farizo KM, Strebel PM, Chen RT et al 1993 Fatal respiratory disease due to Corynebacterium diphtheriae: case report and review of guidelines for management, investigation, and control. Clin Infect Dis 16: 59.

Galazka AM, Robertson SE, Oblapenko GP 1995 Resurgence of diphtheria. Eur J Epidemiol 11: 95.

Harmisch JP, Tronca E, Nolan CM et al 1989 Diphtheria among alcoholic urban adults. Ann Intern Med 111: 71.

Mofred A, Guerin JM, Falfoul-Borsali N et al 1994 Cutaneous diphtheria. Rev Med Interne 15: 515.

Dissecting aneurysm (see Aortic dissection)

Disseminated intravascular coagulation (see Amniotic fluid embolism, Anaemia (intravascular haemolysis), Antithrombin III deficiency, Cancer complications, Coagulation disorders, Diving (decompression sickness), Fibrinolysis, Haemangioma, Heat stroke, Microangiopathic haemolysis and Protein C)

Diving

Diving accidents have become common because of the proliferation of diving activities, both professional and recreational, worldwide. Because of the availability of modern transport, diving sequelae may be seen well away from the original geographical site.

> The most important diving accidents are gas embolism and decompression sickness.
>
> - The most common, however, are ear or sinus damage due to barotrauma.
> - Diving-induced damage may also relate to pre-existing diseases, some of which are contraindications to diving, such as many respiratory, cardiovascular and neurological disorders.
> - Diving may also be a cause of drowning (q.v.).

Diving accidents are usually associated with well-defined risk factors, such as multiple dives, exceeding 'tables', rapid ascent, alcohol or subsequent air travel. A patent foramen ovale is an important risk factor in some patients. Clearly, other factors such as accidents, environmental problems, equipment failure, carelessness and inexperience may also be involved.

Cerebral arterial gas embolism (CAGE) is responsible for about 15% of major problems. It occurs because of rapid ascent with the head up and is due to alveolar overdistension and rupture giving rise to pulmonary barotrauma with embolization to the systemic circulation, if there is a direct communication with the pulmonary vasculature. Neurological changes occur rapidly and may be either dramatic (coma) or subtle (paraesthesiae or mood changes).

Decompression sickness is due to formation of nitrogen bubbles from too rapid an ascent. The nitrogen was dissolved in tissues especially lipids at depth and appropriate staged decompression is therefore essential to prevent its unduly rapid release during ascent. Using sensitive Doppler tests, some bubbles in fact may be detected in virtually all divers, regardless of the care taken with the dive. Intravascular changes of disseminated intravascular coagulation and complement activation may be produced. Symptoms can appear as soon as 1 h or as late as 36 h after the ascent.

- In type 1 (25% of diving accidents), the skin and joints are affected, and the condition is thus called the 'bends'.
- In type 2 (more than half of all major diving accidents), there are neurological changes, including focal and spinal cord signs and respiratory distress (the 'chokes').

Bone necrosis may occur if the process is repeated. There is commonly headache, lethargy and altered sensation.

Treatment priorities are positioning on the left side, oxygen (especially for CAGE), and **recompression** *in a hyperbaric facility. This may usefully be undertaken even up to several hours later.*

Bibliography

Charles MJ, Wirjosemito SA 1989 Flying and diving: still a real hazard. J Hyperbaric Med 4: 23.

Elliot DH, Hallenbeck LM, Bove AA 1974 Acute decompression sickness. Lancet 2: 1193.

Lundgren CEG, Miller JN (eds) 1999 The Lung at Depth. New York: Marcel Dekker.

Melamed Y, Shupak A, Bitterman H 1992 Medical problems associated with underwater diving. N Engl J Med 326: 30.

Moon RE, Camporesi EM, Kisslo JA 1989 Patent foramen ovale and decompression sickness in divers. Lancet 1: 513.

Tetzlaff K, Reuter M, Leplow B et al 1997 Risk factors for pulmonary barotrauma in divers. Chest 112: 654.

Weathersby PK, Survanshi SS, Homer LD et al 1992 Predicting the time of occurrence of decompression sickness. J Appl Physiol 72: 1541.

Weinmann M, Tuxen D, Scheinkestel C et al 1991 Decompression illnesses. SPUMS Journal 21: 135.

Dog bites (see Bites and stings)

Drowning

Drowning and near-drowning are common accidents due to a wide variety of activities at all ages in most societies. Drowning is a major cause of accidental death with an average incidence of 1 per 30 000 of population per year.

In general, the lungs become flooded, though in 10% of patients the lungs are dry and have been protected by intense laryngospasm. The changes in blood volume and composition depend on the amount and tonicity of fluid aspirated. Usually the volume of water aspirated is not large, and serum electrolyte changes are minimal. Fresh water gives hypervolaemia and salt water (5% saline) gives hypovolaemia, but the pathological changes after drowning and the clinical and investigational findings after near-drowning are similar for both fresh and sea water.

> After near-drowning, patients are comatose and apnoeic. Even after resuscitation, central nervous system derangement with confusion, restlessness, delirium and convulsions may persist for some time, due to hypoxic damage with cerebral oedema and even infarction.

Investigations show arterial hypoxaemia, metabolic acidosis, variable serum electrolyte levels, and albuminuria, haematuria and sometimes haemoglobinuria. The chest X-ray generally shows perihilar densities initially, though more florid pulmonary oedema commonly becomes apparent some hours later.

Treatment of near-drowning comprises the following.

- *Aspiration of the upper airway for fluid and foreign bodies should be promptly made, but not aspiration of the tracheobronchial tree as this is ineffective.*
- *The stomach should be aspirated, as the stomach is full and vomiting is common because of the large amount of water that has often been swallowed.*
- *Cardiopulmonary resuscitation is usually required. Even if the resuscitative needs on site are minimal, the patient should be transferred to hospital, because respiratory failure may occur up to 4 h later, with tachypnoea, cough, frothy blood-stained sputum, chest pain and wheeze.*
- *Intensive Care treatment is required for respiratory failure (due to acute pulmonary oedema early or ARDS later), cardiac arrhythmias, metabolic acidosis, cerebral oedema, gastric distension, coagulopathy, hypothermia and infections.*
- *Corticosteroids are of unproven value.*
- *Prophylactic antibiotics are not indicated.*

> **Hypothermia** is usual, because the temperature of even tropical waters is less than that of the body and only a few minutes is required for temperature equilibration (see also Hypothermia).
>
> If the body temperature is <30°C, there is severe depression of the circulation and the patient may appear lifeless; if the temperature is <28°C, ventricular fibrillation occurs. Ventricular fibrillation may also be precipitated by the necessary procedure of intubation, and defibrillation is usually unsuccessful if the temperature is <30°C. At this temperature also, the activity and clearance of drugs is impaired.
>
> *Passive or even active external warming is often inadequate, and core rewarming may then be required.*

The outlook is excellent for victims of near-drowning who have not suffered a cardiac arrest. The survival rate is still 90% if the period of arrest is <5 min, but it is 0% if the period of arrest is >25 min. On average, there is a two-thirds mortality if cardiopulmonary resuscitation is required. Children have a better outcome than adults. The prognosis is also more favourable if there has been hypothermia (core temperature <35°C), but this prognostic criterion is inexact, perhaps since cardiac arrest may have happened during normothermia with cooling occurring only subsequently.

Bibliography

Edwards ND, Timmins AC, Randalls B et al 1990 Survival in adults after cardiac arrest due to drowning. Intens Care Med 16: 336.

Modell JH 1985 Serum electrolyte changes in near-drowning victims. JAMA 253: 557.

Modell JH 1993 Drowning. N Engl J Med 328: 253.

Orlowski JP 1988 Drowning, near-drowning, and ice-water drowning. JAMA 260: 390.

Szpilman D 1997 Near-drowning and drowning classification. Chest 112: 660.

Drug allergy

Drug allergy is uncommon and comprises only 6% of all adverse drug reactions, which overall are, of course, common.

Importantly, drug allergy can occur with only small doses of drug. However, most drug reactions of a seemingly allergic nature are not in fact immune-mediated (i.e. true allergy) but due to other effects often of a chemical nature, e.g. mast cell release.

Drug allergy is separate from

- **drug intolerance** (an adverse pharmacological effect of a drug even at low dose),
- **drug idiosyncrasy** (a non-pharmacological effect due to biochemical alteration in drug metabolism at any dose).

The most common drug allergy is to **penicillin**. This occurs in 1–5% of recipients and is responsible for 90% of all cases of drug allergy and for 90% of cases of fatal anaphylaxis.

Other important drug allergies are seen following:

- anaesthetic agents;
- aspirin;
- diagnostic contrast agents (especially those containing iodine);
- antibiotics (especially beta-lactams);
- hormones;
- dextran;
- opiates;
- echinacea, a popular complementary medicine for cold and flu symptoms.

Most allergic drug reactions take the form of a mild systemic illness, similar to serum sickness (q.v.), with

- fever,
- urticaria,
- arthralgia,
- lymphadenopathy.

The typical onset occurs after 6–12 days and disappears several days after drug cessation.

Anaphylaxis is the potentially fatal manifestation of drug allergy with an onset within minutes. It usually follows parenteral drug administration but can follow oral dosage. Its clinical features include:

- pruritus;
- flushing;
- angioedema of any region but especially the face and larynx;
- hypovolaemia with hypotension and shock.

Drug allergy may be diagnosed when:

- the clinical manifestations are not those of any known pharmacological effect of the drug;
- the drug doses are very small;
- there are allergic symptoms;
- the same reaction occurs with rechallenge;
- it occurs with related drugs.

Skin tests are of most diagnostic value, though less so for penicillin. Until recently there had been no reliable in vitro test, but now serum tryptase (reflecting release of mast cell contents) may be shown to be elevated in blood taken shortly after a major allergic event. Sometimes, IgE antibodies to a specific drug may be detected, but tests involving other immunoglobulins or cell-mediated immunity do not correlate with symptoms.

Treatment includes:

- *cessation of the drug;*
- *specific measures for anaphylaxis (particularly adrenaline);*
- *corticosteroids for an Arthus-type reaction (i.e. serum sickness) or other delayed hypersensitivity reaction (e.g. symptomatic rash);*
- *desensitization which should be considered if the drug is needed to be given again.*

Bibliography

Gorevic P 1985 Drug allergy. In: Kaplan AP (ed)
Allergy. New York: Churchill Livingstone.
p. 473.

Weiss ME 1992 Drug allergy. Med Clin North Am
76: 857.

Drug fever

Drug fever usually occurs without the
diagnostic assistance of other typical signs of
hypersensitivity, such as rash or eosinophilia.

Drug fever is especially seen with the use of:

- antimicrobials (particularly beta-lactams);
- antihypertensives (methyldopa,
  hydralazine);
- anticonvulsants (phenytoin);
- allopurinol;
- isoniazid.

In some cases, the onset of fever may be delayed
for weeks or even months after the drug is first
administered, e.g. methyldopa, phenytoin,
isoniazid.

In the Intensive Care setting, other drugs
which may also produce drug fever include:

- amphotericin;
- diuretics;
- procainamide;
- propranolol;
- quinidine.

Bibliography

Mackowiak PA, LeMaistre CF 1987 Drug fever. Ann
Intern Med 106: 728.

Olson KR, Benowitz NL 1984 Environmental and
drug-induced hyperthermia: pathophysiology,
recognition and management. Emerg Med Clin
North Am 2: 459.

Rosenberg J, Pentel P, Pond S et al 1986
Hyperthermia associated with drug intoxication.
Crit Care Med 14: 964.

Drug–drug interactions

A drug–drug interaction refers to a clinically
significant effect which is different from the
effects seen when the same drugs are given
individually. Such interactions may be clinically
adverse, favourable or neutral.

In hospital practice, 10–20% of all drug
reactions are due to drug–drug interactions. In
addition, adverse reactions are more frequent if
multiple drugs are administered, even when
such an incidence is discounted for the actual
number of drugs. Since the number of drugs
that may be properly prescribed concomitantly,
especially in an Intensive Care Unit, is
enormous and since it is impossible to
remember them all, most drug–drug
interactions are probably undetected.
Comprehensive compendia are now available
covering the interactions of specific drugs.
However, it is best to use an automated
monitoring system, but even then the clinical
significance of a potential interaction is not
necessarily clear.

The number of drug combinations in a
particular patient can be calculated as:

$$no. = n! \div 2\,(n-2)!,$$

where n is the number of drugs and n! is
fractional n (see figure below).

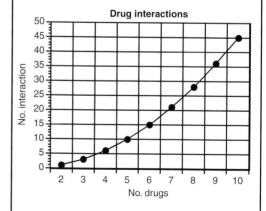

Thus, if 7 drugs are concomitantly
prescribed, there are 21 drug combinations,

each with their own potential to display an interaction.

The incidence of drug–drug interactions has been reported to be 20% if 10 or more drugs are concomitantly prescribed.

The types of drug–drug interaction include:

- pharmacological antagonism or synergy;
- pharmacokinetic changes (e.g. absorption, binding, metabolism, excretion);
- pharmacodynamic changes (e.g. interference at receptor sites).

Clearly multiple drug prescription is inevitable in Intensive Care practice, but combinations should be routinely checked.

A drug–drug interaction is not necessarily a cause for cessation of the drugs involved, as appropriate dosage adjustment may be possible.

Drugs should always be remembered as a potential cause of unusual events. Even new events may occur. Some events may be predicted from in vitro or experimental evidence, and some information is available from case reports.

The most important drug–drug interactions are those which diminish drug efficacy or increase drug toxicity, especially in the seriously ill.

Some drugs have a particular propensity to interact with many other drugs. An interesting recent example has been mibefradil, the first of a new class of calcium antagonists, approved for use in hypertension and angina but now withdrawn worldwide because of the number and diversity of other drugs with which it interacted.

Bibliography
Chrispin PS, Park GR 1997 Unexpected drug reactions and interactions in the critical care unit. Curr Opinion Crit Care 3: 262.

Hansten PB, Horn JR 1989 Drug Interactions. 6th edition. Philadelphia: Lea & Febiger.

Leape LL, Brennan TA, Laird N et al 1991 The nature of adverse events in hospitalized patients: results from the Harvard Medical Practice Study II. N Engl J Med 324: 377.

Peck CC, Temple R, Collins JM 1993 Understanding consequences of concurrent therapies. JAMA 269: 1550.

Zarowitz BJ 1995 Drug–drug interactions in ICU. In: Parker MM, Shapiro MJ, Porembka DT (eds) 1995 Critical Care: State of the Art, Chapter 4. Anaheim: Society of Critical Care Medicine. p 91.

Drugs

The use of drugs as therapeutic agents is one of the cornerstones of the treatment of the seriously ill, as it is in most medical specialties. The non-therapeutic use of drugs is separately considered as **poisoning** (q.v.).

The drugs considered in this book are selected from those which have uncommon but important uses or those whose use may present uncommon problems. These discussions involve

1. **general issues related to drug usage**, including:

- alkaloids;
- autacoids;
- cholinergic crisis;
- drug allergy;
- drug–drug interactions;
- drug fever;
- neuroleptic malignant syndrome;

2. **uncommon problems with common drugs**, including:

- acyclovir;
- adenosine;
- aspirin;
- bismuth;
- bleomycin;
- carbonic anhydrase inhibitors;
- desmopressin;
- heparin;
- lithium;

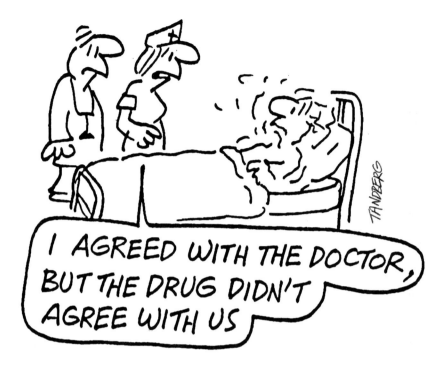

I AGREED WITH THE DOCTOR, BUT THE DRUG DIDN'T AGREE WITH US

3. **uncommon but important drugs**, including:

- amphetamines;
- anticholinergic agents;
- anticholinesterases;
- bacitracin;
- chelating agents;
- cagonists;
- desferrioxamine;
- digoxin-specific antibody;
- liquorice;
- methylene blue;

4. **specific organ-related drug issues**, including:

- drugs and the kidney;
- drugs and the lung.

Bibliography

Adedoyin A, Branch RA 1997 The effect of liver disease on drugs. Curr Opinion Crit Care 3: 255.

Chernow B (ed) 1994 The Pharmacological Approach to the Critically Ill Patient. 3rd edition. Baltimore: Williams & Wilkins.

Chrispin PS, Park GR 1997 Unexpected drug reactions and interactions in the critical care unit. Curr Opinion Crit Care 3: 262.

Crowe AV, Griffiths RD 1997 Nutritional failure and drugs. Curr Opinion Crit Care 3: 268.

Gora-Harper ML, in conjunction with the Society of Critical Care Medicine 1998 The Injectable Drug Reference. Princeton: Bioscientific Resources.

Haddad LM, Shannon MW, Winchester JF (eds) 1997 Clinical Management of Poisoning and Drug Overdose. 3rd edition. Philadelphia: WB Saunders.

Hardman JG, Limbird LE (eds.-in-chief) 1996 Goodman & Gilman's The Pharmacological Basis of Therapeutics. 9th edition. New York: McGraw-Hill.

Karch FE, Lasagna L 1975 Adverse drug reactions: a critical review. JAMA 234: 1236.

Koch-Weser J 1968 Definition and classification of adverse drug reactions. Drug Information Bulletin July/September: 72.

Koch-Weser J 1974 Bioavailability of drugs. N Engl J Med 291: 233 & 503.

Marik P, Varon J 1998 The obese patient in the ICU. Chest 113: 492.

Melmon KL, Morrelli HF, Hoffman BB et al (eds) 1992 Melmon and Morrelli's Clinical Pharmacology: Basic Principles in Therapeutics. 3rd edition. New York: McGraw-Hill.

Misan G (ed.-in-chief) 1998 Australian Medicines Handbook. Adelaide: AMH.

Naranjo CA, Shear NH, Lanctot KL 1992 Advances in the diagnosis of adverse drug reactions. J Clin Pharmacol 32: 897.

Paw H 2000 Handbook of Drugs in Intensive Care. London: Greenwich Medical.

Shann F 1996 Drug Doses. 9th edition. Melbourne: Royal Children's Hospital.

Susla GM, Masur H, Cunnion RE et al 1997 The Handbook of Critical Care Drug Delivery. 2nd edition. Baltimore: Williams & Wilkins.

Thompson DF, Pierce DR 1999 Drug-induced nightmares. Ann Pharmacother 33: 93.

Trujillo MH, Guerrero J, Fragachan C et al 1998 Pharmacologic antidotes in critical care medicine: a practical guide for drug administration. Crit Care Med 26: 377.

Drugs and the kidney

In intensive care units, drug-induced acute renal damage has been calculated to occur in about 15% of patients. Drugs should thus be remembered as potentially contributing to any case of renal failure in the seriously ill, particularly if the cause is not otherwise readily apparent. There are several mechanisms and manifestations of drug-induced nephrotoxicity.

1. **Acute pre-renal renal failure**

Glomerular filtration rate (GFR) is vulnerable to local as well as systemic circulatory changes. Such local changes may be produced by several groups of drugs.

- **Noradrenaline** is a renal vasoconstrictor and can thus reduce GFR, although its effect in this regard can be difficult to distinguish from the effect of the underlying hypotension for which it is being given in the first place. Low-dose dopamine is commonly given in this setting in an attempt to offset the potentially adverse direct effects on the kidney of potent vasoconstictors like noradrenaline.
- **Angiotensin converting enzyme (ACE) inhibitors** cause reversible renal impairment in patients in whom renal autoregulation is active. This autoregulation is effected by efferent arteriole constriction, is produced by angiotensin II (q.v.) and is required to preserve GFR. Clearly ACE inhibitors interfere with this mechanism, which is active in patients with hypovolaemia or with renal artery stenosis (if bilateral or if unilateral with a poorly functioning contralateral kidney). Renal failure in this setting is not structural (i.e. it is not associated with proteinuria, an abnormal urinary sediment or histological changes), but there can be striking hyperkalaemia. Rapid reversal occurs with cessation of the ACE inhibitor and with rehydration.
- **Non-steroidal anti-inflammatory agents (NSAIDs)** can also cause acute renal dysfunction, especially in patients with some degree of underlying renal insufficiency. This occurs because NSAIDs inhibit the synthesis of prostaglandins and because prostaglandins in turn are required to maintain afferent arteriole dilatation and thus GFR in the face of impaired renal blood flow. The adverse effect of NSAIDs in this situation is compounded by any concomitant administration of methotrexate or triamterene.
- **Cyclosporin** causes afferent arteriole constriction and thus the potential for acute renal dysfunction. This effect is increased when NSAIDs or ACE inhibitors are also given.

2. **Acute tubular necrosis**

Acute tubular necrosis (ATN) is the commonest type of drug-induced renal damage in seriously ill patients as well as the commonest type of renal impairment due to circulatory failure. Several drugs are particularly implicated.

- **Aminoglycosides**, especially gentamicin, are the cause of most cases of drug-induced ATN. Although the pathogenetic mechanism is unclear, the risk is increased by hypovolaemia, hypokalaemia, hypomagnesaemia, hyperbilirubinaemia and other nephrotoxic drugs, as well as by the

D

duration and total dose of aminoglycoside given.

- **Amphotericin B** causes renal impairment in most patients given large doses, either daily or cumulative. The risk is increased with diuretics and decreased with added sodium (e.g. 300 mmol per day). The liposomal preparation of amphotericin is much less nephrotoxic though it is very expensive.

- **Cyclosporin** can cause ATN as well as reduced GFR. Nephrotoxicity is one of its main side-effects and is generally manifest as slowly progressive but reversible acute renal failure with hyperkalaemia. As the risk is dose-related, it is increased by drugs which increase blood cyclosporin levels, such as calcium channel blockers (especially diltiazem), ketoconazole, erythromycin.

- **Radiocontrast agents**, either ionic or non-ionic, may cause ATN in patients who are old or dehydrated and especially in patients with diabetes and existing renal impairment. The damage is usually mild, except in patients with severe existing renal impairment. Some protection is afforded by calcium channel blockers and by prostaglandin E1.

3. **Acute interstitial nephritis** (see Tubulointerstitial diseases)

4. **Chronic interstitial nephritis** (see Tubulointerstitial diseases)

5. **Glomerular injury**

Drug-induced glomerular injury is an important cause of the nephrotic syndrome (see Glomerular Diseases).

Bibliography

Bennett WM, Aronoff GR, Golper TA et al 1994 Drug Prescribing in Renal Failure: Dosing Guidelines for Adults. Philadelphia: American College of Physicians.

Hoitsma AJ, Wetzels JFM, Koene RAP 1991 Drug-induced nephrotoxicity: aetiology, clinical features and management. Drug Safety 6: 131.

Drugs and the lung

Many different pulmonary reactions involving a large variety of drugs and poisons may occur.

Although pulmonary reactions are less common than drug-induced reactions involving other organs and systems, they are important because;

- they can be severe and life-threatening;
- they are often reversible if the responsible drug is ceased;
- they can mimic other more common respiratory diseases.

The mechanisms of drug-induced reactions are probably many and among others include immunological (allergic) and pharmacological (idiosyncratic, facultative, toxic) processes.

The diagnosis of a drug-induced pulmonary reaction is usually presumptive.

Clinical suspicion is complemented by a careful history rather than laboratory tests. Even in allergic reactions, serum antibody levels and skin tests are not usually helpful. Rechallenge with the responsible drug would be diagnostically confirmatory but is usually unsafe.

The suspected offending drug should be stopped and most reactions then subside, though some pulmonary infiltrates may take weeks to resolve.

Corticosteroid therapy may hasten the resolution of infiltrative reactions, but other reactions should be treated on their symptomatic merits.

Many reactions are such that the patient should be warned about possible future exposure to the drug.

The types of pulmonary reactions to drugs are as follows.

1. **Bronchospasm**

- Type 1 hypersensitivity

  – antibiotics (especially penicillin);

- antisera;
- iodides (especially contrast media);
- iron-dextran;

- Irritant reflexes

  - acetylcysteine;
  - aerosols (especially cromoglycate);
  - beta-adrenergic blockers;

- Smooth muscle contraction

  - histamine;
  - methacholine;
  - $PGF_2\alpha$;

- Prostaglandin inhibition

  - aspirin;
  - other NSAIDs

2. Interstitial infiltration

- Acute (usually with eosinophilia)

  - azathioprine;
  - gold;
  - isoniazid;
  - nitrofurantoin;
  - para-aminosalicylic acid (PAS);
  - penicillin;
  - sulfonamides;
  - tricyclic antidepressants;

- **Chronic**

  - bleomycin;
  - busulfan;
  - cyclophosph amide;
  - gold;
  - hexamethonium;
  - melphalan;
  - methysergide;
  - nitrofurantoin;
  - oxygen;

- SLE-like

  - digitalis;
  - gold;
  - griseofulvin;
  - hydralazine;
  - isoniazid;
  - methyldopa;

- oral contraceptives;
- penicillin;
- phenytoin;
- procainamide;
- reserpine;
- sulfonamides;
- tetracyclines;
- thiazides.

3. Pulmonary oedema

- Increased hydrostatic pressure

  - adrenaline;
  - iv fluids;
  - propranolol;

- Increased capillary permeability

  - blood transfusion;
  - dextropropoxyphene;
  - heroin;
  - salicylates;
  - thiazides.

4. Pulmonary vascular changes

- Pulmonary hypertension

  - aminorex;
  - talc;

- Vasculitis

  - hydralazine;
  - penicillin;
  - phenytoin;
  - promazine;
  - quinidine;
  - sulfonamides.

5. Respiratory failure

- CNS depression

  - alcohol;
  - anaesthetics;
  - opiates;
  - sedatives;

- Neuromuscular blockade

  - aminoglycosides;
  - muscle relaxants.

6. **Pulmonary haemorrhage**

   – anticoagulants;
   – antiplatelet agents;
   – thrombolytic agents.

7. **Hilar lymphadenopathy**

   – phenytoin.

In addition, a few drugs are occasionally associated with various pleural disorders, particularly eosinophilic effusions.

Bibliography

Albertson TE, Walby WF, Derlet RW 1995 Stimulant-induced pulmonary toxicity. Chest 108: 1140.

Cooper JA, White DA, Matthay RA 1986 Drug-induced pulmonary disease. Am J Respir Dis 133: 321 & 488.

Foucher P, Biour M, Blayac JP et al 1997 Drugs that may injure the respiratory system. Eur Respir J 10: 265.

Heffner JE, Harley RA, Schabel SI 1990 Pulmonary reactions from illicit substance abuse. Clin Chest Med 11: 151.

Morelock SY, Sahn SA 1999 Drugs and the pleura. Chest 116: 212.

Parsons PE 1994 Respiratory failure as a result of drugs, overdoses, and poisonings. Clin Chest Med 15: 93.

Dysentery (see Diarrhoea)

Dysphagia

Acute dysphagia may be due to:

- oesophagitis, which may be caused by:

  – drugs (especially an NSAID tablet lodged in the oesophagus for >5 min);
  – infections (especially due to candida but also CMV or HSV);
  – caustic chemical ingestion.

- local mechanical obstruction;
- bulbar disease;
- Plummer-Vinson (or Paterson–Kelly) syndrome.

This is associated with mucosal atrophy and iron deficiency.

Chronic dysphagia may be due to:

- peptic oesophagitis

  – usually associated with stricture;

- carcinoma;
- diffuse oesophageal spasm;
- achalasia;
- oesophageal ring or diverticulum;
- collagen-vascular disease

  – typically scleroderma.

Dysproteinaemias

Dysproteinaemias comprise multiple myeloma and its variants, namely benign monoclonal gammopathy, cryoglobulinaemia, heavy chain disease and Waldenstrom's macroglobulinaemia (see Multiple myeloma).

Eaton Lambert syndrome (see Myasthenia gravis)

Ebola haemorrhagic fever

Ebola haemorrhagic fever is a severe acute viral illness of tropical Africa. It can also occur in travellers who have visited this region. The reservoir is unknown, and it is transmitted from person to person, including air-borne nosocomial hospital spread.

Of historical interest, it (as well as other conditions) has been postulated as the cause of the plague of Athens in 430 BC.

Ebola haemorrhagic fever is a **viral haemorrhagic fever** (VHF) and is thus related to a number of other types of similar infections, due to Lassa (q.v.), Marburg and Crimean–Congo viruses. Extensive endothelial cell damage is the common pathogenetic mechanism of all the viral haemorrhagic fevers.

Following an incubation period of 6–9 days, there is an acute onset of fever, headache, myalgia, abdominal pain, diarrhoea, rash, bleeding and shock. Diagnosis is made by culture.

There is no specific therapy.

The mortality has been reported to have ranged between 53–88%.

> Special precautionary guidelines have been published, including specific infection control measures.

Bibliography

Bennet D, Brown D 1995 Ebola virus. Br Med J 310: 1344.

Bouree P, Bergman J-F 1983 Ebola virus infection in man. Am J Trop Med Hyg 32: 1465.

Howard CR 1984 Viral hemorrhagic fevers: properties and prospects for treatment and prevention. Antiviral Res 4: 169.

Sanchez A, Ksiazek TG, Rollin PE et al 1995 Reemergence of Ebola virus in Africa. Emerg Infect Dis 1: 3.

Suresh V 1997 The enigmatic haemorrhagic fevers. J R Soc Med 90: 622.

Echinacea (see Angioedema)

Echinococcosis

Echinococcosis (hydatid disease) refers to human infection with the cysts of the dog tapeworm, *Echinococcus granulosus*. Other forms of echinococcus are found in other animals, e.g. foxes, in some parts of the world.

The adult cestode lives in the dog's intestine, and eggs passed in the faeces are ingested by intermediate hosts, usually sheep but occasionally incidentally humans. The cycle is normally completed when dogs eat an infected carcass or offal of one of the intermediate hosts. Hydatid disease is thus most commonly found in sheep-raising countries.

> - Following ingestion by humans, the parasites circulate to any part of the body but especially the liver and the lungs.
> - The cysts then gradually enlarge and can be many centimetres in diameter before giving symptoms of a space-occupying nature.
> - Cyst rupture can give rise to allergic symptoms, including urticaria, bronchospasm or even anaphylaxis.
> - Since the cysts are infective, the rupture can also give rise to disseminated infection and thus new cysts from the contained scolices.

The diagnosis is suggested by X-ray, since the cysts are often calcified. A fluid level may be seen and daughter cysts either free or attached may be identified within the main cyst. Positive serology is sensitive for liver though not lung involvement but is not specific.

*Treatment is generally with **surgery** and/or the **antihelminthic agents**, mebendazole or albendazole.*

Recently, a successful alternative to surgery has been reported, namely percutaneous ultrasound-guided needle aspiration and instillation of a scolicidal solution, such as alcohol or hypertonic saline.

Bibliography
Kammerer WS, Schantz PM 1993 Echinococcal disease. Infect Dis Clin North Am 7: 605.

Ecstasy (see Amphetamines)

Ecthyma

Ecthyma is a skin infection due to group A streptococci and resembling impetigo, except that it is deeper and ulcerated.

> **Ecthyma gangrenosum** (see Gangrene) is a severe local pseudomonal infection. It is seen in critically ill patients who are immunocompromised, usually with haematological malignancy, neutropenia or burns.
>
> While typically caused by pseudomonas, it may sometimes be caused by other Gram-negative bacilli or even fungi. The organisms are present in the adventitia of local vessels.
>
> It presents as a small, round, red, painless macule on the arms, buttocks or groin. This macule then vesiculates and finally sloughs to give a black gangrenous ulcer, with a red halo up to 5 cm in diameter.
>
> If extensive, the condition carries a high mortality despite antibiotic therapy.

Bibliography
Greene SL, Su WP, Muller SA 1984 Ecthyma gangrenosum. J Am Acad Dermatol 11: 781.

Ectopic hormone production (see also Paraneoplastic syndromes)

Ectopic hormone production may arise in a variety of malignancies but most commonly in lung cancer, especially small cell carcinoma. Renal, pancreatic, thymic and carcinoid tumours also commonly produce ectopic hormones.

Such hormones are polypeptides and may include:

- ACTH;
- calcitonin;
- glucagon;
- HCG;
- LH;
- PTH;
- somatostatin;
- vasopressin.

Bibliography
Mallette LE 1991 The parathyroid polyhormones: new concepts in the spectrum of peptide hormone action. Endocr Rev 12: 110.

EDTA (see Chelating agents)

Eisenmenger syndrome

Eisenmenger syndrome arises from congenital cardiac defects in which progressive pulmonary vascular obstruction has caused a predominant right-to-left shunt. These cyanotic congenital heart defects are not treatable surgically, except by transplantation, once pulmonary vascular disease has become irreversible and the Eisenmenger syndrome is produced.

Eisenmenger syndrome typically develops when left-to-right shunts (ASD, VSD, PDA) reverse. This most commonly occurs in ASDs in older patients and is associated with an irreversible plexiform pulmonary arteriopathy, similar to that seen in primary pulmonary hypertension (q.v.).

Bibliography
Borow KM, Karp R 1990 Atrial septal defect: lessons from the past, directions for the future. N Engl J Med 323: 1698.

Nora JJ 1993 Causes of congenital heart disease: old and new modes, mechanisms, and models. Am Heart J 125: 1409.

Wilson NJ, Neutze JM 1993 Adult congenital heart disease: principles and management guidelines. Aust NZ J Med 23: 498 & 697.

Embolism, air (see Diving)

Emphysema

For interstitial emphysema and subcutaneous emphysema, see Barotrauma.

Empyema (see Cavitation and Pleural cavity)

Encephalitis

Encephalitis refers to acute viral infection of the brain. There is commonly associated meningoencephalitis. There is viral replication and consequent inflammation in the brain parenchyma and sometimes in adjacent structures.

Clinical features include:

- delirium;
- fits;
- coma.

If there is associated meningitis, there is also:

- headache;
- neck stiffness;
- fever.

Temporal lobe involvement suggests that the virus is HSV.

The differential diagnosis includes bacterial, fungal or protozoal infections. The specific diagnosis may be made by viral isolation or serology, though this is successful in only about one third of cases. It is however important, since some viral infections, most notably due to HSV, are treatable. Even a delayed diagnosis can be epidemiologically useful.

Examination of the CSF shows lymphocytes, a moderately increased protein and normal glucose.

The viruses most frequently involved are the herpes group (HSV, EBV, CMV, VZV), HIV, arborvirus, enterovirus, picornavirus, measles and mumps. The most common virus is HSV type 1, and it generally responds well to treatment with acyclovir (q.v.). 'Australian encephalitis' is usually caused by the flavivirus (an arborvirus), Murray Valley encephalitis virus (MVE), which despite its name most commonly occurs in Northern Australia. It causes death in about 20% of victims and residual neurological sequelae in another 40%.

Bibliography

Burrow JNC, Whelan PI, Kilburn CJ et al 1998 Australian encephalitis in the Northern Territory: clinical and epidemiological features, 1987–1996. Aust NZ J Med 28: 590.

Whitley RJ 1990 Viral encephalitis. N Engl J Med 323: 242.

Encephalopathy

Encephalopathy refers to acute diffuse cerebral dysfunction due to toxic or metabolic causes.

It is manifest by impaired consciousness, often with fitting or myoclonus. The fitting may be generalized or focal and may be continual, as in epilepsia partialis continua.

Focal neurological signs can also of course be associated with an intracranial mass lesion, which should be excluded if such signs are found. Associated signs of meningeal irritation suggest meningitis or subarachnoid haemorrhage.

There is typically:

- metabolic flap;

- coarse tremor;
- involuntary movements and mouthings;
- abnormal tone.

*Fitting or myoclonic jerks are usefully controlled in most cases with a **benzodiazepine** (e.g. clonazepam iv). Any reversible cause should clearly be treated if possible (e.g. uraemia or sepsis).*

The prognosis is determined partly by the reversibility of the underlying cause and partly by the extent of neurological damage. For example, the encephalopathy of uraemia is usually totally reversible after effective dialysis, whereas the encephalopathy which follows a major hypoxic event such as cardiac arrest may not recover at all. Loss of the pupillary response to light for more than 24 hours is an ominous prognostic sign.

Bibliography

Bolton CF, Young GB, Zochodne DW 1993 The neurological complications of sepsis. Ann Neurol 33: 94.

Brooks BR, Walker DL 1984 Progressive multifocal leukoencephalopathy. Neurol Clin 2: 299.

Celesia GG, Grigg MM, Ross E 1988 Generalized status myoclonicus in acute anoxic and toxic-metabolic encephalopathies. Arch Neurol 45: 781.

Edgren E, Hedstrand U, Kelsey S et al 1994 Assessment of neurological prognosis in comatose survivors of cardiac arrest. Lancet 343: 1055.

Fraser CL, Arieff AI 1988 Nervous system complications in uremia. Ann Intern Med 109: 143.

Endarteritis (see Arteritis)

Endocarditis

Endocarditis refers to infective lesions on the heart valves or endocardium.

- As the organisms involved are usually bacteria, the term bacterial endocarditis is commonly used, though the organisms can sometimes be fungal, rickettsial or chlamydial. The term infective endocarditis (IE) is thus often used.

- Non-infective endocarditis may also be seen in non-bacterial, thrombotic, verrucous or Loeffler's endocarditis.

Acute endocarditis of duration up to six weeks is usually caused by an aggressive pathogen, which has infected normal endocardium following a pyogenic infection with subsequent metastatic suppuration.

The organisms involved are usually *S. aureus* (especially in hospital patients) but also *S. pneumoniae* and Gram-negative bacilli (especially in drug addicts).

Acute endocarditis presents as the sudden onset of:

- fever;
- petechiae (including Janeway lesions and Osler's nodes, which are either autoimmune or embolic and from which organisms may sometimes be cultured);
- a new or changing cardiac murmur;
- disseminated intravascular coagulation;
- systemic emboli, especially to the brain and kidney;
- meningismus.

In drug addicts, the tricuspid valve is commonly involved and the course of the illness is very acute.

Subacute endocarditis is caused by relatively avirulent organisms, which are often endogenous and are disturbed by instrumentation so as to infect an endocardium previously rendered abnormal by congenital or rheumatic lesions.

The organisms usually involved are *S. viridans*, enterococci, and other streptococcal species, which reside in the mouth, urogenital system or gut.

In subacute endocarditis, the features are more insidious and non-specific than in acute endocarditis.

- There has been a previous 'culprit' procedure in two thirds of cases and a prior cardiac lesion with a murmur in over 90%.
- Systemic features include fever, anorexia and malaise.
- Systemic emboli are common and particularly involve the brain, gut, retina, kidney and periphery. Systemic emboli which are large suggest either paradoxical embolization or cardiac emboli from thrombi, tumour or fungal material. Peripheral emboli are manifest as petechiae, lineal subungual splinter haemorrhages, Janeway lesions on the palms, and Olser's nodes on the pulp of the fingers.
- There is anaemia, focal or diffuse glomerulonephritis may occur, and sometimes the emboli may cause a mycotic aneurysm.

Prosthetic valve endocarditis occurs on both mechanical valves and bioprostheses with an incidence of 3% in the first year and 1% per year thereafter.

- Early endocarditis is usually associated with other perioperative complications.
- Late endocarditis is usually procedurally related.

Valvular dysfunction, particularly regurgitation, commonly results.

Investigations for endocarditis show anaemia, leukocytosis (in the acute phase), raised ESR, increased IgG, decreased complement, circulating immune complexes, and commonly positive rheumatoid factor and renal abnormalities. Blood cultures are important and should include methods to detect more fastidious micro-organisms. Cultures taken from arterial blood may sometimes reveal micro-organisms not identified in blood taken by more routine venepuncture. Even so, about 10% of patients remain culture-negative.

The differential diagnosis of endocarditis may sometimes be difficult and includes:

- non-bacterial thrombotic endocarditis;
- rheumatic fever;
- atrial myxoma;
- post-bypass syndromes;
- malignancy (especially carcinoma of the kidney);
- collagen-vascular diseases.

Complications include:

- valvular damage;
- abscess-induced myocardial dysfunction;
- septal invasion with conduction abnormalities;
- cardiac failure;
- pericarditis;
- systemic embolization.

Treatment is with high-dose parenteral antibiotics for 4–6 weeks in native valve endocarditis or 6–8 weeks in prosthetic valve endocarditis.

- *The most commonly used antibiotic is **penicillin** in a dose of 7–10 g (12–18 million U) per day for sensitive organisms and in twice that dose for less sensitive organisms.*
- ***Gentamicin** should be added for synergistic treatment of enterococci (in which case, ampicillin may also be substituted for penicillin).*
- ***Vancomycin** 2 g/day should be used if the patient is sensitive to penicillin or if the responsible organism is methicillin-resistant S. aureus (MRSA).*
- *For sensitive S. aureus, **flucloxacillin** or **dicloxacillin** 12 g/day or cephalothin in the same dose should be used.*
- *For Gram-negative organisms, a **third-generation cephalosporin**, sometimes with gentamicin, should be given.*
- ***Amphotericin** 1 mg/kg daily, preferably with **flucytosine** 10 g daily, is given for fungal endocarditis, but there is still an 80% mortality, so that early surgery is indicated, especially if the lesions are bulky.*
- *For **culture-negative endocarditis**, gentamicin plus flucloxacillin or ampicillin (depending on the likely organism) is given, except in prosthetic valve endocarditis when vancomycin should also be added.*

An antibiotic response should be seen within two days and always within one week. Cultures should become negative, but even if therapy is effective, embolization can still occur for some weeks.

Antithrombotic therapy is sometimes considered in bacterial endocarditis. However, it does not prevent embolization of vegetations and increases the risk of cerebral haemorrhage. It should therefore be used only if such therapy would have been indicated in its own right in the absence of the current endocarditis.

Surgical repair or replacement of the damaged valve is indicated if there is significant circulatory compromise or if the endocarditis is bulky, invasive, staphylococcal, pseudomonal or fungal. There is nowadays a low risk of infection of a new prosthesis.

> **Prophylactic antibiotics** should always be given if a patient with structural heart disease is subjected to a risk procedure.

Structural heart disease includes for this purpose:

- all congenital and valvular heart disease;
- mitral valve prolapse;
- prosthetic valves;
- hypertrophic cardiomyopathy;
- prior endocarditis (regardless of whether an overt lesion was demonstrated or not);
- but not generally ASD (whether corrected or not) and corrected PDA.

Risk procedures include:

- major dental work;
- surgery or invasive investigation of the respiratory, gastrointestinal or urogenital tracts;
- surgery of infected lesions;
- obstetric procedures in the presence of infection.

Unless the patient risk is particularly high, as with prosthetic valves or with previous endocarditis, prophylaxis is not required for **low-risk procedures**, such as:

- dental work without gingival bleeding;
- endotracheal intubation;
- fibreoptic bronchoscopy;
- GI endoscopy without biopsy;
- barium enema;
- liver biopsy;
- urinary catheterization;
- gynaecological examination;
- uncomplicated vaginal or Caesarean delivery, or uterine curettage.

> For **procedures 'above the diaphragm'**,
>
> - the recommended antibiotic prophylaxis is amoxycillin 2–3 g orally 1 h before the procedure (and 1.5 g 6 h after the procedure if the procedure lasts more than 3 h).

- If the patient is sensitive to penicillin or is already on low-dose penicillin prophylaxis for rheumatic fever, erythromycin 1 g or clindamycin 600 mg should be used instead of amoxycillin 2–3 g.
- If oral intake is not possible, iv ampicillin (2 g) or clindamycin (600 mg) should be used 30 min before the procedure.
- In very high-risk patients, ampicillin 2 g iv and gentamicin 120 mg iv or vancomycin 1 g IV should be used.

> For **procedures 'below the diaphragm'**,
>
> - oral or iv amoxycillin (as above) may be used alone if the procedure is low risk and with iv gentamicin if it is high risk.

- Vancomycin should be substituted for amoxycillin in patients sensitive to penicillin.

Since many cases of endocarditis are not in fact related to a defined precipitating event and are probably related to normal activities, such as chewing, it is important that careful dental health be maintained in patients at risk.

The prognosis from endocarditis is still unsatisfactory. There is a 25% overall mortality, rising to 30% if a prosthetic valve is involved and to 50% if the responsible organism is *S. aureus*. The chief causes of death are cardiac failure, embolization and mycotic aneurysms.

Bibliography

Alpert JS, Krous HF, Dalen JE et al 1976 Pathogenesis of Osler's nodes. Ann Intern Med 85: 471.

Bayer AS, Bolger AF, Taubert KA et al 1998 Diagnosis and management of infective endocarditis and its complications. Circulation 98: 2936.

Calderwood SB, Swinski LA, Karchmer AW et al 1986 Prosthetic valve endocarditis. J Thorac Cardiovasc Surg 92: 776.

Dajani AS, Taubert KA, Wilson W et al 1997 Prevention of bacterial endocarditis: recommendations by the American Heart Association. JAMA 277: 1794.

DiNubile MJ 1982 Surgery in active endocarditis. Ann Intern Med 96: 650.

Kaye D 1985 Changing pattern of infective endocarditis. Am J Med 79 (suppl 6B): 157.

Lerner PI, Weinstein L 1966 Infective endocarditis in the antibiotic era. N Engl J Med 274: 199, 259, 323, 388.

Levin HJ, Paulker SG, Salzman EW et al 1992 Antithrombotic therapy in valvular heart disease. Chest 102: S434.

Mansur AJ, Grinberg M, Lemos da Luz P et al 1992 The complications of infective endocarditis. Arch Intern Med 152: 2428.

Stein PD, Alpert JS, Copeland J et al 1992 Antithrombotic therapy in patients with mechanical and biological prosthetic heart valves. Chest 102: S445.

Tornos P, Almirante B, Olona M et al 1997 Clinical outcome and long-term prognosis of late prosthetic valve endocarditis: a 20-year experience. Clin Infect Dis 24: 381.

Tunkel AR, Kaye D 1992 Endocarditis with negative blood cultures. N Engl J Med 326: 1215.

Weinstein L, Rubin RH 1973 Infective endocarditis. Progr Cardiovasc Dis 16: 239.

Endocrinology

Some endocrine disorders are frequently managed in Intensive Care and are well understood there, such as diabetic ketoacidosis and hyperosmolar non-ketosis, hypoglycaemia and diabetes insipidus. Many conditions and issues are less commonly encountered, and are therefore considered in this book, including:

- acromegaly;
- adrenal insufficiency;
- adrenocorticotropic hormone;
- aldosterone;
- angiotensin-converting enzyme;
- calcitonin;
- Conn's syndrome;
- Cushing's syndrome;
- ectopic hormone production;
- euthyroid sick syndrome;
- hirsutism/hypertrichosis;
- hypercalcaemia;
- hyperparathyroidism;
- hyperphosphataemia;
- hyperthyroidism;
- hypocalcaemia;
- hypoparathyroidism;
- hypophosphataemia;
- hypothyroidism;
- multiple endocrine neoplasia;
- myxoedema;
- pituitary;
- renin–angiotensin–aldosterone;
- somatomedin C;
- somatostatin;
- syndrome of inappropriate antidiuretic hormone;
- vasopressin;
- Waterhouse–Friderichsen syndrome;
- Zollinger–Ellison syndrome.

Bibliography

Axelrod L 1976 Glucocorticoid therapy. Medicine 55: 39.

Berl T 1990 Treating hyponatremia: damned if we do and damned if we don't. Kidney Int 37: 1006.

Chernow B (ed) 1994 The Pharmacological Approach to the Critically Ill Patient. 3rd edition. Baltimore: Williams & Wilkins.

Chrousos GP 1995 The hypothalamic–pituitary–adrenal axis and immune-mediated inflammation. N Engl J Med 332: 1351.

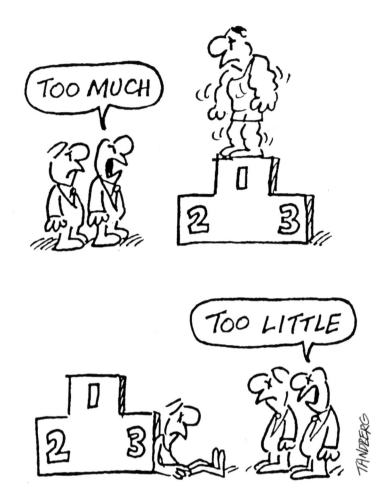

Cook DM, Loriaux DL 1996 The incidental adrenal mass. Endocrinologist 6: 4.

Curry SC, Arnold-Capell P 1991 Nitroprusside, nitroglycerin, and angiotensin-converting enzyme inhibitors. Crit Care Clin 7: 555.

Editorial 1980 Corticosteroids and hypothalamic–pituitary–adrenocortical function. Br Med J 280: 813.

Editorial 1985 The function of adrenaline. Lancet 1: 561.

Ekins R 1992 The free hormone hypothesis and measurement of free hormones. Clin Chem 38: 1289.

Grinspoon SK, Bilezikian JP 1992 HIV disease and the endocrine system. N Engl J Med 327: 1360.

Loriaux DL 1985 The polyendocrine deficiency syndromes. N Engl J Med 312: 1568.

Oster JR, Singer I, Fishman LM 1995 Heparin-induced aldosterone suppression and hyperkalemia. Am J Med 98: 575.

Reichlin S 1993 Neuroendocrine-immune interactions. N Engl J Med 329: 1246.

Rose BD 1986 New approach to disturbances in the plasma sodium concentration. Am J Med 81: 1033.

Salem M, Tainsh RE, Bromberg J et al 1994 Perioperative glucocorticoid coverage: a reassessment 42 years after emergence of a problem. Ann Surg 219: 416.

Tonner DR, Schlechte JA 1993 Neurologic complications of thyroid and parathyroid disease. Med Clin North Am 77: 251.

Wilson JD, Foster DW (eds) 1992 Williams Textbook of Endocrinology. 8th edition. Philadelphia: WB Saunders.

Enterocolitis (see Colitis)

Enteropathogenic *E. coli* (see Diarrhoea)

Envenomation (see Bites and stings)

Environment

Although environmental contact is an inevitable part of human existence, most such contact is not hazardous to health or survival. However, in a variety of uncommon settings, the environment can present particular dangers and some of these will come to the attention of Intensive Care clinicians. In particular, serious illness may be caused by some **chemical exposures** (see Chemical poisoning) and some **physical exposures** (see Cold, Heat, High altitude).

Bibliography

American College of Physicians 1990 Occupational and environmental medicine: the internist's role. Ann Intern Med 113: 974.

Bascom R, Bromberg PA, Costa DL et al 1996 Health effects of outdoor pollution. Am J Resp Crit Care Med 153: 3, 477.

Cugell DW 1992 The hard metal diseases. Clin Chest Med 13: 269.

Nriagu JO, Pacyna JM 1988 Quantitative assessment of worldwide contamination of air, water and soils by trace metals. Nature 333: 134.

Redlich CA, Sparer JS, Cullen MR 1997 Sick building syndrome. Lancet 349: 1013.

Rosenstock L, Cullen M (eds) 1994 Textbook of Clinical Occupational and Environmental Medicine. Philadelphia: Saunders.

Roxe DM, Krumlovsky FA 1988 Toxic interstitial nephropathy from metals, metabolites, and radiation. Semin Nephrol 8: 72.

Eosinopenia (see Eosinophilia)

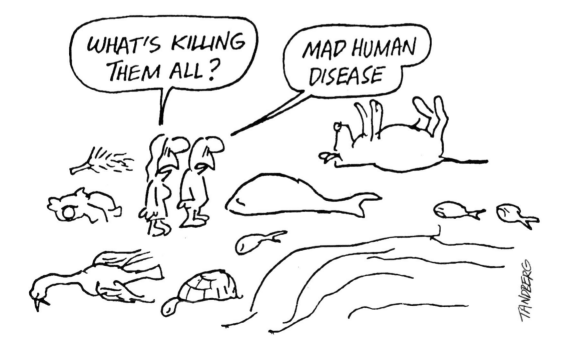

E

Eosinophilia

Eosinophils arise from the granulocyte-macrophage-eosinophil progenitor, which is stimulated by eosinophilopoietin to differentiate into eosinophilic myelocytes, metamyelocytes and finally mature eosinophils.

Most eosinophils (99%) reside in the tissues, especially in the gut mucosa. Eosinophils have prominent granules which contain peroxidase and other proteins such as neurotoxin. They have also a unique membrane enzyme (lysophospholipase), which forms Charcot–Leyden crystals when eosinophils coalesce and fragment.

Eosinophils are attracted by substances (e.g. ECF-A) released from mast cells. They are stimulated by T cells and activated by monocytes, their presumed role being to kill multicellular parasites, an action which is in enhanced by IL-3.

Despite this role, **eosinopenia** (which occurs in some infections and following corticosteroids) is not associated with any specific clinical consequence.

Eosinophilia on the other hand (absolute eosinophil count $>0.44 \times 10^9/L$) is associated with a large variety of clinical disorders. These include:

- allergic disorders
  - especially those involving the lungs or the skin;

- drug reactions
  - especially to chlorpromazine, iodides, sulfonamides;

- infections
  - especially parasitic but occasionally fungal;

- malignancy
  - especially myeloproliferative disorders (including eosinophilic leukaemia);
  - but also other leukaemias and lymphoma;

- pulmonary infiltrates
  - q.v.;

- systemic disorders
  - including connective tissue diseases and granulomatoses;

- **hypereosinophilic syndrome**
  - an uncommon condition of no known aetiology but with an eosinophil count $>1.5 \times 10^9/L$. It is a chronic multi-organ disorder, with cardiomyopathy, recurrent thromboembolism, and central nervous system and sometimes lung and skin involvement.

It responds to **corticosteroids***, but sometimes cytotoxics or leukapheresis may be indicated.*

Bibliography

Fauci A, Harley J, Roberts W et al 1982 The idiopathic hypereosinophilic syndrome. Ann Intern Med 97: 278.

Gleich GJ, Loegering DA 1984 Immunobiology of eosinophils. Annu Rev Immunol 2: 429.

Kita H 1996 The eosinophil: a cytokine-producing cell? J Allergy Clin Immunol 97: 889.

Eosinophilia and lung infiltration

Pulmonary infiltration with eosinophilia (PIE) includes:

- Loeffler's syndrome;
- asthmatic pulmonary eosinophilia;
- tropical eosinophilia;
- eosinophilic pneumonia.

Specific conditions which may also give rise to pulmonary infiltration in association with blood eosinophilia include:

- eosinophilic leukaemia;
- Hodgkin's disease;
- hydatid disease;
- polyarteritis nodosa;
- Churg–Strauss syndrome.

Loeffler's syndrome (simple pulmonary eosinophilia) consists of transient and variable pulmonary infiltrates, associated with a high white cell count (up to $20 \times 10^9/L$) and eosinophil count (up to 20% or more). It is probably an allergic reaction to a variety of possible allergens, particularly helminths.

It generally lasts less than a month, but it may occasionally last up to six months or more. Most cases are clinically silent, but cough and systemic symptoms sometimes occur. Recovery is invariable.

Treatment is not indicated.

Asthmatic pulmonary eosinophilia is characterized by asthma with recurrent, variable and changing shadows on chest X-ray and variable eosinophilia. Most cases are associated with *Aspergillus fumigatus* colonization, and the fungus acts as an antigen. The condition is thus also called **allergic bronchopulmonary aspergillosis**.

Typically, the patient is febrile during acute exacerbations and coughs up brown plugs or bronchial casts containing eosinophils and fungal mycelia. Mucoid impaction may occur with bronchial obstruction due to inspissated mucus. Bronchiectasis and lobar shrinkage may be found.

Precipitins for *Aspergillus fumigatus* are usually present in serum. The course is generally chronic.

*Treatment is as for asthma, with **corticosteroids** usually required. Specific antifungal therapy has been generally unhelpful, except for **itraconazole** in steroid-dependent cases of aspergollosis (q.v.).*

Tropical pulmonary eosinophilia (TPE) is an allergic reaction to mosquito-borne filaria, particularly *Wuchereria bancrofti* but also *Brugia malayi*. Given the frequency of lymphatic filariasis in tropical countries, this allergic response is uncommon, occurring in <1% of infected patients.

The patient presents with episodic fever, cough, wheeze and often systemic symptoms. Particularly in travellers, it may masquerade as refractory asthma. Untreated, alternating recurrences and remissions may persist for years and eventually lead to pulmonary fibrosis.

*Treatment is with **diethylcarbamazine** (DEC), 6 mg/kg daily for 3 weeks.*

Eosinophilic pneumonia is a syndrome of very marked eosinophilia with fever, night sweats, malaise, weight loss, dyspnoea and wheeze. Sometimes, however, it may be asymptomatic. The aetiology is unknown. It mostly affects middle-aged women, many of whom have a past history of atopy.

Chest X-ray characteristically shows bilateral, symmetrical, peripheral pulmonary infiltrates with perihilar sparing (the 'photonegative' picture of acute pulmonary oedema), though commonly there are less characteristic findings, such as patchy interstitial infiltration, lobar consolidation or cavitation.

Diagnosis is made by transbronchial lung biopsy.

*The condition responds dramatically to **corticosteroids**, though relapse after steroid withdrawal may occur.*

Bibliography

Allen JN, Davis WB 1994 Eosinophilic lung diseases. Am J Respir Crit Care Med 150: 1423.

Jederlinic PJ, Sicilian L, Gaensler EA 1988 Chronic eosinophilic pneumonia: a report of 19 cases and a review of the literature. Medicine 67: 154.

Naughton M, Fahy J, FitzGerald MX 1993 Chronic eosinophilic pneumonia. Chest 103: 162.

Ong RKC, Doyle RL 1998 Tropical pulmonary eosinophilia. Chest 113: 1673.

Ottesen EA, Nutman TB 1992 Tropical pulmonary eosinophilia. Annu Rev Med 43: 417.

Ricketti AJ, Greenberger PA, Mintzer RA et al 1983 Allergic bronchopulmonary aspergillosis. Arch Intern Med 143: 1553.

Schatz M, Wasserman S, Patterson R 1981 Eosinophils and immunologic lung disease. Med Clin North Am 65: 1055.

Schuyler MR 1983 Allergic bronchopulmonary aspergillosis. Clin Chest Med 4: 15.

Eosinophilic granuloma (see Histiocytosis X)

Eosinophilic pneumonia (see Eosinophilia and lung infiltration)

Epidermolysis bullosa

Epidermolysis bullosa is a group of over 20 rare genetic and acquired disorders of adhesion molecules of the epidermis and epidermal–dermal junction. They typically appear as blistering after minor trauma. Some conditions are autoimmune and also affect mucosal as well as skin integrity.

Treatment with fluid and electrolyte **resuscitation** *may be required, since blistering can be extensive and cause dehydration and subsequent infection.*

Bibliography
Fine J-D 1986 Epidermolysis bullosa: clinical aspects, pathology, and recent advances in research. Int J Dermatol 25: 143.

Epididymitis

Epididymitis can be due to a variety of micro-organisms. These particularly include:

- chlamydia;
- gonococci;
- meningococci;
- haemophilus;
- salmonella;
- cryptococcus;
- mycobacteria;
- filaria;
- mumps virus.

- In young heterosexual men:
  - it is usually associated with urethritis and conjunctivitis;
  - it is chiefly due to *N. gonorrhoeae* or *C. trachomatis.*

- In homosexual men:
  - it is often associated with urethritis;
  - it is usually due to coliforms or haemophilus.

The differential diagnosis is:

- testicular infection;

  i.e. orchitis (q.v.);

- testicular torsion;
- testicular tumour.

Epidural abscess

An epidural abscess may arise anywhere throughout the length of the epidural space, though it is most usefully classified as cranial or spinal.

Cranial epidural abscess arises from direct spread of infection due to:

- cranial injury;
- wound infection;
- adjacent sinus or mastoid infection.

Since the dura adheres closely to the skull, the size of such an abscess is limited. The most commonly involved organisms are *S. aureus*, enteric Gram-negative bacilli or anaerobes (the latter particularly if the abscess follows sinus or mastoid infection).

The clinical features are those of the underlying condition, together with neck stiffness. Because of its small size, focal neurological signs are uncommon. The exception is V and VI nerve involvement from petrous extension from mastoid disease, with paralysis of the lateral rectus muscle and facial pain (Gradenigo's syndrome). Examination of the CSF shows lymphocytes but no organisms.

Treatment is with **antibiotics** *and surgical* **drainage***.*

Spinal epidural abscess is uncommon and is mostly due to bacteraemia (when it is often associated with vertebral osteomyelitis). Sometimes, it may be due to adjacent infection, as of a wound. The thoracic region is more often involved than the cervical or lumbar. The abscess is usually posterior involving an average of 4–5 spaces.

The organisms most commonly involved are *S. aureus*, followed by Gram-negative bacilli.

Clinical manifestations are described as typically occurring in four phases, namely

- in the first 1–2 days
  - there is back pain and meningismus;
- in the next 4–5 days
  - there is nerve root pain and fever;
- over the next day
  - there is weakness, numbness and incontinence;
- subsequently
  - irreversible paralysis occurs.

The differential diagnosis of a spinal epidural abscess is:

- spinal cord compression, due to tumour or vertebral body disease;
- spinal cord ischaemia;
- transverse myelitis.

The diagnosis is confirmed and its extent delineated by spinal MRI or CT-myelography. Lumbar puncture should not be performed if there is lumbar involvement because of the risk of producing meningitis.

*Treatment is with spinal cord **decompression** and **antibiotics** for 3–4 weeks.*

Bibliography

Baker AS, Ojemann RG, Swartz MN et al 1975 Spinal epidural abscess. N Engl J Med 293: 463.

Jefferson AA, Keogh AJ 1977 Intracranial abscesses. Q J Med 46: 389.

Epstein–Barr virus

Epstein–Barr virus (EBV) infection is limited to nasopharyngeal epithelial cells, B cells and cervical cells in humans. It is well known as the cause of infectious mononucleosis, and it may also be involved in a variety of other conditions, including nasopharyngeal carcinoma in Asians, Burkitt's lymphoma in Africans and several B cell lymphoproliferative disorders.

The virus first infects the cells of the nasopharynx, where it replicates and subsequently infects B cells, within which it is disseminated to other parts of the body. Although B cells carry the viral genome, the virus is not replicated but remains latent for long periods. These B cells can produce a variety of antibodies, including the heterophile antibody, a diagnostic marker of EBV infection, though not in fact an antibody directed to viral antigen but coincidentally to red blood cell antigens of several animals.

About half the population seroconvert by 5 years of age due to asymptomatic infection. When primary infection occurs between 10–20 years, the condition of infectious mononucleosis results. About 15% of seropositive adults shed the virus from the oropharynx, and it is transmitted to others by close contact.

Clinically, infectious mononucleosis is manifest as fever, pharyngitis and lymphadenopathy, often with associated rash (especially if given ampicillin), hepatosplenomegaly and jaundice.

Although the acute illness typically lasts 1–3 weeks, fatigue may last for months.

Haemolytic anaemia, meningoencephalitis and Guillain–Barré syndrome occasionally occur. Chronic EBV infection may occur in some patients. Occasionally, overwhelming infection gives rise to a lymphoproliferative syndrome in immunocompromised hosts.

The diagnosis is confirmed by the typical full blood examination and the presence of serum heterophile antibody which may last for several months. There is an increased number of lymphocytes with >10% being atypical, and often neutropenia and thrombocytopenia. Liver function tests are commonly abnormal.

Treatment is **supportive**. *Acyclovir provides only minimal clinical benefit, but corticosteroids are occasionally useful for complications.*

Bibliography
Tynell E, Aurelius E, Brandell A et al 1996 Acyclovir and prednisolone treatment of acute infectious mononucleosis: a multicenter, double-blind, placebo-controlled study. J Infect Dis 174: 324.

Ergot

Ergot is derived from the fungus, *Claviceps purpurea*, a fungus affecting grasses, especially rye. Infected grain appears large and hard and has brown-black discolouration. Poisoning occurs from the ingestion of affected flour and is referred to as ergotism (St Anthony's fire).

The chief features of this condition are peripheral gangrene due to vascular smooth muscle constriction and fits, possibly leading to death.

Treatment is **symptomatic**.

Ergotism has been reported following normal doses of ergotamine for migraine when combined with erythromycin.

The ergot alkaloid, methysergide, has been reported to cause cardiac valvulopathy, as well as the better known side-effect of retroperitoneal fibrosis. These effects appear to be similar to those which occur in the carcinoid syndrome.

It is of interest that ergot is the source of the synthetic hallucinogen, lysergic acid diethylamide (LSD).

Bibliography
Redfield MM, Nicholson WJ, Edwards WD et al 1992 Valve disease associated with ergot alkaloid use. Ann Intern Med 117: 50.

Erysipelas

Erysipelas is a superficial cellulitis caused usually by group A β-haemolytic streptococci. There is a characteristic red and oedematous appearance, especially of the face, that is demarcated, spreads peripherally and may vesiculate. It is associated with fever and local discomfort.

It has sometime been reported after coronary artery bypass graft surgery as affecting the leg from which the saphenous vein has been removed. In chronic oedematous states, erysipelas may be recurrent.

The diagnosis is made clinically and is supported if possible by culture of fluid from the lesion.

Treatment is with **penicillin**, *which results in improvement within two days, though complete resolution requires several days.*

The main differential diagnosis is two-fold:

- **Erysipeloid**.

This is a non-febrile condition with painful, purple lesions on the hand a few days after handling animal or fish products infected with *Erysipelothrix insidiosa* (or *rhusiopathia*), a Gram-positive bacillus resembling listeria. It may occasionally be complicated by septicaemia.

It is treated with **penicillin**.

- **Acute allergic contact dermatitis** (AECD, see Dermatitis)

- This may affect the face or limbs, in which case it has often been induced by plants.

Bibliography
Grieco MH, Sheldon C 1970 Erysipelothrix rhusiopathiae. Ann NY Acad Sci 174: 523.
Eriksson B, Jorup-Ronstrom C, Karkkoonen K et al 1996 Erysipelas: clinical and bacteriologic spectrum and serological aspects. Clin Infect Dis 23: 1091.

Erythema marginatum

Erythema marginatum is the characteristic rash of rheumatic fever, though it occurs in only 5%

of cases and even then, being transient, it is often missed. It is an evanescent and asymptomatic rash affecting the limbs and trunk, and though it lasts only a few hours it may recur.

Erythema migrans (see Lyme disease)

Erythema multiforme

Erythema multiforme is one of the toxic erythemas.

It is an acute hypersensitivity reaction of skin and mucous membranes, following infections, drugs and some other stimuli.

- Infections may be bacterial (streptococcal, TB), viral (HSV, influenza, mumps), fungal or due to mycoplasma.
- Drugs most commonly include barbiturates, penicillin, sulfonamides, phenytoin.
- Other stimuli include collagen-vascular diseases, malignancy, graft-versus-host reaction.

There is a characteristic inner lesion of a red macule that may vesiculate, ulcerate and in some cases become infected. Surrounding this inner lesion but separated from it by an area of normal skin is an erythematous halo. The entire complex looks like a target. Involvement of the outer lip mucosa is characteristic.

In its severe, disseminated and multisystem form, it is called the **Stevens–Johnson syndrome**.

Treatment should include that of any triggers (e.g. HSV).

- *The use of corticosteroids is debatable, though used early they may be helpful.*
- *Severe cases need supportive care, including fluid resuscitation.*

Bibliography
Tonnesen MG, Soter NA 1979 Erythema multiforme. J Am Acad Dermatol 1: 357.

Erythema nodosum

Erythema nodosum is possibly a delayed hypersensitivity reaction to inflammatory or pharmacological stimuli.

- Inflammatory triggers include streptococcal infection, especially of the upper respiratory tract, TB, sarcoidosis and inflammatory bowel disease.
- Pharmacological triggers include particularly sulfonamides and oral contraceptives.

The condition usually occurs in young women. It appears as red, tender nodules, especially on the legs. It is associated with systemic symptoms of fever, malaise and arthralgia and usually lasts for 3–6 weeks.

The clinical diagnosis is clear-cut, but it should prompt a search for an underlying disease.

Treatment is **symptomatic**, *and should especially include rest. Corticosteroids and potassium iodide are helpful in chronic cases.*

Erythrocytosis (see Polycythaemia)

Erythrocytosis refers to an increased red blood cell (erythrocyte) count, i.e. $>5.80 \times 10^{12}$/L. More valid indices of increased total red cell mass (i.e. polycythaemia) are:

- increased haemoglobin (>180 g/L);
- increased haematocrit (>0.52) – a better index;
- direct isotopic measurement of red cell mass (>36 mL/kg) – probably the best index.

Erythromelalgia (see Thrombocytosis)

Ethylene glycol

Ethylene glycol {1,2-ethanediol, $C_2H_4(OH)_2$ or $HOCH_2.CH_2OH$} is a colourless, odourless, but sweet-tasting and oily liquid. It is the simplest of the glycols, which are organic compounds of the alcohol family but with $(OH)_2$ attached to a carbon structure. It has been widely used since the 1920s as an antifreeze, a brake fluid and in synthetic fibre manufacture.

It may be ingested accidentally or suicidally, but it is most commonly taken deliberately as a cheap substitute for alcohol. Although not toxic itself, its metabolism via alcohol dehydrogenase gives several toxic products, including aldehydes, glycolate, oxalate and lactic acid. Its half-life is about 3 h. Poisoning from ethylene glycol has many similarities with that from methanol.

The minimum lethal dose is about 100 mL in an adult, though recovery has been reported following the ingestion of up to 1 L. A significantly toxic plasma level is >200 mg/L or 3.2 mmol/L.

The clinical features of ethylene glycol poisoning are seen in three stages.

- **Early (4–12 h)**

There are gastrointestinal disturbances:

– with nausea and vomiting;

neurological (meningoencephalitic) disturbances:

– with intoxication (without the smell of alcohol), nystagmus, ophthalmoplegia, myoclonus, decreased reflexes, convulsions and coma.

- **Intermediate (12–24 h)**

There is cardiorespiratory failure:

– with tachycardia, hypertension, tachypnoea and pulmonary oedema.

- **Late (1–3 days)**

There is renal impairment

– with kidney pain and acute tubular necrosis.

Death occurs at this time from multiorgan failure in severely poisoned patients if untreated.

> The diagnosis should be suspected in a patient who is inebriated or comatose with a metabolic acidosis and increased anion gap. There may be an associated neutrophilia, hyperkalaemia and hypocalcaemia.
>
> Urinalysis may show oxalate crystals, as well as haematuria and proteinuria. The presence of calcium oxalate crystals in the urine is characteristic and is more the renal reflection of massive oxalate crystal deposition in tissues throughout the body rather than a manifestation solely of renal clearance of toxic metabolites.

Treatment comprises:

- *gastric lavage;*
- *cardiorespiratory support;*
- *correction of metabolic acidosis (often requiring up to 1000 mmol or more of bicarbonate);*
- *correction of hypocalcaemia;*
- *administration of ethyl alcohol to compete for alcohol dehydrogenase (as for methanol poisoning, q.v.);*
- *administration of **fomepizole** (4-methylpyrazole, 4–MP, Antizol), an expensive new agent recently shown to inhibit alcohol dehydrogenase and thus prevent the production of toxic metabolites, its dosage being 15 mg/kg iv initially followed by 10 mg/kg each 12 h for 48 h followed by 15 mg/kg each 12 h until the plasma ethylene glycol level is <200 mg/L or 3.2 mmol/L;*
- *dialysis or haemofiltration (if the plasma ethylene glycol concentration is >500 mg/L or >8 mmol/L).*

Early diagnosis and treatment is important, because the mortality is high without treatment but virtually nil with treatment.

Bibliography

Brent J, McMartin K, Phillips S et al 1999 Fomepizole for the treatment of ethylene glycol poisoning. N Engl J Med 340: 832.

DaRoza R, Henning RI, Sunshine I et al 1984 Acute ethylene glycol poisoning. Crit Care Med 12: 103.

Hantson Ph, Hassoun A, Mahieu P 1998 Ethylene glycol poisoning treated by intravenous 4-methylpyrazole. Intens Care Med 24: 736.

Jacobsen D, McMartin KE 1997 Antidotes for methanol and ethylene glycol poisoning. J Toxicol Clin Toxicol 35: 127.

Jacobsen D, McMartin KE 1986 Methanol and ethylene glycol poisoning: mechanism of toxicity, clinical course, diagnosis and treatment. Med Toxicol 1: 309.

Karlson-Stiber C, Persson H 1992 Ethylene glycol poisoning: experience from an epidemic in Sweden. J Toxicol Clin Toxicol 30: 565.

Kulig K, Duffy JP, Lenden CH et al 1984 Toxic effects of methanol, ethylene glycol and isopropyl alcohol. Topics in Emerg Med 6: 14.

Parry MF, Wallach R 1974 Ethylene glycol poisoning. Am J Med 57: 143.

Shannon M 1998 Toxicology reviews: fomepizole – a new antidote. Pediatr Emerg Care 14: 170.

Euthyroid sick syndrome

The assessment of thyroid function is difficult in the seriously ill patient. This is because a variety of abnormalities of thyroid function tests may be found which seemingly reflect hypothyroidism, even in the absence of intrinsic thyroid disease. This state has thus been referred to as the euthyroid sick syndrome, and it may reflect the neuroendocrine effects of cytokines. It can occur very early in the course of serious illness, especially sepsis.

Many aspects of serious illness affect thyroid function tests, including:

- systemic illness

  - perhaps mediated by TNFα;

- some specific conditions

  - especially starvation and diabetes mellitus;

- several commonly used drugs

  - notably dopamine, which decreases all thyroid function indices;
  - also corticosteroids, amiodarone and radiographic contrast media, which decrease total T3;

- selenium deficiency

  - related to the impaired peripheral deiodination of T4 to form T3.

In the euthyroid sick syndrome, abnormalities of most thyroid function tests are found.

- **Total T4**:

  - is typically low, because of low TBG or impaired protein binding;
  - occasionally, it may even be increased, because of increased TBG.

- **Free T4**:

  - is normal if directly measured;
  - though if calculated it can be misleadingly low.

- **Total T3 and free T3**:

  - are typically also low, because of decreased peripheral conversion of T4 to T3.

- **TSH**:

  - is normal or low, even in the presence of a low T4 and T3.
  - This may be due to euthyroidism, to hypothalamic or pituitary depression, or to dopamine, which impairs the TSH response to TRH.
  - The TSH is of course low if there is secondary hypothyroidism.
  - It is also decreased by starvation and corticosteroids, as well as by dopamine.
  - The TSH may be abnormally increased for several weeks before returning to normal following recovery from serious illness.

The clinical significance of these abnormalities of thyroid function tests is uncertain. While the low T3 may be homeostatic and thus possibly beneficial, a low T4 is associated with an increased mortality, though it is presumably only a marker as replacement therapy does not improve survival.

In general, the normal ranges for thyroid function tests which have been established in well subjects are inappropriate for the assessment of seriously ill patients.

Nevertheless, the diagnosis of genuine hypothyroidism is important because it is curable, though the erroneous treatment of a euthyroid patient is potentially dangerous.

The most practical approach is to rely on the TSH level, which if elevated generally indicates hypothyroidism and if low generally indicates euthyroidism.

While hypothyroidism will not be overdiagnosed in this way, it may be underdiagnosed if one of the other causes of a low TSH is present, as described above. Laboratory tests thus need to be complemented by clinical features, including past history, goitre, hypothermia or associated autoimmune disorders.

If there is clinical hypothyroidism, especially if the TSH is high, thyroxine should be given.

Bibliography

Berger MM, Reymond MJ, Shenkin A et al 2001 Influence of selenium supplements on the post-traumatic alterations of the thyroid axis. Intens Care Med 27: 91.

Docter R, Krenning EP, De Jong M et al 1993 The sick euthyroid syndrome: changes in thyroid hormone serum parameters and hormone metabolism. Clin Endocrinol 39: 499.

Kaptein EM, Spencer CA, Kamiel MB et al 1980 Prolonged dopamine administration and thyroid hormone economy in normal and critically ill subjects. J Clin Endocrinol Metab 51: 387.

Ramsay I 1985 Drug and non-thyroid induced changes in thyroid function tests. Postgrad Med J 61: 375.

Surks MI, Chopra IJ, Mariash CN et al 1990 American Thyroid Association guidelines for use of laboratory tests in thyroid disorders. JAMA 263: 1529.

Wartofsky L, Burman KD 1982 Alterations in thyroid function in patients with systemic illness:"The euthyroid sick syndrome". Endocrinol Rev 3: 164.

Exfoliative dermatitis

Exfoliative dermatitis (erythroderma) can complicate a number of dermatological and systemic problems, including psoriasis (especially following steroid withdrawal), atopic dermatitis, contact dermatitis, ichthyosis, drug eruptions and lymphoma. Its most generalized form is called the **Stevens–Johnson syndrome** (see Erythema multiforme).

The **staphylococcal scalded skin syndrome** (SSSS) is a form of exfoliative dermatitis, which is produced by the exfoliative toxin of *S. aureus*. It is sometimes called toxic epidermal necrolysis (TEN) type I. The toxin produces an intraepidermal cleavage plane.

There is a diffuse tender scarlatiniform rash with bullae and an associated fever.

Treatment of SSSS is with **flucloxacillin** *or* **dicloxacillin** *(or vancomycin if the organism is methicillin-resistant) and resuscitation, and corticosteroids are possibly helpful in some cases.*

The mortality is less than 5%.

SSSS needs to be distinguished from **toxic epidermal necrolysis** (TEN) type II, which is usually a drug reaction and probably autoimmune-mediated. It is a rare but severe form of Stevens–Johnson syndrome, and is thus the most severe cutaneous drug reaction. Its initial report by Lyell in 1956 described it as a 'scalded skin syndrome', and subsequently it was sometimes referred to as Lyell's syndrome.

It is a severe epidermal necrosis with blistering and a burns-like appearance. The cleavage plane is at the epidermal–dermal junction, i. e. deeper than for type I.

It is usually associated with allopurinol, anticonvulsants, minocycline, NSAIDs, or sulfonamides, though it can also occur in graft-versus-host disease and in mycoplasma infection.

*Treatment of TEN type II is as a **burn**, and corticosteroids should be avoided. Plasma exchange has sometimes been recommended, but there is doubt about its efficacy.*

The mortality is 25–50%, and death is due either to sepsis or to organ involvement (especially the gut or lungs).

Bibliography

Kim P, Goldfarb P, Gaisford T et al 1983 Stevens–Johnson syndrome and toxic epidermal necrolysis. J Burn Care Rehabil 4: 93.

Lyell A 1967 A review of toxic epidermal necrolysis in Britain. Br J Dermatol 79: 662.

Melish ME, Glasgow LA, Turner MD 1972 The staphylococcal scalded-skin syndrome: isolation and partial purification of the exfoliative toxin. J Infect Dis 125: 129.

Nicolis GD, Helwig EB 1973 Exfoliative dermatitis: a clinicopathologic study of 135 cases. Arch Dermatol 108: 788.

Roujeau JC, Kelly JP, Naldi L et al 1995 Medication use and the risk of Stevens–Johnson syndrome or toxic epidermal necrolysis. N Engl J Med 333: 1600.

Schwartz RA 1997 Toxic epidermal necrolysis. Cutis 59: 123.

Sehgal VN, Gangwani OP 1987 Fixed drug eruption: current concepts. Int J Dermatol 26: 67.

Thestrup-Pedersen K, Halkier-Sorensen L, Sogaard H et al 1988 The red man syndrome: exfoliative dermatitis of unknown etiology. J Am Acad Dermatol 18: 1307.

Exophthalmos (see Hyperthyroidism)

Exotic pneumonia

Exotic pneumonia is the term applied to pulmonary infection due to an unusual organism.

This unusual organism may be either:

- common, though not as a respiratory pathogen; or
- uncommon and infectious by virtue of an unusual environment.

The **'common'** organisms include:

- some viruses and rickettsiae;
- bacteria, such as atypical mycobacteria and actinomyces;
- fungi, such as aspergillus and cryptococcus;
- protozoa, such as toxoplasma.

These organisms cause pneumonia mainly in compromised hosts. In these patients, the diagnostic net has to be cast somewhat wider than usual if one of the more expected organisms is not readily isolated.

The **'uncommon'** organisms include:

- bacteria giving rise to melioidosis, nocardiosis, plague, anthrax, tularaemia;
- many fungi which have restricted geographical distribution, such as histoplasma, coccidioidomycosis and blastomyces.

These organisms are generally identifiable, provided there is a high level of clinical suspicion of unusual pathogens in patients who may have acquired their infection in an unfamiliar environment, usually as travellers.

Extrinsic allergic alveolitis (see

Hypersensitivity pneumonitis)

Factitious disorders

A factitious (i.e. artificial) disorder is one which generally mimics a known disease state but which is self-inflicted, usually in a conscious and manipulative way. It is thus related to, but separate from, other self-inflicted problems, such as drug overdose or trauma (self-mutilation). These latter conditions are not only much more common but usually also much more readily identifiable.

A number of factitious disorders may sometimes be encountered in seriously ill patients, particularly in those with personality disorders. There is often associated drug abuse, but the separation from real specific disease can sometimes be difficult.

The most important factitious disorders include:

- bleeding;
- dermatitis;
- diarrhoea;
- fever;
- hyperthyroidism;
- hypoglycaemia.

Familial hypocalciuric hypercalcaemia (see

Hyperparathyroidism)

Fanconi's syndrome

Fanconi's syndrome consists of increased renal excretion of glucose, amino acids (see Aminoaciduria), phosphate and uric acid, due to abnormal proximal renal tubular reabsorption.

It occurs in:

- tubulointerstitial diseases (especially allergic interstitial nephritis, such as that due to beta-lactam antibiotics or outdated tetracycline);
- heavy metal poisoning (such as from lead or cadmium);

- Sjögren's syndrome occasionally.

It can lead to osteomalacia.

The serum phosphate, bicarbonate and often calcium are low, and the alkaline phosphatase increased, while levels of vitamin D and parathyroid hormone (PTH) are normal.

*Treatment is with **vitamin D**, **phosphate** and **bicarbonate**.*

Bibliography

Brenton DP, Isenberg DA, Cusworth DC et al 1981 The adult presenting Fanconi syndrome. J Inh Metab Dis 4: 211.

Farmer's lung (see Hypersensitivity pneumonitis)

Fasciitis

There are a number of forms of **fasciitis**.

- **Necrotizing fasciitis** (see Gangrene)
- **Eosinophilic fasciitis**. This superficially resembles scleroderma. The skin is actually normal, but the subcutaneous fascia contains an inflammatory infiltrate.

The aetiology is unknown, but it has been reported following severe muscular exertion. There is marked eosinophilia with a raised ESR. Rheumatoid serology is negative.

*The condition is self-limited, though improvement is hastened by low-dose **corticosteroids**.*

- **Local fasciitis**. These include Dupuytren's, plantar fasciitis, diabetic stiff hand syndrome.

- **Fournier's gangrene** (see Gangrene)

Felty's syndrome

Felty's syndrome consists of seropositive rheumatoid arthritis with splenomegaly and neutropenia.

Clinical manifestations often also include fever, weight loss, hepatomegaly, lymphadenopathy, skin pigmentation and ulceration.

Investigations typically show a white cell count of $1.5–2.0 \times 10^9$/L with a neutropenia of $0.5–1.0 \times 10^9$/L.

Neutropenia due to other rheumatic diseases, such as SLE, or to marrow depressant therapy, such as gold, needs to be excluded.

Sometimes the neutropenia is severe (i.e. $<0.5 \times 10^9$/L). It may thus be associated with recurrent infections, especially of the lungs and skin, and particularly with Gram-negative bacilli, staphylococci and streptococci.

The pathogenetic mechanisms of neutropenia are probably multiple and include impaired granulopoiesis, which may be T-cell mediated, increased peripheral destruction and increased margination.

Thrombocytopenia is common but is not usually marked.

Treatment is required if the condition is severe.

- *While **corticosteroids** may be useful symptomatically, they may exacerbate infection.*
- ***Splenectomy** may be considered, but continued improvement in the neutrophil count occurs in only about 30% of patients after such surgery.*
- *Disease-modifying drugs such as **gold** may be useful.*
- *Cytokine therapy with **G-CSF** offers new potential.*

Bibliography
Goldberg J, Pinals RS 1980 Felty syndrome. Semin Arthritis Rheum 10: 52.
Spivak JL 1977 Felty's syndrome: an analytical review. Johns Hopkins Med J 141: 156.

Fetal haemoglobin

Fetal haemoglobin (HbF) contains 2-alpha and 2-gamma chains (i.e. it is designated alpha-2 gamma-2). In normal adult haemoglobin, the gamma chains have changed to beta chains, and there is usually only $<2\%$ of residual fetal haemoglobin. Its persistence in larger amounts is chiefly seen in thalassaemia (q.v.).

HbF is also seen in the syndrome of 'hereditary persistence of fetal haemoglobin', an autosomal dominant condition resulting from several gene abnormalities. Homozygotes have 100% HbF and heterozygotes 50%. Whereas traditionally this condition was considered to be asymptomatic, more recently some cases have been found to be anaemic.

Fever (see Pyrexia)

Fever of unknown origin (see Pyrexia)

Fibrinolysis

Fibrinolysis is the process which removes thrombotic material and remodels acute lumenal obstruction, thus restoring vascular patency. Like other plasma enzyme cascades, the fibrinolytic sequence comprises:

- an inactive precursor;
- an active enzyme;
- stimulatory and inhibitory influences;
- substrate;
- end-products.

> Fibrinolysis is one of the four inter-related enzyme cascades (the other three being the coagulation, kinin and complement systems) which are responsible for integrating many of the bodily responses to injury and which are all triggered by activation of factor XII.

Plasminogen activator is released as tissue plasminogen activator (t-PA) locally from damaged endothelial cells and also from a variety of other tissues. Activator converts the inactive circulating precursor, plasminogen, to the active enzyme, plasmin, a broad protease but with a special appetite for fibrin (and also to a lesser extent fibrinogen and other coagulation factors). Other substances may also activate plasminogen, including natural agents, such as urokinase (the plasminogen activator in urine) or exogenous products (such as bacteria-derived streptokinase).

The effect of plasminogen activator and of plasmin are modulated by the circulating inhibitors, plasminogen activator inhibitor (PAI, especially PAI-1) and by antiplasmin (especially α_2-antiplasmin, α_2-AP).

Plasmin lyses fibrin by combining with its lysine-binding site, a site which may be blocked by α_2-AP and by substances resembling lysine, such as epsilon aminocaproic acid (EACA). When fibrin is laid down in a thrombus, circulating plasminogen is incorporated into this clot. It is this plasminogen which is preferentially activated to plasmin by t-PA, partly because it is protected from circulating inhibitors.

Clinical disease arises from disturbed fibrinolysis, either thrombosis from impaired fibrinolysis or haemorrhage from enhanced fibrinolysis.

Impaired fibrinolysis may be due to:

- decreased t-PA synthesis and/or release;
- increased PAI-1;
- abnormal or deficient plasminogen (rarely).

Impaired fibrinolysis is one of the potential causes of a hypercoagulable state.

Enhanced fibrinolysis is uncommon. Its presence is reflected in raised levels of fibrin/fibrinogen degradation products.

It gives rise to a haemorrhagic diathesis which is treatable with EACA.

- **Primary fibrinolysis** is rare and may include congenital α_2-AP deficiency. It is systemic.
- **Secondary fibrinolysis** is the more common pathological abnormality and may be either systemic or local.

Systemic secondary fibrinolysis may be seen:

- in acute promyelocytic leukaemia;
- after congenital heart surgery;
- in primary amyloidosis;
- in disseminated intravascular coagulation (the most common situation and one in which it is often compensatory).

Local secondary fibrinolysis is most frequently seen after prostatectomy. It may also be involved in some cases of bleeding from the gums, stomach, large bowel, uterus and perhaps subarachnoid space.

Bibliography

Collen D, Lijnen HR 1991 Basic and clinical aspects of fibrinolysis and thrombolysis. Blood 78: 3114.
Prins MH, Hirsh J 1991 A critical review of the evidence supporting a relationship between impaired fibrinolytic activity and venous thromboembolism. Arch Intern Med 151: 1721.

Fish envenomation (see Bites and stings (marine vertebrates))

Flushing

The causes of flushing are:

- **acne rosacea**

This is an acneiform eruption on the face, associated with flushing and sometimes with rhinophyma. It is of unknown cause. Eventually, the erythema can be persistent. It is aggravated by heat, cold, sun and wind and may be associated with gastritis.

*Treatment is with oral **tetracycline**. **Isotretinoin** may be used in severe cases, though recently severe depression has sometimes been reported in young patients receiving this drug.*

- **alcohol**

This is because acetaldehyde, the metabolite produced by alcohol dehydrogenase, is a vasodilator.

- anaphylaxis
- carcinoid tumour
- cluster headache
- drugs

These include especially calcitonin, disulfiram (with alcohol), desmopressin (DDAVP) in high-dose, nifedipine, pentamidine.

- **fever**
- **food**

This occurs with some types of food poisoning, including mushrooms (q.v.) and scombroid (q.v.),

- **mastocytosis** (see Urticaria)

- **menopause**

In this, flushing (or flashing) is associated with declining oestrogen levels in about 80% of women. The flushing is probably hypothalamic in origin and is associated with a feeling of heat, then sweating and a rise in surface temperature but a fall in core temperature.

Bibliography
Pochi PE 1983 Hormones, retinoids and acne. N Engl J Med 308: 1024.

Folic acid deficiency (see also Megaloblastic anaemia and Neural tube defects)

Folic acid together with vitamin B_{12} is required for the metabolism of single carbon units and thus for DNA synthesis.

Folic acid deficiency arises from:

- a poor or unusual diet;
- small bowel disease (because 80% of folic acid is absorbed in the small intestine);
- alcoholism;
- chronic renal failure;
- haemolysis;
- pregnancy;
- drugs which interfere with folic acid metabolism (e.g. anti-tuberculous agents, ethanol, methotrexate, phenytoin, sulfasalazine, trimethoprim).

Folic acid deficiency is associated with a megaloblastic anaemia, often with thrombocytopenia but without the features of pernicious anaemia.

Concomitant iron deficiency is frequent, thereby blocking megaloblastosis, but typical hypersegmented neutrophils are still apparent.

There is an increased incidence of **neural tube defects** in babies of mothers who are either folic acid deficient or who fail to take folic acid supplementation during pregnancy.

Since the serum folate may fall rapidly, e.g. within two weeks, in the absence of intake, but the body stores are not yet depleted, the RBC folate level best reflects overall folic acid deficiency. The serum B_{12} level should always be measured, as concomitant deficiency of vitamin B_{12} is frequent.

Treatment is usually with a daily oral dose of 1 mg, though as little as 200 µg is in fact generally adequate. If the diagnosis is correct, treatment gives haematological improvement within a few days.

Folliculitis

Folliculitis is inflammation of the hair follicle giving rise a small pustule. It is usually caused by *S. aureus* or occasionally by *P. aeruginosa*.

Treatment is local, unless the process is extensive, in which case antibiotics are indicated.

Food poisoning

Although food poisoning is a very common condition, its presentation in Intensive Care is uncommon and moreover it may take a number of unusual forms. The types of food poisoning considered in this book include:

- botulism;
- Chinese-restaurant syndrome;
- ciguatera;

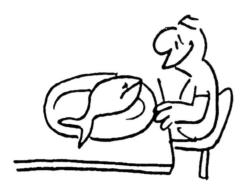 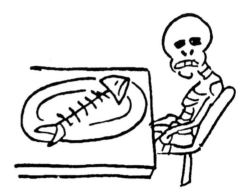

- mushroom poisoning;
- scombroid.

In addition, some aspects of food poisoning are of an infectious nature and are considered more generally (e.g. see Diarrhoea and Norwalk virus).

Bibliography
Haddad LM, Shannon MW, Winchester JF (eds) 1997 Clinical Management of Poisoning and Drug Overdose. 3rd edition. Philadelphia: WB Saunders.

Hughes JM, Merson MH 1976 Fish and shellfish poisoning. N Engl J Med 295: 1117.

Morse DL, Guzewich JJ, Hanrahan JP et al 1986 Widespread outbreaks of clam- and oyster-associated gastroenteritis: role of Norwalk virus. N Engl J Med 314: 678.

Olson KR (ed) 1998 Poisoning and Drug Overdose. 3rd edition. Norwalk: Appleton & Lange.

Trujillo MH, Guerrero J, Fragachan C et al 1998 Pharmacologic antidotes in critical care medicine: a practical guide for drug administration. Crit Care Med 26: 377.

Formaldehyde

Formaldehyde (methanal, HCHO) is a colourless, flammable, pungent and irritating gas. It is the simplest aldehyde and is derived from the oxidation of methanol. It is an organic compound extensively used in the chemical industry, in which it is the base for some explosives, tanning agents and disinfectants. Formalin is a 37% aqueous solution of formaldehyde.

Local damage and systemic toxicity result from its ingestion.

There is no specific treatment.

Fournier's gangrene (see Gangrene)

Friedreich's ataxia (see Cerebellar degeneration)

Frostbite (see also Hypothermia)

When the environmental temperature is less than freezing, atmospheric water vapour becomes ice-crystals (i.e. frost) without first becoming a liquid (i.e. dew).

Frostbite refers to the freezing of tissues, with intracellular ice formation giving rise to mechanical disruption of cells, cellular dehydration, deranged cellular metabolism, haemolysis, thrombosis and gangrene. The tissues start to freeze from about $-2°C$.

Frostbite arises from cold environmental temperature, often with wind, and usually with various risk factors. Risk factors include:

- lack of food or clothing;
- excess exercise;
- illness;
- injury;
- dehydration;
- psychosis;

- alcohol;
- mechanical constriction.

It affects mainly the extremities, which appear cold, white, hard, waxy and pulseless and are affected to a varying depth. The process begins with stinging and is followed by aching and finally numbness.

Reperfusion injury during rewarming may contribute to some of the damage of frostbite.

The complications of frostbite are:

- local or systemic infection;
- gangrene;
- local neurological damage;
- pain, stiffness, wasting, scarring, loss of the subcutaneous fat pad and deformity in the affected part.

Treatment consists of **emergency rewarming**. *The core temperature should be restored if necessary and the affected part thawed rapidly (e.g. with water warmed to 42°C). This may give rise to blistering, which is associated with skin hyperaemia and can be painful and lead to necrosis. Movement should be avoided*

- *Tetanus toxoid and perhaps antibiotics should be given.*
- *Many forms of adjuvant pharmacological therapy, including vasodilators, antithrombotics, anti-inflammatory agents and free radical scavengers,*

have been explored, but they have not been subjected to formal clinical trial.

The prognosis is worse if the cold injury has been of long duration, if the thawing process is slow, and in particular if refreezing occurs. Refreezing is such a serious issue because of resultant enhanced tissue damage that rewarming should be deferred if there is any risk of refreezing occurring.

Prevention of frostbite comprises measures both to maintain core temperature and to prevent local exposure, though these simple but effective principles may not always be achievable. The risk is particularly increased in winter sports and especially if exercise is curtailed because of exhaustion, injury or equipment breakdown.

Furunculosis

149

Furunculosis (boils) refers to deep, inflammatory nodules around hair follicles. They are staphylococcal and can lead to bacteraemia and even metastatic abscesses, endocarditis and/or shock, especially in immunocompromised patients. They may be associated with nasal carriage of the organism or with poor hygiene.

Treatment is by **drainage** *if the lesion is fluctuant and with* **antibiotics** *if there is associated cellulitis or systemic features.*

Gamma-hydroxybutyric acid

Gamma-hydroxybutyric acid (GHB) occurs naturally in the central nervous system and was synthesized in the 1960s. It has been variously used or studied as an anaesthetic, an adjunct in alcohol or opiate withdrawal, a treatment for narcolepsy, an agent to reduce tissue oxygen demand in resuscitation and sepsis, and a stimulator of growth hormone (particularly for body builders). Because of its ability to impair consciousness and to provide associated relaxation, euphoria, disinhibition and increased sensuality, it has recently become a popular but illegal drug of abuse particularly at parties and has been labelled in the press as the 'date rape' drug.

Intoxication can cause profound unconsciousness, with flaccid paralysis, hypothermia, bradycardia, hypotension and respiratory depression. Recovery occurs within a few hours.

Laboratory tests are normal, except that other drugs may have also been taken concomitantly.

*Treatment is generally **supportive**, with particular care to protect the airway.*

- *Atropine is useful for bradycardia.*
- *Neither naloxone nor flumazenil have any reversal effect, but physostigmine may be effective.*

Bibliography

Henderson RS, Holmes CM 1976 Reversal of the anaesthetic action of sodium gamma-hydroxybutyrate. Anaesth Intens Care 4: 351.

Li J, Stokes SA, Wockener A 1998 A tale of novel intoxication: a review of the effects of gamma-hydroxybutyric acid with recommendations for management. Ann Emerg Med 31: 729.

Viera AJ, Yates SW 1999 Toxic ingestion of gamma-hydroxybutyric acid. South Med J 92: 404.

Ganciclovir (see Acyclovir)

Gangrene

Most cases of gangrene involve the lower limb and are due to peripheral ischaemia from atherosclerotic disease. However, some are due to:

- embolism;
- infection;
- thromboangitis obliterans (Buerger's disease);
- trauma;
- vasculitis.

Infectious gangrene (gangrenous cellulitis) is a severe type of skin infection which takes a number of forms. These include:

- necrotizing fasciitis, both streptococcal and non-streptococcal;
- progressive bacterial synergistic gangrene;
- pyoderma gangrenosum;
- pseudomonal gangrenous cellulitis;
- necrotizing cutaneous mucormycosis.

---

1. **Necrotizing fasciitis** may be either streptococcal or non-streptococcal.

Streptococcal infection is caused by group A streptococci which may uncommonly cause a rapid-onset cellulitis, with skin necrosis and subcutaneous gangrene. It usually affects a limb and typically follows surgical or traumatic injury, though diabetes, varicella infection and immunosuppression are also important predisposing factors.

Invasive group A streptococcal infections occur in about 1 in 10 000 of the population per year in developed countries and are complicated by necrotizing fasciitis in 5–10% of cases. A spate of such cases in the UK recently received much dramatic publicity, with detailed descriptions of the destruction caused by the 'new, flesh-eating' germ. The resurgence of such infections does not appear to have a clonal basis, as the responsible strains are genetically heterogeneous.

The affected part is initially blue, but then dark fluid-filled bullae appear, which subsequently rupture revealing non-crepitant gangrene. The lesion is painful and appears like a deep burn. There is also associated systemic toxicity, usually phlebitis, commonly bacteraemia and/or myositis, and sometimes the 'toxic strep syndrome' (q.v.).

The mortality is high (about 30%) despite penicillin and surgery, so that early diagnosis is important. The extent and depth of the necrosis can best be determined by CT or MRI.

Non-streptococcal infection is usually polymicrobial and is seen after abdominal infection or in diabetics. The organisms involved include Gram-negative bacilli, anaerobes and enterococci (i.e. enteric pathogens).

The intra-abdominal process tends to extend rapidly to the abdominal wall, with local pain and crepitus and systemic toxicity.

The chief differential diagnosis is a clostridial infection or perhaps a spider bite.

If the male genitalia are involved, the condition is called **Fournier's gangrene**.

Treatment is with **antibiotics** *(aminoglycoside and metronidazole), extensive surgical* **debridement**, *general* **support**, *and probably* **hyperbaric oxygen**.

2. **Progressive bacterial synergistic gangrene** (Meleney's progressive synergistic gangrene) is usually associated with a pre-existing lesion, including a colostomy.

There is a painful non-crepitant ragged ulceration, with an inner rim of gangrene, a middle rim of purple erythema and an outer rim of pink oedematous skin. The process tends to extend only slowly.

The infection is usually polymicrobial and involves microaerophilic streptococci, together with either Gram-negative bacilli or *S. aureus*.

Treatment usually requires extensive surgical **debridement** *and systemic* **antibiotics**.

3. **Pyoderma gangrenosum** (q.v.).

4. **Pseudomonal gangrenous cellulitis** comprises a circumscribed non-crepitant largely painless lesion, with a necrotic centre and erythematous halo.

It is seen in patients with burns or who are immunocompromised. It has a rapid onset and produces systemic toxicity.

5. **Necrotizing cutaneous mucormycosis** is a non-painful, non-crepitant lesion consisting of a necrotic centre with a purple heaped margin.

It is usually found in diabetics as a slowly progressive lesion which does not produce systemic toxicity.

Bibliography

Bessman AN, Wagner W 1975 Nonclostridial gas gangrene. JAMA 233: 958.

Bisno AL, Stevens DL 1996 Streptococcal infections of skin and soft tissue. N Engl J Med 334: 240.

Brown RD, Davis NL, Lepawski M et al 1994 A multicentre review of the treatment of major truncal necrotising infections with and without hyperbaric oxygen therapy. Am J Surg 167: 483.

Davies HD, McGeer A, Schwartz B et al 1996 Invasive group A streptococcal infections in Ontario, Canada. N Engl J Med 335: 547.

Elliott DC, Kufera JA, Myers RAM et al 1996 Necrotizing soft tissue infections: risk factors for mortality and strategies for management. Ann Surg 224: 672.

Giuliano A, Lewis F, Hadley K et al 1977 Bacteriology of necrotizing fasciitis. Am J Surg 134: 52.

Green RJ, Dafoe DC, Raffin TA 1996 Necrotizing fasciitis. Chest 110: 219.

Jarrett P, Rademaker M, Duffill M 1997 The clinical spectrum of necrotising fasciitis. Aust NZ J Med 27: 29.

Riegels-Nielsen P, Hesselfeldt-Nielsen J, Bang-Jensen E et al 1984 Fournier's gangrene. J Urol 132: 918.

Stevens DL 1992 Invasive group A Streptococcus infections. Clin Infect Dis 14: 2.

Stevens DL 1999 The flesh-eating bacterium. I Infect Dis 179 (suppl 2): S366.

Stone HH, Martin JJ 1972 Synergistic necrotizing cellulitis. Ann Surg 175: 702.

Unsworth IP, Sharp PA 1984 Gas gangrene: an 11-year review of 73 cases managed with hyperbaric oxygen. Med J Aust 140: 256.

Weinstein L, Barza MA 1973 Gas gangrene. N Engl J Med 289: 1129.

Gas gangrene (see Clostridial infections)

Gas in soft tissues

Gas in soft tissues may be due to:

- **Anaerobic cellulitis** due to clostridial infection, usually produced by *C. perfringens* (see Clostridial infections).
- **Necrotizing fasciitis** (see Gangrene), especially polymicrobial cellulitis. This is seen particularly in diabetics or perineal infection. Gram-negative enteric bacilli (especially *E. coli* and klebsiella) are usually present, and anaerobes (bacteroides) are common.
- **Trapped air**, which usually arises from a procedural, surgical or traumatic injury, though it may sometimes be caused by a compressed gas injury or by deep hydrogen peroxide irrigation. Gas from trapped air does not spread, unless it connects with a tension pneumothorax.

Bibliography

Bessman AN, Wagner W 1975 Nonclostridial gas gangrene. JAMA 233: 958.

Giuliano A, Lewis F, Hadley K et al 1977 Bacteriology of necrotizing fasciitis. Am J Surg 134: 52.

Unsworth IP, Sharp PA 1984 Gas gangrene: an 11-year review of 73 cases managed with hyperbaric oxygen. Med J Aust 140: 256.

Weinstein L, Barza MA 1973 Gas gangrene. N Engl J Med 289: 1129.

Gastric emptying

For solid food, the normal half-time of gastric emptying is <1 h. For liquids, the half-life in the stomach is normally about 20 min, but this can be greatly increased in the seriously ill.

In Intensive Care patients, gastroparesis (i.e. delayed gastric emptying) of varying degree occurs in a large of number of conditions, though it is most typically seen in diabetes.

Gastroparesis may respond to treatment with **prokinetic** *drugs, such as metoclopramide, cisapride or domperidone.*

Gastrinoma (see Zollinger–Ellison syndrome)

Gastroenteritis (see Diarrhoea)

Gastroenterology

Gastrointestinal dysfunction of a general nature is very common in the seriously ill, and some would say it is virtually invariable. On the one hand, the gut is a target organ of many systemic insults, and on the other hand, the gut may itself contribute to adverse systemic responses by mechanisms such as cytokine release, enzyme spill or bacterial translocation.

Less common specific gastrointestinal disorders are also sometimes encountered, and those considered in this book include:

- achlorhydria;
- angiodysplasia;
- anorectal infections;
- cholangitis;
- cholestasis;
- colitis;
- Crohn's disease;
- diarrhoea;
- dysphagia;
- enterocolitis;
- food poisoning;
- gastric emptying;
- gastroenteritis;
- gingivitis;
- glossitis;
- inflammatory bowel disease;
- malabsorption;
- Mallory–Weiss syndrome;
- mouth diseases;
- pancreatitis;
- parotitis;
- Plummer–Vinson syndrome;
- pneumatosis coli;
- short bowel syndrome;
- stomatitis;
- tongue;
- ulcerative colitis;
- Whipple's disease.

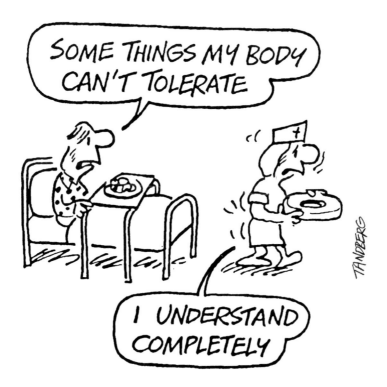

Bibliography

Barie PS, Fischer E, Eachempati SR 1999 Acute acalculous cholecystitis. Curr Opin Crit Care 5: 144.

Blaser MJ, Smith PD, Ravdin JL et al (eds) 1995 Infections of the Gastrointestinal Tract. New York: Raven Press.

Doe WF 1993 The immunology of the gut. In: Peters PJ, Rosen FS, Walport M (eds) Clinical Aspects of Immunology. 4th edition. Oxford: Blackwell. p 2079.

Go VLW et al (eds) 1993 The Pancreas: Biology, Pathobiology and Diseases. New York: Raven Press.

Johnston DE, Kaplan MM 1993 Pathogenesis and treatment of gallstones. N Engl J Med 328: 412.

Powell LW, Piper DW (eds) 1995 Fundamentals of Gastroenterology. 6th edition. Sydney: McGraw-Hill.

Shearman DJC, Finlayson NDC 1989 Diseases of the Gastrointestinal Tract and Liver. 2nd edition. Edinburgh: Churchill Livingstone.

Sherlock S, Dooley J 1993 Diseases of the Liver and Biliary System. 9th edition. Oxford: Blackwell.

Sleisenger MH, Fordtran JS (eds) 1993 Gastrointestinal Disease: Pathophysiology, Diagnosis and Management. 5th edition. Philadelphia: WB Saunders.

Germ warfare (see Anthrax and Warfare agents)

Giant cell arteritis (see Arteritis)

Gingivitis (see Mouth diseases)

Glomerular diseases

Glomerular diseases are mostly immunological in origin, and their distinction is made on renal biopsy. They are responsible for either nephritic and/or nephrotic clinical pictures.

The **nephritic response** comprises:

- haematuria;
- proteinuria;

- hypertension;
- renal impairment.

There is an active urine sediment, with red cell, white cell and granular casts, including abnormal or dysmorphic red blood cell shapes.

The nephritic picture may be produced by either focal or diffuse glomerular disease.

- **Focal disease** involves <50% of glomeruli. It includes:

  - IgA nephropathy;
  - thin basement membrane disease;
  - SLE;
  - Alport's syndrome (hereditary nephritis with deafness and cataracts).

- **Diffuse disease** involves >50% of glomeruli. It includes:

  - rapidly progressive or crescentic glomerulonephritis (including Goodpasture's syndrome);
  - membrano-proliferative (mesangiocapillary) glomerulonephritis;
  - fibrillary glomerulonephritis;
  - post-infectious glomerulonephritis;
  - SLE;
  - vasculitis.

The **nephrotic response** comprises:

- marked proteinuria (>3 g/day), due to podocyte damage;
- hypoalbuminaemia;
- oedema;
- hypercoagulability;
- hyperlipidaemia.

The urine sediment shows fatty casts, sometimes with haematuria.

The nephrotic picture may be produced by:

- **membranous nephropathy** (30%);
- **minimal change disease** (20%);
- **focal segmental glomerulosclerosis** (FSGS) (15%);

- **systemic disorders** (25%), including:

  - diabetes;
  - amyloid;
  - pre-eclampsia;
  - autoimmune diseases (especially SLE);
  - infection;
  - malignancy;
  - drugs (NSAIDs, captopril, gold, lithium, mercury, penicillamine);

- **membrano-proliferative glomerulonephritis** (occasionally);
- **post-infectious glomerulonephritis** (occasionally).

Bibliography

Abraham PA, Keane WF 1984 Glomerular and interstitial disease induced by nonsteroidal anti-inflammatory drugs. Am J Nephrol 4: 1.

Balow J 1985 Renal vasculitis. Kidney Int 27: 954.

Balow JE, Austin HA, Tsokos GC et al 1987 Lupus nephritis. Ann Intern Med 106: 79.

Kincaid-Smith P 1980 Analgesic abuse and the kidney. Kidney Int 17: 250.

Llach F 1985 Hypercoagulability, renal vein thrombosis, and other thrombotic complications of the nephrotic syndrome. Kidney Int 28: 429.

Morgan DB, Dillon S, Payne RB 1978 The assessment of glomerular function: creatinine clearance or plasma creatinine? Postgrad Med J 54: 302.

Muirhead N 1999 Management of idiopathic membranous nephropathy: evidence-based recommendations. Kidney Int 70 (suppl): S47.

Nolin L 1999 Courteau M. Management of IgA nephropathy: evidence based recommendations. Kidney Int 70 (suppl): S56.

Ronco PM, Flahault A 1994 Drug-induced end-stage renal disease. N Engl J Med 331: 1711.

Glossitis (see Mouth diseases)

Glucagonoma

Glucagonoma is an alpha–cell tumour of the pancreas which gives rise to a characteristic syndrome of hyperglycaemia with weight loss, anaemia and a distinct dermatitis. Most such tumours occur in the tail of the pancreas, most are malignant and most occur in older women. Hepatomegaly is common because of metastases, and sometimes there is associated multiple endocrine neoplasia (MEN) (q.v.).

The dermatitis is referred to as **necrolytic migratory erythema** and is sufficiently characteristic for dermatologists to be responsible for most diagnoses of glucagonoma. The initial skin lesion is a reddish macule which then vesiculates and finally sloughs leaving an area of local hypopigmentation. These lesions are seen especially on the buttocks, groin and distal extremities. Sometimes the entire sequence of lesions can be found simultaneously. There is a characteristic histology, with inflammatory cells in clefts. The skin lesions occur early in the course of the disease, even before metastases, and disappear within a few days of successful resection. A generalized decrease in serum amino acid levels may be responsible for this unusual dermatitis.

Investigations show a plasma glucagon level usually 10–20 times normal.

*Surgical **resection** is often possible, as the tumour is slowly growing.*

- *Otherwise, **cytotoxic** therapy is appropriate.*
- ***Octreotide** may be dramatically helpful in some patients.*
- *Successful **liver transplantation** has been reported.*

Bibliography
Leichter SB 1980 Clinical and metabolic aspects of glucagonoma. Medicine 59: 100.

Glucose-6-phosphate dehydrogenase deficiency (see also
Anaemia–haemolysis)

Glucose-6-phosphate dehydrogenase (G6PD) deficiency is one of the most common worldwide disorders, perhaps because it may originally have given some protection against malaria. The gene for the G6PD isoenzymes is on the X chromosome, therefore the disease affects especially men. However, even heterozygote women may have a significant deficiency, explained by the Lyon–Beutler hypothesis of random X inactivation in different cells. This phenomenon has also provided the theoretical basis for the use of G6PD as a valuable marker in confirming the monoclonal pathobiology of most cancers.

G6PD is a dimer, with each component having a molecular weight 55 kD. There are over 200 molecular variants, which increase the proportion of inactive monomers and thus give rise to the biochemical defect.

G6PD catalyses the conversion of NADP+ to NADPH, a potent reducing agent and protector of red blood cells against oxidative damage. G6PD deficiency is thus associated with vulnerability to haemolysis. Severe disease is also associated with impaired neutrophil function and thus proneness to infection.

The clinical picture (referred to as **favism**, because of its classical precipitation by the ingestion of fava beans) may take one of three forms, namely:

- **Class 1** (the least common) with chronic haemolytic anaemia;
- **Class 2** (of intermediate frequency) with episodic haemolysis and associated with severe deficiency;
- **Class 3** (the commonest) with haemolysis following a significant oxidative insult and associated with moderate deficiency.

A G6PD screening test is available, but direct assay is required for definitive diagnosis.

Treatment comprises:

- ***avoidance of culprit drugs** (namely antimalarials (classically primaquine), chloramphenicol, nitrofurantoin, sulfonamides, high-dose aspirin);*
- ***resuscitation** and circulatory support, including transfusion in the presence of acute favism (severe disseminated intravascular coagulation and haemolysis),*
- *possibly high-dose **vitamin E**.*

Bibliography
Beutler E 1990 The genetics of glucose-6-phosphate
dehydrogenase deficiency. Semin Hematol 27: 137.

Glycogen storage diseases

Glycogen storage diseases are of several types, all associated with a positive family history and a specific biochemical defect giving rise to impaired glycogenolysis. The best known example is **McArdle's disease** (type V), which is due to myophosphorylase deficiency and is associated with weakness, poor exercise tolerance and myoglobinuria.

Other biochemical defects affect different organs, especially the brain, heart and liver. There may be hepatomegaly, hypoglycaemia, hyperlipidaemia, hyperuricaemia, lactic acidosis, impaired growth, cyclical neutropenia and bacterial infection. If dietary compliance is poor, chronic renal disease, inflammatory bowel disease, hepatic adenoma, amyloid, gout or osteoporosis may result.

Bibliography
Layzer RB 1985 McArdle's disease in the 1980s. N
Engl J Med 312: 370.
Pears JS, Jung RT, Hopwood D et al 1992 Glycogen
storage disease diagnosed in adults. Quart J Med
82: 207.
Talente GM, Coleman RA, Alter C et al 1994
Glycogen storage disease in adults. Ann Intern
Med 120: 218.

Goodpasture's syndrome

Goodpasture's syndrome comprises pulmonary haemorrhage and glomerulonephritis, associated with autoantibodies to basement membranes of alveoli and glomeruli. Since the renal component can sometimes occur alone, an additional pulmonary injury may be required for full expression of the symptom-complex, such as viral infection or toxic exposure (including smoking).

Clinical features are usually seen in young men, and the initial presentation is usually haemoptysis. The interstitial and alveolar haemorrhage may be considerable enough to cause anaemia. There is an active nephritic picture (see Glomerular diseases) with rapidly progressive renal failure.

Chest X-ray shows a patchy and variable pulmonary infiltrate, initially due to haemorrhage and later to fibrosis. Renal biopsy shows a necrotizing proliferative glomerulonephritis, commonly with crescentic formation. Occasionally, the renal involvement is only mild and focal.

The diagnosis is based on the demonstration of anti-GBM antibodies in serum and on biopsy of the lung or more commonly kidney, the latter showing the characteristic immunofluorescent finding of IgG deposition along the glomerular basement membrane.

*Treatment with corticosteroids even in high dose is ineffective. The mainstay of current treatment is **plasmapheresis** (which removes antibodies), with or without immunosuppression with corticosteroids and cytotoxics, usually cyclophosphamide (to prevent new antibody formation). Plasmapheresis is conducted with 4 L exchanges daily for 1 week. Plasmapheresis interrupts both the haemoptysis and the impending renal failure. However, it does not reverse renal failure if oliguria is established, and it is reported to carry a substantially increased risk of superinfection.*

Until recently, the mortality was high with fatal pulmonary haemorrhage commonly occurring early and end-stage renal disease supervening in 80% of survivors within 1 y. This is because although anti-GBM antibodies disappear spontaneously within 1 y and recurrence is unusual, irreversible damage has occurred during this time unless there is effective treatment. For the same reason, any consideration of transplantation should be deferred until the antibodies have disappeared.

Idiopathic pulmonary haemosiderosis is a rare disease indistinguishable from the pulmonary component of Goodpasture's syndrome and occurring mainly in children. It is often fatal, although the prognosis appears very variable.

There is no clearly effective therapy.

Bibliography

Green RJ, Ruoss SJ, Kraft SA et al 1996 Pulmonary capillaritis and alveolar hemorrhage: update on diagnosis and management. Chest 110: 1305.

Kefalides NA 1987 The Goodpasture antigen and basement membranes: the search must go on. Lab Invest 56: 1.

Kelly PT, Haponik EF 1994 Goodpasture syndrome: molecular and clinical advances. Medicine 73: 171.

Leatherman JW, Davies SF, Hoidal JR 1984 Alveolar hemorrhage syndromes: diffuse microvascular lung hemorrhage in immune and idiopathic disorders. Medicine 63: 343.

Turner N, Mason PJ, Brown R et al 1992 Molecular cloning of the human Goodpasture antigen demonstrates it to be the $\alpha3$ chain of type IV collagen. J Clin Invest 89: 592.

Young KR 2000 Diagnostic pitfalls in alveolar hemorrhage syndromes. Pulm Perspectives; 17: 11.

Gout

Gout is a crystal-induced synovitis. It is characterized by recurrent attacks of acute arthritis, usually associated with an increased plasma urate. The mechanism of inflammation if neutrophil ingestion of sodium urate crystals with consequent release of inflammatory mediators.

Uric acid has no known biological function but is a product of purine metabolism.

The mechanisms for hyperuricaemia are:

- **metabolic** (with increased uric acid production)

  - primary (sometimes associated with a specific enzyme defect of purine metabolism);
  - secondary (especially associated with increased nucleic acid turnover, e.g. in the tumour-lysis syndrome – q.v.).

- **renal** (with decreased excretion of uric acid)

  - primary;
  - secondary (including chronic renal disease, lead nephropathy, drug-induced renal disease due to cyclosporin, diuretics, low-dose salicylates).

Uric acid completely dissociates at a normal pH to give urate anion. If the plasma concentration is >400 μmol/L, there is supersaturation with sodium urate, which therefore precipitates, the crystals then being ingested by neutrophils. The normal plasma urate concentration is 100–500 μmol /L.

The clinical features of gout are well known. A typical attack of the sudden onset of pain in a single joint, usually in the lower extremity. Within a few hours, the joint becomes red, hot, swollen and extremely painful. The process is self-limited and usually subsides within a few days. Half of the cases occur at the first metatarsophalangeal joint (podagra), but the process is polyarticular in 10–15% of cases. Acute gout may be associated with fever.

The disease may then enter an interval period, with recurrent attacks at variable intervals. The next attack usually occurs within two years. In some patients, a chronic phase subsequently occurs, perhaps after 10–20 y, with persistent symptoms. In chronic gout, there may be a polyarthritis involving both upper and lower limbs, with urate deposits (tophi) on tendons, around joints, in the ear and sometimes in deeper structures.

There is a high incidence of renal disease associated with chronic tophaceous gout, even greater than that associated with diabetes mellitus. However, the renal disease is usually due to associated hypertension, and gouty nephropathy is usually mild, though tubulointerstitial urate deposits may be found.

There is a 10–15% incidence of renal calculi, though it is worth noting that most uric acid stones are in fact from acid urine and not from gout, hyperuricaemia or hyperuricuria.

Concomitant diseases are also common, including:

- diabetes mellitus, in up to 80% of cases;
- obesity;
- hyperlipidaemia.

Associated cardiovascular disease is thus very frequent.

The diagnosis of gout is usually readily made on the basis of the clinical features, together with an increased plasma urate. However, the plasma urate is an insensitive test and the level may even fall to some extent during the acute attack. The urinary urate (even >6 mmol/day) is non-specific. Acutely there may be leukocytosis. The diagnosis may be confirmed if necessary by examination of synovial fluid for urate crystals. Histological examination of tophi shows that the chalky material consists of crystal masses.

If there is any suspicion of septic arthritis, examination of synovial fluid is mandatory. This is particularly important to consider, since septic arthritis may precipitate an acute attack of gout in that joint and cause diagnostic confusion.

Treatment of **acute disease** *traditionally has been with* **colchicine***, 0.5 mg orally hourly until relief or a total of 3–5 mg has been given or side-effects have occurred. Colchicine however has been largely superseded because of its marked gastrointestinal side-effects.*

- **Indomethacin** *is in fact just as effective, 50–75 mg being given initially, followed by 25–50 mg tds for 5–7 days. Other NSAIDs are also effective.*
- **Corticosteroids** *either oral or intra-articular may be considered if NSAIDs are contraindicated or ineffective, but the diagnosis should always be reviewed before their use in case septic arthritis has been overlooked.*

In **chronic disease***, the plasma urate should be decreased either by enhancing urinary excretion (by probenecid, 500 mg qid, or sulfinpyrazone, 100 mg qid) or more usually by inhibiting biosynthesis (by* **allopurinol***, 50–100 mg/day initially, increasing over several weeks to 100–300 mg/day in divided doses, depending on the plasma urate level). Allopurinol occasionally produces marked side-effects, including drug fever, rash, hepatitis, vasculitis and rarely a severe toxic syndrome comprising all these features, together with eosinophilia and renal dysfunction.*

- *Low doses of colchicine (e.g. 0.5 mg bd) may also be used in maintenance therapy.*
- *Renal calculi should be treated with enhanced urine flow and alkalinization.*

Hyperuricaemia if asymptomatic does not require treatment.

Pseudogout is due to the deposition of crystals containing calcium pyrophosphate dihydrate (CPPD, apatite). This can give a syndrome resembling gout, though it can also mimic osteoarthritis and even rheumatoid arthritis. It requires examination of synovial fluid for its definitive diagnosis.

Bibliography

Beck LH 1986 Requiem for gouty nephropathy. Kidney Int 30: 280.

Boss GR, Seegmiller JE 1979 Hyperuricemia and gout: classification, complications and management. N Engl J Med 300: 1459.

Dieppe PA, Huskisson EC, Crocker P et al 1976 Apatite deposition disease: a new arthropathy. Lancet 1: 266.

Emmerson BT 1996 The management of gout. N Engl J Med 334: 445.

Hadler NM, Franck WA, Bress NM et al 1974 Acute polyarticular gout. Am J Med 56: 715.

McGill NW 1997 Gout and other crystal arthropathies. Med J Aust 166: 33.

Pascual E 2000 Gout update: from lab to the clinic and back. Curr Opin Rheumatol 12: 213.

Simkin PA 1977 The pathogenesis of podagra. Ann Intern Med 86: 230.

Graves' disease (see Hyperthyroidism)

Growth hormone (see Acromegaly)

Guillain–Barré syndrome (see Neuropathy)

Haemangioma (see also Telangiectasia)

Haemangioma is a benign vascular tumour, either congenital or acquired. It may occur at virtually any site, and because of its vascular fragility it is subject to easy bleeding, either spontaneously or as a result of minor trauma.

Giant haemangiomas (as in the liver, i.e. Kasabach–Merritt syndrome) may cause disseminated intravascular coagulation, haemolysis and thrombocytopenia.

Haematology

The general principles related to bleeding, thromboembolism, anticoagulation, the use of blood products and the complications of haematological malignancies are well understood in Intensive Care practice.

On the other hand, although specific individual haematological disorders are usually uncommon in Intensive Care patients, the great frequency with which haematological problems in general are encountered in the seriously ill reflects the large variety of such conditions which needs to be considered by Intensive Care clinicians.

These conditions include:

- agranulocytosis;
- anaemia;
- anticardiolipin antibody;
- antiphospholipid syndrome;
- antithrombin III;
- basophilia;
- coagulation disorders;
- dysproteinaemias;
- eosinophilia;
- erythrocytosis;
- fetal haemoglobin;
- fibrinolysis;
- haemoglobin disorders;
- haemolysis;
- haemophilia;
- hypersplenism;
- idiopathic thrombocytopenic purpura;
- lupus anticoagulant;
- lymphadenopathy;
- lymphocytosis;
- lymphopenia;
- megaloblastic anaemia;
- methaemoglobinaemia;
- microangiopathic haemolysis;
- neutropenia;
- neutrophilia;

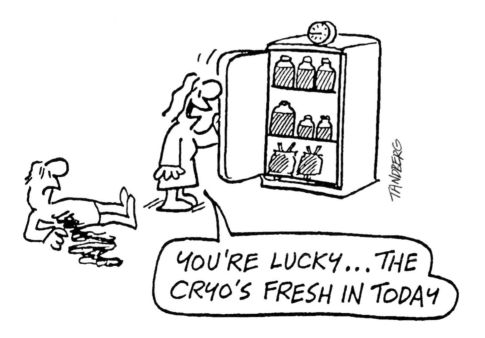

YOU'RE LUCKY... THE CRYO'S FRESH IN TODAY

- pancytopenia;
- pernicious anaemia;
- petechiae;
- plasminogen;
- platelet function disorders;
- polycythaemia;
- protein C;
- protein S;
- purpura;
- reticulocytes;
- sickle cell anaemia;
- sideroblastic anaemia;
- splenomegaly;
- storage disorders;
- thalassaemia;
- thrombasthenia;
- thrombocytopenia;
- thrombocytosis/thrombocythaemia;
- thromboembolism;
- thrombophilia;
- vitamin K deficiency;
- von Willebrand's disease.

Bibliography

Arya S, Hong R, Gilbert EF 1985 Reactive hemophagocytic syndrome. Pediatr Pathol 3: 129.

Barrett-Connor E 1972 Anemia and infection. Am J Med 52: 242.

Bohnsack JF, Brown EJ 1986 The role of the spleen in resistance to infection. Annu Rev Med 37: 49.

Bolan CD, Alving BM 1990 Pharmacologic agents in the management of bleeding disorders. Transfusion 30: 541.

Collen D, Lijnen HR 1991 Basic and clinical aspects of fibrinolysis and thrombolysis. Blood 78: 3114.

Colman N, Herbert V 1980 Hematologic complications of alcoholism: overview. Semin Hematol 17: 164.

Colman RW, Hirsh J, Marder VJ et al (eds) 1982 Hemostasis and Thrombosis: Basic Principles and Clinical Practice. Philadelphia: Lippincott.

Copeman PW 1975 Livedo reticularis: signs in the skin of disturbance of blood viscosity and blood flow. Br J Dermatol 93: 519.

Dalen JE, Hirsh J, Guyatt GH (eds) 2001 Sixth ACCP consensus conference on antithrombotic therapy. Chest 119: no. 1 (Suppl).

Dexter TM 1987 Stem cells in normal growth and disease. Br Med J 295: 1192.

Doll DC, List AF 1992 Myelodysplastic syndromes. Semin Oncol 19: 1.

Editorial 1982 Nitrous oxide and acute marrow failure. Lancet 2: 856.

Editorial 1992 Peripheral stem cells made to work. Lancet 339: 648.

Greenberg CS, Sane DC 1990 Coagulation problems in critical care medicine. In: Lumb PD, Shoemaker WC (eds). Critical Care: State of the Art, Chapter 9. Fullerton: Society of Critical Care Medicine. p 187.

Hirsh J, Levine MN 1992 Low molecular weight heparin. Blood 79: 1.

Kushner I, Rzewnicki DL 1994 The acute phase response: general aspects. Baillieres Clin Rheumatol 8: 513.

Lieschke GJ, Burgess AW 1992 Granulocyte colony-stimulating factor and granulocyte-macrophage colony-stimulating factor. N Engl J Med 327: 28 & 99.

Metcalf D 1993 Hematopoietic regulators: redundancy or subtlety? Blood 82: 3515.

Moake JL 1990 Common hemostatic problems and blood banking in critical care medicine. In: Lumb PD, Shoemaker WC (eds). Critical Care: State of the Art, Chapter 8. Fullerton: Society of Critical Care Medicine. p 161.

Nachman RL 1992 Thrombosis and atherogenesis: molecular connections. Blood 79: 1897.

Ogawa M 1993 Differentiation and proliferation of hemopoietic stem cells. Blood 81: 2844.

Provan D, Henson A (eds) 1998 ABC of Clinical Haematology. London: BMJ Publishing.

Rapaport SI 1983 Preoperative hemostatic evaluation: which tests, if any? Blood 61: 229.

Rose WF 1987 The spleen as a filter. N Engl J Med 317: 704.

Salama A, Mueller-Eckhardt C 1992 Immune-mediated blood cell dyscrasias related to drugs. Semin Hematol 29: 54.

Schafer AI 1984 Bleeding and thrombosis in the myeloproliferative disorders. Blood 64: 1.

Silverstein RL, Nachman RL 1992 Cancer and clotting – Trousseau's warning. N Engl J Med 327: 1163.

Sox HC, Liang MH 1986 The erythrocyte sedimentation rate: guidelines for rational use. Ann Intern Med 104: 515.

Weitz JI 1997 Low-molecular-weight heparins. N Engl J Med 337: 688.

Haematuria

Haematuria is a striking clinical finding, but in fact as little as 1 mL/L can cause a visible colour change, and much lower concentrations can be detected chemically (by dipstick test).

Abnormal urinary tract blood loss is considered to be:

- >1 RBC per high-power field on urine microscopy (>3 RBCs in women);
- >10 000 RBCs per mL of urine.

Haematuria is usually without clots, perhaps because of the local action of urokinase.

Haematuria needs to be distinguished from other causes of red or red-brown urine. These include most importantly:

- **haemoglobinuria** (from haemolysis – q.v.),
- **myoglobinuria** (from rhabdomyolysis – q.v.),

but in these the colour remains in the supernatant after standing or centrifugation.

Red urine may also be caused by:

- drugs

  - such as rifampicin, phenothiazines, sulfasalazine;

- porphyria;
- ingestion of some vegetables

  - e.g. beetroots.

More brownish urine:

- may contain bilirubin or melanin;
- may be caused by drugs

  - such as methyldopa, metronidazole or nitrofurantoin.

Haematuria

- with marked proteinuria suggests glomerulonephritis,
- with pyuria suggests urinary tract infection.

Macroscopic haematuria, with a urinary red cell count of $>10^6$/mL of glomerular origin (i.e. with dysmorphic red cells), is often indicative of a rapidly progressive glomerulonephritis with crescent formation.

Isolated haematuria may be either renal or extra-renal.

- **Renal causes** may be:

  - glomerular, as in glomerulonephritis or following heavy exercise,
  - extra-glomerular, as with calculi, carcinoma, trauma, vascular disease, haemorrhagic disease, cystic disease.

- **Extra-renal causes** include disorders of the:

  - ureter (calculi);
  - bladder (infection, tumour, trauma, cyclophosphamide);
  - prostate (benign hypertrophy, carcinoma);
  - urethra (infection, trauma).

Many instances of haematuria, especially if transient, have no demonstrable cause.

Appropriate investigations include examination of the urine and urinary sediment, renal ultrasound examination, possibly intravenous pyelography and possibly cystoscopy.

Bibliography

Cronin RE, Kaehny WD, Miller, PD et al 1976 Renal cell carcinoma: unusual systemic manifestations. Medicine 55: 291.

Froom P, Ribak J, Benbassat J 1984 Significance of microhaematuria in young adults. Br Med J 288: 20.

Haemochromatosis

Haemochromatosis is a common inherited disease, with a prevalence of 12% for heterozygotes or carriers and of 3.6/1000 for homozygotes. Some heterozygotes (25%) have minor abnormalities of iron metabolism but no clinical disease. Even many homozygotes (50%) do not have clinical disease.

It is an autosomal recessive disease with the abnormal gene located close to the HLA region on chromosome 6. The *HFE* gene has recently been identified and cloned, and its C282Y mutation has been found to be responsible for most familial cases of the disease. The defect gives rise to excess iron absorption, with greatly increased iron stores in the body and deposition in parenchymal cells, particularly of the liver, heart, pancreas and testes.

> Haemochromatosis is the primary, idiopathic or hereditary form of **iron overload disease**. Secondary iron overload syndromes occur in the iron-loading anaemias (q.v.), such as thalassaemia and hereditary spherocytosis. Mild iron overload also occurs in alcoholism.

Symptoms usually commence between 30 and 60 years of age. They occur later and much less frequently in women because of menstruation and pregnancy. There is lethargy, weakness, arthralgia (and later arthritis), abdominal pain, loss of libido and impotence.

On examination, there is hepatomegaly, greyish skin pigmentation, arthropathy and testicular atrophy. Advanced disease may be complicated by diabetes mellitus, cirrhosis, hepatocellular carcinoma and cardiac failure.

> The diagnosis should be considered:
>
> - in any case of liver disease of unknown cause;
> - in the presence of a positive family history;
> - when there is a syndrome of fatigue, diabetes, arthritis and cardiac failure.

Appropriate laboratory investigations are as follows.

- The serum iron level is not helpful, since it may be increased in the presence of hepatic cell destruction from any cause.
- The serum iron-to-iron binding capacity ratio (i.e. transferrin saturation) is the earliest

and most useful abnormal test, as it is increased, often to 80–90% (normal <55%).

- The serum ferritin may be increased (>400 μg/L in men and >200 μg/L in women) if there is clinical disease.
- If either the serum transferring saturation or the serum ferritin is abnormal, liver biopsy should be performed even in asymptomatic patients to:

  – confirm the diagnosis,
  – assess the presence of cirrhosis,
  – measure the iron concentration (hepatic iron index becomes >2.0).

- Liver function tests are often abnormal, but there is usually no jaundice.
- Imaging of the liver with CT or MRI may be helpful.

While population screening is not cost-effective, all first- and second-degree relatives of any index case should be tested. Clearly, siblings have a 25% chance of being homozygous. HLA typing while not diagnostically useful may be helpful in family studies, because the case is probably normal if neither HLA haplotype is shared with the index case. Testing should be commenced at the age of 10 years and continued three yearly until the age of 70 years.

*Treatment is with life-long **venesection** which removes iron via haemoglobin (500 mL of blood contains 250 mg of iron). Since the patient often has 10–20 g of excess iron in the body, 50 units of blood may have to be removed (i.e. one unit each 1–2 weeks for 1–2 years). Thereafter, 3–5 venesections per year will maintain the iron stores at a low level without inducing iron deficiency, for which the best end-points are haemoglobin of 110 g/L and low-normal ferritin levels. Dietary restriction of iron intake is unhelpful, but alcohol intake should be minimized, and care should be taken with vitamin C intake since this enhances iron absorption.*

There is a 50% average mortality within 20 years. With treatment:

- the prognosis is normal if there is no cirrhosis;

- skin pigmentation and cardiac failure improve;
- diabetes mellitus improves but does not disappear;
- gonadal failure and arthritis may sometimes improve;
- cirrhosis does not regress entirely and indeed primary liver cancer may still occur. Its development is best screened for with an alphafetoprotein level (q.v.) and annual imaging of the liver with ultrasound.

Bibliography

Adams PC, Kertesz AE, Valberg LS 1991 Clinical presentation of hemochromatosis. Am J Med 90: 445.

Burke W, Thomson E, Khoury MJ et al 1998 Hereditary hemochromatosis: gene discovery and its implications for population-based screening. JAMA 280: 172.

Burt MJ, George DK, Powell LW 1996 Haemochromatosis – a clinical update. Med J Aust 164: 348.

Challoner T, Briggs C, Rampling MW et al 1986 A study of the haematological and haemorrheological consequences of venesection. Br J Haematol 62: 671.

Editorial 1979 Serum-ferritin. Lancet 1: 533.

Finch CA 1982 The detection of iron overload. N Engl J Med 307: 1702.

Finch CA, Huebers H 1992 Perspectives in iron metabolism. N Engl J Med 306: 1520.

Olynyk JK 1999 Hereditary haemochromatosis: diagnosis and management in the gene era. Liver 19: 73.

Powell LW, Bassett ML 1998 Haemochromatosis: diagnosis and management after the cloning of the HFE gene. Aust NZ J Med 28: 159.

Valberg LS, Ghent CN 1985 Diagnosis and management of hereditary hemochromatosis. Annu Rev Med 36: 27.

Haemodilution (see Anaemia)

Haemoglobin disorders

Haemoglobin disorders (haemoglobinopathies) are a diverse group of disorders providing one mechanism of red blood cell abnormality and thus anaemia due to increased red blood destruction (haemolysis – see Anaemia). There are over 100 types of haemoglobinopathy and many are asymptomatic.

Haemoglobin requires the complex globin assembly of 2 alpha and 2 beta chains, which must then be coordinated with haem synthesis. The alpha genes are on chromosome 16 and the non-alpha genes are on chromosome 11. Haemoglobin A (HbA) contains two beta chains, HbF contains two gamma chains and HbA_2 contains two delta chains.

Genetic defects may cause amino acid substitution (as in sickle cell anaemia) or incoordinated assembly (as in thalassaemia). The resultant abnormal haemoglobin may be unstable, bind oxygen incorrectly, oxidize or crystallize.

1. Thalassaemia

Thalassaemia is encountered worldwide, perhaps because heterozygotes had some survival advantage, e.g. enhanced malarial resistance (as with sickle cell anaemia and glucose 6-phosphate dehydrogenase deficiency). Thalassaemia arises from a variety of genetic defects which cause mismatching of globin chains with resultant molecular aggregation, cell deformity, and metabolic and immunological abnormalities of the red blood cell membrane.

Beta thalassaemia is the common form of the disease and is due to impaired beta chain production. The chains are thus unmatched and there is a compensatory increase in gamma and delta chains, so that haemoglobin HbF and HbA2 are also present.

Thalassaemia major (Cooley's anaemia) is usually homozygous and is associated with severe disease, consisting of haemolytic anaemia, hepatosplenomegaly, growth retardation and susceptibility to infections. Iron overload results from the inevitable multiple transfusions and may be prevented or treated by desferrioxamine (deferoxamine, DFO) (see Chelating agents). Bone-marrow transplantation from

HLA-identical donors has been performed in over 1000 patients worldwide and has been reported to give an 80% cure rate.

Thalassaemia minor (thalassaemia trait) is usually heterozygous and presents with mild disease.

There are many genetic variants, with abnormalities clinically resembling beta thalassaemia. In alpha thalassaemia, there are excess beta chains and no substitute chains available in the adult for the deficient alpha chains.

The differential diagnosis of thalassaemia is chiefly iron deficiency anaemia, but in thalassaemia the red blood cell count is normal.

The diagnosis of thalassaemia is made on the basis of anaemia, decreased MCV, normal RBC count, peripheral blood film showing hypochromia and microcytosis but with basophilic stippling and nucleated erythrocytes, increased HbA_2 and HbF, and specifically abnormal haemoglobin electrophoresis.

2. Sickle cell anaemia

Sickle cell anaemia occurs in many countries around the world, especially in West Africa (and thus also in Black Americans), the Eastern Mediterranean and India. Like thalassaemia, its wide prevalence and persistence are possibly due to some protection by the trait against malaria.

Sickle cell anaemia is due to the presence of HbS, which has a glutamate residue replaced by valine in the sixth position of the beta chain. HbS in deoxy form has reduced solubility and polymerizes, so that the red blood cell becomes distorted into a sickle shape. This process of sickling occurs especially in the microvasculature and is aggravated by hypoxia, acidosis and increased 2,3-DPG. The process is at least partly irreversible, so that the cells remain damaged even after re-oxygenation and are then prematurely removed by the reticuloendothelial system, giving rise to haemolytic anaemia.

Heterozygotes have 30–50% HbS (i.e. they have HbAS) and are asymptomatic. Homozygotes have 70–98% HbS (i.e. they have HbSS) and have symptomatic disease, with chronic haemolytic anaemia and acute vaso-occlusive crises.

These two complications are responsible for the majority of the morbidity and mortality of the disease.

Clinical features are those of chronic haemolytic anaemia. There is jaundice, and about 50% of patients have pigment gallstones. There is hyposplenism and increased susceptibility to infection. The kidneys show loss of concentrating ability. The central nervous system, eyes, lungs, liver, kidneys, bone marrow and penis may be affected by acute vascular occlusion.

The '**acute chest syndrome**' is associated with pulmonary vascular occlusion and perhaps local infection, and an extensive but asymmetrical 'white-out' on chest X-ray. It is a major cause of morbidity and mortality. It is associated with an increased plasma level of phospholipase A_2.

> **Sickle cell crisis** is an acute, life-threatening and painful vaso-occlusive process, leading to local ischaemia or even infarction. The initiating event is often not apparent. The target organs are especially the kidney and the bone marrow.

The diagnosis is based on the typically abnormal blood film and confirmed by haemoglobin electrophoresis. The white cell count and platelet count are usually elevated.

Treatment of a sickle cell crisis includes rest, hydration, oxygenation, alkali and analgesia.

- *Since severe **pain**, especially that of avascular necrosis in bone marrow, may last for over a week, there is a risk of narcotic addiction.*
- *The frequency of the acute chest syndrome is reduced by hydroxyurea.*

*General **anaesthesia** is normally recommended to be deferred until the HbS level has been lowered to about*

50% by transfusion (or exchange transfusion, so that the haematocrit is not >0.35). In fact, however, there have been reported series of general anaesthetics without complications despite no specific precautions. Pregnancy and even oral contraceptives add to the anaesthetic risk.

In the future, **gene therapy** offers prospects for cure, and in the meantime **bone marrow transplantation** has been successful in some patients.

Haemoglobin C disease results from the replacement of glutamate by lysine at the sixth position on the beta chain. It is thus a variant of sickle cell anaemia, except that it is mild. Heterozygotes are asymptomatic, while homozygotes have mild anaemia with splenomegaly.

Haemoglobin E disease is a further variant in which lysine replaces glutamate at the 26 position on the beta chain. The trait is particularly common in some South East Asian populations. The clinical features are similar to those of HbC disease. Drugs with oxidizing properties such as dapsone should be avoided.

Many other amino acid substitutions have been reported, which give unstable haemoglobins associated with chronic haemolytic anaemia without spherocytosis.

Some haemoglobin variants confer abnormal oxygen binding.

- **Left shift of the haemoglobin oxygen dissociation curve**

  – i.e. increased oxygen affinity is produced by haemoglobin Chesapeake, Rainier or Yakima.

- **Right shift of the haemoglobin oxygen dissociation curve**

  – i.e. decreased oxygen affinity is produced by haemoglobin Kansas.
  – This phenomenon can cause cyanosis.

Bibliography

Charache S, Terrin ML, Moore RD et al 1995 Effect of hydroxyurea on the frequency of painful crises in sickle cell anaemia. N Engl J Med 332: 1317.

Davies SC, Luce PJ, Win AA et al 1984 Acute chest syndrome in sickle-cell disease. Lancet 1: 36.

Embury SH 1986 The clinical pathophysiology of sickle cell disease. Annu Rev Med 37: 361.

Francis RB, Johnson CS 1991 Vascular occlusion in sickle cell disease: current concepts and unanswered questions. Blood 77: 1405.

Piomelli S, Loew T 1991 Management of thalassemia major (Cooley's anemia). Hematol Oncol Clin North Am 5: 557.

Platt OS 1994 Easing the suffering caused by sickle cell disease. N Engl J Med 330: 783.

Schrier SL 1994 Thalassemia: pathophysiology of red cell shapes. Annu Rev Med 45: 211.

Styles LA, Schalkwijk CG, Aarsman AJ et al 1996 Phospholipase A2 levels in acute chest syndrome of sickle cell disease. Blood 87: 2573.

Weatherall DJ 1993 The treatment of thalassemia – slow progress and new dilemmas. N Engl J Med 329: 877.

Haemoglobinopathy (see Haemoglobin disorders)

Haemoglobinuria (see Anaemia and Haematuria)

Haemolysis (see Anaemia and Cold agglutinin disease)

Haemolytic–uraemic syndromes

(see also Thrombotic thrombocytopenic purpura)

The haemolytic–uraemic syndromes comprise childhood and adulthood haemolytic–uraemic syndrome (HUS), as well as the related thrombotic thrombocytopenic purpura (TTP)(q.v.), though not disseminated intravascular coagulation.

These conditions have the common features of:

- microangiopathic haemolysis;
- thrombocytopenia;
- platelet-fibrin thrombi in small vessels;
- renal involvement.

In more chronic situations, the histology may show concentric vascular thickening as in malignant hypertension or scleroderma. While HUS is usually idiopathic, there is sometimes such marked local clustering as to suggest an epidemic, especially in children.

HUS may be associated with:

- pregnancy
  - especially the postpartum state, when it particularly occurs if there has been placental abruption, retained placenta or pre-eclampsia;

- bone marrow transplantation;
- immuno-modulation
  - with cyclosporin and some cancer chemotherapeutic agents, e.g. mitomycin C;

- mucous adenocarcinoma of the gastrointestinal tract;
- antiphospholipid syndrome;
- food poisoning
  - due to enteropathogenic (enterotoxigenic, entero-haemorrhagic) *E. coli*, especially serotype O157:H7, and usually in children (see Diarrhoea). This is an important cause of outbreaks of HUS.

Sometimes, these conditions lead to HUS and sometimes to TTP. Whether its pathogenesis primarily involves endothelial cell or platelet activation is uncertain.

Investigations show thrombocytopenia with increased beta-thromboglobulin (βTG),

haemolysis with raised LDH, neutrophilia, and platelet-fibrin thrombi in small arteries in biopsy material (e.g. bone marrow, kidney). Coagulation is normal and there is no disseminated intravascular coagulation, the complement level is normal, the direct Coombs' test is negative, and the urinary sediments is usually normal.

Treatment should be with **plasmapheresis** *if the condition is severe.*

- *Traditionally, therapy with aspirin and/or corticosteroids has been used, but aspirin in particular should be used with caution because of the risk of bleeding.*
- *Platelet transfusion may also give rise to problems (e.g. thrombotic deterioration), and thus should be used only if the patient is bleeding.*
- *Renal support should be instituted on its normal merits.*
- *Clearly, any culprit drugs should be stopped.*

There is an 80% response to early treatment and complete remission is usual, though the microangiopathic changes may take some months to subside. However, one third of cases suffer a recurrence, though this is usually mild and often asymptomatic, being demonstrated only by new thrombocytopenia and microangiopathic haemolysis. The renal recovery may be delayed and incomplete, especially if the patient is untreated. The mortality is worse postpartum, because it is then often associated with cardiomyopathy, but even in this circumstance survival is substantially better than with TTP.

Bibliography

Beers M, Cameron S 1995 Hemolytic uremic syndrome. Emerg Infect Dis 1: 4.

Kaplan B, Drummond K 1978 The hemolytic–uremic syndrome is a syndrome. N Engl J Med 298: 964.

Remuzzi G 1987 HUS and TTP: variable expression of a single entity. Kidney Int 32: 292.

Wong CS, Jelacic S, Habeeb RL et al 2000 The risk of hemolytic–uremic syndrome after antibiotic treatment of *Escherichia coli* O157:H7 infection. N Engl J Med 342: 1930.

Haemophilia

Haemophilia (classical haemophilia or haemophilia A) is the best known of the hereditary haemorrhagic disorders, because although uncommon (1 in 10 000 males) its effects are striking. It is due to either a quantitative or qualitative defect of factor VIII: C, the gene for which is on the X chromosome. The disease is thus confined to hemizygotic males, while females are carriers.

Factor VIII is a large plasma protein of molecular weight 330kD, plasma concentration 100 μg/L (100%) and half-life 10 h. It acts as a coagulation factor rather than a zymogen and assists the activation of factor X to Xa. The severity of disease is directly related to the plasma concentration, which ranges from virtually undetectable to about 50%.

*Treatment has traditionally been with **factor VIII concentrates**, but recombinant factor VIII is now available. The level should be raised to 25–50% before invasive procedures. Avoidance of aspirin and administration of EACA or DDAVP are helpful.*

Haemophilia B (Christmas disease) is due to factor IX deficiency. Like haemophilia A, it is sex-linked. Factor IX is a plasma protein of molecular weight 57 kD and plasma concentration 5 mg/L. It is a zymogen with a half-life of 24 h.

The management principles are similar to those of haemophilia, except that the concentration required for haemostasis is generally lower (usually 20% is adequate) and the smaller size of factor IX results in a larger distribution volume (being about the size of albumin space).

Bibliography
Bloom AL 1991 Progress in the clinical management of haemophilia. Thromb Haemost 66: 166.
Furie B, Furie BC 1990 Molecular basis of hemophilia. Semin Hematol 27: 270.

Haemoptysis

Haemoptysis, or the expectoration of blood, should always be regarded as potentially serious.

Haemoptysis may range from minor blood-streaking of the sputum to the expectoration of large amounts of frank blood. Most haemoptysis is minor, but even relatively small amounts of blood can be quite startling when mixed with expectorated sputum.

The source of expectorated blood is not always clear from the history. Blood from the mouth, nose or throat, or the upper gastrointestinal tract, may well into the throat and then be coughed up. Patients, and even clinicians, may also have difficulty sometimes in distinguishing between haemoptysis and haematemesis.

Some degree of haemoptysis is common with many acute respiratory infections, though most causes of haemoptysis are serious chronic diseases, such as carcinoma, tuberculosis, bronchiectasis and severe left heart failure (classically in the past due to mitral stenosis).

Although the cause may be apparent from the clinical features and/or chest X-ray, bronchoscopy is usually required to clarify the diagnosis. However, even after extensive investigation, some episodes of haemoptysis are not satisfactorily explained.

The chief causes of haemoptysis are (in approximate order of frequency):

1. acute chest infection (bronchitis, pneumonia);
2. carcinoma (also rarely bronchial adenoma);
3. chronic bronchitis;
4. pulmonary infarction;
5. acute pulmonary oedema (left heart failure);
6. foreign body;
7. bronchiectasis, lung abscess;
8. tuberculosis;
9. systemic bleeding disorder;
10. drug reaction;
11. Goodpasture's syndrome;
12. Wegener's granulomatosis;
13. lymphomatoid granulomatosis.

Treatment is primarily that of the underlying condition. In refractory cases, bronchial artery embolization, endobronchial tamponade or even surgery may be indicated if the responsible lesion can be localized.

Bibliography

Bobrowitz ID, Ramakrishna S, Shim Y-S 1983 Comparison of medical v surgical treatment of major hemoptysis. Arch Intern Med 143: 1343.

Jean-Baptiste E 2000 Clinical assessment and management of massive hemoptysis. Crit Care Med 28: 1642.

Remy J, Arnaud A, Fardou H et al 1977 Treatment of hemoptysis by embolization of bronchial arteries. Radiology 122: 33.

Haemostasis (see Coagulation disorders)

Hamman–Rich syndrome (see Diffuse fibrosing alveolitis)

Hand–Schüller–Christian disease (see Histiocytosis X)

Hantavirus

In 1993, a small epidemic of unusual cases of severe acute respiratory failure was reported in the southwestern USA. Within a month, the causative agent had been identified on serological and genetic evidence as a hitherto unrecognized species of hantavirus (Sin Nombre virus), transmitted to humans via contact with infected deer mice and without human to human passage. Within 8 months, 48 cases in that area had been confirmed, with a mortality of about one third even in young previously healthy patients, and the geographic distribution of cases had begun to widen. Hantavirus had previously only been known as a rodent-borne cause of haemorrhagic fever with renal failure in the Eastern Hemisphere.

Clinical features commence with the features of a non-specific viral illness. It progresses to an acute (adult) respiratory distress syndrome, with acute pulmonary oedema due to increased capillary permeability – the hantavirus pulmonary syndrome (HPS). There is associated septic shock, lactic acidosis and thrombocytopenia.

*Treatment with **mechanical ventilation** appears to be required in about half the cases, together with haemodynamic monitoring and inotropic support. The putative antihantavirus drug, ribavirin, is not effective in HPS.*

Bibliography

Duchin JS, Koster FT, Peters CJ et al 1994; Hantaviral pulmonary syndrome: Clinical description of disease caused by a newly recognized hemorrhagic fever virus in the Southwestern United States. N Engl J Med 330: 949.

Hallin GW, Simpson SQ, Crowell RE, James DS, Koster FT, Mertz GJ, Levy H 1996 Cardiopulmonary manifestations of hantavirus pulmonary syndrome. Crit Care Med 24: 252.

Hughes JM, Peters CJ, Cohen ML et al 1993 Hantavirus pulmonary syndrome: an emerging infectious disease. Science 262: 850.

Schmaljohn C, Hjelle B 1997 Hantaviruses: a global disease problem. Emerg Infect Dis 3: 2.

Shope RE 1999 A midcourse assessment of hantavirus pulmonary syndrome. Emerg Infect Dis 5: 1.

Heat (see also Pyrexia)

Heat injury occurs if the body's thermoregulatory processes are overwhelmed.

- This occurs particularly in association with a high environmental temperature.
- It is aggravated by direct sunlight and high humidity.
- Increased risk occurs with:

  – exercise;
  – dehydration;
  – old age;
  – excess clothing;
  – some drugs, such as phenothiazines and anticholinergics.

The heat-related issues discussed in this book are:

- heat cramps;
- heat exhaustion;
- heat rash;
- heat shock proteins;
- heat stroke;
- hot tubs;
- hyperthermia.

Bibliography

Marr JJ, Geiss PT 1982 Management of heat injury syndromes. In: Shoemaker WC, Thompson WL (eds) Critical Care: State of the Art. Fullerton: Society of Critical Care Medicine. p K1.

Heat cramps

Heat cramps are painful muscular spasms, which can occur even in the presence of a normal body temperature.

They may be prevented with adequate hydration and are treated with massage and stretching.

Heat exhaustion

Heat exhaustion is a more severe form of heat injury than heat cramps. It is associated with a moderate increase in body temperature.

There is fatigue, headache, nausea, cramps and hyperventilation. Dehydration and postural hypotension occur, and the patient, though sweating freely, feels cold, often with associated piloerection.

Treatment consists of rest in a cool and preferably dry environment, with hydration and external ***cooling***.

Heat rash

Heat rash is due to occlusion of sweat ducts, which gives rise to:

- small, clear, asymptomatic vesicles (miliaria crystallina) on exposed skin;
- red, pruritic vesicles (miliaria rubra) on covered skin;
- friction blisters at sites of pressure.

Heat shock proteins

Since adverse environmental exposure may jeopardize the survival of any living organism by producing the major acute changes referred to as stress, a common pattern of defence is set in train, resulting in multiple structural and functional changes in the organism. This stress response is often referred to as the heat shock response, because the original and best studied stressor was hyperthermia. This response is associated with the rapid elaboration of a set of proteins, called heat shock proteins (HSP), and a decrease in other cellular proteins. This response is rapid and reversible and is geared to protecting the essential cellular machinery from irreversible injury, thus promoting both survival during the stress and rapid recovery thereafter.

HSPs are members of a larger family of intracellular proteins which maintain the integrity of the cell's structure and are sometimes referred to as 'molecular chaperones'. HSPs are classified as either large (68–100 kD) or small (15–30 kD). HSP70 is the best characterized family of stress proteins. HSPs are synthesized not only typically after a brief increase in temperature of 3–5°C, but also after other insults such as hypoxia, hypoglycaemia, infection and acute chemical exposure. They have been identified in all major cell structures and are also present at low levels in unstressed cells, so that they thus have a background function, probably in maintaining membrane integrity. Following the cloning of the first gene in 1978, all have now been cloned. Extensive amino acid homology has been found, even between humans and bacteria, even though these two species diverged more than 1.5 billion years ago. The response is thus presumed to be of great antiquity. Perhaps these proteins bind to denatured elements and thus prevent their aggregation and resultant cell damage. In general, the process is protective, because there is a correlation between HSP induction on mild stress and the development of tolerance to thermal or other stress. However, HSP may also provide a mechanism for the induction of autoimmunity (q.v.) via molecular mimicry.

The development of HSP may have relevance in fever and/or sepsis. Thus, the failure to mount a fever is associated with an increased mortality in infections, although any benefit of fever itself has not been demonstrated. In addition, thermal pretreatment (and most recently, post-treatment) has been shown to protect experimentally against pulmonary and neurological damage and consequent mortality in sepsis.

Bibliography

Buchman TG 1994 Manipulation of stress gene expression: a novel therapy for the treatment of sepsis? Crit Care Med 22: 901.

Chu EK, Ribeiro SP, Slutsky AS 1997 Heat stress increases survival rates in polysaccharide-stimulated rats. Crit Care Med 25: 1727.

Delogu G, Bosco LL, Marandola M et al 1997 Heat shock protein (HSP70) expression in septic patients. J Crit Care 12: 188.

Lindquist S 1986 The heat shock response. Annu Rev Biochem 55: 1151.

van Eden W, Young DB (eds) 1996 Stress Proteins in Medicine. New York: Dekker.

Villar J, Ribeiro SP, Mullen JBM et al 1994 Induction of the heat shock response reduces mortality rate and organ damage in a sepsis induced acute lung injury model. Crit Care Med 22: 914.

Heat stroke

Heat stroke is the most severe form of heat injury and is a dangerous complication. It is diagnosed on the basis of core temperature >40°C and hot but dry skin.

It is seen in both epidemics and sporadically in individuals.

- Epidemics occur during heat waves in urban areas, especially among the elderly, debilitated or alcoholic population, even if sedentary

- Individual cases occur in hot environments, either in association with strenuous physical exercise, as in athletes or new military recruits, or in confined areas, such as prisons, military barracks or pilgrim crowds.

Apart from a high environmental temperature often without direct sunlight, the risk increases:

- with drug administration (anticholinergics, phenothiazines, tricyclic antidepressants, monoamine oxidase inhibitors);
- with impairment of the body's ability to dissipate heat (as in a humid environment or with dehydration, cardiac failure or inability to sweat).

Heat stroke has a sudden onset with a rapid rise in body temperature, usually to at least 41°C and typically with the cessation of sweating, so that the skin appears flushed and dry. The upper temperature limit for survival is generally about 44°C. Heat stroke represents a major failure of thermoregulation, though the mechanism of damage is more than direct thermal injury and probably includes the elaboration of mediators such as nitric oxide.

- **Neurological dysfunction** occurs with delirium, coma, fits and decerebrate posture.
- **Circulatory failure** is seen, with marked tachycardia and eventually the abrupt onset of hypotension, pulmonary oedema (especially in the elderly) and shock.
- **Dehydration** and **hypovolaemia** are usual.
- **Associated features** include:

  – hyperventilation;
  – hypokalaemia;
  – metabolic acidosis which may be severe;
  – haemoconcentration;
  – leukocytosis;
  – disseminated intravascular coagulation;
  – hypophosphataemia;
  – renal failure (with proteinuria and microscopic haematuria and possibly subsequent acute tubular necrosis);
  – hepatocellular damage of varying severity;
  – rhabdomyolysis;
  – vomiting and diarrhoea.

> There is thus widespread cellular damage and the presence of a medical emergency.

*Treatment consists of **active cooling** to 39°C within 30 min. Cooling should then be tapered to prevent an overshoot in the process. Cooling may be achieved by the use of either ice-packs or a cooling blanket.*

Requisite supportive therapy includes fluids, electrolytes, circulatory and respiratory support, and attention to any metabolic, haematological and renal dysfunction. The value of heparin is unsubstantiated, and the efficacy of dantrolene has not been confirmed in clinical trials.

The condition has a high mortality (with reports from 10–80%), but it is preventable by avoiding the risk factors referred to above and by the provision of appropriate first-aid.

A similar condition occurring after exposure to triggering agents (classically during general anaesthesia) is referred to as **malignant hyperthermia** (q.v.).

Bibliography

Bouchama A, Cafege A, Devol EB et al 1991 Ineffectiveness of dantrolene sodium in the treatment of heatstroke. Crit Care Med 19: 176.

Bouchama A, al-Sedairy S, Siddiqui S et al 1993 Elevated pyrogenic cytokines in heat stroke. Chest 104: 1498.

Clowes GHA, O'Donnell TF 1974 Heat stroke. N Engl J Med 291: 564.

Costrini A 1990 Emergency treatment of exertional heatstroke and comparison of whole body cooling techniques. Med Sci Sports Exerc 22: 15.

Knochel JP 1989 Heat stroke and related heat stress disorders. Dis Mon 35: 301.

Marr JJ, Geiss PT 1982 Management of heat injury syndromes. In: Shoemaker WC, Thompson WL (eds) Critical Care: State of the Art. Fullerton: Society of Critical Care Medicine. p K1.

Simon HB 1993 Hyperthermia. N Engl J Med 329: 483.

Heavy chains (see Multiple myeloma)

Heavy metal poisoning (see Chelating agents)

HELLP syndrome (see also Pre-eclampsia)

The HELLP syndrome comprises <u>h</u>aemolysis, <u>e</u>levated <u>l</u>iver enzymes and <u>l</u>ow <u>p</u>latelet count. It is a pregnancy-related disease of unknown aetiology, first described in 1982 as a separate subgroup of pre-eclampsia. It has been reported to occur in 2–12% of cases of pre-eclampsia, usually in the more severe cases. It usually occurs in the third trimester, though 30% of patients present within the first 48 h of the post-partum period. In these cases, many have had no evidence of pre-eclampsia prior to delivery.

The clinical features include upper abdominal pain and malaise in virtually all patients. Weight gain, oedema and hypertension are commonly present, but these are not necessarily diagnostic for pre-eclampsia at the time.

> A severe illness follows, with associated:
>
> * shock;
> * ARDS;
> * acute renal failure;
> * subcapsular haematoma of the liver (which may even lead to hepatic rupture);
> * generalized haemorrhage;
> * convulsions;
> * blindness (due to retinal detachment);
> * abruptio placentae (especially if there is acute renal failure and disseminated intravascular coagulation).
>
> These complications occur in 1–15% of cases and are more frequent in the post-partum state.

There is a microangiopathic haemolysis with thrombocytopenia but no laboratory evidence initially of disseminated intravascular coagulation, though this eventually occurs in about 20% of cases. The liver function tests are abnormal.

The differential diagnosis includes:

- acute fatty liver of pregnancy (q.v.);
- other causes of microangiopathic haemolysis (q.v.), e.g. thrombotic thrombocytopenic purpura (TTP), haemolytic–uraemic syndrome (HUS), malignancy;
- mild and asymptomatic gestational thrombocytopenia, seen in 5–8% of normal pregnancies.

*Treatment is with **emergency delivery**, usually by Caesarean section, and Intensive Care management. The liver should be treated as for **hepatic trauma**, with great care with palpation, etc. Difficult hepatic bleeding may require hepatic artery embolization. Laparotomy is sometimes indicated if there appears to be an acute abdominal crisis. **Plasmapheresis** should be considered for persistent haematological abnormality.*

Clearly, the condition carries a significant maternal and fetal risk.

Bibliography

Burrows RF, Kelton JG 1990 Thrombocytopenia at delivery: a prospective survey of 6715 deliveries. Am J Obstet Gynecol 162: 731.

Martin JN, Files FC, Blake PG 1990 Plasma exchange for preeclampsia: I. Postpartum use for persistently severe preeclampsia with HELLP syndrome. Am J Obstet Gynecol 162: 126.

Pousti TJ, Tominaga GT, Scannell G 1994 Help for the HELLP syndrome. Intens Care World 11: 62.

Sibai BM, Ramadan MK, Usta I et al 1993 Maternal morbidity and mortality in 442 pregnancies with hemolysis, elevated liver enzymes and low platelets (HELLP syndrome). Am J Obstet Gynecol 169: 1000.

Van Dam PA, Renier M, Baekelandt M et al 1989 Disseminated intravascular coagulation and the syndrome of hemolysis, elevated liver enzymes, and low platelets in severe preeclampsia. Obstet Gynecol 73: 97.

Weinstein L 1982 Syndrome of hemolysis, elevated liver enzymes and low platelet count: a severe consequence of hypertension. Am J Obstet Gynecol 142: 159.

Hemianopia

Hemianopia refers to loss of half of a visual field. The particular half affected depends on the site of the lesion which has interrupted the optic tract or radiation.

Hemianopia may be caused by:

- cerebral tumour (including pituitary tumours);
- stroke (both haemorrhagic and ischaemic);
- cerebral abscess (parietal, subdural);
- meningitis;
- superior sagittal sinus thrombosis;
- migraine (occasionally).

Bibliography

Morantz RA, Walsh JW (eds) 1994 Brain Tumors. New York: Marcel Dekker.

Henoch–Schönlein purpura (see Purpura)

Heparin

Heparin is one of the most commonly used drugs in clinical medicine. Its most common complication is bleeding.

An uncommon but important and nowadays well recognized complication is **heparin-induced thrombocytopenia** (HITS) (see Thrombocytopenia).

More uncommon complications of heparin therapy include:

- **osteoporosis**

  – associated with prolonged use;

- **hyperkalaemia**

  – due to hypoaldosteronism and usually in the presence of renal failure and/or diabetes;

- **skin necrosis** (q.v.)

  – though this is more commonly seen with warfarin therapy and occurs in protein C deficient patients;

- **increased liver enzymes**

  – transaminitis, with levels that though increased are still usually in the normal range, this phenomenon generally reaching a peak after one week and decreasing despite continuing therapy;

- **interaction with intravenous glyceryl trinitrate (nitroglycerin, GTN)**

  – with consequent resistance to heparin.

Bibliography

Hirsh J, Levine MN 1992 Low molecular weight heparin. Blood 79: 1.

Oster JR, Singer I, Fishman LM 1995 Heparin-induced aldosterone suppression and hyperkalaemia. Am J Med 98: 575.

Hepatic diseases

Most hepatic disorders encountered in the Intensive Care Unit are common and well known. They include hepatic failure (including fulminant hepatic failure, FHF), cirrhosis, portal hypertension, hepatic encephalopathy and hepato–renal syndrome. Some conditions of course are less common and are therefore considered in this book, including:

- biliary cirrhosis;
- Budd–Chiari syndrome;
- hepatic necrosis;
- hepatic vein thrombosis;
- hepatitis;
- hepatoma;
- hepatopulmonary syndrome;
- liver abscess;
- Wilson's disease.

Bibliography

Adedoyin A, Branch RA 1997 The effect of liver disease on drugs. Curr Opinion Crit Care 3: 255.

Better OS 1986 Renal and cardiovascular dysfunction in liver disease. Kidney Int 29: 598.

Calvo CP, Sipman FS, Caramelo C 1996 Renal and electrolyte abnormalities in patients with hepatic insufficiency. Curr Opinion Crit Care 2: 413.

Eckardt K-U 1999 Renal failure in liver disease. Intens Care Med 25: 5.

Editorial 1982 Hepatic osteomalacia and vitamin D. Lancet 1: 943.

Fraser CL, Arieff AI 1985 Hepatic encephalopathy. N Engl J Med 313: 865.

Garcia-Tsao G 1991 Treatment of ascites with single total paracentesis. Hepatology 13: 1005.

LaMont JT, Isselbacher KJ 1973 Postoperative jaundice. N Engl J Med 288: 305.

Lieber CS 1995 Medical disorders of alcoholism. N Engl J Med 333: 1058.

Ludwig J 1993 The nomenclature of chronic active hepatitis: an obituary. Gastroenterology 105: 274.

McClain CJ 1991 Trace metals in liver disease. Semin Liver Dis 11: 321.

Mills PR, Sturrock RD 1982 Clinical associations between arthritis and liver disease. Ann Rheum Dis 41: 295.

Riordan SM, Williams R 1999 Current management of fulminant hepatic failure. Curr Opin Crit Care 5: 136.

Runyon BA 1994 Care of patients with ascites. N Engl J Med 330: 337.

Shearman DJC, Finlayson NDC 1989 Diseases of the Gastrointestinal Tract and Liver. 2nd edition. Edinburgh: Churchill Livingstone.

Sherlock S, Dooley J 1993 Diseases of the Liver and Biliary System. 9th edition. Oxford: Blackwell.

Starzl TE, Demetris AJ, Van Thiel D 1989 Liver transplantation. N Engl J Med 321: 1014, 1092.

Vennes JA, Bond JH 1983 Approach to the jaundiced patient. Gastroenterology 84: 1615.

Wright TL 1993 Etiology of fulminant hepatic failure: is another virus involved? Gastroenterology 104: 640.

Hepatic necrosis (see Hepatitis)

Hepatic vein thrombosis (see

Budd–Chiari syndrome)

Hepatitis

Hepatitis is inflammation of the liver cells. It is produced:

- usually by viral infection (especially hepatitis viruses A–E, CMV, EBV);
- sometimes by drugs or toxins.

Hepatitis may thus be a final common pathway for a variety of different liver insults.

Sometimes, fulminant hepatitis occurs with no definable cause, so that it is likely that there are other as yet unidentified viruses, mutant viruses or toxins capable of producing this syndrome. About 5–20% of cases of acute and chronic hepatitis have no currently identifiable cause, prompting in particular a continuing search for viruses other than the main known five (A–E).

Clinical features of hepatitis are variable and often extensive.

Typically, there are systemic inflammatory symptoms affecting the gut, joints and CNS for 1–2 weeks prior to the onset of more specific local features. The more specific local features include:

- dark urine (in over 90%);
- light stools (in over 50%);
- abdominal discomfort;
- tender smooth hepatomegaly;
- jaundice;
- hepatic fetor (fetor hepaticus).

Investigations show abnormal liver function tests with high transaminase levels as the initial finding. The serum bilirubin rises to a maximum of about 350 μmol /L by 2 weeks, and then decreases over the following 2–4 weeks. The alkaline phosphatase is usually moderately elevated, and there is hypoalbuminaemia and a prolonged prothrombin time in severe cases. The full blood examination is mildly abnormal.

Treatment is frustrating because no modalities alter the course of disease.

- *Bed rest is warranted on the clinical merits of the symptoms, but measures such as diet and vitamins are ineffective and even alcohol is not necessarily contraindicated.*
- *Trials involving corticosteroids, immune globulin, cimetidine and exchange transfusion have shown no efficacy.*
- *Lactulose (30 mL 4 hourly) is commonly given, but its benefit is uncertain.*

- *Transplantation is indicated in severe disease with encephalopathy, except in chronic hepatitis B and C because of the high rate of recurrent viraemia and severe hepatitis.*
- *Predisposition to bacterial infection and coagulopathy need to be attended to.*

The outlook after hepatitis is usually favourable, with an uncomplicated course and complete recovery.

Occasionally, however,

- the disease may **relapse** or become **prolonged** especially with hepatitis B and hepatitis C, and also in the elderly;

- there may be an **acute fulminant course**

  – leading to hepatic coma and even death;
  – usually seen in hepatitis B and hepatitis C;
  – sometimes in hepatitis E in pregnancy;

- **chronic hepatitis**

  – may occur in hepatitis B or C pre-disposing to hepatocellular carcinoma;
  – may occur in hepatitis C predisposing to a carrier state;
  – is manifest by raised serum alanine aminotransferase (ALT) for more than six months and progresses slowly to hepatic fibrosis;
  – may be autoimmune, when it is most commonly ANA positive and corticosteroid-responsive,
  – may be cryptogenic.

Many **concomitant extrahepatic syndromes** have also been reported, most commonly in hepatitis B. There have been associated:

- autoimmune haemolytic anaemia;
- polyarteritis nodosa;
- cryoglobulinaemia especially in chronic HCV infection;
- sicca syndrome especially in chronic HCV infection;
- immune-mediated renal disease in chronic HBV and especially HCV infection.

Hepatitis type A virus (HAV, infectious hepatitis virus) is an RNA virus transmitted by faecal contamination.

The incubation period is usually 3–5 weeks, and there is a viraemia with viral shedding for up to 3 weeks before the appearance of jaundice. The patient is not infectious after 3 weeks of clinical illness unless a relapse occurs. There is no animal reservoir.

Infection gives rise to immunity (an early IgM and a later IgG) and antibodies may be detected in about 50% of the population.

Chronic disease does not occur, and the mortality is <0.2%.

*Pooled **immune globulin** given within 2 weeks of exposure decreases the occurrence of clinical disease.*

Hepatitis type B virus (HBV, serum hepatitis) is a DNA virus usually transmitted by percutaneous inoculation of infected blood, but the virus in fact is present in many bodily fluids, so that for example venereal transmission is also common.

The incubation period is usually 2–6 months and averages 12 weeks. Antibodies to surface antigen (anti-HBs) and to core antigen (anti-HBc) appear early and persist in the carrier state, though only anti-HBs is normally seen in convalescent serum or after vaccination.

Chronic disease occurs in up to 10% of patients, and the mortality is 1.5%.

*Treatment is with **immune globulin** if given within one week of exposure, but the most appropriate management is prevention with **recombinant hepatitis B vaccine**. However, the use of this vaccine has become controversial in some countries following reports of both central and peripheral demyelination after its administration.*

Hepatitis type C virus (HCV, non-A, non-B or post-transfusion hepatitis) is an RNA virus also usually transmitted by percutaneous inoculation or infected blood. It was identified in 1989 and is now recognized as the cause of most cases (perhaps 90%) of transfusion hepatitis, but it may also be responsible for up to 25% of sporadic acute community-acquired hepatitis.

Incubation period is usually 5–10 weeks. Anti-HCv antibodies are present in the acute disease, in the carrier state and in over 50% of cases of hepatocellular carcinoma.

Most patients are asymptomatic, even though they are infectious to others. The disease may remain silent and eventual chronic liver impairment may be its first clinical manifestation. Failure of viral clearance is the most important problem following acute infection and this causes chronic disease in about 75%. Chronic hepatitis in turn commonly leads to cirrhosis or hepatocellular carcinoma. The mortality is probably similar to that of hepatitis B. The mechanism for its hepatocarcinogenesis is uncertain because, unlike HBV, HCV is not incorporated into the host genome.

*Treatment with **immune globulin** acutely and with **interferon alpha** (IFN) in the chronic state are helpful. Combination therapy with ribavirin and IFN appears to be more effective both initially and after relapse than IFN alone, with response to therapy varying with viral genotype.*

End-stage liver disease due to hepatitis C infection is nowadays the most common condition requiring liver transplantation.

Hepatitis type D virus (delta-agent) requires hepatitis B virus (HBV) for its expression. Thus, its route of transmission, incubation period and prophylaxis are as for hepatitis B.

It is associated with more severe disease, with an acute mortality of up to 20% and a chronic disease state in HBV carriers. Anti-HDv antibodies appear late in the course of disease.

Hepatitis type E virus is, like HAV, transmitted via faecal contamination. It is an important course of epidemic hepatitis in developing countries. The immunological status is uncertain.

The incubation period is 2–8 weeks. The mortality of acute disease is up to 2% and up to

15% in pregnancy, but it does not lead to chronic disease.

Hepatitis type F virus (HFV) is a recently described DNA virus. Its role as a formal hepatitis virus remains to be clarified.

Hepatitis type G virus (HGV) is a recently described RNA virus, related to but separate from HCV. It appears to be an important cause of post-transfusion hepatitis, though it may be a coinfection with HCV.

Many **drugs** may cause liver damage, usually via idiosyncratic reactions (see Drug Allergy). The clinical and laboratory features are indistinguishable from viral hepatitis. The 'incubation' period is usually 2–6 weeks, but it can be a short as 1 day or as long as 6 months. Although this form of liver damage may be predictable for high doses of some drugs (e.g. paracetamol), it is not normally dose-dependent, as with halothane, isoniazid, methyldopa, phenytoin, sulfonamides.

Recently, the new anti-Parkinsonism drug, tolcapone, was withdrawn from the market because of reports of serious and sometimes fatal hepatotoxicity, the new 'fourth-generation' quinolone, trovafloxacin/alatrofloxacin, has been reported to cause hepatic damage, including rarely acute hepatic necrosis and hepatic failure.

Drug-induced hepatitis can persist despite stopping the drug. Continuing the drug may be fatal.

Conversely, in patients with liver disease there is impairment of oxidative drug metabolism, a drug clearance mechanism (e.g. for theophylline) which has recently been shown to be improved in such patients by supplemental oxygen. Drug clearance by hepatic conjugation (e.g. for paracetamol) is not improved by oxygen.

Toxins producing hepatic damage similar to viral hepatitis may occur in:

- mushroom poisoning (q.v.), including Kombucha 'mushroom' tea;
- plant alkaloid poisoning;
- Reye's syndrome (q.v.).

A similar picture is also seen in some cases of severe hepatic ischaemia and/or congestion.

Bibliography

Davis GL, Esteban-Mur R, Rustgi V et al 1998 Interferon alfa-2b alone or in combination with ribavirin for the treatment of relapse of chronic hepatitis C. N Engl J Med 339: 1493.

Farrell GC 1998 Acute viral hepatitis. Med J Aust 168: 565.

Farrell GC 1998 Chronic viral hepatitis. Med J Aust 168: 619.

Froomes PRA, Morgan DJ, Smallwood RA et al 1999 Comparative effects of oxygen supplementation on theophylline and acetaminophen clearance in human cirrhosis. Gastroenterology 116: 915.

Gross JB, Persing DH 1995 Hepatitis C: advances in diagnosis. Mayo Clin Proc 70: 296.

Hoofnagle JH 1989 Type D (delta) hepatitis. JAMA 261: 1321.

Johnson RJ, Gretch Dr, Yamabe H et al 1993 Membranoproliferative glomerulonephritis associated with hepatitis C virus infection. N Engl J Med 328: 465.

Kaplowitz N, Aw TY, Simon FR et al 1986 Drug-induced hepatotoxicity. Ann Intern Med 104: 826.

Keays R, Harrison PM, Wendon JA et al 1991 Intravenous acetylcysteine in paracetamol fulminant hepatic failure: a prospective controlled trial. Br Med J 303: 1026.

Krawczynski K 1993 Hepatitis E Hepatology 17: 932.

Lau JY, Wright TL 1995 Molecular virology and pathogenesis of hepatitis B. Lancet 342: 1335.

Lee WM 1997 Hepatitis B virus infection. N Engl J Med 337: 1733.

Liang TJ, Rehermann B, Seeff LB et al 2000 Pathogenesis, natural history, treatment, and prevention of hepatitis C. Ann Intern Med 132: 296.

Linnen J, Wages J, Zhen-Yong ZK et al 1996 Molecular cloning and disease association of hepatitis G virus: A transfusion-transmissible agent. Science 271: 505.

Maddrey WC 1993 Chronic hepatitis. Dis Mon 39: 53.

McCaughan GW, Koorey DJ 1997 Liver transplantation. Aust NZ J Med 27: 371.

McCaughan GW, Strasser SI 2000 Emerging therapies for hepatitis C virus (HCV) infection: the importance of HCV genotype. Aust NZ J Med 30: 644.

McHutchison JG, Gordon SC, Schiff ER et al 1998 Interferon alfa-2b alone or in combination with ribavirin as initial treatment for chronic hepatitis C. N Engl J Med 339: 1485.

Mitra AK 1999 Hepatitis C-related hepatocellular carcinoma. Epidem Rev 21: 180.

Perron AD, Patterson JA, Yanofsky NN 1995 Kombucha 'mushroom' hepatotoxicity. Ann Emerg Med 26: 660.

Riordan SM, Williams R 1999 Current management of fulminant hepatic failure. Curr Opin Crit Care 5: 136.

Shapiro CN 1994; Transmission of hepatitis viruses. Ann Intern Med 120: 82.

Tsukuma H, Hiyama T, Tanaka S et al 1993 Risk factors for hepatocellular carcinoma among patients with chronic liver disease. N Engl J Med 328: 1797.

Various. Hepatitis C 1999 Aust Family Physician 28 (Special Issue).

Wanke CA, Guerrant RL 1987 Viral hepatitis and gastroenteritis transmitted by shellfish and water. Infect Dis Clin North Am 1: 649.

Wright TL 1993 Etiology of fulminant hepatic failure: is another virus involved? Gastroenterology 104: 640.

Zuckerman AJ 1995 The new GB hepatitis viruses. Lancet 345: 1453.

Hepatocellular carcinoma (see Hepatoma)

Hepatoma

Hepatoma (hepatocellular carcinoma) is generally associated with pre-existing liver disease. Typically, this precursor disease is cirrhosis, especially following hepatitis B or C infection or haemochromatosis. Sometimes, hepatoma may follow cirrhosis due to alcohol, α_1-antitrypsin deficiency, methotrxate or schistosomiasis. Occasionally, it may follow hepatic damage without cirrhosis, e.g. after ingestion of aflatoxins, androgens and possibly oral contraceptives.

Hepatoma is seen most commonly in men, typically younger men in Africa, middle-aged men in East Asia, and elderly men in developed countries.

Clinical features of hepatoma include:

- weight loss;
- painful hepatomegaly;
- hepatic friction rub;
- worsening of portal hypertension.

It is commonly associated with paraneoplastic features (q.v.), such as:

- dysfibrinogenaemia;
- hypoglycaemia;
- hypercalcaemia;
- polycythaemia.

Investigations involving liver function tests are usually unhelpful, as they are typically abnormal beforehand, although the AST and/or alkaline phosphatase may be especially abnormal. Imaging and biopsy are required for diagnosis including the extent of the tumour. Angiography is required to assess resectability because, unlike hepatic metastases, hepatoma may have increased vascularity. Although the alpha-fetoprotein level (q.v.) is increased in about 70% of patients, it is neither sufficiently specific nor sensitive for diagnosis, though it may assist with the assessment of progress and possibly with the screening of high-risk patients.

*Treatment is with **resection** if technically feasible.*

- *Otherwise, liver transplantation may be considered, although recurrence within two years is common.*
- *Palliation may be produced by local vascular occlusion or chemotherapy.*

The median survival is only about 6 months. The prognosis is worse if there are metastases (usually to lung or bone) or jaundice, but the five-year survival is up to 30% following resection.

Bibliography

El-Serag HB, Mason AC 1999 Rising incidence of hepatocellular carcinoma in the United States. N Engl J Med 340: 745.

Fan S-T, Lo C-M, Lai ECS et al 1994 Perioperative nutritional support in patients undergoing hepatectomy for hepatocellular carcinoma. N Engl J Med 331: 1547.

Farmer DG, Rosove MH, Shaked A et al 1994 Current treatment modalities for hepatocellular carcinoma. Ann Surg 219: 236.

Margolis S, Homcy C 1972 Systemic manifestations of hepatoma. Medicine 51: 381.

Mitra AK 1999 Hepatitis C-related hepatocellular carcinoma. Epidem Rev 21: 180.

Tsukuma H, Hiyama T, Tanaka S et al 1993 Risk factors for hepatocellular carcinoma among patients with chronic liver disease. N Engl J Med 328: 1797.

Venook AP 1994 Treatment of hepatocellular carcinoma: too many options? J Clin Oncol 12: 1323.

Wands JR, Blum HE 1991 Primary hepatocellular carcinoma. N Engl J Med 325: 729.

Hepatopulmonary syndrome

Hepatopulmonary syndrome (or hepatogenic pulmonary angiodysplasia) was described in 1984 as a condition characterized by cirrhosis, cyanosis and clubbing.

Its pathogenesis is unknown, but it may be due to failure of the liver to preserve the normal balance of pulmonary vasoconstrictor and vasodilator substances. Histologically, there are diffuse precapillary dilatations, arteriovenous malformations and pleural spider naevi.

Clinical features of hepatopulmonary syndrome are dominated by hypoxaemia, which can sometimes be severe. There is dyspnoea, cyanosis and digital clubbing.

On standing, the hypoxaemia is paradoxically worse (orthodeoxia) and there is tachypnoea (platypnoea). These unusual phenomena are generally seen only in occasional patients after pneumonectomy or with recurrent pulmonary embolism.

In mild disease, there are no symptoms.

Examination of the chest is normal.

The chest X-ray is normal. Lung function tests show a decreased diffusing capacity and abnormal ventilation–perfusion relationships (typically shunt).

The differential diagnosis includes the many, much more common causes of pulmonary dysfunction in patients with liver disease, namely:

- diaphragmatic disadvantage;
- pleural effusion;
- atelectasis.

Treatment is uncertain, but indomethacin or possibly octreotide may be helpful.

Liver transplantation causes the condition to reverse eventually, provided it has not become chronic.

In Intensive Care practice, the hepatopulmonary syndrome should be remembered as a cause of hypoxaemia in patients with significant liver disease and a normal chest X-ray.

Bibliography

Herve P, Lebrec D, Brenot F et al 1998 Pulmonary vascular disorders in portal hypertension. Eur Respir J 11: 1153.

Krowka MJ, Cortese DA 1994 Hepatopulmonary syndrome: current concepts in diagnostic and therapeutic considerations. Chest 105: 1528.

Krowka MJ, Wiseman GA, Burnett OL et al 2000 Hepatopulmonary syndrome. Chest 118: 615.

Hereditary haemorrhagic telangiectasia (see Arteriovenous malformations)

Herpesviruses (see Acyclovir)

High altitude

Moderate altitude (1500–2500 m) exists in many regions of the world which are either populated or commonly visited. This altitude is of clinical relevance only in patients with existing cardiopulmonary disease and in the occasional particularly susceptible patient who even then has only mild distress. It is the altitude to which commercial airlines are pressurized (i.e. up to 2440 m or 8000 ft).

High altitude (2500–4000 m) is the usual threshold for permanent habitation. The PaO_2 has fallen to 50 mmHg by 4000 m. This region contains the usual threshold for high-altitude medical problems.

Very high altitude (4000–5500 m) encompasses the limits of permanent habitation and acclimatization. At these heights, the barometric pressure is about half that at sea level and the arterial oxygenation is approximately the normal venous level.

Extreme altitude (5500–8848 m, the height of Mount Everest) is reached only by mountaineering expeditions.

High-altitude medical problems comprise the following entities.

1. Acute mountain sickness

This is especially manifest by headache but also fatigue, dizziness, insomnia and nausea. It is due to cerebral hypoxia. It is experienced by about 70% of subjects at least to some degree and is worse on exercise. It is associated with an impaired ventilatory response to hypoxia. It is not associated with unfitness, but it is assisted by acclimatization. It lasts only a few days.

Its treatment is symptomatic, including **oxygen** *administration. Effective measures include* **acetazolamide** *and* **dexamethasone** *but not* **frusemide**. **Descent** *from altitude is required if the illness is severe.*

2. **Pulmonary oedema**

This is manifest by dyspnoea, fatigue and cough and if severe by cerebral dysfunction. It is associated with exercise and lack of acclimatization. It has an average incidence of only 0.5%, though this can be increased 10-fold or more if ascent is rapid. It generally occurs gradually but always within 2–4 days and is commonly preceded by the less severe features of acute mountain sickness. It has a mortality of about 10%, especially if treatment fails.

It is associated with pulmonary hypertension but a normal pulmonary artery wedge pressure. It is thus a high-flow, protein-rich, oedema process, similar to that seen after the relief of acute pulmonary artery obstruction or in hypertensive encephalopathy. It is associated with an irregular hypoxic pulmonary arteriolar constriction, multiple small thrombi, peripheral vasoconstriction and fluid retention due to increased secretion of antidiuretic hormone.

Treatment requires **descent** *from altitude and the administration of* **oxygen**.

- *Diuretics are not appropriate.*
- *Continuous positive airway pressure/positive end-expiratory pressure (CPAP/PEEP) is effective (ancient Chinese merchants crossing high mountains such as the Himalayas were known to use pursed-lip breathing if breathless).*
- *Intubation and mechanical ventilation may occasionally be required.*
- *Nitric oxide has recently been reported to be of benefit.*
- *Nifedipine has been found to be useful prophylactically in susceptible people.*

3. **Cerebral oedema**

This is manifest by headache, disorientation, ataxia, hallucinations and coma. Papilloedema and retinal haemorrhages are commonly seen. There is increased intracranial pressure and cerebral petechiae.

It occurs in about 20% of patients suffering from pulmonary oedema, though its onset may be delayed for several days. It has a mortality of about 15%, and survivors may suffer from prolonged neurological sequelae.

Treatment requires **descent** *from altitude and the administration of* **oxygen**.

- *Corticosteroids have been used, but their value is not established.*

4. **Miscellaneous conditions**

These include:

- chronic mountain sickness, manifest by fatigue, poor mental function, dyspnoea, polycythaemia and pulmonary hypertension;
- thromboembolism;
- peripheral oedema;
- syncope.

5. **Prior conditions adversely affected by altitude**

These include:

- heart disease;
- chronic obstructive lung disease;
- hypertension;
- obesity;
- sickle cell disease;
- decompression sickness.

Bibliography

Boyer SJ, Blume FD 1984 Weight loss and changes in body composition at high altitude. J Appl Physiol 57: 1580.

Cottrell JJ 1988 Altitude exposure during aircraft flight: flying higher. Chest 92: 81.

Cramer D, Ward S, Geddes D 1996 Assessment of oxygen supplementation during air travel. Thorax 51: 202.

Frayser R, Houston CS, Bryan AC et al 1970 Retinal hemorrhage at high altitude. N Engl J Med 282: 1183.

Hackett PH, Rennie D, Levine HD 1976 The incidence, importance and prophylaxis of acute mountain sickness. Lancet 2: 1149.

Hock RJ 1970 The physiology of high altitude. Sci Am 222: 2, 52.

Houston CS, Dickinson J 1975 Cerebral form of high-altitude illness. Lancet 2: 758.

Hultgren HN 1996 High-altitude pulmonary edema: current concepts. Annu Rev Med 47: 267.

Johnson TS, Rock PB 1988 Acute mountain sickness. N Engl J Med 319: 841.

Penaloza D, Sime F 1971 Chronic cor pulmonale due to loss of altitude acclimatization (chronic mountain sickness). Am J Med 50: 728.

Richalet JP 1995 High altitude pulmonary oedema: still a place for controversy? Thorax 50: 923.

Scherrer U, Vollenweider L, Delabays A et al 1996 Inhaled nitric oxide for high-altitude pulmonary edema. N Engl J Med 334: 624.

Schoene RB 1985 Pulmonary edema at high altitude: review, pathophysiology, and update. Clin Chest Med 6: 491.

Sutton JR, Reeves JT, Wagner PD et al 1988 Operation Everest II: oxygen transport during exercise at extreme simulated altitude. J Appl Physiol 64: 1309.

Ward M, Millege J, West J 1989 High Altitude Medicine and Physiology. Philadelphia: University of Pennsylvania Press.

Waterlow JC, Bunje HW 1966 Observations on mountain sickness in the Colombian Andes. Lancet 2: 655.

West JB, Boyer SJ, Graber DJ et al 1983 Maximal exercise at extreme altitudes on Mount Everest. J Appl Physiol 55: 688.

Hirsutism

Hirsutism refers to increased growth of hair at sites that are normally androgen-dependent, namely the face, chest and abdomen. The term usually applies to women.

Excess androgens may be exogenous (e.g. anabolic steroids) or endogenous. Increased endogenous androgen production may be either functional or neoplastic and occurs in either the adrenal gland or ovary (e.g. polycystic ovary syndrome).

Treatment apart from any that may be available for a specific lesion is either **cosmetic** *or* **suppressive**. *Suppression may be achieved with corticosteroids (e.g. dexamethasone) which inhibit ACTH production, oral contraceptives which inhibit pituitary gonadotrophins, and androgen blockers (cyproterone acetate and spironolactone are the most commonly used agents of this type).*

Hypertrichosis refers to increased hair growth of a non-endocrine nature. It may be:

- familial;
- racial;
- drug-induced (minoxidil, phenytoin, cyclosporin);
- idiopathic.

Bibliography

Kvedar JC, Gibson M, Krusinski PA 1985 Hirsutism: evaluation and treatment. J Am Acad Dermatol 12: 215.

McKenna TJ 1994 Screening for sinister causes of hirsutism. N Engl J Med 331: 1015.

Munro DD, Darley CR 1979 Hair. In: Fitzpatrick TB, Eisen AZ, Wolff K et al (eds) Dermatology in General Medicine. New York: McGraw-Hill. p 395.

Histiocytosis X

Histiocytosis X comprises three related diseases, namely:

- eosinophilic granuloma;
- Hand–Schüller–Christian disease;
- Letterer–Siwe disease.

There is a unique granulomatous infiltration with Langerhans'-like cells resembling monocytes and macrophages (i.e. histiocytes) and containing a foamy eosinophilic cytoplasm with characteristic inclusions (X or Birbeck granules) and positive staining with anti-CD1a monoclonal antibody.

The infiltrate is a monoclonal proliferation, and it affects skin, bone, liver and central nervous system, as well as lung.

Eosinophilic granuloma is the form of histiocytosis X which affects the lungs, in which it is an uncommon cause of a diffuse pulmonary infiltrate. It mostly occurs in Caucasian adults and is strongly associated with smoking.

Clinical features generally comprise cough and dyspnoea, though 25% of patients are asymptomatic. Spontaneous pneumothorax occurs in 10–20% of cases. Systemic involvement is common with up to 20% of patients having involvement of bone or pituitary (with diabetes insipidus).

The chest X-ray shows a diffuse reticular or fine nodular pattern, with 50% of cases also having honeycombing or cysts, many too small to be detected except by CT scanning. Rupture of such a cyst is the cause of propensity to pneumothorax. Lung function tests show decreased gas exchange and ventilatory capacity, as for most pulmonary interstitial diseases, but unlike them there is also airflow obstruction.

The diagnosis is made by open lung biopsy, though it may be suggested by the presence of >5% CD1a-positive cells in BAL fluid.

Treatment of local disease is with curettage if feasible or with irradiation.

*Systematic disease is treated with **corticosteroids** with or without cytotoxic agents (vinblastine). However, treatment is often not required, as the condition is relatively benign, frequently asymptomatic and often remits.*

Hand–Schüller–Christian disease occurs in children as well as adults.It is a multi-system disease affecting bone particularly. Diabetes insipidus is common. Pulmonary involvement may include progressive fibrosis with honeycombing.

Letterer–Siwe disease occurs only in infants.

Bibliography

Cheyne C 1971 Histiocytosis X. J Bone Joint Surg 53: 366.

Crausman RS, Jennings CA, Tuder RM et al 1996 Pulmonary histiocytosis X: pulmonary function and exercise physiology. Am J Respir Crit Care Med 153: 426.

Kambouchner M, Valeyre D, Soler P et al 1992 Pulmonary Langerhans' cell granulomatosis (histiocytosis X). Annu Rev Med 43: 105.

Histocompatibility complex

The major histocompatibility complex (MHC) contains genes responsible for the production of highly polymorphic cell-surface antigens which identify cells as 'self' and which are responsible for presentation of peptide antigens to T lymphocytes. In humans, the MHC is specified by the term HLA and resides on the short arm of chromosome 6.

There are two types of MHC molecules, Class I and II.

- Class I antigens are expressed on virtually all cell types. They consist of two polypeptide chains, a polymorphic heavy chain (44 kD), and a non-polymorphic light chain (11.5 kD), called beta 2-microglobulin. The Class I proteins present peptide fragments of proteins made within the cell, including usually encoded proteins, to CD8+ cells.
- Class II antigens are expressed on only a few cell types, mainly lymphocytes, monocytes and dendritic cells, though in inflammation many other cells can also express these antigens. They consist of two polymorphic polypeptide chains of 34 and 28 kD. The Class II proteins present peptide fragments of endogenous endocytosed proteins to CD4+ cells.

There may be many different alleles at each of the 7 loci in the HLA system. There is a correlation between specific HLA antigens and the presence of a large of number of diseases, with relative risks from 2–3-fold up to 90-fold or more. The mechanism of this association is not understood in detail, but it is likely to be related to the ability of different MHC types to bind and present particular peptide antigens to T lymphocytes.

There is a relative risk of 10-fold or more of the following diseases (in descending order of frequency in each group) in patients with specific HLA antigens:

- **dermatological diseases**

  – dermatitis herpetiformis, pemphigus vulgaris;

- **endocrine diseases**

  – juvenile insulin-dependent diabetes mellitus, congenital adrenal hyperplasia, subacute thyroiditis, Addison's disease;

- **gastrointestinal diseases**

  – gluten-sensitive enteropathy;

- **haematological diseases**

  – haemochromatosis;

- **neurological diseases**

  – narcolepsy;

- **renal diseases**

  – Goodpasture's syndrome, gold and penicillamine nephropathy;

- **rheumatic diseases**

  – ankylosing spondylitis, Reiter's syndrome, reactive arthritis, psoriatic arthritis.

Note that some of these conditions (e.g. haemochromatosis, narcolepsy and most notably congenital adrenal hyperplasia) are not immune-related, and their HLA association may relate to other, non-HLA genes nearby.

Bibliography
Guillet J-G, Lai M-Z, Briner TJ et al 1987 Immunological self, nonself discrimination. Science 235: 865.
Schlossman SF, Boumsell L, Gilks W et al 1994 Update: CD antigens 1993. J Immunol 152: 1.
Tiwari JL, Terasaki PI 1985 HLA and Disease Associations. New York: Springer-Verlag.

Histoplasmosis

Histoplasmosis is a systemic mycosis caused by the fungus, *Histoplasma capsulatum*, which is found in soil and bird droppings worldwide. Infection from aerosolized spores thus occurs when soil or bird or bat droppings are disturbed.

Over 90% of infections are asymptomatic, but primary disease if severe gives an influenza-like illness. A chronic progressive cavitatory disease of the lungs may be seen, particularly in older men. Disseminated disease with multiorgan involvement is seen in occasional patients (one in 50 000) with primary disease and in compromised hosts.

> Histoplasmosis has many similarities in pathogenesis and clinical presentation to tuberculosis. It can also mimic sarcoidosis.

The diagnosis is based on culture of the organism. A positive skin test is not specific for the disease-state, but positive serology may be helpful.

*Treatment is with **amphotericin** if the disease is clinically significant.*

- *Ketoconazole is also effective.*
- *Surgical resection may sometimes be indicated for chronic pulmonary lesions.*

Bibliography
Wheat LJ 1988 Systemic fungal infections: diagnosis and treatment; I. Histoplasmosis. Infect Dis Clin North Am 2: 841.

Horner's syndrome

Horner's syndrome describes the phenomenon of unilateral miosis (pupillary constriction) with ptosis (lid droop) and often anhydrosis and enophthalmos. It is caused by interruption of the ascending sympathetic fibres originating in the hypothalamus and innervating the eye.

> Horner's syndrome may be caused by:
>
> - carotid disease;
> - vertebrobasilar ischaemia;
> - brachial plexus infiltration (particularly due to carcinoma of the lung or breast);
> - syringomyelia;
> - migraine and cluster headache;
> - central venous catheterization.

An ipsilateral Horner's syndrome is seen in the **lateral medullary syndrome**, which is caused by vertebral artery thrombosis. In addition, there is nystagmus, ataxia and dysphagia. Typically, there is also ipsilateral impairment of facial sensation and contralateral loss of the sensation of pain and temperature in the limbs.

Bibliography
Reddy G, Coombes A, Hubbard AD 1998 Horner's
   syndrome following internal jugular vein
   cannulation. Intens Care Med 24: 194.

Hot tubs (see Bathing)

Human bites (see Bites and stings)

Hydatid disease (see Echinococcosis)

Hydrocephalus

Hydrocephalus refers to enlargement of the
cerebral ventricles. It is classified as either
communicating or non-communicating.

Communicating hydrocephalus is the more
common form. It is due to impaired
reabsorption of cerebrospinal fluid by the
arachnoid granulations over the dural venous
sinuses. This may follow previous haemorrhage,
infection or trauma.

Non-communicating hydrocephalus arises
from obstruction in the ventricular system (e.g.
in the aqueduct of Sylvius). Thus, cerebrospinal
fluid flow is impaired and the proximal
ventricles become enlarged.

> Hydrocephalus gives rise to progressive
> dementia, with ataxia and incontinence. The
> diagnosis is made by CT and MR scanning.

Treatment is with **shunting***, usually
ventriculoperitoneal but sometimes ventriculoatrial or
ventriculovenous.*

Complications of ventricular shunting include:

- infection;
- shunt occlusion;
- subdural haemorrhage.

Hydrogen sulfide

Hydrogen sulfide (H_2S) is a colourless,
poisonous gas with the characteristic smell of
rotten eggs and is referred to as 'stink damp'. It
is produced from the natural decay of organic
sulfur-containing substances, and it is also
present in the gas from mineral spas and from
volcanoes. It is also produced as a by-product of
petroleum refining, and it is used extensively in
the chemical industry as an analytic agent.

Its accidental inhalation can be fatal.

Treatment is **symptomatic***.*

Hyperbaric oxygen (see Carbon

monoxide and Gangrene)

Hypercalcaemia

Hypercalcaemia is an important phenomenon,
since:

- it may present a life-threatening crisis;
- it may also be a marker of significant and
  potentially treatable underlying disease.

The causes are

1. Increased gastrointestinal absorption

Normal absorption of calcium is under vitamin
D control and increased absorption thus occurs
from excess vitamin D intake, as well as in the
milk-alkali syndrome (in which there is
associated metabolic alkalosis) and in sarcoidosis.

2. Increased bone reabsorption

Normal absorption is under parathyroid control
and increased reabsorption thus occurs in
hyperparathyroidism, as well as in
hyperthyroidism (in which it is mild and
uncommon), metastatic malignancy, multiple
myeloma, Paget's disease, immobility (though
usually there is associated disease) and as a
paraneoplastic phenomenon (due to ectopic
hormone production or to cytokine release,
such as of IL-1).

3. Increased renal absorption

Normal renal absorption of calcium is under
parathyroid hormone control and increased

absorption thus occurs in hyperparathyroidism, as well as in adrenal insufficiency and sometimes following thiazide administration.

> If the patient is well, the usual cause of hypercalcaemia is hyperparathyroidism.

In **tumour-associated hypercalcaemia**, the malignancy is usually apparent clinically.

- The ectopic hormone produced is parathyroid hormone related protein (PTHrP). Even in bony metastases, there may be a humoral element. PTHrP is synthesized by some squamous cell carcinomas (particularly lung, breast and kidney) but also by some normal tissues, such as the placenta. The intact protein of 173 amino acids can be assayed, though variable fragments are also found. PTHrP may have a morphogenetic role at least in the fetus, because 'knockout' mice show marked developmental defects.
- Vitamin D in the form of the active 1, 25-dihydroxyvitamin D {1, 25 (OH)2D} is also produced ectopically in some tumours (particularly lymphomas) and in some granulomas (particularly sarcoidosis and tuberculosis). This form of vitamin D can now be assayed, though normally the best indicator of vitamin D status is the measurement of 25-hydroxyvitamin D (25OHD).
- Thus, measurement should be made of the PTH level routinely and of the 1, 25 (OH)2D level if lymphoma or sarcoidosis are suspected.

> The major clinical consequence of hypercalcaemia is hypovolaemia from impaired renal reabsorption of salt and water.

Treatment depends on the plasma level.

- If <3.0 mmol/L, no symptoms of dehydration are likely and no treatment is required.

- **If >3.0 and <3.5 mmol/L**, and there are no significant symptoms, treatment of the underlying disease only is required.
- **If >3.5 mmol/L**, or if symptoms are present, specific treatment is required.

*Treatment priorities are **rehydration** and **lowering of the plasma calcium level**.*

- *The most important therapeutic measure is intravenous saline, given as 6–8 hourly litres, with frusemide after urine flow is established. Since dehydration is the most immediately life-threatening complication of hypercalcaemia, diuretics must be used with great care, and fluid volume should be monitored by measuring the cardiac filling pressures. Hypernatraemia should be avoided by intermittently giving isotonic dextrose. Consequent hypokalaemia or hypomagnesaemia should be avoided.*
- ***Corticosteroids*** *are effective in some malignancies, in sarcoidosis and following excess vitamin D.*
- ***Phosphate*** *may be used, provided there is no concomitant hyperphosphataemia, in which case there is the risk of metastatic calcification. A dose of 1–1.5 g/24 h is given iv, but its effect is temporary.*
- ***Bisphosphonates*** *(biphosphonates) (originally developed as calcium- and phosphate-binding detergents to prevent washing machine scale) are generally regarded as the front-line agents. Disodium pamidronate (APD) given in a dose of 90 mg iv over 4 h, with an onset within 12–24 h and a duration of up to 2 weeks, is the agent of choice. Sodium etidronate (dose 500 mg orally once-thrice daily) is rarely used now. APD may cause fever, phlebitis, hypomagnesaemia and hypophosphataemia.*
- ***Calcitonin*** *(q.v.) produces a rapid though incomplete and transient effect and is only occasionally used.*
- ***Mithramycin*** *is a potent though toxic agent (dose 25 μg/kg IV) and is rarely used nowadays.*

Bibliography

Anderson JJB, Toverud SU 1994 Diet and vitamin D: a review with an emphasis on human function. J Nutr Biochem 5: 58.

Beall DP, Scofield RH 1995 Milk-alkali syndrome associated with calcium carbonate consumption. Medicine 74: 89.

Bilerzikian JP 1992 Management of acute hypercalcemia. N Engl J Med 326: 1196.

Cox M, Haddad JG 1994 Lymphoma, hypercalcemia, and the sunshine vitamin. Ann Intern Med 21: 709.

DeLuca HF 1978 Vitamin D metabolism and function. Arch Intern Med 138: 836.

Mallette LE 1991 The parathyroid polyhormones: new concepts in the spectrum of peptide hormone action. Endocr Rev 12: 110.

Mundy GR 1988 Hypercalcemia of malignancy revisited. J Clin Invest 82: 1.

Nussbaum SR 1993 Pathophysiology and management of severe hypercalcemia. Endocrinol Metab Clin North Am 22: 343.

Ralston SH, Gallacher SJ, Patel U et al 1989 Comparison of three intravenous biphosphonates in cancer-associated hypercalcemia. Lancet 2: 1180.

Rodan GA, Fleisch HA 1996 Bisphosphonates: mechanisms of action. J Clin Invest 97: 2692.

Theriault RL 1993 Hypercalcemia of malignancy: pathophysiology and implications for treatment. Oncology 7: 47.

Wysolmerski JJ, Broadus AE 1994 Hypercalcemia of malignancy: the central role of parathyroid hormone-related protein. Annu Rev Med 45: 189.

Hyperparathyroidism

Hyperparathyroidism encompasses several groups of conditions associated with increased circulating levels of parathyroid hormone (PTH).

Primary hyperparathyroidism is usually caused by a single parathyroid adenoma. It can also be caused by diffuse hyperplasia of the chief cells, due either to a parathyrotropic substance or to upwards resetting of the calcium homeostat. Rarely, it may be caused by parathyroid carcinoma. It is one of the important presenting features of MEN type I (q.v.).

Normally, PTH secretion is controlled by the Ca^{++}-sensing receptor, which comprises a receptor on the cell surface coupled to an intracellular part via transmembrane elements characteristic of the G protein-coupled receptor superfamily. A similar receptor is also present on the thyroid C cells, where it controls calcitonin secretion, in the kidney, where it controls calcium and phosphorus exchange, and in the central nervous system, where its role is presently uncertain.

Clinical features of primary hyperparathyroidism are numerous and variable.

- The classical features of the student's triad ('bones, stones and abdominal groans') are in fact uncommon.
- Most patients are asymptomatic, having been discovered during coincidental plasma calcium screening.
- Skeletal features include pain, local tenderness, spontaneous fracture, cystic lesions (osteitis fibrosa cystica) and pseudogout.
- Renal features include nephrolithiasis, nephrocalcinosis, polyuria and dysfunction.
- Abdominal features include pain, constipation, weight loss and pancreatitis.
- Neuromuscular features include weakness, fatigue, apathy, somnolence, depression and hypotonia.
- Cardiovascular features include hypertension and short QT interval.
- Miscellaneous features include calcium deposits in the conjunctiva.

The skeletal features are due to increased PTH, while the other features are chiefly due to the hypercalcaemia.

Diagnosis is based on the demonstration of hypercalcaemia (q.v.) in the presence of an increased serum PTH level. There is associated hypophosphataemia and hyperchloraemia. The urinary calcium is usually increased.

If the urinary calcium is not increased, benign or **familial hypocalciuric hypercalcaemia**

(FHH) should be suspected. This is a rare condition inherited as an autosomal dominant and caused by a defect in the Ca^{++}-sensing receptor in the parathyroid (and kidney).

X-ray, especially of the skull and hands, may show typical changes. In some patients, hypercalcaemia may be masked by concomitant renal disease, liver disease, vitamin D deficiency or magnesium deficiency.

Treatment is **surgical**, *though successful parathyroidectomy requires particular operative experience and skill. There is a risk of postoperative tetany, especially if there is significant bony disease, which causes the 'hungry bone phenomenon' and which requires prompt and often vigorous treatment with calcium and 1,25-dihydroxyvitamin D.*

The subsequent postoperative course may be associated with either hypoparathyroidism or recurrent hyperparathyroidism. Follow-up alone without surgery is acceptable if the hypercalcaemia is mild (<3 mmol/L), the alkaline phosphatase is not elevated and the patient is truly asymptomatic (i.e. there is an absence of even subtle symptoms, including any of a psychiatric nature).

Secondary hyperparathyroidism is a complication of other diseases, especially chronic renal failure. It arises from stimulation of PTH from hypocalcaemia and hyperphosphataemia. Since the hyperparathyroidism is compensatory, hypercalcaemia is uncommon.

The diagnosis is:

- suspected when the serum calcium level in this setting is normal instead of low;
- strengthened if there is specific bone disease (osteitis fibrosa cystica); and
- confirmed if the PTH assay is elevated.

Treatment is of the underlying disease where possible.

- *Phosphate-binding agents (non-aluminium containing) and small doses of vitamin D may be used.*

'Tertiary' hyperparathyroidism is seen in the occasional patient with secondary hyperparathyroidism, in whom a hyperplastic gland is presumed to become autonomous and produce an adenoma which then leads to hypercalcaemia.

It is most convincingly documented by persistent hypercalcaemia after renal transplantation, though even then severe secondary disease may take over a year for the hyperplastic glands to regress.

Parathyroidectomy with removal of all glands and autotransplantation is occasionally required for tertiary hyperparathyroidism.

'Pseudo' hyperparathyroidism is the term used to describe hypercalcaemia presumed to be due to ectopic hormone production in malignancy. Hypercalcaemia in this setting is not in fact commonly due to ectopic PTH production but to parathyroid hormone related protein (PTHrP) (see Hypercalcaemia), and the term is thus usually a misnomer.

Bibliography

Brown EM 1991 Extracellular Ca2+ sensing regulation of parathyroid cell function, and role of Ca2+ and other ions as extracellular (first) messengers. Physiol Rev 71: 371.

Brown EM, Gamba G, Riccardi D et al 1993 Cloning and characterization of an extracellular Ca2+-sensing receptor from bovine parathyroid. Nature 366: 575.

Deftos LJ, Parthemore JG, Stabile BE 1993 Management of primary hyperparathyroidism. Annu Rev Med 44: 19.

Fischer JA 1993 'Asymptomatic' and symptomatic primary hyperparathyroidism. Clin Invest 71: 505.

Heath H 1989 Familial benign (hypocalciuric) hypercalcemia: a troublesome mimic of mild primary hyperparathyroidism. Endocrinol Metab Clin North Am 18: 723.

Heath H, Hodgson SE, Kennedy MA 1980 Primary hyperparathyroidism: incidence, morbidity and potential economic impact in a community. N Engl J Med 302: 189.

Mallette LE 1991 The parathyroid polyhormones: new concepts in the spectrum of peptide hormone action. Endocr Rev 12: 110.

Pocotte SL, Ehrenstein G, Fitzpatrick LA 1991 Regulation of parathyroid hormone secretion. Endocr Rev 12: 291.

Slatopolsky E, Delmez JA 1994 Pathogenesis of secondary hyperparathyroidism. Am J Kidney Dis 23: 229.

Tonner DR, Schlechte JA 1993 Neurologic complications of thyroid and parathyroid disease. Med Clin North Am 77: 251.

Hyperphosphataemia

Hyperphosphataemia is associated with:

- acute and chronic renal failure;
- hypercalcaemia due to increased gastrointestinal absorption;
- secondary hyperparathyroidism;
- pseudohypoparathyroidism;
- the tumour-lysis syndrome (see Cancer complications) or other acute cell lysis (as in burns or rhabdomyolysis).

*Treatment is by **restricting phosphate intake**, which also helps to maintain the serum calcium at a normal level and thus decreases the risks of secondary hyperparathyroidism, osteodystrophy and metastatic calcification in chronic renal failure. Since the necessary dietary restriction to 800–1000 mg daily results in an unpalatable diet, a phosphate-binding antacid may usefully be added, though care should be taken with either magnesium- or aluminium-based antacids. The serum phosphate level should be kept at 1.5–2 mmol/L.*

Bibliography

Coburn JW, Salusky IB 1989 Control of serum phosphorus in uremia. N Engl J Med 320: 1140.

Weisinger JR, Bellorin-Font E 1998 Magnesium and phosphorus. Lancet 352: 391.

Hypersensitivity pneumonitis

Hypersensitivity pneumonitis (extrinsic allergic alveolitis) is an interstitial lung disease produced by the inhalation of organic dusts.

Farmer's lung (due to a thermophilic Actinomyces growing in mouldy hay) is the most common example.

Less common examples are:

- **bird fancier's lung**
  - due to pigeon, budgerigar, hen or parrot proteins;
- **humidifier fever**
  - due to organisms similar to those causing farmer's lung but growing in forced air heating, cooling or humidification systems).

There are many other causes of hypersensitivity pneumonitis, but they are quite uncommon and generally associated with unusual exposures, as follows:

- animal food worker's lung (fish meal);
- bagassosis (mouldy, overheated, sugar cane bagasse);
- bible-printer's lung (mouldy typesetting water);
- blackfat tobacco smoker's lung (blackfat tobacco);
- cheese worker's lung (cheese mould);
- coffee worker's lung (coffee-bean extract);
- corn farmer's lung (corn dust);
- detergent lung (detergents);
- furrier's lung (fox fur);
- malt worker's lung (mouldy barley, malt dust);
- maple bark stripper's lung (mouldy maple bark);
- mummy-handler's lung (mummy wrappings);
- mushroom worker's lung (mushroom compost);
- New Guinea lung (mouldy thatch dust);
- paper mill-worker's lung (mouldy wood pulp);
- paprika splitter's lung (paprika dust);
- pituitary snuff taker's lung (heterologous pituitary powder);
- sequoiosis (mouldy redwood sawdust);
- suberosis (mouldy oak bark, cork dust);
- tea grower's lung (tea plants);
- wheat weevil disease (infected wheat flour);
- woodworker's lung (sawdust).

Unlike asthma, the clinical features of hypersensitivity pneumonitis include:

* marked systemic upset,
  - with fever and malaise, often of a flu-like nature and resulting in a common misdiagnosis of infection,
* respiratory features of a restrictive rather than obstructive nature,
  - with symptoms of cough and dyspnoea but not wheeze, and findings of crackles rather than rhonchi.

The course is usually acute, typically occurring within 6–8 h of exposure to the relevant antigen. It subsides spontaneously if the antigen is removed, but it may be prolonged for weeks if there is continued exposure, as on a farm. In such cases, the onset may sometimes be insidious. Occasionally, a chronic process may be seen with cough and dyspnoea on exertion but no systemic features and often no prior acute episodes identified.

Chest X-ray shows micronodular shadows initially and fibrosis (especially of the upper lobes) later.

The diagnosis is particularly dependent on a history of appropriate exposure. Precipitating antibodies to specific antigen are detectable in acute cases, but positive serology indicates only exposure to antigen and not necessarily disease therefrom. Other causes of interstitial disease should be excluded, though separation from idiopathic diffuse fibrosing alveolitis may be difficult. Lung biopsy in such patients will often show granulomas, which then suggest the correct diagnosis. The BAL fluid has >50% lymphocytes, mostly suppressor-cytotoxic T cells, but these findings are of limited diagnostic specificity.

Avoidance of the offending antigen usually results in complete symptomatic remission, though corticosteroids may be required in cases which are severe or chronic.

Bibliography
Bernardo J, Center DM 1981 Hypersensitivity pneumonia. Dis Mon 27: 1.

Hypersplenism (see also Splenomegaly)

Hypersplenism refers to a diverse group of conditions associated with **splenomegaly** from any cause and consequent removal of the formed elements of the blood. The splenomegaly is most commonly congestive and due to portal or splenic vein obstruction, as in hepatic cirrhosis or cardiac failure. It may also occur from direct infiltration, as in:

* lymphoma;
* myeloproliferative disorders;
* collagen-vascular disorders;
* granulomatous disease;
* infectious diseases;
* Felty's syndrome.

Clinically, there is haemolytic anaemia, although even massive splenomegaly does not always cause a decreased red blood cell mass, since there may be considerable haemodilution. Other formed elements, particularly platelets, may also be removed. The bone marrow is typically hyperplastic, unless there is a primary haematological disorder.

Treatment may require splenectomy, including any accessory spleen(s), if clinical disease is substantial. Corticosteroids or radiotherapy may sometimes be helpful.

Bibliography
Bohnsack JF, Brown EJ 1986 The role of the spleen in resistance to infection. Annu Rev Med 37: 49.
Rose WF 1987 The spleen as a filter. N Engl J Med 317: 704.

Hyperthermia (see Pyrexia)

Hyperthyroidism

Hyperthyroidism can have a number of causes.

189

1. **Graves' disease** refers to autoimmune thyroid disease characterized by diffuse toxic goitre and caused by the production of antibodies to TSH receptors (and thus loss of endogenous TSH control). Other associated features of an autoimmune nature may sometimes be seen, particularly including ophthalmopathy and pretibial myxoedema.

The classical clinical picture of Graves' disease, often seen in a young woman, includes

1. symptoms of:

- palpitations;
- tremor;
- sweating;
- weight loss;
- irritability and insomnia;

2. signs of:

- smooth non-tender goitre;
- proptosis and lid lag, with occasionally the more severe eye involvement of exophthalmos or even ophthalmoplegia;
- hyperdynamic circulatory state;
- tremor;
- palmar erythema;
- clubbing (rarely).

Investigations show increased T4 and T3 and suppressed TSH levels. If there is associated hypoproteinaemia and thus decreased TBG, the free T4 level needs to be measured (or calculated). Hyperthyroidism is excluded by a normal TSH level, unless the patient has a TSH-secreting pituitary tumour (see below).

*Treatment options include **antithyroid drugs** (carbimazole, propylthiouracil), **subtotal thyroidectomy** or **radioiodine**, the choice varying between centres. Some clinicians treat with antithyroid drugs for 12–18 months, following which about 50% of patients are in remission and need no further treatment, while about 50% relapse and need surgery or radioiodine. Some clinicians instead favour initial ablation therapy with radioiodine (except in young women), followed by replacement therapy.*

Beta blockade, sedation, rest, adequate nutrition and long-term follow-up are also important.

2. **Toxic nodular goitre** arises in a pre-existing goitre, in which eventual autonomy of thyroid hormone production occurs.

3. **Toxic adenoma** (Plummer's nodule) may be a variant of toxic nodular goitre but may also occur within an atrophic gland.

4. **Drug-induced hyperthyroidism** can occur following the deliberate ingestion of T4 or T3. More practically, it can follow the administration of iodine-containing medications, especially amiodarone, which can produce a variety of abnormalities of thyroid function, including hyperthyroidism (which is reported to occur in 10% of patients on a low iodine intake). In this condition, there is an isolated increase in T4 and not T3.

5. **Excess TSH** from a pituitary tumour can cause hyperthyroidism. In this setting, there may be headache and the eye signs are different, since they include field defects. There are no associated autoimmune phenomena. Rarely, increased TSH may be produced but without resultant hyperthyroidism, because of thyroid hormone resistance.

Hyperthyroidism may present in a number of less common forms.

1. **Occult hyperthyroidism** is seen especially in elderly patients, in whom its first clinical manifestation is cardiac. Thus, arrhythmias (especially atrial fibrillation), angina and cardiac failure are the usual features.

This is an important phenomenon, because it is one of the specifically treatable causes of cardiac disease.

The diagnosis is confirmed by an elevated T3 and decreased TSH, but the T4 level is not necessarily elevated.

2. **Atypical hyperthyroidism** refers to the condition when one single, perhaps atypical,

clinical feature predominates, such as myopathy or personality change.

3. **Drug-suppressed hyperthyroidism** occurs especially during concomitant beta-blocker administration. Beta-blockers mask many of the prominent clinical features of hyperthyroidism, including tremor, sweating and circulatory changes, though they do not influence weight loss, personality changes, goitre, eye signs or laboratory tests.

---

4. **Thyroid storm** refers to a severe exacerbation of hyperthyroidism with fever, dehydration, shock and extreme restlessness. It usually follows concomitant infection, but it may follow trauma or the abrupt withdrawal of antithyroid drugs. If the underlying hyperthyroidism was not previously known, it may be difficult to detect in the presence of severe infection or trauma, but it may be suspected if the physiological response to the current insult appears excessive.

It is confirmed by the finding of increased T4 or T3 and suppressed TSH levels.

*The condition requires urgent **resuscitation** and treatment of the precipitating disease.*

- *__Antithyroid__ treatment is given as propylthiouracil (100 mg qid nasogastrically, followed by sodium iodide 0.5 g iv bd).*
- *__Beta-blockers__ should be used and also **corticosteroids** in very severe cases.*

---

5. **Malignant exophthalmos** refers to severe sight-threatening eye involvement.

The hyperthyroidism is treated on its normal merits, although radioiodine has recently been reported to exacerbate ophthalmopathy.

- *First-line treatment for exophthalmos is with **corticosteroids**, but occasionally surgical decompression of the orbit may be required.*
- *Recently **plasmapheresis** has been reported to be helpful.*

Bibliography

Carter JA, Utiger RD 1992 The ophthalmopathy of Graves' disease. Annu Rev Med 43: 487.

Cooper DS 1986 Which anti-thyroid drug? Am J Med 80: 1165.

DeGroot LJ, Quintans J 1989 The causes of autoimmune thyroid disease. Endocr Rev 10: 537.

Franklyn J, Sheppard M 1992 Radioiodine for thyrotoxicosis: perhaps the best option. Br Med J 305: 727.

Khir ASM 1985 Suspected thyrotoxicosis. Br Med J 290: 916.

Lazar MA 1993 Thyroid hormone receptors: multiple forms, multiple possibilities. Endocr Rev 14: 184.

Magner JA 1990 Thyroid-stimulating hormone: biosynthesis, cell biology, and bioactivity. Endocr Rev 11: 354.

Ramsay I 1985 Drug and non-thyroid induced changes in thyroid function tests. Postgrad Med J 61: 375.

Shupnik MA, Ridgway EC, Chin WW 1989 Molecular biology of thyrotropin. Endocr Rev 10: 459.

Smallridge RC 1992 Metabolic and anatomic thyroid emergencies: a review. Crit Care Med 20: 276.

Stockigt JR 1993 Hyperthyroidism secondary to drugs and acute illness. Endocrinologist 3: 67.

Surks MI, Chopra IJ, Mariash CN et al 1990 American Thyroid Association guidelines for use of laboratory tests in thyroid disorders. JAMA 263: 1529.

Tonner DR, Schlechte JA 1993 Neurologic complications of thyroid and parathyroid disease. Med Clin North Am 77: 251.

Waldstein SS, Slodki SJ, Kaganiec GI 1960 A clinical study of thyroid storm. Ann Intern Med 52: 626.

Woeber KA 1992 Thyrotoxicosis and the heart. N Engl J Med 327: 94.

Hypertrichosis (see Hirsutism)

Hyperuricaemia (see Gout)

Hyperviscosity (see Multiple myeloma)

Hypocalcaemia

The plasma calcium represents <1% of the total body calcium, and of this only the ionized fraction (normally about 50%) influences physiological events. Since in Intensive Care hypoalbuminaemia is common, the ionized or free calcium level can be normal despite a low total serum calcium.

> True hypocalcaemia refers to decreased ionized calcium, which may be measured directly. Alternatively, a corrected total calcium (mmol/L) may be calculated approximately as: ionized Ca^{++} = measured total Ca^{++} + {0.02 × (40-serum albumin)}.

Hypocalcaemia is caused by

1. Parathyroid deficiency

This occurs most commonly post-thyroidectomy, but also post-parathyroidectomy (the 'hungry bone' syndrome) or idiopathic (q.v.).

2. Parathyroid hormone resistance

This is seen in pseudohypoparathyroidsim (q.v.), chronic renal failure, malabsorption, hypomagnesaemia, hypermagnesaemia, hyperphosphataemia, drugs (especially phenytoin).

3. Other conditions

These include disorders such as pancreatitis, rhabdomyolysis, osteoblastic metastases.

In the second two groups of causes, PTH levels are increased.

The clinical features of hypocalcaemia comprise those of the underlying disease as well as of the low serum calcium level itself. The latter depend on the rate as well as the severity of the deficiency. They include paraesthesiae, especially around the mouth, restlessness and Trousseau's and/or Chvostek's signs. More chronic hypocalcaemia may give rise to fatigue and muscle aches. The ECG typically shows a prolonged QT interval.

Treatment of acute hypocalcaemia is with **calcium** *iv (e.g. 10 mL of 10% calcium gluconate) or orally (e.g.*

1 g of calcium chloride) three times daily. Clearly, the underlying disease requires treatment.

Bibliography

Cholst IN, Steinberg SF, Tropper PJ et al 1984 The influence of hypermagnesemia on serum calcium and parathyroid hormone levels in human subjects. N Engl J Med 310: 1221.

Lebowitz MR, Moses AM 1992 Hypocalcemia. Semin Nephrol 12: 146.

Zaloga GP 1992 Hypocalcemia in critically ill patients. Crit Care Med 20: 251.

Hypoglycaemia (see Islet cell tumour)

Hypokaleamia (see Conn's syndrome)

Hyponatraemia (see Central pontine myelinolysis and Syndrome of inappropriate antidiuretic hormone)

Hypoparathyroidism

Hypoparathyroidism refers to the failure of the parathyroid gland to secrete parathyroid hormone (PTH). The condition may be either idiopathic or postoperative (i.e. following parathyroidectomy or more commonly thyroidectomy).

Idiopathic hypoparathyroidism may be an isolated defect, sometimes genetic. More commonly, it is associated with:

- antibodies to other endocrine organs

  - and thus often other endocrine failure, especially of the thyroid and adrenal glands;

- mucocutaneous candidiasis

  - when the condition is referred to as polyglandular autoimmunity type I.

A rare type of hypoparathyroidism is the Di George syndrome, with associated lymphopenia and thymic aplasia.

The clinical features of hypoparathyroidism are those of hypocalcaemia (q.v.).

*Treatment is with **vitamin D**, since it has a similar action to PTH and since PTH is not a practical therapeutic agent.*

- *Hypoparathyroidism if acute requires calcium iv (e.g. 10 mL of 10% calcium gluconate) or if less acute calcium chloride 1 g orally tds.*
- *Synthetic vitamin D analogues may be also be used.*

Pseudohypoparathyroidism refers to the syndrome of PTH-resistance, first described by Albright, in which there is hypocalcaemia, hyperphosphataemia, parathyroid hyperplasia and the somatic abnormalities of short stature, moon face and obesity.

The occasional case in which there is normocalcaemia is sometimes referred to as **pseudopseudohypoparathyroidism**.

In fact, several other mechanisms may also cause PTH-resistance, including:

- chronic renal failure;
- malabsorption;
- hypomagnesaemia;
- drugs (especially phenytoin).

Bibliography

Loriaux DL 1985 The polyendocrine deficiency syndromes. N Engl J Med 312: 1568.

Pocotte SL, Ehrenstein G, Fitzpatrick LA 1991 Regulation of parathyroid hormone secretion. Endocr Rev 12: 291.

Tonner DR, Schlechte JA 1993 Neurologic complications of thyroid and parathyroid disease. Med Clin North Am 77: 251.

Hypophosphataemia

Hypophosphataemia may have a large variety of causes. These include:

- primary hyperparathyroidism;
- hypercalcaemia of malignancy;
- phosphate-binding antacids;
- hypertonic carbohydrate feeding;
- renal tubular defects;
- dialysis;
- correction of diabetic ketoacidosis;
- liver disease;
- malabsorption;
- osteomalacia (except in chronic renal failure);
- post-exercise exhaustion;
- heat stroke;
- respiratory alkalosis.

A phosphate level of <0.5 mmol/L is associated with:

- muscular weakness, including diaphragmatic dysfunction;
- rhabdomyolysis;
- 2–3 DPG depletion (and thus a left-shifted oxygen dissociation curve),
- impaired neutrophil function.

A phosphate level of <0.3 mmol/L is additionally associated with:

- impaired red cell glycolysis and thus haemolysis.

*Treatment of significant hypophosphataemia requires **phosphate** ions iv. This is given as sodium/potassium phosphate (13.4 mmol per 20 mL ampoule, i.e. 0.67 mmol/mL) diluted in saline or dextrose. The usual dose is 1 ampoule given over 4–6 h, though half this dose is adequate in milder deficiency and 2–4 times this dose is needed in severe deficiency (i.e. <0.3 mmol/L and especially if <0.16 mmol/L).*

Bibliography

Aubier M, Murciano D, Lecocguic Y et al 1985 Effect of hypophosphatemia on diaphragmatic contractility in patients with acute respiratory failure. N Engl J Med 313: 420.

Coburn JW, Salusky IB 1989 Control of serum phosphorus in uremia. N Engl J Med 320: 1140.

Kingston M, Al-Siba'l MB 1985 Treatment of severe hypophosphatemia. Crit Care Med 13: 16.

Weisinger JR, Bellorin-Font E 1998 Magnesium and phosphorus. Lancet 352: 391.

Hypothermia (see also Drowning)

Hypothermia refers to a state of lowered core temperature below 35°C. Since clinical mercury thermometers do not generally read below 35°C, a reading of 35°C on such a device does not exclude hypothermia and indeed should prompt the measurement of core temperature using a specific low-reading thermometer. Hypothermia, like hyperthermia, is a dangerous complication.

Hypothermia may occur even in temperate weather following immersion or wind chill. Patients who are at extremes of age, who are physically or mentally ill, are injured, or who have impaired consciousness (e.g. from alcohol or drugs) are especially predisposed to hypothermia. Hypoglycaemia, myxoedema, head injury, multiple trauma and drug overdose are commonly encountered causes of secondary hypothermia.

Hypothermia generally has an insidious onset with fatigue, apathy, confusion, incoordination and shivering.

If the temperature falls to <35°C, there is:

- confusion and disorientation.

If the temperature falls to <32°C, there is:

- muscular rigidity;
- progressive metabolic acidosis;
- hypovolaemia;
- coagulopathy;
- dilated pupils;
- potentially fatal arrhythmias, which can be readily precipitated by minor stimuli.

If the temperature falls to <28°C, there is:

- unconsciousness;
- cardiac instability or arrest (usually in ventricular fibrillation);
- apnoea.

---

*Treatment is with a warm, dry and sheltered environment and warm fluids by mouth. If the process is severe, passive or even active **rewarming***

is required, the latter preferably in hospital. Techniques of active rewarming have not been subject to formal comparative evaluation, though many are available. Rewarming with an electric blanket may lead to relapse, though this may not apply to external rewarming with warm air. Core rewarming may be achieved by warmed (i.e. 40°C enteral, parenteral, peritoneal, pleural or dialysis fluids, or by veno–venous bypass using a haemofiltration system.

*Hypothermic **cardiac arrest** can be particularly difficult to treat, since the cold heart is relatively refractory to drugs and electrical stimuli. Normal resuscitation should be continued until the core temperature has been increased to at least 30°C before being deemed unsuccessful. Survival with good cerebral function has been achieved in young patients in hypothermic asystole by using cardiopulmonary bypass.*

Perioperative hypothermia is an important phenomenon and occurs in about one third of surgical patients in the operating theatre. It is due to impaired thermoregulation caused by anaesthesia, together with a cool environment, open body cavities and cold iv fluids. Even mild perioperative hypothermia has been shown to be associated with an increased incidence of bleeding, wound infections and cardiac events, and with increased hospital stay. The likely mechanism of this increased morbidity is hypothermia-induced stress response, with the production of greatly elevated levels of catecholamines, cortisol and other counter-regulatory hormones. This increased morbidity has been shown in controlled trials to be prevented by maintaining normothermia with active warming using forced air.

Sepsis-induced hypothermia is a seeming paradox which occurs in about 10% of patients with a clinical diagnosis of sepsis. Inability to mount a fever in the presence of severe infection is now known to be associated with a doubling of mortality (see Heat shock proteins). This finding is in contrast to an older view that induced hypothermia might be beneficial in sepsis. Hypothermic patients with sepsis have higher plasma levels of interleukin 6 (IL–6), tumour necrosis factor α (TNF-α) and eicosanoids (especially thromboxane A_2 and prostacyclin) than do febrile patients and are more acidotic. Recently, the cyclo-oxygenase inhibitors, ibuprofen, has been reported to improve the prognosis in hypothermic sepsis.

Bibliography

Arons MM, Wheeler AP, Bernard GR et al 1999 Effects of ibuprofen on the physiology and survival of hypothermic sepsis. Crit Care Med 27: 699.

Brauer A, Wrigge H, Kersten J et al 1999 Severe accidental hypothermia: rewarming strategy using a veno-venous bypass system and a convective air warmer. Intens Care Med 25: 520.

Britt LD, Dascombe WH, Rodriguez A 1991 New horizons in management of hypothermia and frostbite injury. Surg Clin North Am 71: 345.

Clemmer TP, Fisher CJ, Bone RC et al 1992 Hypothermia in the sepsis syndrome and clinical outcome. Crit Care Med 20: 1395.

Dexter WW 1990 Hypothermia: safe and efficient methods of rewarming the patient. Postgrad Med 88: 55.

Dowd PM 1987 Cold-related disorders. Prog Dermatol 21: 1.

Easterbrook PJ, Davis HP 1985 Thrombocytopenia in hypothermia: a common but poorly recognised complication. Br Med J 291: 23.

Ku J, Brasel KJ, Baker CC et al 1999 Triangle of death: hypothermia, acidosis, and coagulopathy. New Horizons 7: 61.

Reuler JB 1978 Hypothermia: pathophysiology, clinical settings, and management. Ann Intern Med 89: 519.

Sessler DI 1997 Mild perioperative hypothermia. N Engl J Med 336: 1730.

Varon J, Sadovnikoff N, Sternbach GL 1992 Hypothermia: saving patients from the big chill. Postgrad Med 92: 47.

Walpoth BH, Walpoth-Aslan BN, Mattle HP et al 1997 Outcome of survivors of accidental deep hypothermia and circulatory arrest treated with extracorporeal blood warming. N Engl J Med 337: 1500.

Woodhouse P, Keatinge WR, Coleshaw SR 1989 Factors associated with hypothermia in patients admitted to a group of inner city hospitals. Lancet 2: 1201.

Hypothyroidism

Hypothyroidism refers to the bodily deficiency of thyroid hormone. **Myxoedema** refers to the florid clinical syndrome associated with this. In fact, however, most patients with hypothyroidism have only mild symptoms, and indeed many are asymptomatic.

Hypothyroidism has many causes, though more than 95% are due to intrinsic thyroid disease, from:

- inflammation, especially Hashimoto's thyroiditis;
- previous surgery;
- iodine deficiency or excess;
- drugs, e.g. lithium, amiodarone, other iodine-containing medications;
- local irradiation.

A few cases are due to disease of the:

- pituitary (with TSH deficiency); or
- hypothalamus (with TRH deficiency).

195

The classical clinical features of myxoedema include:

- cold intolerance;
- thick dry skin;
- hoarse voice;
- apathy;
- motor retardation;
- constipation;
- occasionally headache, myalgia, arthralgia, oedema.

However, a single feature may at times predominate. More importantly, the changes may occur so slowly as to be difficult to recognize without assistance (e.g. from an old photograph).

Diagnosis is based on decreased T4 and increased TSH, though marginal abnormalities of these tests commonly occur in asymptomatic patients, in whom diagnosis then remains difficult. The TSH is not elevated if the hypothyroidism is of pituitary or hypothalamic origin. T3 is decreased late in the course of disease and is not a useful test in this setting. Antithyroid antibodies (mainly to thyroid peroxidase, i.e. anti-TPO, and also to thyroglobulin) occur early in autoimmune thyroiditis (see Autoimmune disorders).

*Treatment is with **thyroid replacement**, generally thyroxine 100 μg daily, though it is usually commenced at lower doses, e.g. 50 μg daily.*

Sometimes higher maintenance doses are needed, in which case they should be achieved over some weeks. Increased doses are particularly required during pregnancy. Increased doses are also required during concomitant therapy with agents which alter the bioavailability of T4, such as sucralfate, cholestyramine or soy bean-based feeds (which decrease absorption of T4) and barbiturates, carbamazepine, phenytoin or rifampicin (which increase hepatic metabolism of T4).

On the other hand, in elderly or cardiac patients, initial doses should often be as low as 25 μg daily.

The euthyroid state is achieved when symptoms have receded and the TSH level is normal (the T4 level is not a reliable guide to euthyroidism).

Myxoedema coma is a rare complication of hypothyroidism. It is seen mainly in the elderly and is usually precipitated by infection or exposure. There is hypothermia as well as coma.

*Treatment comprises resuscitation and administration of **T3** 10 μg iv.*

- ***Resuscitation** needs to be undertaken with great care, as fluid overload can easily be produced on the one hand, and repair of hypothermia can require considerably increased fluids on the other hand.*
- *It is wise to administer **corticosteroids** concomitantly, in case there is associated hypopituitarism.*

Bibliography

Bastenie PA, Bonnyns M, Vanhaelst L 1985 Natural history of primary myxedema. Am J Med 79: 91.

DeGroot LJ, Quintans J 1989 The causes of autoimmune thyroid disease. Endocr Rev 10: 537.

Editorial 1986 Subclinical hypothyroidism. Lancet 1: 251.

Jordan RM 1993 Myxedema coma: the prognosis is improving. Endocrinologist 3: 149.

Lazar MA 1993 Thyroid hormone receptors: multiple forms, multiple possibilities. Endocr Rev 14: 184.

Loriaux DL 1985 The polyendocrine deficiency syndromes. N Engl J Med 312: 1568.

Magner JA 1990 Thyroid-stimulating hormone: biosynthesis, cell biology, and bioactivity. Endocr Rev 11: 354.

Mazzaferri EL 1986 Adult hypothyroidism. Postgrad Med 79: 64, 75.

Ramsay I 1985 Drug and non-thyroid induced changes in thyroid function tests. Postgrad Med J 61: 375.

Shupnik MA, Ridgway EC, Chin WW 1989 Molecular biology of thyrotropin. Endocr Rev 10: 459.

Smallridge RC 1992 Metabolic and anatomic thyroid emergencies: a review. Crit Care Med 20: 276.

Surks MI, Chopra IJ, Mariash CN et al 1990 American Thyroid Association guidelines for use of laboratory tests in thyroid disorders. JAMA 263: 1529.

Vance ML 1994 Hypopituitarism. N Engl J Med 330: 1651.

Tonner DR, Schlechte JA 1993 Neurologic complications of thyroid and parathyroid disease. Med Clin North Am 77: 251.

Walsh JP, Stuckey BGA 2001 What is the optimal treatment for hypothyroidism. Med J Aust 174: 141.

Idiopathic pulmonary fibrosis (see Diffuse fibrosing alveolitis)

Idiopathic pulmonary haemosiderosis (see Goodpasture's syndrome)

Idiopathic thrombocytopenic purpura (see also Thrombocytopenia)

Idiopathic thrombocytopenic purpura (ITP) is due to an autoimmune IgG antibody, usually directed against the platelet membrane glycoprotein, GP IIb–IIIa. Sometimes there may be circulating immune complexes, as in HIV infection.

Platelets with bound antibody are vulnerable to trapping and thus destruction via phagocytosis, especially in the spleen. Platelet production in the bone marrow increases by 3–4-fold, but this is only about half the known marrow reserve, perhaps because platelet antibodies react also with megakaryocytes.

The clinical features are usually seen in young women, in whom there is often associated immune thyroid disease. There is no splenomegaly. Sometimes, there is purpura only, but if more severe there is also mucosal bleeding.

The course is usually chronic and relatively benign, except for the occasional occurrence of intracranial haemorrhage. The condition may spontaneously remit, only to relapse in the presence of infection.

Acute ITP typically follows a viral illness and disappears within three months.

The peripheral blood film is normal apart from the appearance of large platelets. These are young, metabolically active and highly functional. An increased titre of platelet associated IgG is usual, but this test though sensitive is non-specific.

Treatment is not required if the platelet count is $>30–50 \times 10^9/L$ and there is no bleeding. Aspirin should clearly be avoided. If treatment is required, corticosteroids are usually effective within a few days.

- *If relapse occurs, splenectomy produces a remission in 75% of cases, with the platelet count rising by the first postoperative day and commonly exceeding normal by the second week.*
- *High-dose human IgG (e.g. 20 g iv daily for 5 days) or plasmapheresis may be effective.*
- *Cytotoxic agents (particularly vincristine), cyclosporin or interferon alpha have also been used. Immunosuppression should clearly be avoided in patients with AIDS.*

Platelet transfusions *are recommended if bleeding is severe, because 6–20 U 2–4 times daily confers clinical benefit, even though there is increased platelet destruction and the platelet count itself may not necessarily rise.*

In pregnancy, the diagnosis of ITP should not be made unless pre-eclampsia has been excluded. Splenectomy is contraindicated because it may precipitate abortion. Some degree of maternal thrombocytopenia is common anyway (8% incidence) and is neither immune-mediated nor clinically significant. Corticosteroids and Caesarean section may be required in cases of confirmed ITP in pregnancy.

An ITP-like syndrome may also be seen in lymphoma or SLE, but in these conditions it is in fact secondary.

Bibliography
Ferrara JLM 1995 The febrile platelet transfusion reaction: a cytokine shower. Transfusion 35: 89.

Immotile cilia syndrome (see Situs inversus)

Immune complex disease

This is a heterogeneous group of diseases in which exogenous or endogenous antigens have combined with antibodies to cause either local or systemic tissue damage.

The amount of **immune complex** formed is related to the relative concentrations of antigen and antibody, the largest amount and in general the largest size of immune complexes being formed when antigen and antibody are present in molar equivalence. Their normal clearance is by the reticuloendothelial system following their transport on red blood cell membranes. This clearance is rapid and does not produce damage.

However, if normal clearance is impaired, such as by complement factor deficiency, immune complexes can be deposited in small blood vessels in any organ or tissue in the body but particularly in the kidney and to a lesser extent in the skin and choroid plexus. Vasoactive substances are then released from circulating basophils and later from tissue mast cells and infiltrated neutrophils, platelets are activated and vascular permeability is enhanced. The immune complexes can then migrate beyond the endothelium to the basement membrane and even into surrounding tissues.

Immune complex disease may be local or systemic.

1. Localized immune complex disease

The prime example of this phenomenon is the **Arthus reaction**. This is an acute haemorrhagic and necrotic local reaction usually in the skin and occurring 2–4 h after the injection of antigen into an immunized animal.

Clinically, such a phenomenon occurs when antigen is localized, so that any reaction with formed antibodies is also localized. This occurs with:

- endogenous antigens which are either structural (e.g. basement membrane) or secreted (e.g. thyroglobulin);
- exogenous antigens which are concentrated locally (e.g. inhaled).

Examples with endogenous antigens include Goodpasture's syndrome, Hashimoto's thyroiditis and pemphigus vulgaris.

Examples with exogenous antigens include hypersensitivity pneumonitis.

2. Systemic immune complex disease

Serum sickness is the prime example of this phenomenon. This is a condition associated with fever, rash, lymphadenopathy, splenomegaly and arthritis about 10 days after a large exposure to foreign antigen. Serum sickness runs a benign and self-limited course over about a week, though occasionally reversible vasculitis or polyneuritis may occur.

A chronic form may develop if the antigen exposure is prolonged or repeated.

Systemic immune complex disease can follow

- infections, e.g. viral (such as hepatitis B), bacterial (such as streptococcal) and parasitic,
- administration of many different drugs which can act as haptens (such as aspirin, gold, penicillamine, penicillin, phenytoin, sulfonamides and thiazides).

Immune complex assays can be useful as markers of progress, but the levels are neither sensitive nor specific. Their presence may also be suggested by evidence of complement activation, with decreased C3 and C4. A more specific test is the immunohistological examination of biopsy material.

Treatment consists of removal of the offending antigen if possible, anti-inflammatory agents (especially antihistamines), corticosteroids, cytotoxics and possibly plasmapheresis. Cephalosporins and methyldopa may offer interesting therapeutic possibilities.

Recent experimental evidence suggests the potential therapeutic value of the cytokines, IL-4 and IL-10, of antibodies to integrins and selectins, and of nitric oxide synthetase inhibition.

Bibliography

Lawley TJ, Bielory L, Gascon P et al 1984 A prospective clinical and immunologic analysis of patients with serum sickness. N Engl J Med 311: 1407.
Schifferli JA, Ng YC, Peters DK 1986 The role of

complement and its receptors in the elimination of immune complexes. N Engl J Med 315: 488.

Wiggins RC, Cochrane CG 1981 Immune-complex-mediated biologic effects. N Engl J Med 304: 518.

Immunodeficiency

Immunodeficiency diseases arise because of a defect either in:

- immunoglobulin production (i.e. B-cell deficiency);
- cell-mediated immunity (i.e. T-cell deficiency).

1. Immunoglobulin deficiency

The best known such condition is X-linked agammaglobulinaemia (q.v.), but many other specific deficiencies of antibody production have been reported, particularly common variable immunodeficiency and selective immunoglobulin deficiency.

- **Common variable immunodeficiency** (CVID) is a non-inherited form of hypogammaglobulinaemia which usually appears in adult life. There is a generalized decrease in all immunoglobulins, presumably due to B-cell dysfunction. There may be multiple pathogenetic mechanisms, but the clinical features are similar to those of agammaglobulinaemia with proneness to infection and to autoimmune diseases. Additional features include chronic lung damage, lymphoid hyperplasia and giardia-induced diarrhoea.

*Treatment is with **replacement therapy** and **antibiotics**, while corticosteroids should be used with caution.*

- **Selective immunoglobulin deficiency** comprises a number of categories, some inherited, and including IgG sub-classes, IgM, IgA and combined defects. Their clinical effects are variable, and they are frequently asymptomatic.

2. Cell-mediated immunodeficiency

This is manifested as impaired delayed hypersensitivity with proneness to infections. Infections are frequent and severe and may be due to many different organisms, especially opportunists (e.g. candida, pneumocystis), Gram-negative bacteria and viruses.

- **Primary deficiencies** are sometimes inherited and include:

  - severe combined immunodeficiency disease (SCID) and its several variants;
  - the Wiskott–Aldrich syndrome, an X-linked disorder with associated eczema, thrombocytopenia and lymphoid cancers;
  - ataxia-telangiectasia, the mutant gene which has recently been identified as being responsible for greatly increased sensitivity to ionizing radiation, so that there is a propensity for chromosomal damage.

- **Secondary deficiencies** are due to other diseases, such as collagen-vascular, inflammatory (especially HIV infection), neoplastic, nutritional or traumatic disorders, or to drugs. Psychological stress has been reported to be a potential cause of increased susceptibility to viral infections in some patients.

Bibliography

Buckley RH, Schiff RI 1991 The use of intravenous immune globulin in immunodeficiency diseases. N Engl J Med 325: 110.

Sneller MC, Strober W, Eisenstein E et al 1993 NIH conference: new insights into common variable immunodeficiency. Ann Intern Med 118: 720.

Van de Meer JWM 1994 Defects in host-defense mechanisms. In: Rubin RH, Young LS (eds) Clinical Approach to Infections in the Compromised Host. 3rd edition. New York: Plenum. p 33.

Yu Z, Lennon VA 1999 Mechanism of intravenous immune globulin therapy in antibody-mediated autoimmune diseases. N Engl J Med 340: 227.

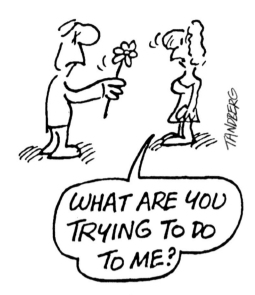

WHAT ARE YOU TRYING TO DO TO ME?

Immunology

Disorders with an immunological aetiology or more commonly with an immunological contribution are frequent in Intensive Care, as in medicine generally. While many such disorders are more logically considered under specific organ-system headings, some immunological conditions and principles of a general character are considered in this book as separate topics, including:

- agammaglobulinaemia;
- angioedema;
- antinuclear antibodies;
- autoimmune disorders;
- cold agglutinin disease;
- complement deficiency;
- cryoglobulinaemia;
- Henoch–Schonlein purpura;
- histocompatibility complex;
- immune complex disease;
- immunodeficiency;
- Jarisch–Herxheimer reaction;
- light chains;
- serum sickness.

Bibliography

Anderson KC, Weinstein HJ 1990 Transfusion-associated graft-versus-host disease. N Engl J Med 323: 315.

Austen KF, Burakoff SJ, Rosen FS et al (eds) 1996 Therapeutic Immunology. Cambridge: Blackwell.

Ballow M, Nelson R 1997 Immunopharmacology: immunomodulation and immunotherapy. JAMA 278: 2008

Barnes PJ, Karin M 1997 Nuclear factor-$\kappa\beta$ – a pivotal transcription factor in chronic inflammatory disease. N Engl J Med 336: 1066

Chrousos GP 1995 The hypothalamic–pituitary–adrenal axis and immune-mediated inflammation. N Engl J Med 332: 1351.

Clark EA, Ledbetter JA 1994 How B and T cells talk to each other. Nature 367: 425.

Cohen JJ 1993 Apoptosis. Immunol Today 14: 126.

Couriel D, Weinstein R 1994 Complications of therapeutic plasma exchange: a recent assessment. J Clin Apheresis 9: 1.

Dwyer JM 1992 Manipulating the immune system with immune globulin. N Engl J Med 326: 107.

Engelhard VH 1994 How cells process antigens. Sci Am 271(2): 54.

Faist E, Wichmann M, Kim C 1997 Immunosuppression and immunomodulation in surgical patients. Curr Opinion Crit Care 3: 293.

Guillet J-G, Lai M-Z, Briner TJ et al 1987 Immunological self, nonself discrimination. Science 235: 865.

Nossal GJV 1987 Current concepts: immunology: the basic components of the immune system. N Engl J Med 316: 1320.

Nossal GJV 1989 Immunologic tolerance: collaboration between antigen and lymphokines. Science 245: 147.

Nossal GJV 1993 Life, death and the immune system. Sci Am 269(3): 20.

Nossal GJV 1994 Negative selection of lymphocytes. Cell 76: 229.

Pardoll DM 1994 Tumour antigens: a new look for the 1990s. Nature 369: 357.

Parker CW 1982 Allergic reactions in man. Pharmacol Rev 34: 85.

Paul WE 1993 Infectious diseases and the immune system. Sci Am 269(3): 57.

Reichlin S 1993 Neuroendocrine-immune interactions. N Engl J Med 329: 1246.

Reimann PM, Mason PD 1990 Plasmapheresis: technique and complications. Intens Care Med 16: 3.

Roberts NJ 1991 Impact of temperature elevation on immunologic defenses. Rev Infect Dis 13: 462.

Shortman K, Scollay R 1994 Death in the thymus. Nature 372: 44.

Smith RM, Giannoudis PV 1998 Trauma and the immune response. J R Soc Med 91: 417.

Van de Meer JWM 1994 Defects in host-defense mechanisms. In: Rubin RH, Young LS (eds) Clinical Approach to Infections in the Compromised Host. 3rd edition. New York: Plenum. p 33.

Von Boehmer H 1994 Positive selection of lymphocytes. Cell 76: 219.

Yu Z, Lennon VA 1999 Mechanism of intravenous immune globulin therapy in antibody-mediated autoimmune diseases. N Engl J Med 340: 227.

Zanetti G, Calandra T 1997 Intravenous immunoglobulins and granulocyte colony-stimulating factor for the management of infection in intensive care units. Curr Opinion Crit Care 3: 342.

Zweiman B, Levinson AI 1992 Immunologic aspects of neurological and neuromuscular diseases. JAMA 268: 2918.

Infections

Infectious diseases are especially relevant to Intensive Care, because sepsis in its various forms is one of the single largest groups of problems encountered.

Many specific infections are therefore commonly encountered and well understood by Intensive Care staff, including nosocomial and community-acquired pneumonia, classical sepsis (many cases of which are also nosocomial), abdominal sepsis, and the systemic inflammatory response syndrome in its various guises (and names). The general principles of microbiological diagnosis, antibiotic prescribing and infection control are also part of front-line Intensive Care.

However, the spectrum of infectious diseases that may potentially be encountered in Intensive Care is very large, and it is the many but less common among these specific infections which are outlined in this book. These include:

- acquired immunodeficiency syndrome;
- actinomycosis;
- amoebiasis;
- anthrax;
- aspergillosis;
- botulism;
- brucellosis;
- cat-scratch disease;
- cholera;
- clostridial infections;
- Creutzfeldt–Jakob disease;
- cryptococcosis;
- cytomegalovirus;
- dengue;
- diphtheria;
- Ebola haemorrhagic fever;
- echinococcosis;
- epididymitis;
- Epstein–Barr virus;
- fasciitis;
- Fournier's gangrene;
- hantavirus;
- histoplasmosis;
- hydatid disease;
- Lassa fever;
- leptospirosis;
- listeriosis;
- Lyme disease;
- malaria;
- melioidosis;
- Norwalk virus;
- orchitis;
- paragonimiasis;
- pediculosis;

Infections

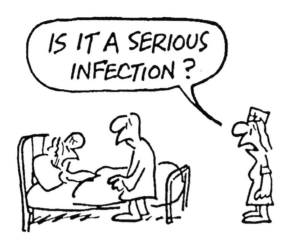

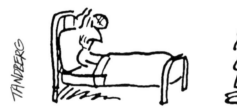

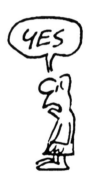

- poliomyelitis;
- Q fever;
- rabies;
- relapsing fever;
- rickettsial diseases;
- scarlet fever;
- schistosomiasis;
- syphilis;
- tetanus;
- toxoplasmosis;
- tuberculosis;
- typhoid fever;
- typhus;
- varicella;
- yellow fever.

Numerous additional issues of more general relevance to infectious diseases are also considered, such as fever, neutropenia, immunocompromise, various drug reactions, and mediators.

Bibliography

Barrett-Connor E 1972 Anemia and infection. Am J Med 52: 242.

Bion JF, Brun-Buisson C (eds) 2000 Infection and critical illness: genetic and environmental aspects of susceptibility and resistance. Intens Care Med 26; Suppl.1.

Bohnsack JF, Brown EJ 1986 The role of the spleen in resistance to infection. Annu Rev Med 37: 49.

Brigden ML, Pattullo AL 1999 Prevention and management of overwhelming postsplenectomy infection – an update. Crit Care Med 27: 836.

Cassell GH, Cole BC 1981 Mycoplasmas as agents of human disease. N Engl J Med 304: 80.

Cohen S, Tyrrell DA, Smith AP 1991 Psychological stress and susceptibility to the common cold. N Engl J Med 325: 606.

Cunha BA (ed) 1998 Infectious Diseases in Critical Care Medicine. New York: Marcel Dekker.

Durand MI, Calserwood SB, Weber MD et al 1993 Acute bacterial meningitis in adults. N Engl J Med 328: 21.

Fisman DN 2000 Hemophagocytic syndromes and infection. Emerg Infect Dis 6: 6.

Gorbach SL, Bartlett JG, Blacklow NR (eds) 1998 Infectious Diseases. 2nd edition. Philadelphia: WB Saunders.

Howard CR 1984 Viral hemorrhagic fevers: properties and prospects for treatment and prevention. Antiviral Res 4: 169.

Keusch GT, Barza MJ, Bennish ML et al (eds) 1998 Year Book of Infectious Diseases 1998. St Louis: Mosby-Year Book.

Mandell GL, Douglas RG, Bennett JE (eds) 1990 Principles and Practice of Infectious Diseases. 3rd edition. New York: John Wiley & Sons.

Meslin F-X 1997 Global aspects of emerging and potential zoonoses: a WHO perspective. Emerg Infect Dis 3: 2.

Paul WE 1993 Infectious diseases and the immune system. Sci Am 269(3): 57.

Peeling RW, Brunham RC 1996 Chlamydiae as pathogens: new species and new issues. Emerg Infect Dis 2: 4.

Rahal JJ 1978 Antibiotic combinations: the clinical relevance of synergy and antagonism. Medicine 57: 179.

Sigurdardottir B, Bjornsson OM, Jonsdottir KE et al 1997 Acute bacterial meningitis in adults. Arch Intern Med 157: 425.

Spach D, Liles W, Campbell G et al 1993 Tick-borne diseases in the United States. N Engl J Med 329: 936.

Tomkins L 1992 The use of molecular methods in the diagnosis of infectious diseases. N Engl J Med 327: 1290.

Whitley RJ 1990 Viral encephalitis. N Engl J Med 323: 242.

Zanetti G, Calandra T 1997 Intravenous immunoglobulins and granulocyte colony-stimulating factor for the management of infection in intensive care units. Curr Opinion Crit Care 3: 342.

Zumla A, James DG 1996 Granulomatous infections: etiology and classification. Clin Infect Dis 23: 146.

Inflammatory bowel disease

Non-specific inflammatory bowel disease comprises ulcerative colitis and Crohn's disease, each with different pathological, clinical and therapeutic aspects, but both requiring distinction from other serious bowel diseases, such as infections or ischaemia. Biological agents targeting the immuno-inflammatory response offer new therapeutic opportunities for these distressing diseases.

1. **Ulcerative colitis** comprises inflammation of colonic epithelium, usually affecting the rectum and distal colon. While there is some minor familial and ethnic clustering, its aetiology is unknown, but it is probable that there are subgroups of separate causation.

Clinical features are seen most commonly in young adults. In the early stages, blood and/or mucus is noted in the stools, and there may even be constipation. In the later stages, there is diarrhoea and systemic features, with fatigue, anorexia, fever and weight loss.

The severity of illness is very variable.

- **Mild disease**

This is seen in most patients (60%), with intermittent diarrhoea (e.g. up to four stools per day) and associated abdominal cramps.

In most such patients (85%), the process remains confined to the rectum (proctitis) or rectum and distal colon (proctosigmoiditis).

There are no systemic features or laboratory abnormalities.

- **Moderate disease**

This occurs in 25% of patients, with involvement of up to half of the colon (left-sided colitis).

There is watery diarrhoea, with blood and mucus (e.g. more than five stools per day), associated with abdominal cramps and rectal urgency.

Some systemic symptoms are usual.

- **Severe disease**

This occurs in 15% of patients, with involvement of the entire colon (extensive or total colitis).

There is constant profuse bloody diarrhoea, with abdominal distension and marked systemic symptoms.

Such patients require hospitalization.

- **Toxic megacolon**

This is the most severe of form of the disease and occurs in about 3% of cases. Since one third of such cases present initially in this way, the differential diagnosis can be difficult, especially as diarrhoea may be minimal at this time and systemic symptoms prominent. There are signs of an acute abdomen, and the patient may become shocked.

The **local complications** of ulcerative colitis include:

- bowel haemorrhage;
- bowel perforation;
- bowel stricture;
- cancer of the colon

  - this is related to the duration, extent and severity of the disease and is responsible for a third of deaths from the disease.

Extra-colonic complications may be prominent and may involve the:

- **eyes**

  - with iritis and/or conjunctivitis and/or episcleritis;

- **joints**

  - with migratory monarticular arthritis of large joints;
  - with an increased incidence of ankylosing spondylitis;

- **liver**

  - with jaundice, cholangitis, fatty liver;
  - occasionally with cirrhosis;

- **skin**

  - occasionally with erythema nodosum;
  - rarely with pyoderma gangrenosum.

The diagnosis is made on sigmoidoscopy, at which the mucosa appears friable and granular. Biopsy excludes Crohn's disease or other specific disorders, and microbiological examination excludes amoebae or pathogenic bacteria. Colonoscopy or barium contrast enema shows the extent of disease.

The differential diagnosis is:

- Crohn's disease;
- irritable bowel syndrome;
- diverticulitis;
- ischaemic colitis;
- bacterial or amoebic gastroenteritis.

Treatment modalities are several.

- *Simple **anti-diarrhoeal** medication (e.g. loperamide, diphenoxylate) may be effective in mild disease, but they should be used with care because of the risk of toxic megacolon.*
- ***Sulfasalazine** is used primarily for maintenance, but it is also useful for mild exacerbations. Although typically given orally, it may also be used in the form of a retention enema.*
- ***Corticosteroids** are used locally in enema form and systemically for moderate or severe disease.*
- ***Immunosuppressive therapy** (azathioprine, cyclosporin) is indicated for severe or refractory disease.*
- ***Surgery** (proctocolectomy) may be required.*

- **Toxic megacolon** *requires resuscitation, fluids and electrolytes, nasogastric aspiration, intravenous cortocosteroids and antibiotics. Anti-diarrhoeal drugs are contraindicated, and indeed they may precipitate this syndrome. As soon as the patient becomes stable, a total **proctocolectomy** is peformed preferably within 48 h.*

The course of illness is very variable. About 10% of patients experience long remissions of up to 15 years, though most (75%) have intermittent exacerbations over many years. About 10% of patients have continuous disease. The 1-year mortality is 5% overall and up to 15–20% in toxic megacolon.

2. **Crohn's disease** is a granulomatous ileocolitis affecting all layers of the bowel and presenting as an enteritis, enterocolitis, colitis or proctocolitis. Like ulcerative colitis, there is some minor familial and ethnic clustering, but its aetiology remains unknown.

Clinical features are also seen mainly in young adults. Chronic indolent symptomatic disease has been present on average for five years before presentation. Mild, watery but not blood-stained diarrhoea and abdominal pain is often diagnosed as irritable bowel syndrome. In some patients, there are systemic features of anorexia, fatigue, weight loss, abdominal mass, fistulae, iritis and anaemia.

Complications include:

- anal fissure;

- bowel fistulae

  – which occur in 50% of patients at some time during the course of the disease;

- peri-rectal abscess;
- fulminant colitis ('toxic megacolon')

  – this can occur but is uncommon;

- increased incidence of both gallstones and renal oxalate calculi

  – particularly in those patients with severe fat malabsorption;
- the eye, joint and skin features seen in ulcerative colitis occur in about 10% of patients.

The differential diagnosis and investigations are as for ulcerative colitis.

Treatment is also similar to that for ulcerative colitis, except that medical therapy is often disappointing and surgery is required in most patients because of either *initial disease or its complications. However, there is a high postoperative recurrence rate, and about half of the patients require re-operation.*

*Recently, a chimeric monoclonal antibody to tumour necrosis factor α, **infliximab**, was reported to enhance greatly the closure of abdominal and perineal fistulae*

Bibliography

Gibson PR, Anderson RP 1998 Inflammatory bowel disease. Med J Aust 169: 387.

Greenberg GR 1992 Nutritional support in inflammatory bowel disease: current status and future directions. Scand J Gastronenterol 192 (suppl): 117.

Kornbluth A, George J, Sachar DB 1994 Immunosuppressive drugs in Crohn's disease. Gastroenterologist 2: 239.

MacDermott RP, Stenson WF 1992 Inflammatory Bowel Disease. New York: Elsevier.

Present DH, Rutgeerts P, Targan S et al 1999 Infliximab for the treatment of fistulas in patients with Crohn's disease. N Engl J Med 340: 1398.

Rachmilewitz D 1992 New forms of treatment for inflammatory bowel disease. Gut 33: 1301.

Sands BE 1997 Biologic therapy for inflammatory bowel disease. Inflamm Bowel Dis 3: 95.

Inhalation injury (see Burns (respiratory complications))

Insect bites and stings (see Bites and stings)

Interstitial lung diseases

The interstitial lung diseases are a group of diffuse pulmonary processes, many of unknown aetiology. They are listed below as a group for comparison, but their individual details are considered separately in this book.

Specific interstitial diseases, such as pneumonia, pulmonary oedema, pneumoconioses and other occupational lung diseases, drug reactions and lung involvement in systemic diseases are usually considered separately.

High-resolution CT scanning is generally the most useful imaging technique in this group of conditions.

The major interstitial lung diseases are:

1. **sarcoidosis**

2. **diffuse fibrosing alveolitis**

   – i.e. idiopathic pulmonary fibrosis, interstitial pneumonitis;

3. **haemorrhagic infiltrates**

   – Goodpasture's syndrome;
   – idiopathic pulmonary haemosiderosis;

4. **pulmonary infiltration with eosinophilia (PIE)**

   – Loeffler's syndrome;
   – asthmatic pulmonary eosinophilia;
   – tropical pulmonary eosinophilia;
   – eosinophilic pneumonia;

5. **angiitis and granulomatosis**

   – Wegener's granulomatosis;
   – lymphomatoid granulomatosis;
   – bronchocentric granulomatosis;

6. **rare pulmonary infiltrative condition**

   – histiocytosis X;
   – pulmonary alveolar proteinosis;
   – pulmonary alveolar microlithiasis;
   – lymphangiomyomatosis;
   – pulmonary amyloidosis.

Bibliography

Chu SC, Horiba K, Usuki J et al 1999 Comprehensive evaluation of 35 patients with lymphangioleiomyomatosis. Chest 115: 1041.

Coultas DB, Zumwalt RE, Black WC et al 1994 The epidemiology of interstitial lung diseases. Am J Respir Crit Care Med 150: 967.

Crystal RG, Bitterman PB, Rennard SI et al 1984 Interstitial lung diseases of unknown cause. N Engl J Med 310: 154, 235.

Kitaichi M, Nishimura K, Itoh H et al 1995 Pulmonary lymphangioleiomyomatosis. Am J Respir Crit Care Med 151: 527.

Moss J (ed) 1999 LAM (lymphangioleiomyomatosis) and Other Diseases Characterized by Smooth Muscle Proliferation. New York: Marcel Dekker.

Prakash UB, Barham SS, Rosenow EC et al 1983 Pulmonary alveolar microlithiasis. Mayo Clin Proc 58: 290.

Reynolds HY 1998 Diagnostic and management strategies for diffuse interstitial lung disease. Chest 113: 192.

Taylor JR, Ryu J, Colby TV et al 1990 Lymphangioleiomyomatosis. N Engl J Med 323: 1254.

Interstitial nephritis (see Tubulointerstitial diseases)

Interstitial pneumonitis (see Diffuse fibrosing alveolitis)

Iron

Iron (Fe, atomic number 26, atomic weight 56) comprises 35% of the Earth's composition, being the chief constituent of the Earth's core and a major constituent (5%) of the Earth's crust, in which it is the fourth most common element after oxygen, silicon and aluminium. It has for centuries been the most used and cheapest metal in all societies. As is well known, iron has an important role in biological functions.

The total body stores of iron are normally about 4.5 g, 65% being present in haemoglobin, a small amount in myoglobin and haem enzymes, and the remainder in stores of both soluble ferritin and insoluble haemosiderin (in liver, spleen and bone marrow). One mL of blood contains about 0.5 mg of iron.

The daily dietary requirement is 10–20 mg, of which about 10% is actually absorbed, with extra requirements for menstruation and pregnancy. The recommended iv dose is 20 μmol/day.

Clinical conditions associated with iron abnormalities include:

- iron deficiency (see Anaemia);
- iron overload (see Haemochromatosis and Haemoglobin disorders);
- iron poisoning (see Desferrioxamine).

Bibliography

Bothwell TH, Charlton RW, Cook JD et al 1979 Iron Metabolism in Man. Oxford: Blackwell.

Conrad ME, Umbreit JN, Moore EG 1994 Iron absorption and cellular uptake of iron. Adv Exp Med Biol 356: 69.

Cook JD, Skikne BS 1989 Iron deficiency: definition and diagnosis. J Intern Med 226: 349.

Editorial 1979 Serum-ferritin. Lancet 1: 533.

Finch CA 1982 Erythropoiesis, erythropoietin, and iron. Blood 60: 1241.

Finch CA 1982 The detection of iron overload. N Engl J Med 307: 1702.

Finch CA, Huebers H 1992 Perspectives in iron metabolism. N Engl J Med 306: 1520.

Hershko C, Peto TEA, Weatherall DJ 1988 Iron and infection. Br Med J 296: 660.

Huebers HA, Finch CA 1987 The physiology of transferrin and transferrin receptors. Physiol Rev 67: 520.

Kuhn LC 1994 Molecular regulation of iron proteins. Baillieres Clin Haematol 7: 763.

Mills KC, Curry SC 1994 Acute iron poisoning. Emerg Clin North Am 12: 397.

Sayers MH, English G, Finch C 1994 Capacity of the store-regulator in maintaining iron balance. Am J Hematol 47: 194.

Iron overload disease (see Haemochromatosis and Haemoglobin disorders)

Irritable bowel syndrome (see Colitis)

Islet cell tumour

Islet cell tumours of the pancreas cause fasting hypoglycaemia, which is associated with abnormally high (i.e. non-suppressed) insulin levels and which displays Whipple's triad.

Whipple's triad consists of hypoglycaemia, which:

- displays typical clinical features (especially neuroglycopenia);
- with an appropriately low blood sugar;
- with relief of symptoms with therapy which restores the blood sugar to normal.

The islet cell tumour is thus an insulinoma. Most such tumours (90%) are single, small and benign. Occasionally, they are multiple (as in multiple endocrine neoplasia – q.v.) or even malignant.

The differential diagnosis includes the other causes of fasting hypoglycaemia, which is also seen in:

- sepsis;
- liver failure;
- severe cardiac failure;
- diffuse malignancy.

The diagnosis is made by the demonstration of appropriate hypoglycaemia after fasting. The blood glucose level should be <2 mmol/L in men or <1.5 mmol/L in women and not just <3 mmol/L (the lower limit of normal), because this level can occur with normal fasting (falls much greater than this are usually prevented by gluconeogenesis and decreased insulin secretion). The usual fast is overnight (i.e. 12 h), which has a diagnostic yield of about 65%. If the fast is increased to 24 h, 48 h and 72 h, the diagnostic yields increase accordingly to 71%, 92% and 98%, respectively. At this time also, the ratio of immunoreactive insulin (IRI) to glucose is abnormally increased.

If the diagnosis is still in doubt, a provocative test with exogenous insulin may be administered (in which case there is a failure of proinsulin or C peptide to fall).

Similar findings can also be produced by some oral hypoglycaemic agents, so that the association of profound fasting hypoglycaemia with hyperinsulinaemia should always prompt a urinary drug screen for sulfonylureas.

If appropriately abnormal fasting hypoglycaemia is associated with a normal IRI: glucose ratio, a non-pancreatic tumour should be sought. Some large mesodermal tumours, such as fibrosarcoma, mesothelioma and rarely haemangiopericytoma, either secrete insulin-like growth factors (IGFs) or metabolize glucose at an excess rate and thus cause marked hypoglycaemia.

Islet cell tumours are potentially curable by surgical **resection**.

Bibliography

Le Quesne LP, Nabarro JDN, Kurtz A et al 1979 The management of insulin tumours of the pancreas. Br J Surg 66: 31.

Jarisch-Herxheimer reaction

The Jarisch–Herxheimer reaction occurs within a few hours of commencing treatment of spirochaetal diseases, particularly leptospirosis, relapsing fever and syphilis. It is due to the release of lipopolysaccharide products from the organism and resembles an immunological reaction. Like sepsis, it is associated with mediator and cytokine release.

There is fever, tachycardia, hypotension, headache and myalgia. It occurs within 8 h and lasts about 12–24 h.

There is no specific treatment, though sometimes supportive care for hypotension may be required.

Interestingly, it has been reported to be decreased by giving antibodies to tumour necrosis factor (anti-TNFα).

Bibliography

Gelfand JA, Elin RJ, Berry FW et al 1976 Endotoxemia associated with the Jarisch–Herxheimer reaction. N Engl J Med 295: 211

Jellyfish envenomation (see Bites and stings (marine invertebrates))

Kaposi's sarcoma (see Acquired immunodeficiency syndrome)

Kartagener's syndrome (see Bronchiectasis and Situs inversus)

Korsakoff syndrome (see Wernicke–Korsakoff syndrome)

Kyphoscoliosis

Kyphoscoliosis refers to a deformity of the vertebral column,

- kyphosis comprising anterior flexion,
- scoliosis comprising lateral curvature with rotation.

The two features are usually combined, and distortion of the thoracic cage results.

Kyphoscoliosis is the most common structural abnormally of the thoracic cage. Most cases (80%) are idiopathic, but some are secondary.

- Idiopathic kyphoscoliosis commences in childhood, usually affecting girls, and often becoming severe during the years of rapid skeletal growth.
- Secondary kyphoscoliosis is associated either with neuromuscular diseases, such as poliomyelitis or syringomyelia, or sometimes with congenital vertebral defects.

Clinical features may comprise dyspnoea on exertion and increased susceptibility to respiratory tract infections or CNS depressant drugs, in addition to the obvious skeletal deformity.

> If kyphoscoliosis is severe, the mechanical distortion of the chest wall and the mechanical disadvantage of the respiratory muscles lead to ventilatory failure.

Investigations in severely affected patients show markedly impaired ventilatory capacity, with decreased vital capacity and total lung capacity. A vital capacity of <45% is associated with an increased risk of respiratory failure. In contrast to the gas exchange abnormalities seen in parenchymal lung disease, there is hypercapnia and a relatively normal alveolar-arterial oxygen tension difference. Pulmonary hypertension and cor pulmonale are usual.

Treatment is with **surgical correction**, *if possible early in the course of disease.*

- *Otherwise, treatment should be directed to those complicating problems which are reversible or preventable (e.g. influenza and pneumococcal vaccination).*
- *Even after chronic respiratory failure has supervened, the outlook may be favourable for many years with home oxygen therapy and mechanical ventilation at night.*

Bibliography
Libby DM, Briscoe WA, Boyce B et al 1982 Acute respiratory failure in scoliosis or kyphosis: prolonged survival and treatment. Am J Med 73: 532.

Lactase deficiency

Lactase deficiency refers to the loss from the intestinal mucosa of the disaccharidase enzyme required to break down the disaccharide, lactose, i.e. glucose-galactose (or sucrose, i.e. glucose-fructose) to monosaccharides which can then be absorbed. Otherwise these sugars remain in the bowel, where their osmotic load takes up water and produces diarrhoea (q.v.). In the lower bowel, additional bacterial digestion produces even smaller but still non-absorbable fragments, thereby increasing the osmotic effect further.

Lactase deficiency may rarely be congenital, but it is usually acquired in later childhood. It is common in peoples of non-Northern European origin, and its management requires removal of dairy foods from the diet.

In normal subjects without lactase deficiency, ingestion of other saccharides can produce similar gastrointestinal effects, e.g.:

- indigestible oligosaccharides from legumes;
- non-absorbable sugar alcohols (mannitol, sorbitol);
- indigestible disaccharides (lactulose).

Lactic acidosis

Lactic acidosis is the most common form of metabolic acidosis associated with an increased anion gap, i.e. $[Na^+] - [Cl^-] - [HCO_3^-] > 13$ mmol/L (or about half this if there is severe hypoalbuminaemia). It is a frequent complication of serious illness and is associated with a mortality of 60–90% despite treatment.

About 1000 mmol of lactic acid is normally produced per day, and this load is greatly increased in sepsis, hypotension or other tissue ischaemia. These are conditions which result in impaired oxidation of pyruvate in mitochondria. Pyruvate is normally metabolized aerobically to CO_2 and water via the tricarboxylic acid (TCA or Krebs) cycle. In anaerobic conditions, pyruvate is metabolized to lactate.

Decreased lactic acid clearance also occurs in hepatic hypoperfusion, since the liver normally converts lactate back to pyruvate with the consequent regeneration of bicarbonate and more importantly also converts lactate to glucose via gluconeogenesis. Since in exercise, lactate production can exceed 300 mmol/h without significant acidosis, it is apparent that in disease lactate acidosis must arise from impaired clearance as well as from increased production.

The lactate/pyruvate ratio is normally about 10:1. It is increased in lactic acidosis and was formerly the basis of a classification for this condition.

A more practical classification, and one with more therapeutic meaning, is into

- **type A** (with apparent tissue hypoxia). This includes shock, hypoxaemia and probably sepsis. This is sometimes referred to as 'shock' lactate, which is an index of tissue hypoxia or hypoperfusion

- **type B** (without apparent tissue hypoxia). This includes:

   – congenital enzyme deficiencies,
   – acquired diseases, such as renal failure, liver failure, pancreatitis, diabetes, sepsis, malignancy,
   – drugs, such as ethanol, methanol, ethylene glycol, sodium nitroprusside, adrenaline, salicylates, metformin.

This is sometimes referred to as a 'stress' lactate which, is an index of hypermetabolism, at least in sepsis.

The clinical features are those of the underlying disease. Particular note must be taken of the presence of tissue hypoxia.

The serum lactate level is increased in lactic acidosis (normal <1–2 mmol/L), but levels >6 mmol/L are required for renal excretion. Arterial or mixed venous samples should be used, so that global rather than regional changes are assessed. There is no direct relationship between blood lactate and hydrogen ion concentrations.

The serum lactate level is normal (though there is still an increased anion gap) in an unusual form of lactic acidosis due to d-lactate accumulation, as in the short bowel syndrome. D-lactate is produced by some bacteria, whereas mammalian tissues produce L-lactate, the laevo isomer which is measured by most analytical methods.

> The arterial PCO_2 is usually low, but the mixed venous PCO_2 is high. This wide venoarterial difference for CO_2 is a better guide to the severity of the problem than the arterial PCO_2. It is due to increased CO_2 production and/or decreased cardiac output.

Treatment is primarily that of the underlying cause. It is important to recognize in any particular case whether increased lactate does or does not indicate hypoperfusion, as it is not only under-resuscitation that has adverse clinical consequences but also over-resuscitation.

*The use of **bicarbonate** is controversial. While it has traditionally been considered reasonable on theoretical grounds to administer it cautiously if the acidosis is severe (i.e. pH <7.20), controlled studies have in fact been unable to show an increased survival following its use or any other evidence to support its administration.*

While metabolic acidosis with a high anion gap is most commonly attributed to lactic acidosis in the critically ill, in some cases unidentified anions appear to be involved. Acquired **pyroglutamic acid** excess, due particularly to paracetamol ingestion, may be one such cause.

Bibliography

Arieff AI 1991 Indications for use of bicarbonate in patients with metabolic acidosis. Br J Anaesth 67: 165.
Bakker J 2001 Lactate: may I have your votes please? Intens Care Med 27: 6.
Cohen RD, Woods HF (eds) 1976 Clinical and Biochemical Aspects of Lactic Acidosis. Oxford: Blackwell.
Cooper DJ, Walley KR, Wiggs BR et al 1990 Bicarbonate does not improve hemodynamics in critically ill patients who have lactic acidosis. Ann Intern Med 112: 492.
Dempsey GA, Lyall HJ, Corke CF et al 2000 Pyroglutamic acidemia: a cause of high anion gap metabolic acidosis. Crit Care Med 28: 1803.
Editorial 1990 The colon, rumen, and d-lactic acidosis. Lancet 336: 599.
Emmett M, Narins RG 1977 Clinical use of the anion gap. Medicine 56: 38.
Forsythe SM, Schmidt GA 2000 Sodium bicarbonate for the treatment of lactic acidosis. Chest 117: 260.
Huckabee WE 1961 Abnormal resting blood lactate: II. Lactic acidosis. Am J Med 30: 840.
James JH, Luchette FA, McCarter FD et al 1999 Lactate is an unreliable indicator of tissue hypoxia in injury and sepsis. Lancet 354: 505.
Kruse JA 1997 Clinical utility and limitations of the anion gap. Int J Intens Care 4: 51.
Malhotra D, Shapiro JI 1996 Pathogenesis and management of lactic acidosis. Curr Opinion Crit Care 2: 439.
Mizock BA 1989 Lactic acidosis. Dis Mon 35: 233.
Nasraway S, Black R, Sottile F 1989 The anion gap in patients admitted to the medical intensive care unit. Chest 96: 287S.
Schelling JR, Howard RL, Winter SD et al 1990 Increased osmol gap in alcoholic ketoacidosis and lactic acidosis. Ann Intern Med 113: 580.
Stacpoole PW 1986 Lactic acidosis: the case against bicarbonate therapy. Ann Intern Med 105: 276.

Lassa fever

Lassa fever is one of the four forms of **viral haemorrhagic fever** transmitted from person to person (see Ebola haemorrhagic fever). It was first recognized in 1970 in Nigeria and is known to have a rodent reservoir, with person to person spread following human ingestion of contaminated food. The pathogenesis involves viral interaction with and damage to endothelial cells and platelets, giving rise to a generalized capillary leak.

The incubation period is 6–21 days, which provides sufficient time nowadays for travel anywhere in the world.

The illness presents initially as influenza-like, with a sore throat, rash and gastrointestinal symptoms. In the second week, encephalopathy, hepatitis and pleurisy are seen. Haemorrhage, renal failure and shock may occur in some patients.

The diagnosis is made by viral culture and serology.

The differential diagnosis includes many other infective diseases, including:

* malaria;
* pneumonia;
* gastroenteritis;
* influenza;
* typhoid.

*Treatment is with **ribavirin** (2 g loading dose, then 1 g qid for 4 days and then 0.5 g tds for 6 days), together with resuscitation and supportive care.*

When first described, the mortality was 50%, but it is nowadays 1–2%. Prolonged weakness is experienced by survivors and 25% have permanent deafness.

Bibliography

Howard CR 1984 Viral hemorrhagic fevers: properties and prospects for treatment and prevention. Antiviral Res 4: 169.

McCormick JB, Webb PA, Krebs JW et al 1987 A prospective study of the epidemiology and ecology of Lassa fever. J Infect Dis 155: 437.

Lateral medullary syndrome (see Horner's syndrome)

Lead

Lead (Pb, atomic number 82, atomic weight 207, melting point 328°C) is a soft, dense malleable, durable and corrosion-resistant great metal. It is probably the oldest known metal, and although not found free in nature it is readily produced from its major source, namely lead sulfide (galena). There are many industrial applications for lead or lead-containing compounds, including plumbing, solder, batteries, ammunition, insulation, shielding, glass and petrol (as the additive tetraethyl lead).

Lead poisoning may thus occur in a wide variety of circumstances, including the home, industry, agriculture and from motor vehicle exhaust fumes.

Much of the risk of lead poisoning has disappeared since lead salts are no longer used as pigments in white exterior paint or in insecticides. Nevertheless, lead may readily accumulate in the body and produce toxicity (referred to as **plumbism**), which takes the form in children particularly of cognitive and behavioural effects and in adults of renal disease.

The maximum recommended exposure is not >50 μg/m^3/8 h and a whole blood level of <60 μg/dL. The free RBC protoporphyrin level may be used as a screening test, since lead blocks haemosynthesis and thus produces an acquired porphyrin disease.

Although the toxic effects are widespread and especially involve the central nervous system, kidneys, bone marrow and gut, there is very variable individual susceptibility.

Acute toxicity in adults classically gives rise to abdominal colic, haemolytic anaemia (a benign variant of sideroblastic anaemia with coarse basophilic stippling of erythrocytes) and encephalopathy (similar to that seen in hypertension). There may be pallor, irritability, a metallic taste in the mouth, a black line at the base of the gums, anorexia and constipation.

Acute toxicity in children causes neurological damage, which may lead to intellectual impairment and if more severe to deafness, blindness and seizures.

Chronic toxicity is manifest by renal failure, hypertension and saturnine gout. Lead nephropathy is a tubulointerstitial nephritis, with an unremarkable urinary sediment, and impaired uric acid excretion and increased serum uric acid out of proportion to the degree of renal impairment. Neurological changes of headache, confusion, visual disturbance and peripheral motor neuropathy (e.g. wrist drop) are seen. Permanent mental loss occurs in about one third of patients. Cardiomyopathy with potentially fatal arrhythmias can follow repeated petrol sniffing.

*Treatment of lead poisoning requires the **chelating agents**, calcium edetate and/or penicillamine (q.v.). A prolonged course is required, but complete recovery is usual, provided there is no neurological damage.*

Bibliography

Alperstein G, Reznik RB, Duggin GG 1991 Lead: subtle forms and new modes of poisoning. Med J Aust 155: 407.

Balestra DJ 1991 Adult chronic lead intoxication: a clinical review. Arch Intern Med 151: 1718.

Carton JA, Maradona JA, Arribas JM 1987 Acute–subacute lead poisoning: clinical findings and comparative study of diagnostic tests. Arch Intern Med 147: 697.

White JM, Selhi HS 1975 Lead and the red cell. Br J Haematol 30: 133.

Leptospirosis

Leptospirosis is due to infection with the small spirochaete, *Leptospira interrogans*. The organism is endemic in animals in the tropics, both domestic and wild, in which the infection is often asymptomatic and the organism is shed in the urine. Human infection is incidental and occurs after contact of abraded skin or mucous membranes within infected material. In warm and moist conditions, the organism can survive for weeks outside the body. There is an obvious occupational risk for abattoir workers, farmers and veterinarians and a less apparent one from a number of outdoor recreational activities.

Following an incubation period of 7–12 days, there is an acute non-specific febrile illness, which is often severe and lasts for 4–7 days. However, the clinical manifestations are variable, and infection may also be subclinical. Typically, there is bradycardia, rash, conjunctivitis, stiff neck and muscle tenderness. There is occasional hepatosplenomegaly and lymphadenopathy. Leptospirae are present in the blood during this phase.

After improvement lasting 1–3 days, recurrent fever and meningitis occur which then last up to some weeks.

Specific syndromes at this stage include the following.

- **Weil's disease**

This is the most severe form of the illness. It is seen in 5–10% of patients and presents with jaundice, uraemia, encephalopathy, anaemia. Sometimes, there is rhabdomyolysis and vasculitis.

- **Aseptic meningitis**

Initially this mimics viral meningitis, but eventually the CSF shows a lymphocytosis, markedly increased protein level and normal glucose.

- **Pretibial fever** (Fort Bragg fever)

There is splenomegaly and raised, red, painful lesions on the shins. The diagnosis is made from positive culture or serology.

The differential diagnosis is an acute viral illness.

*Treatment is primarily with **supportive** measures, but **antibiotics** (doxycycline for 7 days or possibly penicillin) probably shorten the duration of disease and decrease its severity.*

There is no satisfactory prevention. The mortality is 3–6%, and survivors recover completely.

Bibliography

Turner LH 1973 Leptospirosis. Br Med J 1: 537.

Leukocytoclastic vasculitis (see Urticaria)

Leukoencephalopathy (see Demyelinating diseases)

Lewisite (see Chelating agents and Warfare agents)

Lice (see Pediculosis)

Light chains (see Multiple myeloma)

Lightning

The electrical discharge in lightning comprises an estimated 20 million or more volts DC with a current of up to 20 000 amps, although the duration is <500 msec.

> Lightning may strike an individual in several different ways, namely:
>
> - directly;
> - as a splash or flash from a nearby object of high resistance;
> - via contact with a primary object;
> - from the adjacent ground via the legs as a stride potential;
> - via telephone lines.

Burns (flash burn over the outside of the body, which may even rip clothing apart), electrical injury or blast injury may be produced. The electrical injury is usually minor, and the blast injury is equivalent to blunt trauma.

The injuries are thus neurological, musculoskeletal, cardiovascular, cutaneous and ophthalmological. Direct strike may of course cause immediate death, though an electrically induced respiratory arrest may be reversible for up to 24 h.

- **Neurologically**, there may be confusion and paralysis. Most patients suffer at least some loss of consciousness. Fixed dilated pupils can be due to local eye damage and not necessarily to brainstem death. From telephone contact, there may be headache, deafness and tinnitus.
- **Cardivascular effects** include any arrhythmia and particularly asystole. Vasoconstriction can be marked, even to the point of tissue ischaemia.

- The **skin** may show a Lichtenberg flower, a delicate branching lesion which is not a burn and disappears within 24 h. Localized deep burns may also be seen.
- **Eye** damage most commonly results in later development of cataract.

The mortality is 20–30% in humans struck by lightning. There is thus one death per year from this cause per 10 million population. Importantly, long-term sequelae independent of the direct consequences of the injury, including psychiatric illness and cataracts, occur in about two thirds of survivors.

Bibliography
Browne B, Gaasch W 1992 Electrical injuries and lightning. Emerg Med Clin North Am 2: 211.
Hiestant D, Colice G 1988 Lightning-strike injury. J Intens Care Med 3: 303.

Liquorice

Liquorice is derived from the perennial herb, *Glycyrrhiza glabra*, and comprises glycyrrhizic acid (etymologically meaning sweat root). It is obtained from the roots of the plant and is similar to anise.

It has long been used for flavouring and in medicines to disguise unpleasant components. It is also a popular confection and has been used in chewing tobacco. Medically, liquorice has been prescribed in peptic ulcer disease and in Addison's disease.

Since liquorice is **salt-retaining**, its excessive use (e.g. >0.45 kg/week) can give rise to oedema or to pseudoprimary aldosteronism and thus secondary hypertension (see Conn's syndrome).

It can also give rise to **hypokalaemic periodic paralysis**, although more commonly this condition occurs due to:

- potassium loss from the kidney or gut;
- diuretic or corticosteroid use;
- thyrotoxicosis.

Bibliography

Blachley JD, Knochel JP 1980 Tobacco chewer's hypokalemia: licorice revisited. N Engl J Med 302: 784.

de Klerk GJ, Nieuwenhuis MG, Beutler JJ 1997 Hypokalaemia and hypertension associated with use of liquorice flavoured chewing gum. Br Med J 314: 751.

Listeriosis

Listeriosis is caused by the aerobic Gram-positive bacillus, *Listeria monocytogenes*, a saprophyte found widely in soil, plants and animals. It is relatively resistant to heat, including pasteurization, and can grow even in refrigerated food. It is thus often food-borne.

Despite its ubiquitous nature, human disease is in fact uncommon. It is, however, an important cause of neonatal sepsis and of adult meningitis.

> **Meningitis** particularly occurs in the elderly or in compromised hosts. It is clinically similar to other forms of meningitis, except that:
>
> - tremor and ataxia are more common;
> - encephalitis especially of the pons may sometimes be seen.

Other less common forms of infection include:

- isolated bacteraemia;
- occasional focal lesions;
- an influenza-like illness in pregnancy, with associated amnionitis and fetal damage.

The diagnosis is made from bacterial identification, as there is no routine serological test (though an anti-listeriolysin-O test has recently been developed). The organism may sometimes be difficult to identify, as it can have coccoid forms and may therefore sometimes be confused with streptococci.

Since listeriosis presents to Intensive Care as meningitis, specific diagnosis is important because the third-generation cephalosporins which are commonly used in most forms of meningitis are not appropriate for the treatment of this organism.

*Treatment is with **ampicillin** 2 g iv 4 hourly for 10 days beyond the subsidence of fever. This is longer than is usual for bacterial meningitis and is required because of the frequency of relapse following shorter courses.*

- *Penicillin, erythromycin, tetracycline, cotrimoxazole and vancomycin are also effective.*
- *Gentamicin is synergistic with ampicillin in vitro but probably not in vivo, whereas cotrimoxazole is synergistic with ampicillin in vivo and thus provides a clinically effective combination.*

Bibliography

Calder JAM 1997 Listeria meningitis in adults. Lancet 350: 307.

Durand ML, Calderwood SB, Weber DJ et al 1993 Acute bacterial meningitis in adults. N Engl J Med 328: 21.

Gellin BG, Broome CV 1989 Listeriosis. JAMA 261: 1313.

Hearmon CJ, Ghosh SK 1989 *Listeria monocytogenes* meningitis in previously healthy adults. Postgrad Med J 65: 74.

Nieman RE, Lorber B 1980 Listeriosis in adults: a changing pattern. Rev Infect Dis 2: 207.

Southwick PS, Purich DL 1996 Intracellular pathogenesis of listeriosis. N Engl J Med 334: 770.

Lithium

Lithium (Li, atomic number 3, atomic weight 7, melting point 179°C) is the lightest solid element. It was discovered in 1817 and is a soft, white substance which floats on water (SG 0.53). Although it has a variety of industrial uses, it is best known for its use as lithium carbonate, its is used in a dose of manic-depressive illness, first described in 1949 in Australia. In this condition, it is used in a dose of 900–2400 mg/day in divided doses to give a trough therapeutic plasma level of about 1 mmol/L.

Lithium is a reactive element with a large variety of biological effects. Of particular relevance to its psychopharmacological effects is its inhibition at therapeutic plasma levels of a second messenger system in the central nervous system. At higher levels, it decreases adenyl cyclase and thus cAMP. It is distributed in the total body water and excreted solely by the kidney, where like sodium it undergoes glomerular filtration though not distal tubular reabsorption (so that its excretion is not enhanced by diuretics like thiazides). However, like sodium, with which it competes, it is reabsorbed from the proximal tubule, so that its plasma level is increased in states of sodium depletion (and also with NSAIDs).

Lithium has a low therapeutic index, and acute toxicity may be seen with plasma levels >2 mmol/L. Moreover, side-effects are common at any level.

Adverse experiences of lithium are manifest as:

- **renal**

  - with nephrogenic diabetes insipidus, seen to some degree in about 20% of patients and treated with a thiazide or preferably amiloride;
  - interstitial nephritis or nephrotic syndrome, both uncommon but requiring permanent cessation of lithium;

- **neurological**

  - with intention tremor, drowsiness, confusion, fits, coma, hyperreflexia, ataxia, dysarthria, blurred vision, tinnitus, focal neurological signs;

- **neuropsychiatric**

  - impaired memory, cognition and creativity, though these complaints may be no more than cessation of hypomania;

- **thyroid**

  - with non-toxic goitre or hypothyroidism, these abnormalities being seen in 5% of patients, particularly women with thyroid antibodies, and requiring thyroid replacement therapy though not cessation of lithium;

- **cardiovascular**

  - with arrhythmias, especially conduction defects;
  - hypotension;
  - T-wave inversion on ECG, a benign change;
  - vasculitis;

- **dermatological**

  - with acne;
  - precipitation or exacerbation of psoriasis;
  - stress alopecia;

- **haematological**

  - with raised white cell count, due to increased neutrophil turnover and mass;

- **gastrointestinal**

  - with nausea, vomiting and diarrhoea;

- **metabolic**

  - with mild hypercalcaemia;

- **general**

  - with oedema and weight gain;

- **teratogenic**

  - with congenital heart disease (as with rubella).

---

*The treatment of lithium toxicity is an **emergency**, since high plasma levels may cause permanent neurological damage or death. Therapy is supportive, with sodium and water replacement and enhancement of urinary lithium excretion by alkalinization and osmotic diuresis. Renal replacement therapy is required if toxicity is severe, though recovery is delayed despite the return to normal of plasma lithium levels, since the intracellular effects themselves are slow to reverse.*

Bibliography

Cade JFJ 1949 Lithium salts in the treatment of psychotic excitement. Med J Aust 2: 349.

Kulig K 1992 All lithium overdoses deserve respect. J Emerg Med 10: 757.

Mitchel JE, MacKenzie TB 1982 Cardiac effects of lithium therapy in man: a review. J Clin Psychiatry 43: 47.

Walker RG 1993 Lithium nephrotoxicity. Kidney Int 42 (suppl): S93.

Livedo reticularis

Livedo reticularis refers to blue-red mottling of the skin which characteristically takes a fishnet pattern reflecting the underlying vascular anatomy. It is thus a vascular disorder, though its cause is in practice usually unknown.

Idiopathic livedo reticularis occurs chiefly in young to middle-aged women and is typically precipitated by cold or stasis. Symptoms are minimal but may include numbness or tingling.

Treatment is not required.

Secondary livedo reticularis occurs in a number of conditions, including:

- antiphospholipid syndrome;
- immune vasculitis;
- endocarditis;
- thrombocythaemia;
- hyperviscosity syndromes;
- cholesterol embolization.

Livedo vasculitis is a related but more serious condition, with a course which is either chronic or relapsing.

There is microvascular occlusion with pain and ulceration, especially affecting the lower limbs. The cerebral circulation may be involved with resultant cerebrovascular ischaemia.

Antithrombotic therapy is recommended.

Bibliography

Burton JL 1988 Livedo reticularis, porcelain-white scars, and cerebral thromboses. Lancet 1: 1263.

Copeman PW 1975 Livedo reticularis: signs in the skin of disturbance of blood viscosity and of blood flow. Br J Dermatol 93: 519.

Klein K, Pittelkow M 1992 Tissue plasminogen activator for the treatment of livedoid vasculitis. Mayo Clin Proc 67: 923.

Schroeter AL, Diaz-Perez JL, Winkelmann RK et al 1975 Livedo vasculitis (the vasculitis of atrophie blanche): immunohistopathologic study. Arch Dermatol 111: 188.

Liver abscess

Liver abscess is the most common intra-abdominal visceral abscess. It may arise from either local or systemic infection.

Local causes include:

- cholangitis;
- direct extension;
- portal venous transmission following abdominal surgery or PTCA.

Systemic causes are bacteraemias. In turn, liver abscess may give rise to bacteraemia or metastatic infection elsewhere.

> Clinical features of liver abscess may be subtle and include only fever and leukocytosis. Sometimes, there may be abnormal local signs or liver dysfunction.

Although the plain X-ray may show an associated right pleural effusion or even an air–fluid level within the liver, imaging with ultrasound or CT is usually required. Sometimes, there may be difficulty in distinguishing a liver abscess from other types of intrahepatic mass, such as cyst or neoplasm.

> The micro-organisms involved in liver abscess are usually Gram-negative enteric bacilli, as for peritonitis or other intra-abdominal abscesses. Often the condition is polymicrobial. Blood cultures may assist the microbiological diagnosis. An amoebic aetiology should be suspected if the abscess is a single right-sided lesion in a traveller.

Treatment is nowadays by **percutaneous drainage***, together with appropriate* **antibiotics***.*

The progress and prognosis depend on the underlying cause.

Bibliography

Branum GD, Tyson GS, Branum MA et al 1990 Hepatic abscess: changes in etiology, diagnosis and management. Ann Surg 212: 655.

Rustgi AK, Richter JM 1989 Pyogenic and amebic abscess. Med Clin North Am 73: 847.

Loeffler's syndrome (see Eosinophilia and lung infiltration)

Lung tumours

Primary malignant tumours of the lung are:

- predominantly, bronchogenic carcinoma (lung cancer);
- less commonly, mesothelioma, pulmonary lymphoma, melanoma, sarcoma;
- less malignantly, bronchoadenoma (carcinoid tumour, cylindroma, others);
- rarely, papilloma, neurofibroma, haemangiopericytoma, teratoma, plasmacytoma.

Primary benign tumours include chiefly hamartoma and angioma. Many rare tumours (e.g. chemodectoma) have also been reported.

Secondary (malignant) tumours of the lung are probably more common than in other sites. The most frequent sources of the primary tumour are:

- breast;
- gastrointestinal tract;
- urogenital system;
- thyroid;
- connective tissue sarcoma;
- lymphoma.

Primary benign and malignant tumours as well as metastases may also occur in intrathoracic structures other than the lung, such as the mediastinum, chest wall and spine.

The thoracic signs of lung cancer comprise:

- local wheeze;
- unresolving pneumonia;
- pleural effusion;
- recurrent laryngeal or phrenic nerve involvement;
- thoracic inlet (Pancoast) syndrome

  – with shoulder pain, Horner's syndrome and brachial plexus damage;

- supraclavicular lymph node involvement;
- superior vena cava obstruction.

Lung cancer is particularly prone to give systemic, non-metastatic manifestations or paraneoplastic phenomena (q.v.). These include:

- **general disability**

  – tiredness, weakness, anorexia and weight loss;

- **connective tissue disorders**

  – clubbing, hypertrophic pulmonary osteoarthropathy, acanthosis nigricans, dermatomyositis;

- **neuromuscular disorders**

  – myasthenia, cerebellar degeneration, motor and/or sensory neuropathy, dementia;

- **endocrine disorders**

  – hypercalcaemia, Cushing's syndrome, syndrome of inappropriate antidiuretic hormone, carcinoid syndrome, hyperthyroidism, hypoglycaemia;

- **haematological disorders**

  – thrombophlebitis, venous thromboembolism, non-bacterial thrombotic endocarditis, haemolytic anaemia, red cell aplasia, thrombocytopenia.

Bibliography

Bains MS 1991 Surgical treatment of lung cancer. Chest 100: 826.

Belani CP (ed) 1998 International symposium on thoracic malignancies. Chest 113 (suppl): 1S.

Clamon GH, Evans WK, Shepherd FA et al 1984 Myasthenic syndrome and small cell cancer of the lung: variable response to antineoplastic therapy. Arch Intern Med 144: 999.

Hall TC (ed) 1974 Paraneoplastic syndromes. Ann NY Acad Sci 230: 1.

McCaughan BC, Martini N, Bains MS 1985 Bronchial carcinoids. J Thorac Cardiovsc Surg 89: 8.

Menkes MS, Comstock GW, Vuilleumier JP et al 1986 Serum beta-carotene, vitamins A and E, selenium, and the risk of lung cancer. N Engl J Med 315: 1250.

Minna J, Ihde D, Glatstein E 1986 Lung cancer: scalpels, beams, drugs, and probes. N Engl J Med 315: 1411.

Pass HI, Mitchell JB, Johnson DH et al (eds) 2000 Lung Cancer. Philadelphia: Lippincott Williams & Wilkins.

Sugarbaker DJ (ed) 1997 Multimodality therapy of chest malignancies – update '96. Chest 112: 181S.

Yellin A, Rosenman Y, Lieberman Y 1984 Review of smooth muscle tumours of the lower respiratory tract. Br J Dis Chest 78: 337.

Yesner R, Careter D 1982 Pathology of carcinoma of the lung: changing patterns. Clin Chest Med 3: 257.

Lupus anticoagulant (see

Antiphospholipid syndrome)

Lyme disease

Lyme disease is caused by the tick-borne spirochaete, *Borrelia burgdorferi*, and is the most common vector-borne disease in non-tropical developed countries. It was first observed in the town of Lyme in Connecticut in 1975, its causative agent was confirmed in 1983 and its genome sequenced in 1997, and it is now widely observed around the world. Animal reservoirs include numerous wild and domestic animals and birds, and a variety of tick species and perhaps other insect vectors become infected.

Humans are inoculated through the skin giving rise to **erythema migrans**, in which the organism can be identified in nearly 90% of cases. The organism then disseminates to the joints, heart and CNS. The disease has protean manifestations, and probably many cases are unrecognized. Infection occurring during pregnancy may cause fetal damage or fetal death at any stage.

The disease has early and late phases.

- **Stage one**

A distinctive skin lesion is noted 3–20 days after the tick bite, which is itself remembered only by about 20% of patients. The lesion consists of a maculopapule which enlarges to 6–16 cm in diameter and fades after 3–4 weeks. There may be associated systemic systems including myalgia and a stiff neck.

- **Stage two**

This is a disseminated condition seen in some patients and occurring 1 day–8 weeks after the skin lesion. In this condition:

- 80% have arthritis (involving large joints);
- 15% have neurological abnormalities (aseptic meningitis, encephalitis, cranial and peripheral neuropathy, sometimes resembling Guillain–Barré syndrome);
- 16% have cardiac dysfunction (with varying degrees of AV block and myocardial but not valvular dysfunction);
- occasional patients have hepatitis, pneumonitis (resembling ARDS) or ocular involvement.

- **Stage three**

This represents late disease, with persistent infection more than one year later.

The diagnosis is primarily a clinical one, supported by positive serology (though sensitivity and specificity are limited, especially in the early stages). PCR diagnosis is now possible. The differential diagnosis includes:

- erythema marginatum;
- rheumatic fever;
- reactive arthritis;
- rheumatoid arthritis.

False-positive diagnoses are probably frequent, especially in patients with atypical arthritis and fatigue. In addition, false-positive serology can be produced by unrelated conditions, including autoimmune diseases and bacterial infections.

*Treatment is with **tetracycline** (e.g. doxycycline 100 mg bd for 10–30 days) or amoxycillin, penicillin or ceftriaxone*

Prophylactic antibiotics have been shown not to be warranted. Prevention is with protective clothing and removal of ticks from the skin, and with a newly available vaccine for inhabitants of high-risk areas.

Bibliography

Barbour AG, Fish D 1993 The biological and social phenomenon of Lyme disease. Science 260: 1610.

Burgdorfer W, Barbour AG, Benach JL et al 1982 Lyme disease – a tick-borne spirochetosis? Science 216: 1317.

Fraser CM, Casjens S, Huang WM et al 1997 Genomic sequence of a Lyme disease spirochaete, *Borrelia burgdorferi*. Nature 390: 580.

Halperin J, Luft BJ, Volkman DJ et al 1990 Lyme neuroborreliosis: peripheral nervous system manifestations. Brain 113: 1207.

Shadick NA, Philips CB, Logigian EL et al 1994 The long-term clinical outcomes of Lyme disease. Ann Intern Med 121: 560.

Spach D, Liles W, Campbell G et al 1993 Tick-borne diseases in the United States. N Engl J Med 329: 936.

Steere AC, Taylor E, McHugh GL et al 1993 The overdiagnosis of Lyme disease. JAMA 269: 1812.

Steere AC, Sikand VJ, Meurice F et al 1998 Vaccination against Lyme disease with recombinant Borrelia burgdorferi outer surface protein A with adjuvant. N Engl J Med 339: 209.

Lymphadenopathy

Lymphadenopathy of a generalized nature may be due to:

- infectious diseases

  – viral, bacterial, parasitic, fungal;

- haematological malignancies;
- immune disorders;
- miscellaneous conditions, such as

  – Felty's syndrome;
  – sarcoidosis;
  – SLE;
  – drugs (e.g. phenytoin).

Lymphocytosis

Lymphocytosis refers to an increased peripheral blood lymphocyte count of $>4.5\times10^9$/L. It is uncommon, but it is occasionally seen in some infections, such as:

- brucellosis;
- chicken pox;
- measles;
- tuberculosis.

Persistent lymphocytosis suggests the possibility of underlying chronic lymphatic leukaemia.

Atypical lymphocytosis refers to an absolute lymphocytosis with a significant proportion of cells (often about one third) being atypical, i.e. enlarged cells with increased cytoplasm. This most commonly occurs following viral infection, especially infectious mononucleosis. It is also seen with:

- cytomegalovirus;
- toxoplasmosis;
- allergic reactions (e.g. serum sickness);
- some malignancies (e.g. lymphoma).

221

L

It is associated with:

- lymphadenopathy usually;
- splenomegaly often;
- hepatomegaly sometimes;
- signs of meningeal irritation occasionally.

Lymphomatoid granulomatosis

(see Wegener's granulomatosis)

Lymphopenia

Lymphopenia (lymphocytopenia) refers to an absolute lymphocyte count in peripheral blood of $<1.5 \times 10^9$/L. It is seen with:

- severe infections;
- major surgery or trauma;

- uraemia;
- nutritional deficiency;
- lymphoma;
- immune suppression

 – thus it is an important finding in HIV infection.

Bibliography

Castelino DJ, McNair P, Kay TWH 1997 Lymphocytopenia in a hospital population – what does it signify? Aust NZ J Med 27: 170.

Lyssavirus (see Bites and stings (bats), and Rabies)

Magnesium

Magnesium (Mg, atomic number 12, atomic weight 24) is the lightest structural metal and was first isolated in 1808, though it had long been known in compounds. It is widely distributed in nature and is responsible for much of the bitter taste of sea water, which contains 0.13% magnesium chloride. In biology, it is an important cofactor or catalyst for enzyme reactions in carbohydrate metabolism.

The normal plasma level is 0.8–1 mmol/L, of which about 70% is free or ionized and the rest bound to albumin. The total body magnesium is about 1000 mmol (about 25 g), of which the majority is in bone. Magnesium is thus primarily (about 99%) an intracellular cation, being the second most common after potassium. The recommended daily intake is 125–500 mg (5–20 mmol), of which about 40% is absorbed.

Magnesium causes an osmotic diarrhoea, and this is seen following the administration of magnesium-containing antacids or magnesium salts which are popular cathartics.

Magnesium given within the first 24 h has been reported to decrease mortality in acute myocardial infarction by 2.5% (10.3% to 7.8%). This finding, however, was not confirmed in the recent large ISIS-4 trial, though it may be that the magnesium was not given early enough in that trial to replicate previous observations. Magnesium is useful in a number of tachyarrhythmias, especially in torsade de pointes but also in digitalis toxicity and after cardiac surgery, when a dose of 10 mmol (2.5 g of MgSO4 or 5 mL of 50% solution) may be given over 1–2 min. This dose raises the plasma level by about 0.8 mmol/L. A continuous iv infusion of about 5 mmol/h for 24 h may then be used.

Magnesium is also the agent of choice to prevent convulsions in pre-eclampsia (q.v.).

Hypermagnesaemia is uncommon. It is usually seen in patients with renal failure who have been taking magnesium-containing antacids or laxatives. It may give rise to an acquired hypoparathyroidism and thus hypocalcaemia.

> Increased plasma magnesium levels are potentially toxic, though the relation between the plasma level and specific abnormalities is only approximate.

- **2–4 mmol/L**

this is a 'therapeutically increased level', as in pre-eclampsia.

- **>3.0 mmol/L**

there may be drowsiness, headache, lethargy, sweating, flushing and nausea;there may also be diplopia, dysarthria and decreased deep tendon reflexes.

- **>5 mmol/L**

toxicity becomes important and is manifest by hyporeflexia and sometimes abnormal cardiac conduction (i. e. prolonged PR interval, widened QRS complex).

- **>7.5 mmol/L**

there is areflexia, muscle paralysis, narcosis, respiratory failure due to hypoventilation, hypotension and complete heart block.

- **>12.5 mmol/L**

asystole occurs.

*Treatment is with **hydration** and **calcium** (10–20 mL iv of 10% calcium gluconate over 10 min). The reversal of magnesium toxicity by calcium is temporary, and its persistence may require dialysis.*

Hypomagnesaemia, on the other hand, occurs in about 10% of hospital patients and in about 40% of seriously ill patients. However, when ionized magnesium instead of the usual total plasma magnesium is measured, hypomagnesaemia is much less frequent, occurring in perhaps only 15% of seriously ill patients. The relationships between measurements of intracellular, ionized plasma and total plasma magnesium are somewhat loose and of uncertain clinical significance. When daily intake is omitted, the magnesium 'stores' become depleted in about a week and hypomagnesaemia occurs.

Decreased intake is compounded by increased loss. This usually arises from:

- losses via the gut, especially from GI fistulae,
- losses via the kidney (a fractional magnesium excretion in the urine of >2.5% indicates renal magnesium wasting);
- drugs giving increased urinary loss (aminoglycosides, amphotericin, cisplatin, cyclosporin, pamidronate, pentamidine, thiazides);
- diabetic ketoacidosis;
- alcoholism;
- hypothermia;
- burns.

The hypokalaemia associated with diuretic use has concomitant hypomagnesaemia in 40% of cases. Treatment of both is required to correct the hypokalaemia and associated arrhythmias. It is of interest that the potassium-sparing diuretics also conserve magnesium.

> Since magnesium is important in cardiovascular, neurological and endocrine function, its deficiency can give rise to widespread effects and especially tachyarrhythmias, cardiac failure and sudden death. Hypomagnesaemia is one of the causes of a prolonged QT interval and thus torsade de pointes.

Like hypermagnesaemia, hypomagnesaemia can also give rise to an acquired hypoparathyroidism.

Treatment depends on severity.

- *If severe, 10–20 mmol should be given, as 5–10 mL iv of 50% **magnesium sulfate** in 100 mL of 5% dextrose over 10–20 min.*
- *If very severe, up to 40–80 mmol may be given in a similar way.*
- *In chronic mild/moderate deficiency, 25–50 mmol should be given daily.*

- *To prevent deficiency, 5–20 mmol should be given daily, unless there are continuing losses when these too must be taken into account.*

Renal calculi contain magnesium in 15% of cases in the form of struvite (magnesium ammonium phosphate) – see Nephrolithiasis.

Bibliography

Arsenian MA 1993 Magnesium and cardiovascular disease. Progr Cardiovasc Dis 35: 271.

Casscells W 1994 Magnesium and myocardial infarction. Lancet 343: 807.

Cholst IN, Steinberg SF, Tropper PJ et al 1984 The influence of hypermagnesemia on serum calcium and parathyroid hormone levels in human subjects. N Engl J Med 310: 1221.

ISIS-4 (Fourth International Study of Infarct Survival) Collaborative Group 1995 ISIS-4: A randomised factorial trial assessing early oral captopril, oral mononitrate, and intravenous magnesium sulphate in 58 050 patients with suspected acute myocardial infarction. Lancet 345: 669.

Lucas MJ, Leveno KJ, Cunningham FG 1995 A comparison of magnesium sulfate with phenytoin for the prevention of eclampsia. N Engl J Med 333: 201.

McLean RM 1994 Magnesium and its therapeutic uses. Am J Med 96: 63.

Nadler JL, Rude RK 1995 Disorders of magnesium metabolism. Endocrinol Metab Clin North Am 24: 623.

Teo KK, Yusuf S, Collins R et al 1991 Effects of intravenous magnesium in suspected acute myocardial infarction: overview of randomized trials. Br Med J 303: 1499.

Weisinger JR, Bellorin-Font E 1998 Magnesium and phosphorus. Lancet 352: 391.

Whang R, Whang D, Ryan M 1992 Refractory potassium depletion: a consequence of magnesium deficiency. Arch Intern Med 152: 40.

Woods KL, Fletcher S, Roffe C et al 1992 Intravenous magnesium sulphate in suspected acute myocardial infarction: results of the second Leicester Magnesium Intervention Trial (LIMIT-2). Lancet 339: 1553.

Malabsorption

Malabsorption is a commonly used global term encompassing:

- true malabsorption

  - i.e. failure to absorb nutrients due to damage of the small intestinal mucosa;

- maldigestion

  - i.e. due to either deficiency of digestive secretions, especially biliary and/or pancreatic, or to a number miscellaneous causes.

The causes of **true malabsorption** are:

- coeliac disease

  - i.e. gluten-sensitive enteropathy;

- tropical sprue,
- miscellaneous conditions, including

  - ischaemia;
  - extensive bowel resection;
  - lymphoma;
  - amyloid;
  - Crohn's disease;
  - Whipple's disease;
  - parasitic infection;
  - AIDS;
  - irradiation;
  - high altitude;
  - hypogammaglobulinaemia;
  - abetalipoproteinaemia.

The causes of **maldigestion** include:

- chronic pancreatitis or biliary obstruction;
- post-gastrectomy;
- diabetic dysautonomia;
- scleroderma;
- drugs

  - particularly alcohol, colchicine, laxatives.

The clinical features of malabsorption in general comprise:

- steatorrhoea (the passage of light and bulky stools);
- weight loss despite an adequate food intake;
- fatigue;
- the consequences of single or multiple vitamin deficiency.

Investigations show anaemia, hypoalbuminaemia, hypocalcaemia and hypomagnesaemia. In true malabsorption, there is impaired xylose absorption, though this test has largely fallen into disuse. Confirmatory investigations include faecal fat analysis, barium follow-through and small bowel biopsy.

Bibliography

Campbell CB, Roberts RK, Cowen AE 1977 The changing clinical presentation of coeliac disease in adults. Med J Aust 1: 89.

Corsini G, Gandolfi E, Bonechi I et al 1966 Postgastrectomy malabsorption. Gastroenterology 50: 358.

Duggan JM 1997 Recent developments in our understanding of adult coeliac disease. Med J Aust 166: 312.

Fisher RL (ed) 1989 Malabsorption and nutritional status and support. Gastrenterol Clin North Am 18: 467.

Go VLW et al (eds) 1993 The Pancreas: Biology, Pathobiology and Diseases. New York: Raven Press.

Gosh SK, Littlewood JM, Goddard D et al 1977 Stool microscopy in screening for steatorrhoea. J Clin Pathol 30: 749.

Green PHR, Tall AR 1979 Drugs, alcohol and malabsorption. Am J Med 67: 1066.

Marshak RL, Lindner AE 1966 Malabsorption syndrome. Semin Roentgenol 1: 138.

Malaria

Malaria is a parasitic vector-borne disease, still uncontrolled and causing at least 100 million cases and 2 million deaths per year worldwide, mainly in tropical countries. It is also seen in temperate climates in travellers. The geographic range of disease is expected to extend as future global warming enlarges the range of its main vector.

Occasionally, malaria (particularly due to *P. falciparum*) has been seen in people who have never been in an endemic area, and presumably this is either:

- so-called **'airport malaria'** (from an infected mosquito which has hitchhiked aboard a plane from a malarious country), or

- **'autochthonous malaria'** (from a local Anopheles mosquito which has fed on a case of imported disease).

Most disease is caused by *P. falciparum* (46%) and *P. vivax* (43%). The parasite has a complex but well documented life-cycle in humans, following the injection of the sporozoite by a mosquito of the anopheline type which is the definitive host. Malaria can also be transmitted by blood transfusion in countries where the disease is prevalent.

> The incubation period is typically 10 days to 4 weeks, but sometimes it is much longer, particularly in those who have been on suppressive antimalarial drugs or who are semi-immune, in whom clinical disease may occur months or years after leaving an endemic area. The clinical picture is one of high fever (up to 41°C or more), chills, sweating and prostration. Anaemia, jaundice and hepatosplenomegaly are observed. Sometimes, there is renal failure, diarrhoea and coma.
>
> *P. falciparum* gives a continuous or intermittent fever, with obstruction of the microcirculation, especially in the brain, gut and lung (giving an ARDS-like picture). There is hypoglycaemia, intravascular haemolysis and lactic acidosis. *P. vivax* gives a tertian or second daily fever.

The diagnosis is made by detection of the parasites on blood film, though the parasites may be scanty or absent at the time of severe illness and a repeat smear may be needed.

Treatment options have been reduced because drug resistance, most importantly to chloroquine, is now widespread. Normally, acute treatment is with **chloroquine** *0.6 g then 0.3 g in 6 h and 0.3 g daily for two days.*

If the parasites are resistant, alternative agents are quinine 0.6 g orally tds for three days or quinidine gluconate 600 mg iv over 1–2 h then 1 mg/min iv for 2–3 days. Pyrimethamine with a sulfonamide,

tetracycline or clindamycin, or mefloquine should be added. The tissue phase of P. vivax infection requires primaquine (15 mg daily for two weeks) to eradicate extra-erythrocytic or hepatic infection.

In acute malaria, corticosteroids have sometimes been given, but they are unhelpful and may even be deleterious in cerebral malaria.

Prevention requires avoidance of mosquitoes, prophylactic medication and awareness of its possibility for up to a year after potential exposure. Prophylactic agents in chloroquine-resistant areas include doxycycline (100 mg per day) or mefloquine (250 mg per week), depending on the region. A malaria vaccine is currently being developed.

Bibliography

Iqbal KM, Ahmed N, Aziz L 2000 Malaria: its severe form and its management. Crit Care & Shock 3: 69.

Mai NTH, Day NPJ, Chuong LV et al 1996 Post-malaria neurological syndrome. Lancet 348: 917.

Martens P, Hall L 2000 Malaria on the move. Emerg Infect Dis 6: 2.

Public Health Committee Report 1993 Malaria Prophylaxis. Canberra: NH&MRC.

Wyler DJ 1983 Malaria – resurgence, resistance, and research. N Engl J Med 308: 875.

Zucker JR 1996 Changing patterns of autochthonous malaria transmission in the United States. Emerg Infect Dis 2: 37.

Malignant hyperthermia

Malignant hyperthermia (MH) is a rare and striking complication of general anaesthesia, in which it occurs in about 1 in 50000 adult cases and more commonly in children. It was first recognized in 1960 in Melbourne. It is usually associated with the use of suxamethonium and volatile agents (especially halothane) and mostly occurs during induction, though occasionally it may appear as late as the recovery period. Previous anaesthetics may not have caused the syndrome. It can even sometimes occur in the non-anaesthetic situation, such as in stress or exercise.

The aetiology is a genetically determined biochemical defect of muscle metabolism, seen in families who are otherwise normal. Although the condition is inherited as an autosomal dominant in severe cases, there is genetic heterogeneity with recessive inheritance in milder forms of the disease. The regulation of intracellular calcium ions in muscle is abnormal, so that neuronal stimulation and muscle depolarization lead to excessive calcium egress into the cytoplasm, dysregulation of the many calcium-mediated cell processes and thus muscle hypermetabolism.

It sometimes occurs in patients with various forms of muscle disease, such as myopathy, muscular dystrophy or the neuroleptic malignant syndrome.

Clinical features comprise the rapid onset of:

- rapidly increased core temperature;
- tachyarrhythmias;
- hypercapnia despite tachypnoea;
- metabolic acidosis;
- muscular rigidity;
- mottled skin and cyanosis;
- excessive bleeding;
- shock;
- coma.

There is hyperkalaemia, myoglobinuria, increased lactate, increased creatine kinase, and the hypercapnia is out of proportion to a seemingly adequate ventilation.

Treatment involves cooling, hyperventilation, oxygenation and therapy for abnormalities of electrolytes (e.g. hyperkalaemia) and acid–base (e.g. metabolic acidosis).

*Most importantly, specific therapy is available with **dantrolene**, which decreases calcium ion release from the sarcoplasmic reticulum and thus decreases muscle contractility. It is given in a dose of 1–2 mg/kg iv and repeated in 5–10 min to give an initial dose of 2–3 mg/kg. This dosage is usually very effective, but it may need to be repeated 4 hourly and occasionally total dosage up to 10 mg/kg over 48–72 h may be required. An important but uncommon side-effect of dantrolene is severe hepatitis.*

The untreated mortality is 30% but this is greatly reduced with prompt and appropriate treatment. After recovery, patient and family counselling should be undertaken, including advice about any future anaesthesia.

Bibliography

Denborough MA, Lovell RR 1960 Anaesthetic deaths in a family. Lancet 2: 45.
Kolb ME, Horne ML, Martz R 1982 Dantrolene in human malignant hyperthermia: a multicenter study. Anesthesiology 56: 254.
MacLennon DH, Phillips MS 1992 Malignant hyperthermia. Science 256: 789.
Nelson TE, Flewellen EH 1983 The malignant hyperthermia syndrome. N Engl J Med 309: 416.

Mallory–Weiss syndrome

Mallory–Weiss syndrome refers to a mucosal or submucosal tear of the lower oesophagus, usually associated with retching or vomiting, particularly if it has been held back.

Boerhaave's syndrome refers to a complete oesophageal rupture under similar circumstances.

A Mallory–Weiss tear is reported to be responsible for 5–10% of cases of upper gastrointestinal bleeding.

In Intensive Care, it is an important cause of acute mediastinitis.

Manganese

Manganese (Mn, atomic number 25, atomic weight 55) is a hard white brittle metal, first recognized in 1774 and mainly used as an alloy in steel.

It is an essential trace element in animals and plants, but it is toxic in excess. It is a required cofactor in many enzyme systems and is also required for the action of vitamin K. The most obvious effect of its lack is thus vitamin K deficiency (q.v.). Manganese deficiency has also been associated with osteoarthritis.

It is present in many fruits, nuts and cereals. It is normally excreted in the bile and therefore can accumulate in the body in the presence of cholestasis.

The required daily intake is 150–2000 μg orally and the recommended iv dose is 5 μmol/day. These doses should be decreased if there is biliary obstruction.

Marfan's syndrome

Marfan's syndrome is an inherited disorder of connected tissue which causes extensive physical abnormalities. The basic defect is in the gene for fibrillin, a glycoprotein of 350 kD, which is a structural component of the microfibrils associated with elastin. There is thus disruption of collagen and elastic fibres in many structures, most importantly in the cardiovascular system, but also in the eye and musculoskeletal system.

> The four groups of clinical features of Marfan's syndrome are:
>
> - abnormally long limbs (dolichostenomelia) and fingers (arachnodactyly), chest wall abnormalities (kyphoscoliosis, pectus excavatum), increased risk of spontaneous pneumothorax and high arched palate;
> - aortic dilatation, with proneness to aortic regurgitation and aortic dissection;
> - mitral valve prolapse;
> - ectopia lentis, which is an upward displacement of the lens, usually bilateral and occurring in up to 80% of subjects. It is due to disrupted ciliary zonular fibres and may be associated with myopia and an increased risk of retinal detachment.

The diagnosis is based on the presence of at least two of the groups of clinical features and is strong if three or four groups are present. Clinical examination and even chest X-ray may be normal, and echocardiography is required to detect significant cardiovascular lesions. Annual echocardiographic screening is often recommended.

*Prophylactic **beta blockers** are indicated if there is aortic root dilatation.*

- *There should be rigorous control of any hypertension.*
- *Surgical replacement of the ascending aorta and aortic valve is indicated for marked aortic regurgitation.*

Pregnancy in Marfan's syndrome predisposes to aortic dissection.

Marine vertebrate and invertebrate stings (see Bites and stings)

Mast cells (see Basophilia)

Mastocytosis (see Urticaria)

Mediastinal diseases

Acute mediastinitis usually follows oesophageal perforation or rupture. Vomiting may damage the lower oesophagus with either a Mallory–Weiss tear and haemorrhage or a complete perforation giving rise to Boerhaave's syndrome with pneumomediastinum and left pleural effusion and/or pneumothorax. Oesophageal perforation may also be caused by a procedure, foreign body or carcinoma. Occasionally, mediastinitis may be due to spread of infection from adjacent chest structures or to infection of a mediastinal cyst.

The clinical features include fever, dysphagia and chest pain. Typically, the patient appears well initially (i.e. up to 48 h) but then becomes seriously ill.

*Treatment comprises appropriate **antibiotic** therapy (with anaerobic cover) and surgical **drainage** of any abscess.*

Chronic mediastinitis is usually associated with a progressive fibrotic process.

The cause is unknown, but it may be related to other fibrosing diseases, especially retroperitoneal fibrosis, but also Riedel's thyroiditis, Dupuytren's contracture, Peyronie's disease and sclerosing cholangitis. Methysergide therapy for migraine has been implicated in some cases. Sometimes the disease is localized (e.g. to the hilar region).

There is no effective therapy.

Other mediastinal diseases include chiefly cysts and tumours. The most common, in order, are:

- neurogenic tumours (especially neurofibroma);
- cysts (especially bronchogenic or pericardial);
- thymoma (more often benign than malignant);
- teratoma (also more often benign than malignant);
- lymphoma;
- retrosternal thyroid.

However, many different types of lesions may occur in the mediastinum, and their nature depends greatly on their site.

- **Superior mediastinum**

  - thymoma;
  - teratoma;
  - lymphoma;
  - retrosternal thyroid or parathyroid mass;
  - cystic hygroma;
  - aortic aneurysm;
  - haemangioma;
  - abscess;
  - lymphadenopathy;
  - oesophageal lesion.

- **Anterior mediatinum**

  - thymoma;
  - teratoma;
  - lymphoma;

  - retrosternal thyroid or parathyroid mass;
  - pericardial or pleuropericardial cyst;
  - cystic hygroma;
  - hernia through the sternocostal or retrosternal hiatus (foramen of Morgagni);
  - neoplasm (germ cell, mesenchymal).

- **Middle mediastinum**

  - aortic aneurysm or other great vessel abnormality;
  - bronchogenic or pleuropericardial cyst;
  - lymphoma;
  - lipoma;
  - mediastinitis;
  - tumour (trachea, lymph nodes, cardiac);
  - hernia through the sternocostal or retrosternal hiatus (foramen of Morgagni).

- **Posterior mediastinum**

  - neurogenic tumour (neurofibroma);
  - gastro-oesophageal or bronchogenic cyst;
  - oesophageal lesion (tumour, diverticulum);
  - meningocele;
  - aortic aneurysm;
  - hernia through the vertebrocostal or posterolateral hiatus (foramen of Bochdalek);
  - thoracic spine disease.

The clinical features of mediastinal disease may include pain, dysphagia, hoarseness, stridor, cough, haemoptysis and dyspnoea.

Physical examination may reveal Horner's syndrome (q.v.), superior vena cava obstruction, enlarged cervical lymph nodes or pleural effusion.

Investigations include chest X-ray and particularly CT scanning, and sometimes tomography, aortography, bronchoscopy and mediastinoscopy.

Bibliography

Abolnik I, Lossos IS, Breuer R 1991 Spontaneous pneumomediastinum. Chest 100: 93.

Azarow KS, Pearl RH, Zurcher R et al 1993 Primary mediastinal masses. J Thorac Cardiovasc Surg 106: 67.

Estrera AS, Landay MJ, Grisham JM et al 1983 Descending necrotizing mediastinitis. Surg Gynecol Obstet 157: 545.

Schowengerdt CG, Suyemoto R, Main FB 1969 Granulomatous and fibrous mediastinitis. J Thorac Cardiovasc Surg 57: 365.

Strollo DC, de Christenson MLR, Jett JR 1997 Primary mediastinal tumors. Chest 112: 511 & 1344.

Mediastinitis (see Mediastinal diseases)

Mediterranean fever (see Pyrexia)

Medullary sponge kidney (see Renal cystic disease)

Medullary thyroid cancer (see Calcitonin)

Megaloblastic anaemia

Megaloblastic anaemia refers to anaemia characterized by macrocytes on the peripheral blood film and megaloblastic erythroid hyperplasia in the bone marrow. There is a defect of DNA synthesis and thus cell division, so that larger cells are produced.

This defect is due most commonly to folic acid or vitamin B_{12} deficiency, but it may also be produced by drugs (e.g. nitrous oxide for >6 h). It may sometimes be a genetic disorder.

The morphological changes are not confined to the bone marrow and are seen at other sites of rapid cell turnover, such as the gut mucosa. Both folic acid and vitamin B_{12} are required for the metabolism of single carbon units, and both are thus required dietary nutrients.

The diagnosis is suggested from the clinical features and the presence of macrocytosis. It is most readily confirmed nowadays by electronic cell counters which provide a sensitive index of macrocytosis (i.e. MCV >98 fL).

However, macrocytosis is not specific, in that it also occurs in non-megaloblastic disorders, such as:

- alcoholism;
- liver disease;
- anti-metabolite therapy.

It can also be masked by concomitant iron deficiency or thalassaemia.

The peripheral blood film typically also shows hypersegmented neutrophils (5 or more lobes), occasional nucleated red blood cells and sometimes neutropenia or thrombocytopenia. The levels of folic acid and B_{12} should be measured.

Folic acid deficiency is seen with

- inadequate intake

  – alcoholism, malnutrition, pregnancy;

- impaired absorption

  – intestinal disease;

- certain drugs

  – methotrexate, phenytoin, pyrimethamine, trimethoprim.

Folic acid deficiency can occur rapidly, since the body contains stores for only two weeks.

*Treatment is with **folic acid** 1 mg/day or with folinic acid if the deficiency is secondary to specific blocking drugs.*

Vitamin B_{12} deficiency is seen:

- classically in pernicious anaemia

  – q.v.;

- in other causes of impaired absorption, such as

  – post-gastrectomy;
  – pancreatic disease;

- ileal disease;
- infection with the fish tapeworm;
- drugs (alcohol, colchicine, neomycin);

- also in extreme and prolonged malnutrition,
- following loss of coenzymes

  - e.g. after nitrous oxide,

- in rare congenital disorders.

Bibliography

Editorial 1982 Nitrous oxide and acute marrow failure. Lancet 2: 856.

Pruthi RK, Tefferi A 1994 Pernicious anemia revisited. Mayo Clin Proc 69: 144.

Melatonin

Melatonin is a serotonin derivative, secreted by the pineal gland when the retina fails to perceive light. Its name derives from the fact that it lightens amphibian skin by aggregating melanophores (i.e. the opposite effect to that of melanocyte-stimulating hormone, MSH – see Adrenocorticotropic hormone), though such an effect has not been shown in humans.

It was not discovered until 1958 but has been widely studied since. Its secretion is circadian and thus provides the body with an internal clock in synchrony with the natural day and night. It may thus influence the function of the brain, psyche, thyroid and gonads.

Melatonin is available as an over-the-counter drug in many countries and it has become very popular in people with a variety of sleep disorders, since unlike sedatives it induces normal REM sleep. A recent small study showed it to be effective in a dose of 3 mg in improving sleep quality and preventing sleep deprivation in patients in the traditionally difficult Intensive Care environment.

Bibliography

Garfinkel D, Laudon M, Zisapel N 1995 Improvement in sleep quality in elderly people by controlled-release melatonin. Lancet 346: 541.

Lewis KS, McCarthy RJ, Rothenberg DM 1999 Does melatonin decrease sedative use and time to extubation in patients requiring prolonged mechanical ventilation? Anesth Analg 88: S123.

Shilo L, Dagan Y, Smorjik Y et al 2000 Effect of melatonin on sleep quality of COPD Intensive Care patients. Chronobiol Int 17: 71.

Webb SM, Puig-Domingo M 1995 Role of melatonin in health and disease. Clin Endocrinol 42: 221.

Wurtman RJ, Moskowitz MA 1977 The pineal organ. N Engl J Med 1329: 1383.

Meleney's progressive synergistic gangrene (see Gangrene)

Melioidosis

Melioidosis is caused by an unusual pseudomonas-like organism, *Burkolderia pseudomallei* (formerly called *Pseudomonas pseudomallei*), a Gram-negative aerobic bacillus found in water and soil in tropical areas up to 20° of latitude either side of the Equator and in particular in Southeast Asia. The organism is enzootic in animals, but these are not a source of direct transmission to humans, nor does person-to-person transmission occur. The organism enters the skin via an abrasion or the lungs via aerosol.

Infection is also seen in travellers, even those who have long left an endemic area.

There are three patterns of infection, namely subclinical, acute and chronic.

- **Subclinical infection**

This is presumably common, because positive serology is found in up to 30% of populations at risk. There may be an asymptomatic pulmonary infiltrate in some patients.

- **Acute infection**

This comprises a local pustule, pneumonia or septicaemia.

The pustule appears after an incubation period of two days and is usually self-limited, though it may lead to septicaemia. Pneumonia is the most common clinical form and ranges from mild to fulminating. The most severe form is associated with necrosis, cavitation and septicaemia. Septicaemia is similar to other Gram-negative septicaemias and can lead to septic shock or metastatic abscess formation.

- **Chronic infection**

This comprises suppuration, particularly in the lungs and typically with upper lobe cavities. It may thus resemble tuberculosis.

Recrudescent disease of any form may appear many years later and is usually precipitated by:

- diabetes;
- immune suppression;
- infection;
- liver disease;
- trauma.

The diagnosis is made by specific culture, though identification may be difficult and thus delayed. Positive serology in a traveller may assist.

Optimal treatment is not established because of variable susceptibility of the organism.

- *It is commonly aminoglycoside-resistant, and treatment is traditionally with chloramphenicol, tetracycline or cotrimoxazole.*
- *Newer antipseudomonal agents (e.g. ceftazidime) are of value on their sensitivity merits.*
- *The duration of treatment is at least a month and in chronic cases up to 6 months.*

Mortality is up to 50% if septicaemia is present.

Bibliography

Koponen M, Zlock D, Palmer D et al 1991 Melioidosis: forgotten, but not gone! Arch Intern Med 151: 605.

Mendelson's syndrome (see Aspiration)

Meningococcaemia (see Waterhouse–Friderichsen syndrome)

Meningoencephalitis (see Encephalitis)

Mercury

Mercury (Hg, atomic number 80, atomic weight 201, melting point $-39°C$, SG 13.5) is a metal of the zinc group. It is the only metal which is liquid at room temperature, and it was well known to the ancients. Although native mercury occurs in nature, most is readily obtained from the red sulfide (cinnabar), which though rarer than copper or zinc is more abundant than many other common metals, such as tin.

Mercury is a reactive substance which forms metal alloys readily to reproduce an amalgam. Its uses in thermometers, barometers, sealed electrical switches, vapour lamps and dentistry are well known. It has also been used in fungicides and pharmaceuticals. Mercury is also widely used in industrial processes, the effluent from which can result in biological concentrations via the chain of bacteria to fish to man. The maximum recommended exposure is not >0.1 mg/m^3 or 0.05 mg/m^3/8 h.

Mercurous chloride (calomel) and mercuric chloride (corrosive sublimate) have antiseptic proprieties, but mercury-containing therapeutic agents, such as these, diuretics and ointments, are not nowadays used. Mercury poisoning thus usually arises from industrial accidents. Industrial exposure may be indirect, as in the Minamata accident in Japan in the early 1950s when factory effluent into a local bay affected fishermen and their families together with their household cats and the nearby seabirds. Toxicity has also occurred in farmers eating instead of planting grain seed treated with mercury-containing fungicide.

Acrodynia (pink disease) occurs in children from eating house paint containing mercury-based, antimould preparations. For the first half of the 20th century, it occurred in children given worm cures or teething powders containing mercury in the form of calomel. Its name derived from the bright pink colour of the child's extremities, which were also painful. The patient was also miserable, lethargic and photophobic.

Acute toxicity arises from soluble mercury compounds, which are generally also corrosive. There is nausea, abdominal pain, bloody diarrhoea and renal failure.

Chronic toxicity usually arises from a mercury salt which has been inhaled or absorbed through the skin (the latter for example as mercury nitrate in felt hat manufacture giving the 'mad hatter' syndrome).

- Oral manifestations include salivation, a metallic taste, stomatitis, a blue line on the gums and loose teeth. Anorexia and weight loss may occur.
- Mental effects may include personality change. Weakness, blindness, peripheral neuropathy, paralysis, coma and death may result.
- Acute tubulointerstitial disease may be produced.
- A lichenoid skin reaction with purple, flat, irregular papules resembling idiopathic lichen planus may occur from mercury and indeed from a number of drugs.

Bibliography
Black J 1999 The puzzle of pink disease. J R Soc Med 92: 478.

Mesothelioma (see Asbestos)

Metabolic acidosis (see Lactic acidosis)

Metabolism and nutrition

Many disorders of metabolism, such as the major acid–base and electrolyte abnormalities, and many aspects of nutrition, such as enteral and parenteral nutrition, are part of the 'bread and butter' of Intensive Care practice. Numerous other issues and conditions which are less frequently encountered are considered in this book, including:

- beriberi;
- chromium;
- copper;
- Fanconi's syndrome;
- folic acid deficiency;
- glucose-6-phosphate dehydrogenase deficiency;
- glycogen storage diseases;
- haemochromatosis;
- hypercalcaemia;
- hyperphosphataemia;
- hypocalcaemia;
- hypophosphataemia;
- iron;
- lactase deficiency;
- lactic acidosis;
- magnesium;
- manganese;
- porphyria;
- pseudohyperkalaemia;
- pseudohyponatraemia;
- scurvy;
- selenium;
- trace elements;
- vitamin deficiency;
- zinc.

Bibliography
Anderson JJB, Toverud SU 1994 Diet and vitamin D: a review with an emphasis on human function. J Nutr Biochem 5: 58.
Chandra RK 1992 Effect of vitamin and trace-element supplementation on immune responses and infection in elderly patients. Lancet 340: 1124.
Crowe AV, Griffiths RD 1997 Nutritional failure and drugs. Curr Opinion Crit Care 3: 268.
DeLuca HF 1978 Vitamin D metabolism and function. Arch Intern Med 138: 836.

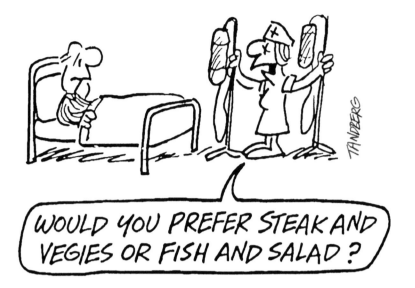

WOULD YOU PREFER STEAK AND VEGIES OR FISH AND SALAD ?

Dent CE, Smith R 1969 Nutritional osteomalacia. Q J Med 38: 195.

Editorial 1982 Hepatic osteomalacia and vitamin D. Lancet 1: 943.

Fisher RL (ed) 1989 Malabsorption and nutritional status and support. Gastrenterol Clin North Am 18: 467.

Kellum JA 1998 Recent advances in acid-base physiology applied to critical care. In: Vincent J-L (ed) Yearbook of Intensive Care and Emergency Medicine 1998. Berlin: Springer. p 577.

Marik P, Varon J 1998 The obese patient in the ICU. Chest 113: 492.

Nasraway S, Black R, Sottile F 1989 The anion gap in patients admitted to the medical intensive care unit. Chest 96: 287S.

Rose BD 1994 Clinical Physiology of Acid–Base and Electrolyte Disorders. 4th edition. New York: McGraw-Hill.

Schelling JR, Howard RL, Winter SD et al 1990 Increased osmol gap in alcoholic ketoacidosis and lactic acidosis. Ann Intern Med 113: 580.

Methaemoglobinaemia (see

Methylene blue)

Methaemoglobinaemia can be either inherited or acquired. The diagnosis of methaemoglobinaemia may be readily confirmed using any of the sophisticated blood gas machines which have become widely available recently and which include dyshaemoglobins among their measured parameters.

Inherited methaemoglobinaemia is a haemoglobinopathy due to a deficiency of the enzymes required to maintain iron in its reduced or ferrous state. Iron in its ferric form does not bind oxygen, so that cyanosis occurs in methaemoglobinaemia at levels of 10% or more (in contrast to the requirement of about 30% of deoxyhaemoglobin before cyanosis is apparent). Symptoms of anaemia become apparent at methaemoglobin levels >25%.

Acquired methaemoglobinaemia is seen following exposure to many agents,

- classically with nitrites,
- nowadays, most commonly after the therapeutic use of nitric oxide, particularly in relation to cardioplumonary bypass,
- also with drugs such as dapsone, glyceryl trinitrate, primaquine, sulfasalazine and vitamin K analogues.

Bibliography
Charache S 1986 Methemoglobinemia – sleuthing for a new cause. N Engl J Med 314: 776.

Dotsch J, Demirakca S, Hamm R et al 1997 Extracorporeal circulation increases nitric oxide induced methemoglobinemia in vivo and in vitro. Crit Care Med 25: 1153.

Hall AH, Kulig KW, Rumack BH 1986 Drug- and chemical-induced methemoglobinemia: clinical features and management. Med Toxicol 1: 253.

Schweitzer SA 1991 Spurious pulse oximeter desaturation due to methemoglobinemia. Anesth Intens Care 19: 988.

Warren JB, Higenbottam T 1996 Caution with the use of inhaled nitric oxide. Lancet 348: 629.

Methanol

Methanol (methyl alcohol, CH_3OH, 'wood alcohol') is the simplest aliphatic alcohol, with uses in industry and possibly as a future fuel. It is occasionally taken as a substitute for ethyl alcohol, since it causes mild inebriation. Most cases are sporadic, although mini–epidemics are seen following the consumption of contaminated illicit liquor.

There is considerable variability in the potentially lethal dose.

- Usually 70–100 mL is fatal.
- Death has been reported after as little as 6 mL.
- Total lack of any symptoms has been reported after as much as 500 mL.

Blindness can occur following the ingestion of as little as 4 mL.

The minimum toxic level of methanol is 50 mg/dL.

It is absorbed, distributed and metabolized similarly to ethyl alcohol. Although methanol itself is excreted in the lungs and kidneys, most is metabolized by alcohol dehydrogenase to formaldehyde (HCOH) and then by aldehyde dehydrogenase to formic acid (HCO.OH). These substances and especially the latter are toxic, since they are very reactive, being able to bind proteins and inhibit oxidative metabolism. The further metabolism of formate to carbon dioxide requires folic acid. The oxidation of methanol is 7-fold slower than that of ethanol, so that complete excretion takes several days.

Although not toxic in itself, toxicity from its metabolites occurs after a latent period of several hours. Typically, although methanol is rapidly absorbed, there is a lag period of 12–24 h (range 1–72 h) before toxicity is apparent. The longer delay is especially seen if there has been concomitant ethanol ingestion.

- **Visual impairment** is the most prominent clinical feature, and indeed it occurs to some degree in all cases. Eye damage includes hyperaemia of the optic disc, papilloedema and retinal oedema and even fixed dilated pupils and often total permanent blindness.
- **Neurological signs** include headache, drowsiness, vertigo, and if severe, fits and coma. There is CT evidence of cerebral oedema and patchy infarction, particularly of the putamen. Permanent motor dysfunction of a Parkinsonian type may be seen.
- **Gastrointestinal symptoms** are common and include nausea, vomiting, severe abdominal pain (possibly pancreatic in origin), actual pancreatitis and haemorrhagic gastritis.
- **Metabolic acidosis** is typically present and can be severe. It is partly due to lactic acidosis associated with circulatory impairment, but mostly it is due to the production of formic acid. The metabolic acidosis is usually uncompensated because of respiratory depression, manifest typically by slow 'fish-like' gasping. There is an increased anion gap (due to the presence of formate) and an increased osmolar gap.

Treatment priorities are two-fold, namely:

- *correction of acidosis;*
- *alteration of metabolism.*

Other modalities such as gastric lavage (unless very early) and charcoal administration are not effective.

---

1. *Treatment of the acidosis is urgent. The metabolic acidosis in this setting is relatively refractory to bicarbonate. Thus, dialysis is indicated if the acidosis is persistently severe and/or if the serum methanol concentration is >0.5 g/L. Dialysis increases the removal of methanol 3-fold. While*

haemodialysis is very effective, peritoneal dialysis or haemoperfusion are not.

2. **The metabolism of methanol should be decreased** *(by ethanol) and* **the metabolism of formate increased** *(by folic acid).*

- *The value of* **ethanol** *(ethyl alcohol) derives from its competition for the enzyme, alcohol dehydrogenase, so that the degradation of methanol and the accumulation of toxic metabolites are slowed. Ethanol has a greater affinity than methanol for this enzyme and saturates it at a concentration of 1–1.5 g/L (22–33 mmol/L). This blood alcohol level is 2–3 times the maximum legal level permitted for driving and causes marked intoxication in at least a third of subjects.*

The required blood level is achieved with a loading dose of 0.7 g/kg, equivalent to about 500 mL of 10% alcohol iv over 1 h or 125 mL of 43% alcohol orally (i.e. 4 'drinks'). This level is maintained by about 10–15% of the loading dose given hourly.

In patients who are heavy drinkers or if dialysis is used, this maintenance requirement needs to be increased 2–3-fold. The administration of ethanol in this way may need to be modified in patients with pre-existing neurological, cardiac or liver damage. During dialysis, maintenance may also be achieved by adding 1 g/L of alcohol to the dialysate.

Since the administration of fomepizole (4-methylpyrazole, Antizol), an expensive new agent recently shown to inhibit alcohol dehydrogenase and thus prevent the production of toxic metabolites, has been used successfully in ethylene glycol poisoning (q.v.), it may also be similarly useful in methanol poisoning.

- *The administration of* **folate** *(e.g. 50–100 mg iv 4 hourly) may be helpful in increasing the metabolism of formate.*

The prognosis of methanol poisoning is related to the degree of metabolic acidosis, with a 50% mortality in patients who have a serum bicarbonate <10 mmol/L.

Bibliography

Burns MJ, Graudins A, Aaron CK et al 1997 Treatment of methanol with intravenous 4-methylpyrazole. Ann Emerg Med 30: 829.

Jacobsen D, McMartin KE 1986 Methanol and ethylene glycol poisoning: mechanism of toxicity, clinical course, diagnosis and treatment. Med Toxicol 1: 309.

Jacobsen D, McMartin KE 1997 Antidotes for methanol and ethylene glycol poisoning. J Toxicol Clin Toxicol 35: 127.

Kruse JA 1992 Methanol poisoning. Intens Care Med 18: 391.

Kulig K, Duffy JP, Lenden CH et al 1984 Toxic effects of methanol, ethylene glycol and isopropyl alcohol. Topics in Emerg Med 6: 14.

Palatnick W, Redman LW, Sitar DS et al 1995 Methanol half-life during ethanol administration: implications for management of methanol poisoning. Ann Emerg Med 26: 202.

Methylene blue

Methylene blue is a bright, blue-green organic dye of the phenothiazine family. It was discovered in 1876 and is manufactured from aniline material, most commonly from an organic diazo group. Methylene is a carbene, a class of reactive molecules with divalent carbon atoms (i.e. only two of four potential bonds are formed with other atoms). The generic formula of a carbene is R1-C-R2. Methylene is the most reactive of the carbenes and can attack almost every organic compound.

Methylene blue is used as a dye, a biological stain and a chemical indicator.

> Clinically, methylene blue is used as a reducing agent in the treatment of methaemoglobinaemia (q.v.).

Methaemoglobinaemia (q.v.) occurs when the iron in haemoglobin is in the oxidized or ferric form and thus (like carboxyhaemoglobin) cannot bind oxygen. This occurs following exposure to many agents, particularly nitrites, but also drugs such as dapsone, glyceryl trinitrate, primaquine, sulfasalazine and vitamin K analogues.

Methylene blue is given as an iv infusion of 1000 mg in 100 mL from which 1–2 mg/kg is administered over 5 min. Extravasation should be avoided because of the risk of local tissue necrosis. Cyanosis is immediately reversed, though relapse may occur some hours later due to the release from tissues of further oxidizing agent, so that the further administration of methylene blue may be needed, usually the same dose hourly, up to a total dose of 7 mg/kg if needed. A continuous iv infusion of 1 mg/kg/h may be used but is not generally recommended. If the concentration of methaemoglobin is very high (e.g. 60%), exchange transfusion with or without dialysis is recommended.

Methylene blue is not effective in glucose–6-phosphate dehydrogenase (G6PD) deficiency (q.v.), because it must first be reduced to leuko-methylene blue in red blood cells by NADPH (and NADPH requires G6PD for its formation).

The potential value of methylene blue in septic shock has recently been explored, on the basis that the free radical, nitric oxide (NO), may be an important mediator of the refractory vasodilatation in that condition and methylene blue is of value in nitrate toxicity. Haemodynamic improvement has been observed, though at the expense of hypoxaemia, so that survival data must be awaited before any clinically useful conclusion can be made about the utility of this new pharmacological approach.

Bibliography
Blass N, Fung D 1976 Dyed but not dead: methylene blue overdose. Anesthesiology 45: 458.
Gachot B, Bedos JP, Veber B et al 1995 Short-term effects of methylene blue on hemodynamics and gas exchange in humans with septic shock. Intens Care Med 21: 1027.
Hall HA, Kulig KW, Rumack BH 1986 Drug and chemical-induced methaemoglobinaemia; clinical features and management. Med Toxicol 1: 253.

Microangiopathic haemolysis

Microangiopathic haemolysis refers to the finding on peripheral blood film of fragmented and bizarre-shaped red blood cells with associated haemolysis.

The abnormal red blood cell morphology is caused by shear stress from intravascular obstruction, such as:

- local fibrin deposits;
- arteriovenous shunt;
- intracardiac shunt;
- classically cardiac valve disease or mechanical prostheses, especially the older Starr–Edwards models.

Microangiopathic haemolysis may also be associated with:

- vasculitis;
- metastatic cancer;
- thrombotic thrombocytopenic purpura;
- haemolytic–uraemic syndrome;
- meningococcaemia;
- rickettsial diseases;
- abnormal haemodynamic jets;
- cyclosporin.

If it is severe, it may be associated with thrombocytopenia and even disseminated intravascular coagulation.

Treatment is primarily of that of the underlying disease.

Bibliography
Nand S, Bansal VK, Kozeny G et al 1985 Red cell fragmentation syndrome with the use of subclavian hemodialysis catheters. Arch Intern Med 145: 1421.

Miller Fisher syndrome (see

Neuropathy (Guillain–Barré syndrome))

Mites (see Pediculosis)

Mixed connective tissue disease

Mixed connective tissue disease (MCTD) is a clinical syndrome with features common to a number of rheumatic diseases and not specific for any single diagnostic category. It may or may not be a separate disease entity, and some cases have been regarded as variants of SLE (q.v.), though without the typical serology.

Clinical features are very variable and involve chiefly women, though with an age range from 5–80 y. All patients have arthralgia, most with an arthritis resembling rheumatoid arthritis but non-deforming, with swollen fingers as in scleroderma and with a rash as in SLE. Asymptomatic pulmonary involvement is common, but renal involvement is uncommon. Proximal myopathy resembling polymyositis may be seen. Many patients have neuropsychiatric symptoms.

Investigations typically show leukopenia, raised ESR, increased IgG, positive rheumatoid factor and high titre of antinuclear antibodies. The most typical antibody is to an RNP antigen. Unlike in SLE, LE cells and DNA antibodies are not usually seen and complement levels are usually normal.

Treatment is with **NSAIDs** *in mild disease but otherwise with* **corticosteroids**.

Bibliography

Prockop DJ 1992 Mutations in collagen genes as a cause of connective-tissue diseases. N Engl J Med 326: 540.

Monkey bites (see Bites and stings)

Monosodium glutamate (see Chinese-restaurant syndrome)

Motor neurone disease (see Amyotrophic lateral sclerosis)

Mouth diseases

Mouth diseases include:

- gingivitis;
- glossitis;
- stomatitis;
- parotitis.

1. **Gingivitis**

Gingivitis is commonly of dental origin. The organisms involved are usually anaerobic upper respiratory tract flora (peptostreptococci, fusobacteria, bacteroides). In hospital patients, Gram-negative bacilli and staphylococci may also be involved. Uncommon causes include viruses or actinomyces. Gingivitis may also be associated with

- stomatitis;
- sinusitis;
- Vincent's angina

  – i.e. trench mouth;

- Ludwig's angina

  – i.e. sublingual cellulitis;

- peritonsillar abscess

  – sometimes called quinsy;

- haemorrhage
  – seen in bleeding disorders or scurvy;

- hyperplasia

  – classically occurring with phenytoin or more recently with cyclosporin and calcium channel blockers (of the dihydropyridine group, such as nifedipine, amlodipine, felodipine), and generally slowly reversible following cessation of the drug.

Persistent gingivitis should be remembered as a risk factor for subacute bacterial endocarditis.

---

2. **Glossitis**

Glossitis occurs in a number of forms.

A. **Atrophic glossitis**

This is seen in vitamin deficiency (niacin, riboflavin, B_{12}, folate). It is commonly associated with

- angular cheilitis, namely fissuring at the corners of the mouth. This is also and more commonly associated with dribbling of saliva. It may become secondarily infected.

- cheilosis, namely vertical fissuring of the lips. This also is commonly due to other causes, such as local irritation, solar damage and drugs, such as isotretinoin.

B. **Black hairy tongue**

This is a benign hyperplasia of the filiform papillae of the tongue. It is associated with bacterial overgrowth of chromogenic bacteria due to prolonged antibiotic therapy. It may also be caused by tobacco and certain foods. It is offensive both in appearance and odour.

C. **Xerostomia**

This refers to a dry mouth due to decreased saliva. This is seen typically in Sjögren's syndrome, but it may also be seen following irradiation for head and neck cancer and in chronic sialadenitis.

D. **Benign migratory glossitis** ('geographic tongue')

This is caused by an irregular loss of papillae of the tongue and is manifest as raised white areas containing red patches.

E. **Strawberry tongue**

This is seen in scarlet fever.

F. **Leukoplakia**

This is a pre-malignant condition, manifest as white patches on the tongue. It is traditionally caused by tobacco, but it is also seen in AIDS.

G. **Macroglossia**

This refers to enlargement of the tongue and is seen acromegaly, amyloidosis, lymphangioma, myxoedema.

H. **Miscellaneous disorders** of the tongue include:

- candidiasis due to inhaled corticosteroids;
- herpetic and other ulceration;
- malignancy;
- XII nerve paralysis.

3. **Stomatitis**

Although stomatitis may be due to local disease, it can more importantly be a manifestation of systemic disease, particularly a generalized dermatosis. In this setting, the mucous membrane is clearly different from skin, in that it has no stratum corneum or appendages and has salivary glands instead of sweat glands. Important forms of stomatitis associated with systemic disease of this type include:

- erythema multiforme and Stevens–Johnson syndrome;
- pemphigus;
- generalized candidiasis;
- graft-versus-host disease;
- Reiter's syndrome;
- SLE.

Other forms of stomatitis include:

- aphthous ulceration;
- Behçet's syndrome;
- hereditary haemorrhagic telangiectasia (Osler–Weber–Rendu syndrome);
- HSV infection
  - usually HSV type 1, but sometimes HSV type 2 in sexually active young adults;
- other viruses
  - coxsackie which gives herpangina, and VZV and EBV which have additional clinical features;
- **Peutz–Jeghers** syndrome. This is an autosomal dominant condition manifest by macules in and around the mouth and often associated with gastrointestinal polyps. These lesions are hamartomas, but they can bleed or obstruct. There may be an associated ovarian tumour.

4. **Parotitis**

Parotitis is the prominent clinical feature of mumps. In hospital patients, it is more commonly bacterial (especially staphylococcal), but it may be caused by other infections (e.g. parainfluenza virus). It may also be seen in:

- sarcoidosis;
- tumour;

- Sjögren's syndrome;
- cat-scratch disease;
- following drugs.

Bibliography

Moreland LW, Corey J, McKenzie R 1988 Ludwig's angina. Arch Intern Med 148: 463.

Pruett TL, Simmons RL 1984 Nosocomial gram-negative bacillary parotitis. JAMA 251: 252.

Utsunomiya J, Gocho H, Miyanaga T et al 1975 Peutz–Jeghers syndrome: its natural course and management. Johns Hopkins Med J 136: 71.

Multifocal motor neuropathy (see Amyotrophic lateral sclerosis)

Multiple endocrine neoplasia

The multiple endocrine neoplasia (MEN) (or multiple endocrine adenomatosis, MEA) syndromes refer to several patterns of multiple endocrine abnormalities inherited as autosomal dominant conditions. They are relatively rare, with a prevalence of about 1:20–25000.

MEN type I (MEN1) comprises pituitary, parathyroid and pancreatic adenomas (or hyperplasia), though pancreatic tumours may be malignant. Clearly, MEN1 may clinically present as one of these tumours alone, though in this case there is less than a 10% chance of a particular patient in fact having MEN1. Carcinoid tumours may also occur. Hyperparathyroidism is the commonest clinical manifestation.

The mutation is of the tumour suppressor gene, *MEN1*, located on the long arm of chromosome 11 in 1988 and cloned in 1997. Its penetrance is high, with virtually all carriers of the mutation developing clinical disease before the age of 40 years. However, over 200 different mutations of this large gene have been described, so that genetic screening is complicated.

*Effective management requires early diagnosis of the component tumours and their surgical **resection**, especially for parathyroid and pancreatic tumours.*

MEN type II (MEN2) comprises:

- thyroid medullary carcinoma

  - a rare type of thyroid cancer, which arises in the parafollicular cells and which secretes thyrocalcitonin;

- phaeochromocytoma

  - which is often bilateral and may be malignant;

- parathyroid hyperplasia.

MEN2 is subdivided into two groups, namely:

1. MEN2A, which comprises thyroid medullary cancer, plus phaeochromocytoma in half the cases, plus hyperparathyroidism in 15% of cases;

2. MEN2B, which comprises thyroid medullary cancer and phaeochromocytoma, plus other unusual features, including mucosal neuromas and gastrointestinal ganglioneuromatosis.

The mutation is of the *RET* proto-oncogene. Its penetrance is moderate, with about half the carriers of the mutation developing clinical disease before the age of 60 years. Genetic screening is relatively straightforward, since the responsible mutations are tightly clustered.

Treatment of identified carriers is with prophylactic thyroidectomy in childhood.

Bibliography

Brandi ML 1991 Multiple endocrine neoplasia type 1: general features and new insights into etiology. J Endocrinol Invest 14: 61.

Burgess JR 1999 Multiple endocrine neoplasia type 1: current concepts in diagnosis and management. Med J Aust 170: 605.

Chandrasekharappa SC, Guru SC, Manickam P et al 1997 Positional cloning of the gene for multiple endocrine neoplasia-type 1. Science 276: 404.

Eng C 1999 RET proto-oncogene in the development of human cancer. J Clin Oncol 17: 380.

Learoyd DL, Delbridge LW, Robinson BG 2000 Multiple endocrine neoplasia. Aust NZ J Med 30: 675.

Mallette LE 1991 The parathyroid polyhormones: new concepts in the spectrum of peptide hormone action. Endocr Rev 12: 110.

Robinson BG 1994 Multiple endocrine neoplasia –
who should be screened? Med J Aust 160: 739.
Schimke RN 1990 Multiple endocrine neoplasia:
how many syndromes? Am J Med Genet 37: 375.

Multiple myeloma

Multiple myeloma (plasma cell myeloma) is a
relatively slowly growing malignant tumour
arising in a clone of plasma cells. Since normal
plasma cells synthesize immunoglobulins as
matched heavy and light chains, malignant
plasma cells commonly secrete an abnormal
monoclonal immunoglobulin (paraprotein) with
a single heavy chain class and a single light chain
type giving the classical M protein spike on
serum electrophoresis. Commonly, there are
excess kappa or lambda light chains (which
appear in the urine as Bence Jones proteins,
q.v.). Sometimes, there can be no heavy chains
at all (with resultant hypogammaglobulinaemia
associated with the Bence Jones proteinaemia)
or excess heavy chains (either gamma, alpha or
mu, giving one of the heavy chain diseases) or
neither chain at all (giving
panhypogammaglobulinaemia).

Normal plasma cell function is depressed in
patients with multiple myeloma, resulting in
immunocompromise. The bone marrow is
infiltrated with resultant pancytopenia, the bone
itself can be eroded by plasmacytomas, and
extramedullary infiltration is common in liver,
spleen, lymph nodes, gut, subcutaneous tissues,
pleural cavity, nasopharynx and nasal sinuses.

A variety of other clinical problems may be
produced, including:

- **hypercalcaemia** (q.v.);
- **renal disease**;
- **hyperviscosity**, especially due to IgA and
  IgM variants. The abnormal protein
  aggregates red blood cells, and headache,
  retinopathy and cardiac failure may result.
  Sometimes, the abnormal proteins are
  precipitated by cold (i.e. these are
  cryoglobulins – see below) and Raynaud's
  phenomenon results;

- **bleeding** may result from interference with
  platelets and coagulation factors, particularly
  factors I, II and VIII.

The diagnosis is made biochemically,
histologically and radiologically.

- Biochemically, there is typically Bence Jones
  protein in the urine and/or a monoclonal
  spike on serum electrophoresis. No M
  protein is seen in 25% of patients, but most
  of these still have Bence Jones proteins in the
  urine.
- Histologically, typical changes are seen in
  bone marrow or tissue biopsy material.
- Radiologically, lytic bone lesions may be
  seen.

*Treatment is with **radiotherapy** for local lesions and
cytotoxic therapy for systemic disease. Recently,
several aggressive and complex cytotoxic regimens have
improved the response rate.*

- *Trials of both autologous and allogeneic bone
  marrow transplantation have been reported, but
  there have been significant problems with both
  techniques.*
- *Hyperviscosity is treated with plasmapheresis.*
- *Hypercalcaemia is treated on its usual merits
  (q.v.).*
- *Skeletal problems, particularly bone pain, may be
  relieved by the second-generation bisphosphonate,
  pamidronate (APD) (see Hypercalcaemia).*
- *Infectious complications may require
  immunoglobulin replacement.*
- *Dialysis may be indicated for renal failure.*

If a response is achieved, there is a mean
survival of about three years in good health.
Occasionally, very long survival is seen. The
prognosis is worse in the presence of anaemia,
hypercalcaemia, multiple osteolytic bone lesions
or paraproteins in large amounts.

There are several variants of multiple myeloma.

1. **Solitary plasmacytoma** may be seen,
especially of bone.

2. **Waldenstrom's macroglobulinaemia** is a
variant due to an IgM clone.

3. **Heavy chain disease**, with gamma, alpha or mu fragments, tends to behave as a chronic haematological malignancy.

4. **Benign monoclonal gammopathy** (so-called) may be seen in older patients. Eventually, classical myeloma develops in about 20% of patients within about 10 years if the gammopathy is IgG, and other lymphoproliferative disorders develop in about 50% of patients if the gammopathy is IgM.

5. **Cryoglobulinaemia** occurs when the abnormal plasma proteins are precipitated by cold.

There are three types of cryoglobulinaemia.

- Type 1 is due to a monoclonal immunoglobulin – IgM, IgG, IgA, or BJ in descending order of frequency.
- Type 2 is a mixed condition.
- Type 3 is associated with polyclonal immunoglobulins.

Types 2 and 3 probably represent immune complex diseases, in which the immune complexes are precipitated by cold. Most cryoglobulins in this setting have rheumatoid factor activity and can produce a large variety of effects, including inflammation, platelet aggregation, clotting factor consumption, microvascular obstruction, hyperviscosity, bleeding, vascular purpura, Raynaud's phenomenon, renal dysfunction and neurological changes. Commonly, there is an underlying autoimmune disease or chronic hepatitis (HBV or even more frequently HCV infection).

*Treatment with **plasmapheresis** is effective, but corticosteroids and cytotoxics are not helpful.*

6. **Amyloidosis** comprises a number of disorders characterized by the accumulation in tissues of protein in fibrillar form (i.e. amyloid). The protein is laid down in beta-pleated sheets, so that it is insoluble, resistant to proteolysis and phagocytosis, typically stains with Congo red and is birefringent under polarizing light.

Several different proteins can be modified in this way and different secondary structures result, giving distinct pathophysiological and clinical manifestations for each.

A. **Primary amyloidosis** is produced by light chain Ig fragments (molecular weight 5–25 kD) similar to Bence Jones proteins. Deposits occur especially in muscle (e.g. tongue and heart), skin (especially of the upper part of the body), liver, spleen, gut, kidneys (with nephrotic syndrome), joints and peripheral nerves.

The clinical manifestations are related to the type of local involvement. Bleeding occasionally occurs because of either the trapping of factor X or from increased fibrinolysis. Median survival has been reported to be 18 months.

*No therapy is consistently effective, but **corticosteroids** and **melphalan** have been reported to be helpful in some patients and more so than other therapies such as colchicine.*

B. **Secondary amyloidosis** is a reactive process to chronic inflammation, especially pyogenic infections, tuberculosis and rheumatoid arthritis. The protein, amyloid A (AA, molecular weight of 8.5 kD) is derived from a normal acute phase reactant in plasma, called serum amyloid A (SAA, molecular weight 84–200 kD and cleaved by monocytes). Since deposits of amyloid occur only in some patients with chronic inflammation, different patterns of monocyte degradation of SAA may be responsible for the individual variation.

Deposits are seen mostly in liver, spleen, kidneys and adrenals, and the main clinical feature is the nephrotic syndrome.

*Treatment is with **colchicine** which blocks SAA secretion.*

C. **Miscellaneous amyloidosis** occurs in several forms, including hereditary (as in familial Mediterranean fever, due to amyloid A production), senile and local forms.

Bibliography

Attal M, Harousseau J-L, Stoppa A-M et al 1996 A prospective, randomized trial of autologous bone marrow transplantation and chemotherapy in multiple myeloma. N Engl J Med 335: 91.

Bataille R 1996 Management of myeloma with bisphosphonates. N Engl J Med 334: 529.

Bjorkstrand B, Ljungman P, Svensson H et al 1996 Allogeneic bone marrow transplantation versus autologous stem cell transplantation in multiple myeloma. Blood 88: 4711.

Brouet JC, Clouvel JP, Danon F et al 1974 Biologic and clinical significance of cryoglobulins. Am J Med 57: 775.

Dauel TF, Dauth J, Mellstedt H et al 1985 Waldenstrom's macroglobulinaemia. Lancet 2: 311.

Dowd PM 1987 Cold-related disorders. Prog Dermatol 21: 1.

Frankel AH, Singer DRJ, Winearls CG et al 1992 Type II essential mixed cryoglobulinemia: presentation, treatment and outcome in 13 patients. Q J Med 82: 101.

Gertz MA, Kyle RA 1991 Secondary systemic amyloidosis. Medicine 70: 246.

Gertz MA, Kyle RA, Greipp PR 1991 Response rates and survival in primary systemic amyloidosis. Blood 77: 257.

Greipp PR 1992 Advances in the diagnosis and management of myeloma. Semin Hematol 29: 24.

Hamblin TJ 1986 The kidney in myeloma. Br Med J 292: 2.

Joshua DE, Gibson J 2000 Multiple myeloma – evolving concepts of biology and treatment. Aust NZ J Med 30: 311.

Kintzer JS, Rosenow EC, Kyle RA 1978 Thoracic and pulmonary abnormalities in multiple myeloma. Arch Intern Med 138: 727.

Kisilevsky R, Benson MD, Frangione B et al (eds) 1994 Amyloid and Amyloidosis. New York: Parthenon.

Kyle RA 1993 "Benign" monoclonal gammopathy. Mayo Clin Proc 68: 26.

Kyle RA, Gertz MA, Greipp PR et al 1997 A trial of three regimens for primary amyloidosis. N Engl J Med 336: 1202.

McGrath MA, Penny R 1976 Paraproteinemia: blood hyperviscosity and clinical manifestations. J Clin Invest 58: 1155.

Norden CW 1980 Infections in patients with multiple myeloma. Arch Intern Med 140:1150.

Pepys MB 1988 Amyloidosis: some recent developments. Q J Med 67: 283.

Solomon A, Weiss DT, Kattine AA 1991 Nephrotoxic potential of Bence Jones proteins. N Engl J Med 324: 1845.

Multiple sclerosis

Multiple sclerosis (MS) is a condition of chronic patchy demyelination which occurs in the white matter in zones called plaques. These are of varying site and size within the CNS.

Its aetiology is unknown, but it may be an autoimmune response to viral infection, possibly via molecular mimicry with a homologous sequence within the myelin protein. It mostly occurs in young adults who are predisposed because of certain genetic haplotypes, but these influences are only partly characterized. Environmental factors are presumably also important, because of the excess of cases occurring in temperate zones and in urban areas (and perhaps also in the more affluent). Its overall prevalence is about 50 per 100 000 population.

> The clinical features of multiple sclerosis are characterized by fluctuating neurological signs, attributable to multiple sites of involvement.
>
> Both its initial onset and subsequent relapses typically occur over a few days. Subsequently, there is stable dysfunction for a few weeks, followed by gradual but usually partial recovery.

Initial symptoms particularly comprise:

- **motor changes**
  - weakness, clumsiness, stiffness;
- **sensory changes**
  - paraesthesiae;
- **visual disturbances**, particularly
  - **optic neuritis**, which is manifest by impaired visual acuity, with a central scotoma, loss of pupillary reaction to light and sometimes an oedematous disc on ophthalmoscopy; optic neuritis may sometimes occur as an isolated condition, in which case it is probably a forme fruste of MS;

– **internuclear ophthalmoplegia**, which is caused by demyelination of the medial longitudinal bundle; on lateral conjugate gaze, there is thus impaired adduction of the following eye and nystagmus in the leading or abducting eye.

- **vestibular disturbance**;
- **incontinence** and/or **impotence**;
- **psychiatric disturbances**.

The later course of the disease is very variable, with exacerbations at irregular intervals over long periods but eventually with persistent signs of spastic weakness, uncoordination and incontinence. Various clinical patterns are recognized, particularly relapse–remission and chronic progressive patterns. Many cases have quite a benign course, and even permanent remission may occasionally be seen.

The diagnosis is based on clinical criteria, but it should be substantiated by special tests, particularly MRI (which shows typical demyelination plaques in over 90% of cases). The CSF shows increased IgG, with oligoclonal banding. The responses to evoked potentials are abnormal. A normal MRI and CSF and the absence of eye signs and incontinence should suggest an alternative diagnosis.

Treatment is of limited efficacy.

- *Corticosteroids (except as pulsed, high-dose, intravenous methylprednisolone for relapse), cytotoxics, plasmapheresis, immune globulin and hyperbaric oxygen have all been shown to be ineffective.*
- *New drugs, especially **beta-interferon**, are showing promise in clinical trials, but their long-term value is still uncertain. They appear to be of most value in patients with frequent attacks and no more than moderate disability.*
- *Symptoms of spasticity may be improved with baclofen or diazepam and symptoms of urinary urgency with propantheline.*
- *Elective surgery carries an increased risk of relapse, but pregnancy is normally well tolerated.*

Bibliography

Anderson DW, Ellenberg JH, Leventhal CM et al 1992 Revised estimate of the prevalence of multiple sclerosis in the United States. Ann Neurol 31: 333.

Dhib-Jalbut S, McFarlin DE 1990 Immunology of multiple sclerosis. Ann Allergy 64: 433.

Ebers GC 1985 Optic neuritis and multiple sclerosis. Arch Neurol 42: 702.

Editorial 1991 Where to hit MS. Lancet 337: 765.

Kilpatrick TJ, Soilu-Hanninen M 1999 New treatments for multiple sclerosis. Aust NZ J Med 29: 801.

McDonald WI 1992 Multiple sclerosis: diagnostic optimism. Br Med J 304: 1259.

Pender MP 1996 Recent advances in the understanding, diagnosis and management of multiple sclerosis. Aust NZ J Med 26:157.

Pender MP 2000 Multiple sclerosis. Med J Aust 172: 556.

Ron MA, Feinstein A 1992 Multiple sclerosis and the mind. J Neurol Neurosurg Psychiatry 55; 1.

Muscular dystrophies

Muscular dystrophies comprise a group of hereditary disorders of muscle, characterized by progressive weakness and wasting. The major types are described below, but the many types can now be classified in some detail according to the genes involved and thus the protein affected.

1. Duchenne's (pseudohypertrophic) dystrophy

This is an X-linked recessive disorder and is therefore seen in boys of mothers who are carriers. Genetic screening is available. It particularly involves the muscles of the pelvic girdle, resulting in a waddling gait. Most patients have succumbed by their mid-20s to either respiratory failure and/or associated cardiomyopathy.

*No treatment has generally been effective, though **corticosteroids** have recently been shown to be helpful. Non-invasive nocturnal ventilation may be useful in advanced disease.*

2. Facioscapulohumeral dystrophy

This is an autosomal dominant condition which is very slowly progressive from adolescence onwards. It primarily involves the muscles of the face and shoulder girdle. There is no associated cardiomyopathy, so that a normal life-span is common.

3. **Myotonic dystrophy** (dystrophia myotonia)

This is also an autosomal dominant condition, with an onset usually in adolescence. It primarily involves the muscles of the face (including eyelids) and neck and the small muscles of the hands and feet.

As its name implies, myotonic dystrophy is associated with myotonia, i.e. delayed muscular relaxation. Myotonia is also seen in:

- **myotonia congenita** (a benign myopathy);
- periodic paralysis (due to hyperkalaemia) (q.v.).

Pathophysiologically, the muscle membrane has decreased permeability to chloride ion, and there is a characteristic EMG.

Myotonic dystrophy is associated with baldness, cardiomyopathy, cataracts, glucose intolerance, dysphagia and gonadal atrophy. Often, the condition is mild and the course slow.

Treatment with **phenytoin** *or* **procainamide** *can help the myotonia but not the weakness.*

Bibliography

Griggs RC, Moxley RT, Mendell JR et al 1993 Duchenne dystrophy: randomized, controlled trial of prednisone (18 months) and azathioprine (12 months). Neurology 43: 520.

Harper PS 2001 Myotonic Dystrophy. London: WB Saunders.

Moser H 1984 Duchenne muscular dystrophy: pathogenetic aspects and genetic prevention. Hum Genet 66: 17.

Mushroom poisoning

Mushroom poisoning is a worldwide problem because of the difficulty in identifying the many species which grow in the wild. Commercially available mushrooms, however, are cultured. Poisoning also occurs because of the 'recreational' use of mushrooms for their hallucinogenic properties. In fact, only about 1% of mushrooms are poisonous.

The term 'mushroom' is non-scientific and refers to the edible type of fungus, whereas the equally lay term 'toadstool' refers to any poisonous variety. Mushrooms are the umbrella-shaped, fleshy, fruiting body of fungi of the order Agaricales in the class Basidiomycetes. In the ground, the fungal mycelia may live for hundreds of years as an underground mat of threads, from which a new crop of fruiting sporophores arises each season.

Within the order Agaricales are both

- the family Agaricaceae, which includes *Agaricus campestris* (the common field mushroom) and *Agaricus bisporus* (the common commercial variety),
- the family Amanitaceae, which includes many poisonous varieties and in particular the genus Amanita which has about 100 species within it. The most common poisonous mushroom is *Amanita phalloides*, called the 'death cap', which is responsible for 90% of fatal mushroom poisonings worldwide. It is mostly associated in a symbiotic relationship with older oak and other deciduous trees.

Mushroom poisoning usually occurs in the autumn. There have been many famous deaths of this nature in history, including the Euripides family, the Roman Emperor Claudius, Pope Clement II, Charles VI of France and of course Barbar the elephant's royal predecessor.

Several syndromes may be produced by mushroom poisoning. The most common syndromes are:

- cytotoxic;
- neurotoxic.

Cytotoxins are primarily amatoxins, cyclic octapeptides from the Amanita genus. They are very potent, with as little as 50 g (or one mushroom), containing about 5 mg of toxin, possibly being fatal. They inhibit protein synthesis, giving rise to cell membrane destruction.

Symptoms arise after a latent period 6–24 h, by which time the patient may have forgotten having eating a mushroom. There is abdominal pain, nausea and vomiting, but these symptoms usually subside by 24 h or so. Despite clinical improvement, liver enzymes become abnormal by 48 h. Between 2–4 days, hepatic and renal failure occur.

Optimal treatment is uncertain.

* *Gastric lavage and charcoal are recommended if the diagnosis is made early.*
* *The administration of high-dose penicillin for three days inhibits hepatocyte uptake of the toxin.*
* *Thioctic acid has been reported to be helpful.*
* *Dialysis is indicated on its normal merits for renal support but does not remove toxin.*
* *Liver transplantation has been used in some severely affected patients.*
* *If alcohol is taken during the first three days, a disulfiram-like reaction may be seen.*

The mortality is about 20%.

Neurotoxins are varied in type and less commonly fatal.

Symptoms appear within 2 h, last for 6–12 h and resolve spontaneously. They comprise chiefly muscarinic effects (with anticholinergic features of sweating, salivation and gastrointestinal upset), hallucinations (which may be LSD-like) or disulfiram-like reactions (with flushing, tachycardia and tachypnoea, following alcohol).

Atropine may be given for muscarinic effects but not if there are associated hallucinations as it may worsen these. Hallucinations are best treated with diazepam.

The presence of the rapid and brief neurotoxic reaction does not exclude the possibility of associated amatoxin ingestion and thus later cytotoxic damage.

Bibliography

Barbato MP 1993 Poisoning from accidental ingestion of mushrooms. Med J Aust 158: 842.
Klein AS, Hart J, Brems JJ et al 1989 Amanita poisoning: treatment and the role of liver transplantation. Am J Med 86: 187.
Mitchell DH 1980 Amanita mushroom poisoning. Annu Rev Med 31: 51.
Rumack BH, Spoerke DG eds 1994 Handbook of Mushroom Poisoning: Diagnosis and Treatment. 2nd edition. Boca Raton: CRC Press.

Mustards (see Warfare agents)

Myasthenia gravis

Myasthenia gravis is a condition of muscle weakness due to impaired neuromuscular transmission.

It is caused by autoantibodies to a subunit of the acetylcholine receptor on the post-junctional muscle membrane. It occurs primarily in younger women or older men. In about 10% of cases, there is an associated thymic tumour (thymoma).

> There is typically a gradual onset of muscle fatigue, characteristically with increasing weakness with repetitive use. It may range in severity from mild and local to severe and generalized. It particularly involves the muscles innervated by the cranial nerves (eyes, face, jaw, pharynx and voice). Typically, there is diplopia and ptosis.

The diagnosis is made on the basis of the EMG and confirmed with edrophonium (Tensilon, a short-acting anticholinesterase). After edrophonium 10 mg iv, dramatic improvement in muscle power occurs within 60 s and lasts for a few minutes. Acetylcholine antibodies are present in about 90% of cases, and there may be other associated autoimmune diseases, in particular thyroid disease. A CT scan is required to assess the presence of an associated thymoma.

Treatment modalities include:

- **anticholinesterase** *therapy (in particular pyridostigmine). Dosage requirements vary considerably and range from 15 mg 8 hourly to 120 mg 4 hourly orally (60 mg orally being equivalent to 2 mg iv). However, excess dosage can give a cholinergic crisis (q.v.), which is associated with muscarinic side-effects.*
- **corticosteroids**. *These are of value if the response to anticholinesterase is unsatisfactory or the patient is very sick. There is an 80% response rate within 2 weeks.*
- **cytotoxic agents** *(usually azathioprine). These may enhance the steroid response.*
- **plasmapheresis** *or* **immune globulin**. *These are used for an acute crisis and for perioperative support.*
- **thymectomy**. *Even in the absence of a thymoma, this gives a 70% response rate. It is best considered early in the course of disease.*

Two variants of myasthenia gravis may be seen.

1. Drug-induced myasthenia

This may be caused by aminoglycosides. Weakness of this type may be caused even in normal subjects, as well as increased weakness in myasthenics. Penicillamine therapy for rheumatoid arthritis may be associated with myasthenia.

Needless to say, prolonged neuromuscular junction abnormalities are common after long infusions of neuromuscular blocking drugs, particularly in patients with liver and kidney dysfunction. While this phenomenon is usually due to the persistence of long-acting metabolites (e.g. of vecuronium), a myasthenia-like syndrome has also been reported and is probably due to damage to the neuromuscular junction.

2. Myasthenic syndrome (Eaton Lambert syndrome)

This is a paraneoplastic phenomenon (q.v.). It is caused by the binding of antibodies to the presynaptic membrane of the neuromuscular junction.

Although there is typical muscular weakness and fatigue, there is paradoxical improvement with repeated use. It is exacerbated by muscle relaxants and may be improved with successful treatment of the underlying carcinoma (usually of the lung).

It sometimes responds to pyridostigmine, corticosteroids and/or plasmapheresis.

Bibliography

Berrouschot J, Baumann I, Kalischewski P et al 1997 Therapy of myasthenic crisis. Crit Care Med 25: 1228.

Clamon GH, Evans WK, Shepherd FA et al 1984 Myasthenic syndrome and small cell cancer of the lung: variable response to antineoplastic therapy. Arch Intern Med 144: 999.

Gracey DR, Divertie MB, Howard FM 1983 Mechanical ventilation for respiratory failure in myasthenia gravis. Mayo Clin Proc 58: 597.

O'Neill JH, Murray NM, Newsom-Davis J 1988 The Lambert–Eaton myasthenic syndrome. Brain 111: 577.

Segredo V, Caldwell J, Matthay M et al 1992 Persistent paralysis in critically ill patients after long-term administration of vecuronium. N Engl J Med 327: 524.

Seybold ME 1983 Myasthenia gravis: a clinical and basic science review. JAMA 250: 2516.

Sokoll M, Gergis S 1981 Antibiotics and neuromuscular function. Anesthesiology 55: 148.

Swift TR 1981 Disorders of neuromuscular transmission other than myasthenia gravis. Muscle Nerve 4: 334.

Tonner DR, Schlechte JA 1993 Neurologic complications of thyroid and parathyroid disease. Med Clin North Am 77: 251.

Wright EA, McQuillen MP 1971 Antibiotic-induced neuromuscular blockade. Ann NY Acad Sci 183: 358.

Mycetism (see Mushroom poisoning)

Mycetoma (see Aspergillosis)

Mycoplasma hominis (see Pregnancy)

Mycoplasma pneumoniae (see Cold agglutinin disease)

Mycotic aneurysms

Mycotic aneurysms arise from destruction of the arterial wall following infection. This process may be produced by:

- direct bacterial invasion of the arterial wall;
- deposition of immune complexes in the arterial wall;
- embolic occlusion of vasa vasorum.

Although the arterial wall damage is an acute process, it may not become clinically evident until long after the original infection has subsided.

A mycotic aneurysm is thus the sterile end-result of a previous infection.

- It may occur in any artery, including the sinus of Valsalva and the pulmonary artery (e.g. following iv heroin use).
- The antecedent infection is a bacteraemia, especially if associated with acute or subacute bacterial endocarditis. The most common organism involved is *S. aureus*.

Clinical features include:

- a pulsatile mass (which may be tender and which usually is noted in a palpable artery, e.g. brachial, femoral or popliteal);
- local pressure problems;
- an abdominal bruit;
- a sudden haemorrhage;
- rupture of a sinus of Valsalva into the right heart giving a left-to-right shunt and a continuous murmur.

*Treatment is **surgical**, if the aneurysm is accessible. Prophylactic surgical excision is recommended, because rupture is a major complication which can be fatal.*

Myelitis (see Demyelinating diseases)

Myelopathy

Myelopathy may be either:

- local; or
- associated with encephalopathy (q.v.), as an encephalomyelopathy.

Isolated myelopathy is due to local spinal cord damage, such as that due to:

- disc protrusion;
- infection;
- nutritional deficiency (particularly due to vitamin B_{12});
- radiation.

Myoglobinuria (see Rhabdomyolysis)

Myopathy

Myopathy is a general term indicating a muscle disorder. It may be either primary or secondary.

Primary myopathies include:

- genetic disorders
  - glycogen storage diseases;
  - lipid storage myopathy;
  - mitochondrial diseases;
- malignant hyperthermia (q.v.);
- muscular dystrophy (q.v.);
- myasthenia gravis (q.v.)
  - in fact a neuromuscular disease;
- periodic paralysis (q.v.);
- poliomyelitis (q.v.)
  - in fact a denervating disease.

Secondary myopathy may be caused by:

- inflammation;

- toxic/metabolic disorders

  - alcoholism;
  - drugs (antimalarials, colchicine, zidovudine, and especially fluorinated corticosteroids, even in standard doses);
  - endocrine disorders (adrenal, parathyroid and thyroid disorders of either excess or deficiency);
  - metabolic disturbances (hypophophataemia, hypokalaemia, hypocalcaemia, hypomagnesaemia);

- trauma

  - rhabdomyolysis;
  - severe exertion.

Acute necrotizing myopathy is one of the less common forms of critical illness neuromuscular abnormality (CINMA) – see Critical illness neuropathy. It may be seen in Intensive Care patients who have received prolonged neuromuscular blockade with any of the non-depolarizing agents, commonly with concomitant corticosteroids. It was thus first recognized as a complication of severe asthma, and those paralyzed for more than 24 h may be at particular risk. Experimental evidence suggests that it may be due to marked enhancement of steroid-induced myopathy by pharmacological denervation. It may be a cause of prolonged ventilator dependence.

This condition may be difficult to distinguish from critical illness polyneuropathy (with which it may also coexist). A less well understood variant is **critical illness myopathy**. This is seen in patients with sepsis and/or multi-organ failure and may have a similar pathogenesis to critical illness polyneuropathy.

Myopathy due to disuse atrophy may of course occur following any serious illness, particularly if it is prolonged.

Electrophysiological studies and histology may be required to clarify these conditions in an individual patient (see also Neuropathy).

Bibliography

Batchelor PM, Taylor LP, Thaler HT et al 1997 Steroid myopathy in cancer patients. Neurology 48: 1234.

Chad DA, Lacomis D 1994 Critically ill patients with newly acquired weakness: the clinicopathological spectrum. Ann Neurol 35: 257.

De Jonghe B, Cook D, Sharshar T et al 1998 Acquired neuromuscular disorders in critically ill patients: a systematic review. Intens Care Med 24: 1242.

Hansen-Flaschen J 1997 Neuromuscular complications of critical illness. Pulmonary Perspectives 14(4): 1.

Hund E 1999 Myopathy in critically ill patients. Chest 27: 2544.

Layzer RB 1985 McArdle's disease in the 1980s. N Engl J Med 312: 370.

Nates JL, Cooper DJ, Day B et al 1997 Acute weakness syndromes in critically ill patients – a reappraisal. Anaesth Intens Care 25: 502.

Segredo V, Caldwell JE, Matthay MA et al 1992 Persistent paralysis in critically ill patients after long-term administration of vecuronium. N Engl J Med 327: 524.

Tonner DR, Schlechte JA 1993 Neurologic complications of thyroid and parathyroid disease. Med Clin North Am 77: 251.

Myositis

Myositis, or inflammation of muscle, may be seen in several settings.

1. **Autoimmune diseases**

- mixed connective tissue disease;
- Sjögren's syndrome.

2. **Infective**

- clostridial,
- streptococcal

  - Group A streptococci may sometimes cause a potentially fatal gangrenous myositis and/or necrotizing fasciitis (see Gangrene).
  - This is the severe end of the spectrum which ranges from superficial skin infection (impetigo) to deeper infections (such as cellulitis or erysipelas).

– *Treatment requires surgical **drainage** and/or **debridement**, as well as **antibiotics**.*

- tropical

  – Pyomyositis is common in the tropics and in AIDS.
  – It is usually due to *S. aureus*.
  – The muscle abscess is usually best diagnosed with CT scanning.

- viral

  – most widely known with influenza virus;
  – also with adenovirus, coxsackievirus, echovirus, HIV.

3. **Myositis ossificans**

- This is post-traumatic.

4. **Polymyositis**

- q.v.

5. **Inclusion body myositis**

- see Polymyositis.

6. **Myositis associated with vasculitis**

- About 50% of cases of vasculitis have histological evidence of associated myositis, though mostly such muscle involvement is asymptomatic.

Bibliography
Miller FW 1994 Classification and prognosis of inflammatory muscle disease. Rheum Dis Clin North Am 20: 811.

Myotonia (see Muscular dystrophy)

Myxoedema (see Hypothyroidism)

Myxoma (see Cardiac tumours)

Nails

Nails, especially finger nails, can show a large variety of physical abnormalities, many of which are associated with systemic diseases.

- **Onychomycosis** is usually associated with paronychia and is commonly fungal in origin, though it may be caused by staphylococci or pseudomonas (in which case green nails are sometimes seen). It especially occurs in the immunocompromised.
- **Onycholysis** refers to separation of the nail plate from the nail bed. It may follow drugs (tetracycline, quinolones especially when associated with ultraviolet light), dermatoses (e.g. psoriasis), peripheral vascular disease, thyroid disease and trauma.
- **Koilonychia** refers to spoon-shaped nails and is seen typically in iron deficiency anaemia but also in haemochromatosis.
- **Clubbing** of the nails may be inherited or may be idiopathic. Most commonly, it arises from malignancy or chronic inflammation in the lungs or mediastinum. Clubbing of a single digit may follow a local vascular abnormality, such as an AV fistula.
- **Leukonychia** indicates white streaking of the nails and is seen in psoriasis, systemic infections and poisoning (arsenic, thallium).
- **Yellow discolouration** of the nails is seen in jaundice, chronic respiratory infections, amyloid, thyroid disease and AIDS.
- **Brown discolouration** of the nails is seen following the use of some antimalarial or cytotoxic drugs.
- **Splinter haemorrhages**, while purportedly typical of subacute bacterial endocarditis, are usually in fact traumatic in origin.
- **Onychodystrophies** refer to a large variety of alterations of nail shape, surface or colour. They are especially seen in the elderly, in whom for example, brittle or longitudinally-ridged nails may be seen.
- **Pitting** of the nails is typical in psoriasis (q.v.) though not pathognomonic.
- **Atrophy** or **hypertrophy** of the nails may occasionally be seen as congenital conditions.

Bibliography

Daniel CR 1983 Diseases of the nails. In: Cann HF (ed) Current Therapy. Philadelphia: WB Saunders. p 653.

Necrolytic migratory erythema (see Glucagonoma)

Necrotizing cutaneous mucormycosis (see Gangrene)

Necrotizing pneumonia (see Cavitation)

Nephrolithiasis

Nephrolithiasis (renal calculous disease) occurs in about 5% of the population. The calculi may be composed of a variety of substances.

1. **Calcium oxalate**, an octahedron, occurs with or without calcium apatite (70% of calculi). Such stones form when:

- the urine volume is small;
- there is increased urinary calcium or oxalate

  - increased oxalate intake with ingestion of some foods, such as chocolate, peanuts, leafy vegetables, strong tea;
  - increased oxalate absorption in inflammatory bowel disease or the short bowel syndrome;
  - increased oxalate turnover in pyridoxine deficiency;

- there is decreased urinary inhibitors

  - such as citrate, glycoprotein, magnesium.

2. **Struvite**, magnesium ammonium phosphate, is typically in the shape of a coffin lid and sometimes forms a staghorn (15% of calculi). Such stones form particularly in urinary tract infections when ammonia production is increased from urease secreted by bacteria. These are typically proteus, though other

Gram-negative bacilli and staphylococci may also be involved.

3. **Uric acid** calculi occur in the shape of radiolucent diamonds (10% of calculi).

4. **Calcium phosphate** produces an amorphous stone (2% of calculi).

5. **Cystine** produces hexagons (1% of calculi). These occur in cystinuria, which an autosomal recessive condition.

Clinical consequences of renal calculi include:

- pain;
- urinary tract obstruction;
- urinary tract obstruction infection;
- haematuria.

Sometimes, the patient may present with:

- renal impairment;
- ileus;
- hypovolaemia.

The differential diagnosis of calculi, particularly if radiolucent, includes sloughed renal papilla, clot, tumour or uric acid stone. A diagnosis of renal tubular acidosis (q.v.) is supported by the presence of diffuse tiny nephrocalcinosis and metabolic acidosis with a normal anion gap and high urinary pH. Definitive diagnosis usually requires an intravenous pyelogram.

*Treatment requires **removal of the stone**, unless it is passed spontaneously. Removal options include retrograde basket extraction or lithotripsy, though in severe cases a nephrostomy may be required first.*

Antibiotics are required if there is concomitant infection.

Bibliography

Coe FL, Parks JH, Asplin JR 1992 The pathogenesis and treatment of kidney stones. N Engl J Med 327: 1141.

Curhan GC, Willett WC, Rimm EB et al 1997 Family history and risk of kidney stones. J Am Soc Nephrol 8: 1568.

NIH Consensus Development Panel 1988 Prevention and treatment of kidney stones. JAMA 260: 977.

Singer A, Das S 1989 Cystinuria: a review of the pathophysiology and management. J Urol 142: 669.

Stewart C 1988 Nephrolithiasis. Emerg Med Clin North Am 6: 617.

Wilson DM 1990 Clinical and laboratory evaluation of renal stone patients. Endocrinol Metab Clin North Am 19: 773.

Nephrology

Most renal disorders encountered in Intensive Care are very well known, especially the various conditions associated with acute and chronic renal failure, acute tubular necrosis, dialysis, transplantation, trauma, and acid–base, fluid and electrolyte disturbances. Nevertheless, a variety of other, less common aspects of renal disease can be relevant to Intensive Care practice and are considered in this book. They include:

- aminoaciduria;
- beta$_2$-microglobulin;
- drugs and the kidney;
- glomerular diseases;
- haematuria;
- myoglobinuria;
- nephrolithiasis;
- proteinuria;
- renal artery occlusion;
- renal cortical necrosis;
- renal cysts;
- renal tubular acidosis;
- renal vein thrombosis;
- tubulointerstitial diseases.

Bibliography

Arieff AI, Massry SG, Barrientos A et al 1973 Brain water and electrolyte metabolism in uremia: effects of slow and rapid hemodialysis. Kidney Int 4: 177.

Arieff AI, Guisado R, Massry SG et al 1976 Central nervous system pH in uremia and the effects of hemodialysis. J Clin invest 58: 306.

Bennett WM, Aronoff GR, Golper TA et al 1994

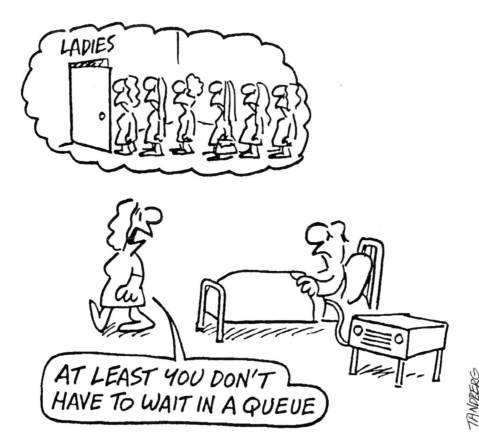

AT LEAST YOU DON'T HAVE TO WAIT IN A QUEUE

Drug Prescribing in Renal Failure: Dosing Guidelines for Adults. Philadelphia: American College of Physicians.

Caruana RJ 1987 Heparin free dialysis: comparative data and results in high risk patients. Kidney Int 31: 1351.

Cronin RE, Kaehny WD, Miller, PD et al 1976 Renal cell carcinoma: unusual systemic manifestations. Medicine 55: 291.

Dossetor JB 1966 Creatininemia versus uremia: the relative significance of blood urea nitrogen and serum creatinine in azotemia. Ann Intern Med 65: 1287.

Fraser CL, Arieff AI 1988 Nervous system complications of uremia. Ann Inter Med 109: 143.

Hoitsma AJ, Wetzels JFM, Koene RAP 1991 Drug-induced nephrotoxicity: aetiology, clinical features and management. Drug Safety 6: 131.

Hruska KA, Teitelbaum SL 1995 Renal osteodystrophy. N Engl J Med 333: 166.

Keshaviah P, Shapiro FL 1982 A critical examination of dialysis-induced hypotension. Am J Kidney Dis 2: 290.

Kincaid-Smith P 1980 Analgesic abuse and the kidney. Kidney Int 17: 250.

Massry SG, Glassock RJ (eds) 1994 Textbook of Nephrology. 3rd edition. Baltimore: Williams & Wilkins.

Mathew T 1988 Recurrence of disease after renal transplantation. Am J Kidney Dis 12: 85.

Morgan DB, Dillon S, Payne RB 1978 The assessment of glomerular function: creatinine clearance or plasma creatinine? Postgrad Med J 54: 302.

Raskin NH, Fishman RA 1976 Neurologic disorders in renal failure. N Engl J Med 294: 143.

Ronco PM, Flahault A 1994 Drug-induced end-stage renal disease. N Engl J Med 331: 1711.

Schrier RW 1992 An odyssey into the milieu interieur: pondering the enigmas. J Am Soc Nephrol 2: 1549.

Schwartz WB, Relman AS 1967 Effects of electrolyte

disorders on renal structure and function. N Engl J
Med 276: 383, 452.

Sherman RA, Eisinger RP 1982 The use (and
misuse) of urinary sodium and chloride
measurements. JAMA 247: 3121.

Stamm WE, Hooton TM 1993 Management of
urinary tract infections in adults. N Engl J Med
329: 1328.

Nephrotic syndrome (see Glomerular diseases)

Neural tube defects (see Arnold–Chiari malformation, Bathing, Folic acid deficiency and Syringomyelia)

Neurofibromatosis

Neurofibromatosis arises from dysplasia of the
neural and cutaneous ectoderm. It is inherited as
an autosomal dominant condition. The genes
(*NF-1* and *NF-2*) are on separate chromosomes,
NF-1 being responsible for 90% of cases and
NF-2 for 10%.

It is the most common neurocutaneous
disorder, with a prevalence of 1 in 3000 of the
population.

The most common form of neurofibromatosis is
referred to as **von Recklinghausen's disease**.
This comprises cafe au lait spots (which may be
present from birth), freckles in skin folds,
neurofibromas, plexiform neuromas, bilateral
hamartomas of the iris, neurological impairment
and bone involvement.

The neurofibromas are derived from all the
nerve elements, including the nerve cells, sheath
cells and connective tissue. Histologically, they
are therefore multicellular and while not
encapsulated they are well circumscribed.

They appear as soft pedunculated lesions from
puberty onwards. They are skin-coloured or
purplish and may be pruritic. Although they
may be become malignant (with sarcomatous

change especially in non-cutaneous sites), more
commonly they may eventually compress
surrounding structures. In the gut, a
neurofibroma may be one of the causes of polyp
formation.

The less common form of neurofibromatosis is
associated with bilateral acoustic neuromas.
There may also be meningioma or spinal cord
neurofibroma (which is usually subdural and
found in the thoracic region). Sometimes, there
may be associated glioma, cataracts or skin
lesions.

Neurofibromatosis may sometimes present with
skin lesions in a single dermatome or with an
associated phaeochromocytoma and thus
hypertension.

Treatment is with **excision** *of symptomatic lesions.*
Ketotifen *may be useful both for symptoms and to
decrease tumour growth.*

Genetic counselling should be undertaken.

Bibliography
Martuza RL, Eldridge R 1988 Neurofibromatosis 2
(bilateral acoustic neurofibromatosis). N Engl J
Med 318: 684.

Riccardi VM 1981 Von Recklinghausen's
neurofibromatosis. N Engl J Med 305: 1617.

Neuroleptic malignant syndrome

The neuroleptic malignant syndrome is a rare,
non-dose-related, idiosyncratic reaction which
may occur potentially to any antipsychotic
agent, though usually to phenothiazines. Its
pathogenesis is unclear, but it probably
represents dysfunction of the hypothalamus and
basal ganglia due to dopamine antagonism.

It is associated with fever, rigidity, fluctuating
consciousness and autonomic instability. These
clinical features generally evolve over a few
days.

Laboratory investigations usually show elevated
CK levels, renal impairment due to
myoglobinuria and dehydration, and abnormal
liver function tests.

The mortality has been reported to be possibly as high as 20%, but the condition is too rare to calculate a true mortality.

Treatment comprises drug cessation and general supportive measures.

Bromocriptine, *a dopamine agonist, and* **dantrolene**, *a direct-acting muscle relaxant (see Malignant hyperthermia), are probably helpful.*

There is a high incidence of recurrence if the culprit drug is resumed, so that alternative psychiatric therapy is required.

Bibliography

Caroff SN, Mann SC 1993 Neuroleptic malignant syndrome. Med Clin North Am 77: 185.

Guze BH, Baxter LR 1985. Neuroleptic malignant syndrome. N Engl J Med 313: 163.

Kornhuber J, Weller M 1994 Neuroleptic malignant syndrome. Curr Opin Neurol Neurosurg 7: 353.

Rosenberg MR, Green M 1989 Neuroleptic malignant syndrome: review of response to therapy. Ach Intern Med 149: 1927.

Shaw A, Mathews EE 1995 Postoperative neuroleptic malignant syndrome. Anesthesiology 50: 246.

Neurology

This book does not include the more common neurological disorders seen in Intensive Care, such as those related to cerebrovascular disease, trauma, headache, epilepsy or meningitis, but rather the large number of less frequently encountered neurological conditions, many of which raise important issues of diagnosis or management. They include:

- amnesia;
- amyotrophic lateral sclerosis;
- anorexia nervosa;
- Arnold–Chiari malformation;
- Bell's palsy;
- benign intracranial hypertension;
- central pontine myelinolysis;
- cerebellar degeneration;
- Charcot–Marie–Tooth disease;
- critical illness polyneuropathy;
- delirium;
- dementia;
- demyelinating disease;
- encephalitis;
- encephalopathy;
- epidural abscess;
- Guillain–Barré syndrome;
- hemianopia;
- Horner's syndrome;
- hydrocephalus;
- leukoencephalopathy;
- meningoencephalitis;
- motor neurone disease;
- multiple sclerosis;
- muscular dystrophies;
- myasthenia gravis;
- myelitis;

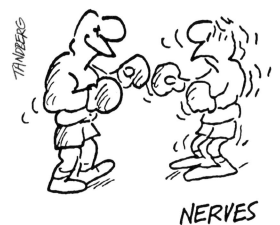

NERVES   "CURED"

- myelopathy;
- myopathy;
- neuropathy;
- ophthalmoplegia;
- optic neuritis;
- papilloedema;
- periodic paralysis;
- polyneuropathy;
- ptosis;
- restless legs;
- retinal haemorrhage;
- retrobulbar neuritis;
- syringomyelia;
- tardive dyskinesia;
- tinnitus;
- vertigo;
- Wernicke–Korsakoff syndrome.

Bibliography

Arieff AI, Massry SG, Barrientos A et al 1973 Brain water and electrolyte metabolism in uremia: effects of slow and rapid hemodialysis. Kidney Int 4: 177.

Arieff AI, Guisado R, Massry SG et al 1976 Central nervous system pH in uremia and the effects of hemodialysis. J Clin Invest 58: 306.

Bhardwaj A, Williams MA, Hanley DF (eds) 1997 Critical Care of Stroke. In: New Horizons. Baltimore: Williams & Wilkins and SCCM. 5: no. 4.

Bolton CF 1996 Sepsis and the systemic inflammatory response syndrome: Neuromuscular manifestations. Crit Care Med 24: 1408.

Bolton CF 1996 Neuromuscular conditions in the intensive care unit. Intens Care Med 22: 841.

Caplan LR, Brass LM, DeWitt LD (et al) 1990 Transcranial Doppler ultrasound: present status. Neurology 40: 696.

Chang CWJ 1999 Neurologic complications of critical illness and transplantation. Curr Opin Crit Care 5: 112.

Charness ME, Simon RP, Greenberg DA 1989 Ethanol and the nervous system. N Engl J Med 321: 442.

Chiappa KH, Ropper AH 1982 Evoked potentials in clinical medicine. N Engl J Med 306: 1140, 1205.

Ciavarella D, Wuest D, Strauss RG et al 1993 Management of neurologic disorders. J Clin Apheresis 8: 242.

Fraser CL, Arieff AI 1988 Nervous system complications of uremia. Ann Intern Med 109: 143.

Hansen-Flaschen J 1997 Neuromuscular complications of critical illness. Pulmonary Perspectives 14(4): 1.

Knochel J 1982 Neuromuscular manifestations of electrolyte disorders. Am J Med 72: 521.

Lyons MK, Meyer FB 1990 Cerebrospinal fluid physiology and the management of increased intracranial pressure. Mayo Clin Proc 65: 684.

Mandel JL 1989 Dystrophin: the gene and its product. Nature 339: 584.

Marton KI, Gean AD 1986 The spinal tap: a new look at an old test. Ann Intern Med 104: 840.

Miller DH, Raps EC (eds) 1999 Critical Care Neurology. Woburn: Butterworth–Heinemann.

Moore PM 1989 Diagnosis and management of isolated angiitis of the central nervous system. Neurology 39: 167.

Morantz RA, Walsh JW (eds) 1994 Brain Tumors. New York: Marcel Dekker.

Moskowitz MA 1991 The visceral organ brain. Neurology 41: 182.

Raskin NH, Fishman RA 1976 Neurologic disorders in renal failure. N Engl J Med 294: 143.

Rosenberg RN 1981 Biochemical genetics of neurologic disease. N Engl J Med 305: 1181.

Rosenberg RN 1998 Atlas of Clinical Neurology. Current Medicine 1998. Oxford: Butterworth–Heinemann.

Schwartzman RJ, McLellan TL 1987 Reflex sympathetic dystrophy: a review. Arch Neurol 44: 555.

Sherman DG, Dyken ML, Fisher M et al 1992 Antithrombotic therapy for cerebrovascular disorders. Chest 102: S529.

Strandgaard S, Paulson OB 1984 Cerebral autoregulation. Stroke 15: 413.

Strange K 1992 Regulation of solute and water balance and cell volume in the central nervous system. J Am Soc Nephrol 3: 12.

Swift TR 1981 Disorders of neuromuscular transmission other than myasthenia gravis. Muscle Nerve 4: 334.

Tonner DR, Schlechte JA 1993 Neurologic complications of thyroid and parathyroid disease. Med Clin North Am 77: 251.

Wall PD, Melzack RE 1994 Textbook of Pain. 3rd edition. Edinburgh: Churchill Livingstone.

Zweiman B, Levinson AI 1992 Immunologic aspects of neurological and neuromuscular diseases. JAMA 268: 2918.

Neuropathy

Neuropathy is usually a polyneuropathy. Sometimes, it may be a mononeuropathy or an asymmetrical mononeuropathy multiplex. It may be either motor or sensory or more commonly both motor and sensory. Mononeuropathy is commonly due to a local cause.

The types of polyneuropathy include:

1. genetic neuropathies;
2. toxic neuropathies;
3. inflammatory neuropathies;
4. systemic disease-induced neuropathies;
5. critical illness neuropathy;
6. diabetic neuropathy;
7. Guillain–Barré syndrome (GBS) and its variants;
8. multi-focal motor neuropathy.

1. **Genetic neuropathies** include:

- Charcot–Marie–Tooth disease (q.v.).

2. **Toxic neuropathies** may be produced by:

- drugs

  - such as amiodarone, cytotoxics, gold, hydralazine, isoniazid, nitrofurantoin, phenytoin;

- heavy metals

  - such as arsenic and lead in particular;

- poisons, mainly industrial chemical agents

  - such as acrylamide, hexacarbons, organophosphates, rapeseed oil, trichloroethylene.

3. **Inflammatory neuropathies** may occur in:

- AIDS, diphtheria, leprosy.

4. **Systemic disease-induced neuropathies** can be produced by:

- malignancy

  - as a paraneoplastic phenomenon, especially in carcinoma of the breast, lung or ovary, or in multiple myeloma;

- collagen-vascular diseases;
- alcoholism;
- nutritional deficiency;
- sarcoidosis;
- Lyme disease;
- porphyria;
- uraemia;
- vitamin B_{12} deficiency.

5. **Critical illness neuropathy**

Critical illness neuropathy/polyneuropathy (CIP) is the most common and best recognized of the critical illness neuromuscular disorders (CINMA). It comprises axonal degeneration of peripheral nerves seen in patients with sepsis and/or multi-organ failure (MOF) of prolonged duration. It may therefore represent the neurological manifestation of MOF. It is not generally apparent until after at least a week of critical illness.

This condition was first described in the early 1980s, but no specific aetiology has yet been demonstrated. In patients with multiorgan failure prospectively examined electrophysiologically, the incidence has been found to be as high as 70%. However, the overall incidence in Intensive Care patients appears to vary greatly, and even mild clinical features are found in only about half of those suspected on EMG of having CIP.

Motor features are generally more prominent than sensory or autonomic, with generalized weakness and wasting due to muscle denervation. There is symmetrical flaccid paresis, particularly of the lower limbs, with reduced deep tendon reflexes. In severe cases, breathing and swallowing can be affected. There is relative preservation of cranial nerve function.

The diagnosis can of course be difficult, because of the limitations of neurological examination in Intensive Care patients receiving sedation and muscle relaxants and because of the many other causes of neurological dysfunction seen in such patients. The EMG shows an axonal polyneuropathy and there is abnormal spontaneous muscle activity typical of denervation. Conduction velocities are normal, whereas they are reduced in demyelination (as in Guillain–Barré syndrome).

CIP needs to be distinguished in particular from an acute myopathy, such as that typically seen in Intensive Care patients who have had prolonged neuromuscular blockade and/or corticosteroids (see Myopathy).

If the phrenic nerve is involved, prolonged ventilator dependence may result.

The mortality is reported to be about 60%, but clearly this is also the mortality of the severe underlying conditions. The motor disturbances of CIP are not always reversible, even with prolonged rehabilitation.

6. Diabetic neuropathy

A neuropathy may be found in about 60% of patients with either insulin-dependent or non-insulin-dependent diabetes mellitus. The precise mechanism of production of this neuropathy is unclear.

Polyneuropathy is seen in about half of these cases. There is symmetrical distal mainly sensory involvement. It is often subclinical, but mild symptoms are sometimes seen. These are especially paraesthesiae of the lower limbs, occasionally with sensory loss and even weakness and decreased reflexes. The condition is worse at night and can be very painful. In some patients, it eventually becomes severe, with associated autonomic involvement, including urinary retention, faecal incontinence, impotence and postural hypotension.

Mononeuropathy is seen in about a third of cases. Like diabetic polyneuropathy, it is also often subclinical. Symptoms when seen relate usually to the carpal tunnel syndrome.

Occasionally, other nerves are involved, either singly or combined, such as:

- cranial (especially VII, III and VI);
- ulnar;
- femoral;
- sciatic;
- peroneal;
- lateral femoral cutaneous;
- thoracic roots.

Sometimes, diabetic amyotrophy may be produced, with painful wasting and weakness of the proximal muscles of the lower limbs.

The EMG in diabetic neuropathy typically shows the abnormal nerve conduction of denervation. CSF examination shows a moderately increased protein.

The neuropathy may be improved with good diabetic control. Pain may be alleviated in some cases by carbamazepine or tricyclic antidepressants.

7. **Guillain–Barré syndrome** (GBS) is an acute idiopathic polyneuritis (acute inflammatory demyelinating polyradiculoneuropathy). It is the most common type of acute neuromuscular paralysis. There is patchy inflammation and demyelination of peripheral nerves, with axonal degeneration in some severe cases.

The aetiology is presumed to be immunological, since antibodies may be found to myelin and there is an increased serum concentration of IL-2 receptors indicating T cell activation. The trigger of the putative immune attack is unknown, as is its specific molecular target. Although there is an increased incidence in Hodgkin's disease and SLE, the majority of patients have had an infective illness in the previous two months, with particularly severe disease following diarrhoea due to *Campylobacter jejuni* and with a small increased risk following influenza vaccination.

Clinical features comprise the acute onset of predominantly motor dysfunction commencing in the legs and ascending to the trunk, arms, face and even bulbar muscles over a few days. Typically, the conditions progresses for 1–4 weeks and is followed by gradual improvement over weeks to months. Complications particularly include:

- respiratory failure;
- dysautonomia;
- inappropriate ADH syndrome;
- the consequences of prolonged Intensive Care with associated instrumentation.

The diagnosis is made clinically and is supported by nerve conduction studies (although these may be initially normal) and by CSF findings of a raised protein level (which may not be apparent for over a week) but usually no cells.

A discrete sensory level, asymmetrical features or mononuclear cells in the CSF suggest an alternative diagnosis of either an inflammatory or neoplastic nature.

*The treatment of affected patients requires complex and prolonged care. Corticosteroids are not helpful, but **plasmapheresis** and **immune globulin** (ivIG) have both been shown in clinical trials to be effective if given early, presumably because they modulate the inflammatory process responsible for the nerve injury rather than promoting nerve regeneration or remyelination. They are of similar efficacy and have no demonstrable additive benefit when combined.*

- *Plasmapheresis should be commenced early, with 3.5 L exchanges second daily for five occasions. The course may need be repeated after two weeks, if there is a relapse.*
- *Immune globulin is given in a dose 0.5 g/kg daily for five days. It is certainly less complicated than plasma exchange and is probably as effective.*

The mortality is now <5%, but recovery is slow and some patients have persistent weakness (especially those with preceding *C. jejuni* infection).

Variants of Guillain–Barré syndrome include:

- **chronic relapsing polyneuropathy**. This is a recurrent form of GBS. It can be associated with neurofibromatosis and with some HLA types.

It is steroid-responsive.

- **chronic inflammatory demyelinating polyneuropathy** (CIDP). This is a more slowly progressive condition, with a poorer recovery.

It may respond to corticosteroids, immune suppression, immune globulin or plasmapheresis.

- **Miller Fisher syndrome**. This refers to the presence of a triad of ataxia, ophthalmoplegia and areflexia, in the absence of significant limb weakness.

8. **Multi–focal motor neuropathy** (see Amyotrophic lateral sclerosis).

The types of mononeuropathy include the following:

- **Carpal tunnel syndrome**;
- **Brachial plexus neuropathy**;
- **Isolated palsies**.

These are usually due to a local disease (or sometimes diabetes) and involve the radial, ulnar, peroneal or lateral femoral cutaneous nerves.

- **Cranial neuropathies**

If multiple, they are usually paraneoplastic (though sometimes they may be diabetic).

Individual cranial neuropathies may be caused as follows.

I

- meningioma;
- meningitis;
- post-viral;
- trauma;

II

- optic atrophy (often nutritional);
- optic neuritis (see above);
- tumour (craniopharyngioma, glioma, pituitary);

III, IV, VI

- see Ophthalmoplegia;

V

- trigeminal neuralgia (tic douloureux);
- disorders of the posterior cranial fossa or base of skull (the most common causes of a V nerve lesion);

VII

- Bell's palsy;
- lesions of the pons or cerebellopontine angle;
- sarcoidosis;
- Guillain–Barré syndrome;
- hemifacial spasm (it and related disorders are now being usefully treated with botulinum toxin);

VIII

- acoustic neuroma;
- aminoglycoside toxicity;
- brainstem lesions;
- Ménière's disease;
- meningitis;
- vestibular neuronitis;

IX, X, XI

- brainstem lesions;
- cervical infection, trauma or tumour;
- jugular foramen syndrome;
- motor neurone disease;

XII

- cervical infection, trauma or tumour,
- motor neurone disease.

Bibliography

Ashbury AK 1988 Understanding diabetic neuropathy. N Engl J Med 319: 577.

Ashbury AK, Cornblath DR 1990 Assessment of current diagnostic criteria for Guillain-Barré syndrome. Ann Neurol 27 (suppl): S21.

Berek K, Margreiter J, Willeit J et al 1996 Polyneuropathies in critically ill patients: a prospective evaluation. Intens Care Med 22: 849.

Bleck TP 1996 The expanding spectrum of critical illness polyneuropathy. Crit Care Med 24: 1282.

Bolton CF 1996 Sepsis and the systemic inflammatory response syndrome: neuromuscular manifestations. Crit Care Med 24: 1408.

Bolton CF, Gilbert JJ, Hahn AF et al 1984 Polyneuropathy in critically ill patients. J Neurol Neurosurg Psychiatry 47: 1223.

Bromberg MB, Feldman EL, Albers JW 1992 Chronic inflammatory demyelinating polyradiculoneuropathy. Neurology 42: 1157.

Chad DA, Lacomis D 1994 Critically ill patients with newly acquired weakness: the clinicopathological spectrum. Ann Neurol 35: 257.

Dalakas MC, Engel WK 1981 Chronic relapsing (dysimmune) polyneuropathy: pathogenesis and treatment. Ann Neurol 9 (suppl): 134.

De Jonghe B, Cook D, Sharshar T et al 1998 Acquired neuromuscular disorders in critically ill patients: a systematic review. Intens Care Med 24: 1242.

Dyck PJ, Kratz KM, Karnes JL et al 1993 The prevalence by staged severity of various types of diabetic neuropathy, retinopathy, and nephropathy in a population-based cohort: the Rochester Diabetic Neuropathy Study. Neurology 43: 817.

Feasby TE, Hughes RA 1998 *Campylobacter jejuni*, antiganglioside antibodies, and Guillain–Barré syndrome. Neurology 51: 340.

Fisher M 1956 An unusual variant of acute idiopathic polyneuritis (syndrome of ophthalmoplegia, ataxia and areflexia). N Engl J Med 255: 57.

Fuller GN, Jacobs JM, Guiloff RJ 1993 Nature and incidence of peripheral neuropathy syndromes in HIV infection. J Neurol Neurosurg Psychiatry 56: 372.

Halperin J, Luft BJ, Volkman DJ et al 1990 Lyme neuroborreliosis: peripheral nervous system manifestations. Brain 113: 1207.

Hansen-Flaschen J 1997 Neuromuscular complications of critical illness. Pulmonary Perspectives 14(4): 1.

Harrison MS 1962 "Epidemic vertigo" – "vestibular neuronitis": a clinical study. Brain 85: 613.

Hillbom M, Wennberg A 1984 Prognosis of alcoholic peripheral neuropathy. J Neurol Neurosurg Psychiatry 47: 699.

Hughes RAC 1991 Ineffectiveness of high-dose intravenous methylprednisolone in Guillain-Barré syndrome. Lancet 338: 1142.

Hughes RA, van der Meche FG 2000 Corticosteroids for treating Guillain-Barré syndrome. Cochrane Database Systematic Review 2: CD001446.

Hund EF, Fogel W, Krieger D et al 1996 Critical illness polyneuropathy: Clinical findings and outcomes of a frequent cause of neuromuscular weaning failure. Crit Care Med 24: 1328.

Lasky T, Terracciano GJ, Magder L et al 1998 The Guillain-Barré syndrome and the 1992–1993 and 1993–1994 influenza vaccines. N Engl J Med 339: 1797.

Leijten FSS, De Weerd AW, Poortvliet DCJ et al
1996 Critical illness polyneuropathy in multiple
organ dysfunction syndrome and weaning from the
ventilator. Intens Care Med 22: 856.

Moore P, Owen J 1981 Guillain–Barré syndrome:
incidence, management and outcome of major
complications. Crit Care Med 9: 549.

Morantz RA, Walsh JW (eds) 1994 Brain Tumors.
New York: Marcel Dekker.

Nakamo KK 1978 The entrapment neuropathies.
Muscle Nerve 1: 264.

Nates JL, Cooper DJ, Day B et al 1997 Acute
weakness syndromes in critically ill patients – a
reappraisal. Anaesth Intens Care 25: 502.

Pestronk A 1991 Motor neuropathies, motor neuron
disorders, and antiglycolipid antibodies. Muscle
Nerve 14: 927.

Plasma Exchange/Sandoglobulin Guillain–Barré
Syndrome Trial Group 1997 Randomised trial of
plasma exchange, intravenous immunoglobulin,
and combined treatments in Guillain–Barré
syndrome. Lancet 349: 225.

Rees JH, Soudain SE, Gregson NA, Hughes RAC
1995 *Campylobacter jejuni* infection and
Guillain–Barré syndrome. N Engl J Med 333:
1374.

Ropper AH 1988 Campylobacter diarrhea and
Guillain–Barré syndrome. Arch Neurol 45: 655.

Ropper AH 1992 The Guillain–Barré syndrome. N
Engl J Med 326: 1130.

Segredo V, Caldwell JE, Matthay MA et al 1992
Persistent paralysis in critically ill patients after
long-term administration of vecuronium. N Engl J
Med 327: 524.

Sweet WH 1986 The treatment of trigeminal
neuralgia (tic douloureux). N Engl J Med 315:
174.

van der Meche FGA, Schmitz PIM 1992 The Dutch
Guillain–Barré Study Group: A randomized trial
comparing intravenous immune globulin and
plasma exchange in Guillain–Barré syndrome. N
Engl J Med 326: 1123.

Williams AC, Sturman S, Kelsey S et al 1986 The
neuropathy of the critically ill. Br Med J 293: 790.

Windebank AJ, Blexrud MD, Dyck PJ et al 1990
The syndrome of acute sensory neuropathy:
clinical features and electrophysiologic and
pathologic changes. Neurology 40: 584.

Zochodne DW, Bolton CF, Wells GA et al 1987
Critical illness polyneuropathy: A complication
of sepsis and multiple organ failure. Brain 110:
819.

Neutropenia

Neutropenia refers to an absolute neutrophil count in peripheral blood of $<2 \times 10^9$/L. Often it is $<1 \times 10^9$/L; in severe cases, it is $<0.5 \times 10^9$/L. However, in some ethnic populations, neutrophil counts as low as 1×10^9/L may in fact be normal.

The causes of neutropenia are:

- decreased production;
- increased removal;
- sequestration.

Decreased production is due usually to:

- drugs, the most common cause – see below;
- viral infection;
- bone marrow hypoplasia or infiltration;

or less commonly to

- folic acid or vitamin B_{12} deficiency;
- Felty's syndrome;
- cachexia.

Genetic, cyclic and chronic benign forms of neutropenia due to decreased production sometimes occur.

Increased removal from the circulation occurs:

- in immune disease

  – especially Felty's syndrome;

- with drugs (see below).

Sequestration of neutrophils occurs

- in splenomegaly;
- with toxic margination

  – best known in Gram-negative sepsis.

Drugs which impair granulopoiesis may do so via cytotoxic, immunological or idiosyncratic mechanisms. Most cases recover within two days to two weeks.

- **Cytotoxic effects** are produced by a wide variety of agents. These include:

  – cancer chemotherapeutic agents (most commonly),
  – benzene and related compounds.

- **Immunological mechanisms** are invoked by:

  – beta-lactam antibiotics;
  – hydralazine;
  – procainamide;
  – quinidine.

- **Idiosyncratic mechanisms** are involved with:

  – analgesics (especially NSAIDs, classically phenylbutazone but also indomethacin);
  – antibiotics (ampicillin, chloramphenicol);
  – antihistamines;
  – antithyroid drugs;
  – cimetidine;
  – phenytoin;
  – procainamide;
  – quinidine;
  – ranitidine;
  – sulfonamides;
  – tranquillizers (especially phenothiazines and most recently clozapine).

Clinically, the neutropenia may be found coincidentally or because of an infection. Such infections may produce diminished signs because of the absence of pus, and they typically respond poorly to antibiotics. They particularly involve the skin, respiratory tract and urinary tract, and they are due to an increased risk of infection by those pathogens which normally colonize the body's surfaces.

*Treatment is primarily of the underlying problem, but occasional cases respond to **corticosteroids** or even **lithium**.*

- *Granulocyte colony-stimulating factor (G-CSF) is effective in many types of neutropenia.*
- *Antibiotics in this setting need to be bactericidal. Antibiotic regimens need to be carefully considered,* *because prolonged use of broad-spectrum agents can lead to colonization and infection by resistant organisms, including fungi.*

Bibliography

Dale D, Guerry D, Wewerka J et al 1979 Chronic neutropenia. Medicine 58: 128.

Jones RN 1999 Contemporary antimicrobial susceptibility patterns of bacterial pathogens commonly associated with febrile patients with neutropenia. Clin Infect Dis 29: 495.

van der Klauw MM, Wilson JH, Stricker BH 1998 Drug-associated agranulocytosis. Am J Haematol 57: 206.

Vincent PC 1986 Drug-induced aplastic anemia and agranulocytosis. Drugs 31: 52.

Neutrophilia

Neutrophilia refers to an increased peripheral blood neutrophil count of $>7.5 \times 10^9$/L.

Neutrophilia is a very common finding and may be produced by several mechanisms, namely:

1. **increased production and/or release**, due to

   – inflammatory diseases;
   – malignancy;
   – lithium;
   – cytokine administration (e.g. G-CSF, GM-CSF);

2. **decreased exit from the circulation**, due to

   – physical activity;
   – corticosteroids;

3. **decreased sequestration and/or margination**, due to

   – physical activity;
   – corticosteroids;
   – adrenergic influences.

This third mechanism causes a pseudo-neutrophilia, because the blood pool of neutrophils is not in fact increased.

Any treatment is of the underlying disorder.

Non-respiratory thoracic disorders

Non-respiratory thoracic disorders considered in this book are those related to abnormalities of the:

- chest wall (q.v.);
- diaphragm (q.v.);
- mediastinum (q.v.);
- pleural cavity (q.v.).

Norwalk virus

Norwalk virus is the commonest cause (40%) of non-bacterial gastroenteritis worldwide. It was named following an outbreak in Norwalk, Ohio in 1968. It is acquired from food, especially seafood, water or other persons (with a variable transmission rate reported between 4–43%). There is a year-round risk. Following an incubation period of 24–48 h during which time the proximal small bowel becomes infected, there is nausea, watery diarrhoea and systemic symptoms which last another 24–48 h.

The diagnosis is made by electron microscopy or radioimmunoassay of antigen in faeces.

The differential diagnosis includes other Norwalk like-viruses, enteroviruses, hepatitis, and in children rotavirus.

*Treatment is with **fluid replacement**.*

Nutrition (see Metabolism and nutrition)

O

Obstetrics and gynaecology

Several aspects of women's health are of relevance to Intensive Care, particularly obstetric disasters and gynaecological illnesses of a septic or multi-organ nature. Those considered in this book include:

- abortion;
- acute fatty liver of pregnancy;
- amenorrhoea;
- amniotic fluid embolism;
- HELLP syndrome;
- ovarian hyperstimulation syndrome;
- pneumonia in pregnancy;
- pre-eclampsia;
- pregnancy;
- salpingitis;
- trauma in pregnancy.

Bibliography

Australian Drug Evaluation Committee 1999 Prescribing Medicines in Pregnancy. 4th edition. Canberra: Australian Government Printing Service.

Australian Society for the Study of Hypertension in Pregnancy 1993 Management of hypertension in pregnancy: consensus statement. Med J Aust 158: 700.

Batagol R 1996 Drugs and Breast Feeding. Melbourne: CSL Pharmaceuticals.

Briggs GG, Freeman RL, Yaffe SJ (eds) 1990 Drugs in Pregnancy and Lactation. 3rd edition. Baltimore: Williams & Wilkins.

Brooks DC, Sznyter LA 1998 Pregnancy. In Scientific American Surgery, Section VII Special Problems in Perioperative Care, Chapter 11. New York: Scientific American.

Chestnut DH 1989 Critical care in obstetric practice. In: Fuhrman BP, Shoemaker WC (eds) Critical Care: State of the Art, Chapter 7. Fullerton: Society of Critical Care Medicine. 121.

Clark SL, Cotton DB, Hankins GDV et al 1997 Critical Care Obstetrics. Oxford: Blackwell.

Cope I 1991 Medicines in pregnancy. Med J Aust 155: 214.

Council on Scientific Affairs, American Medical

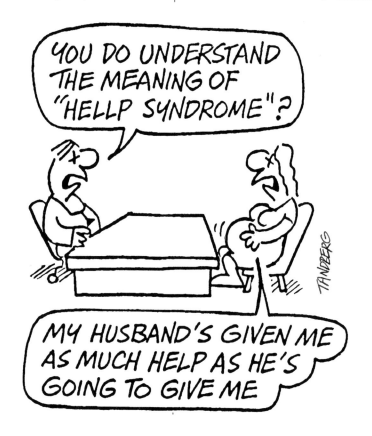

Association 1983 Fetal effects of maternal alcohol use. JAMA 249: 2517.

Jamal S, Maurer JR 1994 Pulmonary disease and the menstrual cycle. Pulmonary Perspectives 11: 3.

Lim V, Katz A, Lindheimer M 1976 Acid–base regulation in pregnancy. Am J Physiol 231: 1764.

Newmark ME, Penry JK 1980 Catamenial epilepsy: a review. Epilepsia 21: 281.

Rizk NW, Kalassian KG, Gilligan T et al 1996 Obstetric complications in pulmonary and critical care medicine. Chest 110: 791.

Sanson B-J, Lensing AWA, Prins MH et al 1999 Safety of low-molecular-weight heparin in pregnancy: a systematic review. Thromb Haemost 81: 668.

Wood CE 1996 Menorrhagia: a clinical update. Med J Aust 165: 510.

Occupational lung diseases

Lung damage from inhalation of dusts, fumes or other injurious substances may occur in many occupations in most societies. There is a vast number of such substances, and the consequences of their inhalation range from minor to severe. Fortunately, most substances to which the population is exposed are not harmful, and those that are injurious are probably well recognized nowadays, so that appropriate preventive measures can be taken.

It is worth noting that in general, occupational diseases are not pathologically unique. They are the same as their counterparts due to other causes and are distinguished primarily by their history.

> The major occupational lung diseases comprise the following:
>
> - pneumoconiosis;
> - occupational asthma;
> - hypersensitivity pneumonitis;
> - acute lung irritation;
> - occupational pulmonary infections;
> - occupational pulmonary neoplasms;
> - miscellaneous occupational lung diseases.

1. **Pneumoconiosis** refers to the permanent accumulation of inhaled dust in the lungs, together with the tissue reaction to its presence.

A dust is an aerosol of solid, inanimate particles, and their size should be less than 10 μm to be retained in the lung. This size is somewhat unusual, especially in nature, and requires the disruptive forces of industrial processes. Moreover, only a few specific dusts among the many produced give rise to clinical disease. In addition, associated damage due to smoking is very common and may outweigh any effect of inhaled dust.

> The chief pneumoconioses are due to:
>
> - coal dust;
> - silica;
> - asbestos.

Coal dust and **silica** give rise to simple pneumoconiosis with few or no symptoms or lung function abnormalities, but the chest X-ray shows diffuse, multiple, rounded opacities, often primarily affecting the upper lobes. If the silica is inhaled as very fine particles, a diffuse interstitial fibrosis rather than a nodular pathology may result.

For reasons that are unclear but may be immunological, some patients develop complicated pneumoconiosis in the form of **progressive massive fibrosis** with large fibrotic lesions, often with cavities and usually in the upper lobes. Symptoms of dyspnoea and cough now appear. The progressive massive fibrosis of silicosis and of coal workers' pneumoconiosis may be complicated by tuberculosis or rheumatoid arthritis (Caplan's syndrome), respectively.

Asbestos (q.v.) may produce progressive, diffuse fibrosis, at which stage symptoms appear. Lung function changes, particularly decreased gas transfer, precede both symptoms and radiographic changes.

In addition to producing a pneumoconiosis (asbestosis), asbestos also predisposes to:

- calcified pleural plaques;
- diffuse pleural fibrosis;
- bronchogenic carcinoma;
- pleural and peritoneal mesothelioma.

Pneumoconioses are also produced by:

- other silicates (e.g. talc and kaolin, but not cement or fibreglass);
- aluminium;
- barium sulfate;
- iron oxide;
- tin oxide;
- tungsten carbide;
- beryllium (q.v.) (beryllium also gives rise to diffuse granuloma formation).

2. **Occupational asthma** may be caused by exposure to substances which are allergenic, pharmacologically active or directly irritant to the bronchial tree.

Animal danders, vegetable, flower and grain dusts, wood dusts, cotton dusts, isocyanates, latex, soldering flux, insecticides, gases (e.g. sulfur dioxide) and various chemicals and proteolytic enzymes may be incriminated.

Many patients have no past history or family history of asthma or atopy, and symptoms may sometimes be atypical in that wheeze is not always prominent. Typically, the symptoms are worse at work and subside at weekends ('Monday morning asthma') and on holidays, but eventually they may become chronic.

3. **Hypersensitivity pneumonitis** (q.v.).

4. **Acute lung irritation** (q.v.).

5. **Occupational pulmonary infections** include:

- tuberculosis
    - in health workers and miners with silicosis;
- Q fever
    - in farmers, veterinarians and abattoir workers;

- hydatid disease
    - in sheep farmers.

6. **Occupational pulmonary neoplasms** include:

- carcinoma of the lung
    - following exposure to asbestos, uranium mining, arsenic, nickel, chromate, beryllium, mustard gas and probably other substances;
- mesothelioma
    - following exposure to asbestos (q.v.).

7. **Miscellaneous occupational lung diseases** include:

- byssinosis
    - a condition found in textile workers inhaling cotton, flax or hemp dust;
    - with cough, chest tightness, dyspnoea and wheeze, especially on Mondays;
    - with an obstructive pattern on spirometry but a normal chest X-ray;
- pulmonary infiltration due to hair sprays
    - sometimes picturesquely called thesaurosis;
- paraquat lung
    - a lethal, proliferative and destructive reaction following ingestion of this toxic weed killer (q.v.).

Bibliography

Bernardo J, Center DM 1981 Hypersensitivity pneumonia. Dis Mon 27: 1.

Berry G 1995 Environmental mesothelioma incidence, time since exposure to asbestos and level of exposure. Environmetrics 6: 221.

Chan-Yeung M, Malo J-L 1995 Occupational asthma. N Engl J Med 333: 107.

Davidoff F 1998 New disease, old story. Ann Intern Med 129: 327.

Ho A, Chan H, Tse KS et al 1996 Occupational asthma due to latex in health care workers. Thorax 51: 1280.

Mitchell CA 1997 Occupational lung disease. Med J Aust 167: 498.

Schwartz DA 1987 Acute inhalational injury. Occup Med 2: 297.

van Kempen V, Merget R, Baur X 2000 Occupational airway sensitizers. Am J Ind Med 38: 164.

Octreotide (see Acromegaly, Carcinoid syndrome, Diarrhoea, Glucagonoma and Hepatopulmonary syndrome)

Oncofetal antigen (see Alpha-fetoprotein and Carcinoembryonic antigen)

Ophthalmoplegia

Ophthalmoplegia refers to weakness of the ocular muscles due to damage to the III, IV and/or VI cranial nerves.

- If **unilateral**, it is commonly due to an orbital lesion. It may also be associated with:
  - an intracavernous carotid artery aneurysm,
  - diabetes,
  - recent viral infection.
- If **bilateral**, it may be caused by:
  - cavernous sinus thrombosis,
  - midbrain lesion (usually ischaemic),
  - multiple sclerosis,
  - myasthenia gravis,
  - Wernicke's encephalopathy.

Clinical features are manifest as follows:

- III nerve damage causes weakness of upward, downward and inward eye movement, associated with ptosis and a dilated pupil;
- IV nerve damage causes weakness of downward and inward eye movement;
- VI nerve damage causes weakness of outward eye movement.

Optic neuritis (see Multiple sclerosis)

Orchitis

The major causes of **orchitis** are:

- mumps;
- varicella;
- typhoid;
- Coxsackie virus B infection;
- filariasis.

In post-pubertal males, mumps causes orchitis in about 10% of patients and is then followed in half by infertility and testicular atrophy.

Orchitis should be distinguished from:

- epididymitis (q.v.);
- testicular torsion;
- testicular tumour.

Organophosphates (see Warfare agents)

Osler–Weber–Rendu disease (see Arteriovenous malformations)

Ovarian hyperstimulation syndrome

Ovarian hyperstimulation syndrome (OHSS) is a serious multisystem complication of ovulation induction, first described in 1984. Ovarian stimulation by exogenous hormone administration is used to produce the oocytes needed in IVF and GIFT programmes, and OHSS is thus an inadvertent iatrogenic condition.

The pathogenesis of OHSS is presumably an exaggeration of the normal ovulation process, with mediator release, increased capillary permeability, and fluid shift from the intravascular space into the serous cavities. There is thus hypovolaemia and haemoconcentration.

267

OHSS occurs in about 20% of ovarian inductions, with the majority of cases being mild and only about 1% being severe. It occurs a few days after the start of the luteal phase and usually lasts only a week or so.

OHSS is classified as:

- mild disease

  – Grade 1 (abdominal discomfort and distension);
  – Grade 2 (nausea, vomiting and diarrhoea);

- moderate disease

  – Grade 3 (ascites);

- severe disease

  – Grade 4 (ascites, pleural effusion and dyspnoea);
  – Grade 5 (hypovolaemia, hypotension, oliguria, coagulopathy).

In the full-blown picture, there is thus:

- shock;
- multiorgan failure (acute respiratory distress syndrome, renal failure, liver dysfunction);
- thrombosis and/or haemorrhage.

Treatment is required for all except mild cases, which are self-limiting within about two weeks. Appropriate treatment comprises urgent Intensive Care management, with fluid resuscitation, circulatory monitoring, albumin administration, and abdominal and pleural paracenteses.

Specific pharmacological treatment is not available, as antihistamines and prostaglandin inhibitors have been disappointing, though recently ACE inhibitors have shown promise.

Bibliography

Brinsden PR, Wada I, Tan SL et al 1995 Diagnosis, prevention and management of ovarian hyperstimulation syndrome. Br J Obstet Gynaecol 102: 767.

Golan A, Ron-El R, Herman A et al 1989 Ovarian hyperstimulation syndrome: an update review. Obstet Gynecol Surv 44: 430.

Myrianthefs P, Ladakis C, Lappas V et al 2000 Ovarian hyperstimulation syndrome (OHSS): diagnosis and management. Intens Care Med 26: 631.

Tassone M, Kuhn R, Talbot JM 1997 Ovarian hyperstimulation syndrome. Aust NZ J Obstet Gynaecol 37: 5.

Williamson K, Mushambi MC 1994 Ovarian hyperstimulation syndrome. Br J Anaesth 3: 731.

Oxytocin (see Desmopressin)

Paget's disease

Paget's disease of bone is a local disorder with considerable histological complexity.

Although its aetiology is uncertain, there is some familial clustering and variable ethnic prevalence (e.g. it is found in up to 3% of older patients in North America and Western Europe but not in Asia). This epidemiology, together with the finding of intranuclear inclusion bodies resembling paramyxovirus nucleocapsids and reacting against measles, RSV or other related viruses, suggests that the disease may be due to an infectious agent acquired some years before.

Histologically, there is a mixed osteolytic/osteoblastic process, the latter becoming predominant later in the disease. In addition to increased bone reabsorption with abnormal osteoclasts, there is osteoblastic activity with new bone formation, typically a mosaic of both lamellar and woven bone. A loose fibrous stroma with prominent vessels replaces the bone marrow. The entire process may be different in different bones at the same time.

The clinical features of a focal bone disorder of this type clearly depend on its site and extent.

- Although commonly asymptomatic, there may be local deformity, local pain, local hyperaemia or pathological fracture. Specific local symptoms include deafness, neural compression or renal calculi (if there has been hypercalcuria).
- Systemically, there may be a hyperdynamic state, if more than 30% of the skeleton is involved. These features are usually seen in middle-aged or elderly patients.
- Occasionally, there may be neoplastic change, either benign giant cell tumour (which is locally destructive) or osteosarcoma (of the osteolytic type). Most osteosarcomas in adults arise in patients with Paget's disease.

Investigations include abnormal X-ray findings, especially in the skull, with lytic lesions surrounded by a somewhat irregular margin. Even if the X-ray is normal, there may be increased uptake on isotope bone scans. There is increased urinary hydroxyproline (reflecting collagen reabsorption) and increased plasma type I procollagen fragments (reflecting collagen synthesis). Although the serum alkaline phosphatase is increased, the urinary calcium is generally normal, unless the patient is confined to bed. Hypercalcaemia is also uncommon (despite an increased calcium and phosphate flux which may rise up to 20-fold without changes in plasma levels), and this too occurs usually only with immobilization such as with bed rest.

Treatment is often not required. Symptoms respond to NSAIDs for clinically significant disease. Specific inhibition of osteoclast formation and function may be obtained with calcitonin, bisphosphonates or plicamycin (mithramycin).

- *Calcitonin has been available for about 20 years and improves most clinical features except deafness. It is given as 50–100 U sc daily or second daily on a long-term basis, since relapse follows its cessation. Although its onset of action is prompt, the fall in alkaline phosphatase, sometimes even to normal values, may take some weeks. Occasional side-effects include nausea, flushing, abnormal taste and local bone pain. More importantly, antibodies develop in some patients, who thus become resistant unless the synthetic human form of calcitonin is then used.*
- *Bisphosphonates include aledronate, pamidronate and etidronate (see Hypercalcaemia). These too may exacerbate local pain, but improvement tends to be sustained for many months after cessation of therapy.*
- *Plicamycin is given in a dose of 15 μg/kg per day for 10 days. These are much lower doses than are used for cancer chemotherapy, so that although nausea or thrombocytopenia may occur, bone marrow, liver and renal toxicity do not occur. Again, prolonged remissions may be produced.*

Paget's disease of nipple comprises a reddish scaly and often ulcerated plaque, involving the nipple and areola and associated with an underlying carcinoma.

It is unilateral and mostly seen in women. However, extramammary lesions of a similar nature can be seen in either sex, involving apocrine gland sites, especially in the perineum or axilla. These too usually reflect an underlying carcinoma.

Bibliography

Singer FR 1991 Clinical efficacy of salmon calcitonin in Paget's disease of bone. Calcif Tissue Int 49 (suppl 2): S7.

Singer FR 1995 Paget's disease of bone. In: De Groot LJ (ed) Endocrinology. Philadelphia: p 1259.

Singer FR, Minoofar PN 1995 Bisphosphonates in the treatment of disorders of mineral metabolism. Adv Endocrinol Metab 6: 259.

Palmar erythema

Palmar erythema describes a dark reddish-purple area on the palm of the hand, usually over the hypothenar eminence.

> It is typically associated with hepatic cirrhosis, but it is also seen in chronic active hepatitis, thyrotoxicosis and rheumatoid arthritis.

Pancreatitis

Acute pancreatitis is well known to be precipitated by alcohol or biliary disease.

> Less common causes of acute pancreatitis include:
>
> * hypercalcaemia;
> * hyperlipoproteinaemia;
> * abdominal trauma
>
>   – including surgery;
>
> * infections
>
>   – particularly mumps, salmonella;
>
> * drugs
>
>   – especially azathioprine, cytosine arabinoside, frusemide, oestrogens, sulfonamides, tetracycline, thiazides.

The treatment of severe acute pancreatitis is well known in Intensive Care practice and its elements have recently been critically reviewed (see bibliography).

Chronic pancreatitis is also well known to be associated with:

* alcoholism;
* biliary disease.

It may less commonly follow abdominal trauma.

Bibliography

Baron TH, Morgan DE 1999 Acute necrotizing pancreatitis. N Engl J Med 340: 1412.

Go VLW et al (eds) 1993 The Pancreas: Biology, Pathobiology and Diseases. New York: Raven Press.

Green PHR, Tall AR 1979 Drugs, alcohol and malabsorption. Am J Med 67: 1066.

Layer P, Yamamoto H, Kalthoff L et al 1994 The different courses of early- and late-onset idiopathic and alcoholic chronic pancreatitis. Gastroenterology 107: 1481.

Marshall JB 1993 Acute pancreatitis: a review with an emphasis on new developments. Arch Intern Med 153: 1185.

Marshall JC 1999 Surgical approaches to the management of acute severe necrotizing pancreatitis. Curr Opin Crit Care 5: 159.

Rotstein OD 1999 Surgical approach #1 to severe necrotizing pancreatitis. Curr Opin Crit Care 5: 160.

Starr MG 1999 Surgical approach #2 to severe necrotizing pancreatitis. Curr Opin Crit Care 5: 162.

Steer ML, Meldolesi J 1987 The cell biology of experimental pancreatitis. N Engl J Med 316: 144.

Steer ML, Waxman I, Freedman S 1995 Chronic pancreatitis. N Engl J Med 332: 1482.

Wyncoll DL 1999 The management of severe acute necrotizing pancreatitis: an evidence-based review of the literature. Intens Care Med 25: 146.

Pancytopenia

Pancytopenia refers to the presence of combined anaemia, neutropenia and thrombocytopenia (see Anaemia). Sometimes, the causative process may affect only one or two cell lines.

If the bone marrow has been infiltrated, viable stem cells may circulate and relocate in sites of fetal haemopoiesis. This is referred to as extramedullary haemopoiesis and is associated with a leukoerythroblastic blood film.

Any cytopenia (affecting 1, 2 or all 3 cell lines) or a leukoerythroblastic blood film provides an indication for bone marrow examination.

Papilloedema

Papilloedema or swelling of the optic disc is seen classically in conditions of increased intracranial pressure. Papilloedema also occurs in:

- malignant hypertension;
- hypercapnia;
- optic neuritis (q.v.).

Bibliography
Lyons MK, Meyer FB 1990 Cerebrospinal fluid physiology and the management of increased intracranial pressure. Mayo Clin Proc 65: 684.

Paragonimiasis

Paragonimiasis occurs following the ingestion of fresh water crustaceans infected with lung flukes from the genus paragonimus. It occurs predominantly in tropical Asia, Africa and Central America.

The flukes migrate from the duodenum via the peritoneal cavity and diaphragm to the lung, where they form a nodule with a necrotic centre surrounded by an inflammatory capsule. After 5–6 weeks, the fluke lays eggs and the capsule ruptures into the bronchial tree, giving sputum containing blood, inflammatory cells and eggs.

The patient often appears well, but sometimes there may be night sweats, chronic cough and pleuritic pain. The effects of a space-occupying lesion are noted if the parasite migrates to other sites, e.g. CNS.

Chest X-ray shows a transient pulmonary infiltrate as in Loeffler's syndrome, and cavities or pleural effusion may subsequent appear. There is an eosinophilia.

The diagnosis is made following identification of typical eggs in sputum or faeces (since sputum is often swallowed).

The differential diagnosis is primarily tuberculosis. The illness can thus present as AFB-negative presumed tuberculosis.

*Treatment is with **praziquantel**.*

Bibliography
Pachucki CT, Levandowski RA, Brown VA et al 1984 American paragonimiasis treated with praziquantel. N Engl J Med 311: 582.

Paraneoplastic syndromes

Paraneoplastic syndromes occur in malignancies and comprise a variety of local and systemic features not associated with any direct effect of the original cancer, either its primary tumour or its metastases.

They may occur before the cancer itself has been identified and may thus be an early marker of an undetected cancer. They disappear after successful treatment of the underlying cancer, and any reappearance thus signifies a relapse or recurrence.

The most important paraneoplastic syndromes comprise:

- **dermatoses**;
- **ectopic hormone production**;
- **neurological changes**.

A variety of other conditions, such as cachexia, disseminated intravascular coagulation and thromboembolism are commonly associated with malignancies, but these are not usually included among the paraneoplastic syndromes.

1. **Dermatoses**

There are a number of dermatoses specifically suggestive of underlying malignancy. These include:

- **hyperpigmentation**

    – due to ACTH production;

- **flushing**

    – due to carcinoid syndrome (q.v.);

- **proliferative skin lesions**

    – as in multiple seborrhoeic keratosis due to secretion of growth factors;

- **necrolytic migratory erythema**

    – due to glucagonoma (q.v.).

Other, non-specific, dermatoses are also commonly associated with malignancy.

- **Psoriasis–like lesions** can be associated with metastatic squamous cell carcinoma.
- **Hypertrichosis lanuginosa** can be associated with disseminated carcinoma and consists of fine downy hair in a previously hairless region. It may also be associated with ichthyosis or acanthosis nigricans.
- **Pyoderma gangrenosum** (q.v.) may be associated with myeloproliferative disorders, as well as with chronic inflammatory disease.
- **Generalized pruritus** may be associated with polycythaemia vera or lymphoma. Although commonly associated with drugs or scabies, it may also reflect serious non-malignant disease, such as thyrotoxicosis, cholestasis or chronic renal disease.
- **Painful red skin plaques with fever and neutrophilia** (Sweet's syndrome) may be associated with myeloproliferative disorders. More often, it is associated with arthritis, and it is also seen after bowel bypass surgery.
- The skin and internal organs may suffer **concomitant insult** from a potentially cancerous agent, such as arsenic (q.v.).

2. **Ectopic hormone production** (q.v.)

A large variety of biologically active substances may be produced by neoplastic cells. These include particularly a variety of polypeptide hormones, such as ACTH, ADH, calcitonin, glucagon, growth hormone, HCG, LH, MSH, PTH and somatostatin. Corticosteroids, prostaglandins and renin may also be secreted. Corticosteroids, prostaglandins and renin may also be secreted.

The most frequently encountered clinical feature from ectopic hormone production is inappropriate ADH syndrome (q.v.). Cushing's syndrome, erythrocytosis, hypercalcaemia, hyperpigmentation, hypoglycaemia may also be produced. The haematological findings of eosinophilia and raised ESR may also be sometimes related to ectopic hormone production.

3. **Neurological changes**

Neurological abnormalities are common and can precede any symptoms directly due to the cancer itself. The mechanisms are uncertain, and there can be a variety of overlapping syndromes. The cancers most commonly involved are lung and ovary but also gastrointestinal tract and breast.

The neurological abnormalities encountered involve:

- **brain**

    – progressive multifocal leukoencephalopathy;
    – subacute cerebellar degeneration;
    – brainstem or limbic encephalitis;

- **spinal cord**

    – degeneration of anterior horn cells;
    – subacute necrotizing myelopathy;

- **peripheral nerve**

    – sensory or mixed neuropathy;

- **neuromuscular junction**

  – myasthenia gravis or related conditions (e.g. Eaton Lambert syndrome);

- **muscle**

  – polymyositis;
  – myopathy;
  – neuromyopathy.

Bibliography

Cascino TL 1993 Neurologic complications of systemic cancer. Med Clin North Am 77: 265.

Clamon GH, Evans WK, Shepherd FA et al 1984 Myasthenic syndrome and small cell cancer of the lung: variable response to antineoplastic therapy. Arch Intern Med 144: 999.

Cohen PR, Kurzrock R 1987 Sweet's syndrome and malignancy. Am J Med 82: 1220.

Cohen PR, Talpaz M, Kurzrock R 1988 Malignancy-associated Sweet's syndrome; review of the world literature. J Clin Oncol 6: 1887.

Cronin RE, Kaehny WD, Miller, PD et al 1976 Renal cell carcinoma: unusual systemic manifestations. Medicine 55: 291.

Fitzpatrick TB, Eisen AZ, Wolff K et al (eds) 1979 Dermatology in General Medicine. New York: McGraw-Hill.

Hall TC (ed) 1974 Paraneoplastic syndromes. Ann NY Acad Sci 230: 1.

Jemec GBE 1986 Hypertrichosis lanuginosa acquisita. Arch Dermatol 122: 805.

Mallette LE 1991 The parathyroid polyhormones: new concepts in the spectrum of peptide hormone action. Endocr Rev 12: 110.

McLean DI 1986 Cutaneous paraneoplastic syndromes. Arch Dermatol 122: 765.

O'Neill JH, Murray NM, Newsom-Davis J 1988 The Lambert–Eaton myasthenic syndrome. Brain 111: 577.

Peterson K, Rosenblum MK, Kotanides H et al 1992 Paraneoplastic cerebellar degeneration. Neurology 42: 1931.

Ruther U, Nunnensiek C, Bokemeyer C (eds) 1998 Paraneoplastic Syndromes. Basel: Karger.

Paraquat

Paraquat (1,1-dimethyl-4,4-bipyridylium) is a potent phytotoxic herbicide, used worldwide in agriculture since the early 1960s. Most cases of human poisoning have occurred from accidental or deliberate ingestion (rather than from inhalation or skin absorption), with as little as 10 mL of the 20% concentrate being potentially lethal. The granular form is considered less toxic.

Although paraquat causes marked local irritation (e.g. of skin, eyes or gastrointestinal tract), its most dramatic effects are systemic, with renal failure, liver damage and in particular pulmonary oedema. Although these complications may be rapidly fatal, more typically death occurs in a few weeks from severe pulmonary fibrosis.

Rapid diagnosis is dependent on an accurate history, and confirmation is by a qualitative urine test or plasma radioimmunoassay.

Urgent treatment is with **gastric lavage** *and* **prevention of further absorption** *using Fuller's Earth (30% solution 250 mL 4 hourly), with magnesium sulfate as a purgative to hasten the faecal removal of the paraquat–Fuller's Earth complex.*

- *Various measures to enhance removal of absorbed paraquat, such as diuresis, dialysis and haemoperfusion, and possible antidotes, such as corticosteroids and free radical scavengers, have been ineffective.*
- *Recently,* **propofol** *has been found to be protective in experimental animals.*
- **Lung transplantation** *has been reported, though recurrence of 'paraquat lung' has also been observed in such cases.*

Bibliography

Ariyama J, Shimada H, Aono M et al 2000 Propofol improves recovery from paraquat acute toxicity in vitro and in vivo. Intens Care Med 26: 981.

Ng LL, Naik RB, Polak A 1982 Paraquat ingestion with methaemoglobinaemia treated with methylene blue. Br Med J 284: 1445.

Suzuki K, Takasu N, Arita S et al 1991 Evaluation of severity indexes of patients with paraquat poisoning. Hum Exp Toxicol 10: 21.

Parotitis (see Mouth diseases)

Paroxysmal nocturnal haemoglobinuria (see Anaemia)

Pediculosis

Pediculosis is produced by one of two ectoparasites which infect the skin and cause a marked itch. These are:

* *Sarcoptes scabiei*, a burrowing mite, and
* *Pediculus humanus*, a blood-sucking louse.

Infection occurs in one of three forms, i.e. capitis, corporis and pubis.

Scabies is the more common infestation, except in overcrowding or wartime when lice become more common. Infection occurs from person to person transmission or from fomites. The eggs hatch in about one week, and the parasites have a life-span of about one month.

Phthiriasis, the 'lousy disease' of antiquity in which lice ate away the flesh of the unfortunate victim as a fatal punishment from the gods, has not been reported for more than a century and may never have existed as such.

Many local treatments are available, including **lindane** *and over-the-counter* **pyrethrins**.

The human body louse is also the vector for transmission of Bartonella quintana, the aetiological agent in **trench fever**. This presents as acute periodic fever with headache and painful shins. Trench fever has recently been noted to have returned to industrialized societies, particularly in homeless people.

Bibliography
Bondeson J 1998 Phthiriasis: the riddle of the lousy disease. J R Soc Med 91: 328.

Pelvic inflammatory disease (see Salpingitis)

Pemphigus

Pemphigus vulgaris is a vesiculobullous disease, presumably of autoimmune origin, since antibodies may be found to the epidermal desmosome adhesion protein, plakoglobulin.

From a local lesion usually in the mouth, it may progress to involve extensive areas of skin and mucous membrane. The affected epidermis can be dislodged by lateral digital pressure (Nikolsky's sign, which is also seen in the staphylococcal scalded skin syndrome – see Exfoliative dermatitis. The bullae ulcerate and then heal slowly with hyperpigmentation. Histologically, there is loss of epidermal cell cohesion (acantholysis).

The differential diagnosis includes the other vesiculobullous diseases (q.v.).

Treatment is with **corticosteroids**, *which may be life-saving if the disease is extensive, in which case fluid and protein loss also need to be repaired. Plasmapheresis, cyclosporin, other immunosuppressive drugs and gold may also help.*

Variants of pemphigus include

* **Pemphigus vegetans**, which consists of raised wart-like plaques, which respond to dapsone,
* **Pemphigus foliaceus**, seen in sun-exposed areas and sometimes merging with SLE,
* **Paraneoplastic pemphigus**, associated with malignancy,
* **Bullous pemphigoid**, in which recurrent crops of subepidermal bullae, often with secondary infection, occur in older patients. The condition often begins with urticaria and pruritus. Mucosal involvement can sometimes occur. If this includes the conjunctiva, blindness may result.

Bibliography
Jolles S, Hughes J, Whittaker S 1998 Dermatological uses of high-dose intravenous immunoglobulin. Arch Dermatol 134: 80.
Korman N 1987 Bullous pemphigoid. J Am Acad Dermatol. 21: 1089.
Provost TT 1982 Pemphigus. N Engl J Med 306: 1224.

Penicillamine (see Chelating agents)

Periodic breathing (see Sleep disorders of breathing)

Periodic paralysis (see also Liquorice)

Periodic paralysis is due to an abnormal potassium flux across muscle cell membranes. The serum potassium may be either increased, decreased or normal, thus classifying the condition into three types. All are autosomal dominant conditions.

Muscle weakness, usually generalized, occurs rapidly and lasts for hours to days. Typically, there are recurrent attacks, but they vary greatly in frequency and severity.

> A similar condition also occurs in chronic hypokalaemia from any other cause (e.g. gut loss).

All types of periodic paralysis usually respond to ***acetazolamide***, *250 mg 6 hourly.*

Bibliography
Griggs R, Ptacek L 1992 The periodic paralysis. Hosp Pract 27: 123.
Knochel J 1982 Neuromuscular manifestations of electrolyte disorders. Am J Med 72: 521.

Pernicious anaemia

Pernicious anaemia is an autoimmune-induced vitamin B_{12} deficiency. Normally, vitamin B_{12} binds to intrinsic factor, a 45 kD glycoprotein secreted by the gastric parietal cells. This complex then binds to specific sites in the distal ileum from where it is absorbed.

In pernicious anaemia, there is an autoimmune antibody to intrinsic factor, and thus vitamin B_{12} deficiency occurs due to impaired absorption. Commonly, the condition is associated with other autoimmune phenomena, especially thyroid disease.

Clinical features in addition to anaemia include glossitis and neurological disease. The neurological disease is referred to as subacute combined degeneration and comprises peripheral neuropathy as well as spinal cord involvement. It is manifest by paraesthesiae and initially loss of sensations passing through the posterior columns, i.e. loss of vibration sense and proprioception, but the sensations of touch and temperature are preserved until the disease is advanced. There is thus ataxia and spastic weakness. Patients can also suffer from neuropsychiatric impairment, especially memory loss and depression.

Treatment is with ***vitamin B_{12}*** *1000 μg parenterally weekly for six weeks, then monthly for life.*

If the anaemia is severe, transfusion may be considered, but this needs to be administered with great care as volume overload is easily produced in these patients.

Bibliography
Pruthi RK, Tefferi A 1994 Pernicious anemia revisited. Mayo Clin Proc 69: 144.

Peroneal muscular atrophy (see Charcot–Marie–Tooth disease)

Petechiae

Petechiae are the smallest haemorrhagic lesions on the skin and mucous membranes and are manifest as non-blanching red-purple dots.

> Petechiae have three mechanisms of causation, namely:
> - thrombocytopenia (q.v.);
> - platelet function defect (q.v.);
> - microvascular damage (i.e. vascular purpura).

Vascular purpura is especially associated with serious infections, such as septicaemia (see Purpura).

Peutz–Jeghers syndrome (see Mouth diseases)

Phaeochromocytoma

Phaeochromocytoma is the only lesion of the adrenal medulla. It is a vascular and secretory tumour associated with the production of hypertension and thus detected mainly in such patients.

- Traditionally, there is paroxysmal hypertension, but this is seen in only 40% of patients and the majority in fact have sustained hypertension.
- An occasional patient may even present with paradoxical hypotension, especially of a postural nature, from excess beta stimulation and hypovolaemia.
- There is associated headache, sweating and tachycardia, with a hypermetabolic state (including glucose intolerance, weight loss and leukocytosis).

Phaeochromocytoma may sometimes be associated with the MEN syndrome type 2 (q.v.), in which case it is often bilateral. Occasionally, the tumours are found extra-abdominally, e.g. in the thoracic para-aortic region. Most phaeochromocytomas (90%) are benign. Some are clinically undiagnosed during life.

The diagnosis should be considered in young patients with hypertension, in paroxysmal hypertension or if there are associated symptoms.

The differential diagnosis particularly includes:

- hypertension with associated anxiety;
- posterior fossa lesions which can stimulate the medullary sympathetic–adrenal axis.

The diagnosis is confirmed by the demonstration of increased metabolites in the plasma or urine. The most convenient test has been 24 h urinary secretion of VMA (vanillylmandelic acid) and catecholamines, but the 24 h urinary excretion of metanephrine is more reliable and elevated plasma catecholamine levels are the most sensitive. Specific provocative or inhibitory tests of catecholamine secretion can be hazardous. Direct imagining of the tumour with CT scanning is required to demonstrate the actual site of lesions >5 mm in diameter.

*Treatment requires careful pre-operative preparation with **alpha blockade** (using phenoxybenzamine) for blood pressure control, followed if necessary by **beta blockade** (using e.g. propranolol) for heart rate control. Following normalization of blood pressure, heart rate and blood volume, **surgery** may be undertaken, though great care needs to be taken with sudden hypertension during surgical handling of the tumour, followed by hypotension after its removal. Thus, sodium nitroprusside and noradrenaline infusions need to be prepared for use, as well as parenteral beta-blocker and intravenous fluids.*

Rarely, a **phaeochromocytoma crisis** may occur, which produces features similar to those of a number of other conditions, including cerebral trauma, monoamine oxidase inhibitor crisis or abrupt cessation of clonidine.

It is treated with phentolamine or sodium nitroprusside infusion for blood pressure control, followed by beta blockade.

Bibliography

Bravo EL, Gifford RW 1984 Pheochromocytoma: diagnosis, localization and management. N Engl J Med 311: 1298.

Daly PA, Landsberg L 1992 Phaeochromocytoma: diagnosis and management. Bailliere's Clin Endocrinol Metab 6: 143.

Editorial 1985 The function of adrenaline. Lancet 1: 561.

Golub MS, Tuck ML 1992 Diagnostic and therapeutic strategies in pheochromocytoma. Endocrinologist 2: 101.

Sutton MG, Sheps SG, Lie JT 1981 Prevalence of clinically unsuspected pheochromocytoma. Mayo Clin Proc 56: 354.

Whalen RK, Althausen AF, Daniels GH 1992 Extra-adrenal pheochromocytoma. J Urol 147: 1.

Phosgene (see Warfare agents)

Phrenic nerve (see Diaphragm)

Phthiriasis (see Pediculosis)

Physical exposure

The physical exposures considered in this book are those to:

- cold, in relation to

    - frostbite;
    - hypothermia;

- heat, in relation to

    - heat cramps;
    - heat exhaustion;
    - heat stroke;
    - heat rash;
    - heat shock proteins;
    - hot tubs;
    - hyperthermia;

- high altitude.

Each of these topics is considered individually.

Pigmentation disorders

1. Hypopigmentation

- **Albinism**. This is an uncommon condition, in which several types of genetic defect of melanin production may be inherited as an autosomal dominant.
- **Hypomelanosis**. This refers to decreased pigmentation following recent skin trauma or inflammation (including eczema, leprosy, psoriasis, syphilis).

- **Vitiligo**. This refers to patchy depigmentation following loss of melanin and/or melanocytes, especially on the face or limbs. These lesions may coalesce so as to become extensive. The same process may also destroy pigment cells in the retina. Vitiligo is particularly associated with endocrine disorders, such as Addison's disease, diabetes, pernicious anaemia and thyroid disease.

2. Hyperpigmentation

A. Local hyperpigmentation

- **Acanthosis nigricans**. This refers to pigmented papillomatous lesions resembling dirt lines and especially seen in skin folds.

It may be associated with:

- obesity;
- autoimmune disease;
- endocrine disease

    - flexural brown thickening of the skin suggests hyperinsulinaemia;

- malignancy

    - especially abdominal adenocarcinoma;
    - occasionally squamous cell carcinoma of the cervix.

It may also be seen as a familial trait.

- **Freckles**, or solar lentigines. These may be seen after local trauma or inflammation or in neurofibromatosis.
- **Melasma** (chloasma). This occurs on the face and is seen with oral contraceptives, pregnancy or liver disease.

B. Diffuse hyperpigmentation

- **Systemic diseases**. These include:

    - Addison's disease;
    - haemochromatosis;
    - drugs (amiodarone, antimalarials, cytotoxic agents, oral tanning agents, phenothiazines, tetracycline).

277

- **Non-melanin** hyperpigmentation. This may be due to deposition of:

  – carotene;
  – haemoglobin;
  – foreign substances, such as heavy metals (arsenic, silver).

Bibliography

Grimes PE 1995 Melasma: etiologic and therapeutic considerations. Arch Dermatol 131: 1453.

Hendrix JD, Greer KE 1992 Cutaneous hyperpigmentation caused by systemic drugs. Int J Dermatol 31: 458.

Mosher DB, Fitzpatrick TB, Ortonne J-P 1979 Abnormalities of pigmentation. In: Fitzpatrick TB, Eisen AZ, Wolff K et al (eds) Dermatology in General Medicine. New York: McGraw-Hill. p 568.

Orlow SJ 1997 Albinism: an update. Semin Cutan Med Surg 16: 24.

Pituitary

The **hypothalamic–pituitary axis** is the major junction between the body's two chief pathways for integrated systemic responses, namely the nervous and endocrine systems.

The richly innervated hypothalamus provides the link with the CNS. Since it is outside the blood–brain barrier, it can also sense circulating substances, such as cortisol, glucose and sodium. In addition, it has amine, opioid and peptide receptors. It is thus well placed to house the major homeostatic centres for control of osmolality, temperature, thirst and appetite.

It provides the link with the endocrine system via secretion of stimulatory or inhibitory peptides into the hypophyseal-portal venous system and thus into the anterior pituitary. These peptides include AVP/ADP, CRH, dopamine, GHRH, GnRH, somatostatin, TRH.

The **anterior pituitary** secretions, if abnormally increased or decreased, are usually manifest via abnormalities of the target gland. If the pituitary abnormality is caused by a tumour,

there may also be local symptoms, particularly of a visual nature. Pituitary apoplexy is an emergency condition which can complicate any pituitary tumour (see Acromegaly).

The most common deficiency of anterior pituitary secretion is global, i.e. panhypopituitarism. This is usually due to a tumour, particularly a chromophobe adenoma. Other tumours, such as craniopharyngioma or occasionally metastases, or sometimes other space-occupying lesions, such as granulomas, may be responsible for global pituitary deficiency.

Sheehan's syndrome refers to the rare entity of pituitary deficiency following postpartum shock, though hypophysitis may be a more common cause of pituitary deficiency in the postpartum period.

Pituitary reserve is best tested currently via the response of the pituitary hormones and target hormones to releasing hormones.

Treatment of pituitary deficiency is traditionally with ***target gland hormone replacement*** *(adrenal, gonadal, thyroid), since pituitary hormones themselves are generally inconvenient to administer clinically.*

The exception is ***human growth hormone***, *which is easily given by daily subcutaneous injection. Its indication in adults is controversial, though it is licensed in several countries for use in growth hormone deficiency. It is now made by recombinant technology and is thus safe, though it is very expensive.*

(see Adrenal insufficiency and Hypothyroidism)

The **posterior pituitary** comprises the terminal parts of the hypothalamic neurones. It is here that vasopressin (AVP or ADH) is secreted, having migrated along the axons from the hypothalamus where it was synthesized.

Vasopressin secretion responds to small changes (e.g. 1%) in osmolality and to larger changes (e.g. 10%) in blood pressure or blood volume. As little as 1% increase in plasma osmolality causes sufficient vasopressin secretion to increase the urine osmolality by 200 mOsm/kg. This response is sensitive in either direction in normal subjects, but it becomes substantially impaired in older patients and in cardiac failure.

The chief disorders of vasopressin are:

- diabetes insipidus

  - i.e. ADH deficiency;

- the syndrome of inappropriate antidiuretic hormone (q.v.)

  - i.e. ADH excess.

(see also Desmopressin)

Bibliography

Bills DC, Meyer FB, Laws ER et al 1993 A retrospective analysis of pituitary apoplexy. Neurosurgery 33: 602.

Burke CW 1992 The pituitary megatest: outdated? Clin Endocrinol 36: 133.

Chrousos GP 1995 The hypothalamic–pituitary–adrenal axis and immune-mediated inflammation. N Engl J Med 332: 1351.

Dash RJ, Gupta V, Suri S 1993 Sheehan's syndrome. Aust NZ J Med 23: 26.

Editorial 1980 Corticosteroids and hypothalamic–pituitary–adrenocortical function. Br Med J 280: 813.

Elster AD 1993 Modern imaging of the pituitary. Radiology 187: 1.

Hoffman DM, Ho KKY 1999 Growth hormone deficiency in adults: to treat or not to treat. Aust NZ J Med 29: 342.

Loriaux DL 1985 The polyendocrine deficiency syndromes. N Engl J Med 312: 1568.

Magner JA 1990 Thyroid-stimulating hormone: biosynthesis, cell biology, and bioactivity. Endocrinol Rev 11: 354.

Molitch ME, Russell EJ 1990 The pituitary 'incidentaloma'. Ann Intern Med 112: 925.

Robertson GL 1987 Physiology of ADH secretion. Kidney Int 32 (suppl 21): S20.

Shupnik MA, Ridgway EC, Chin WW 1989 Molecular biology of thyrotropin. Endocr Rev 10: 459.

Vance ML 1994 Hypopituitarism. N Engl J Med 330: 1651.

Vokes TJ, Robertson GL 1988 Disorders of antidiuretic hormone. Endocrinol Metab Clin North Am 17: 281.

Pituitary apoplexy (see Acromegaly)

Placental abruption (see Trauma in pregnancy)

Plasmacytoma (see Multiple myeloma)

Plasminogen

Plasminogen is the inactive circulating precursor of the fibrinolytic system. Its molecular weight is 90 000 and its plasma concentration is about 200 μg/mL (2.4 μM).

Its role is described in Fibrinolysis (q.v.).

Platelet function defects

Platelet function defects refer to qualitative platelet abnormalities, as opposed to the quantitative platelet abnormality of thrombocytopenia.

279

> They present as a bleeding disorder with prolonged bleeding time but normal platelet count.

Platelet function defects may be congenital or acquired.

1. Congenital

- absence of platelet membrane receptors, due to the rare conditions

  - glycoprotein IIb–IIIa (Glanzmann's thrombasthenia);
  - glycoprotein Ib–Ix (Bernard–Soulier) disease;

- platelet granule deficiency, i.e. α- and δ-storage pool disease (also rare);
- von Willebrand's disease (q.v.)

2. Acquired

- storage pool defect

  - in myeloproliferative disorders;

P

- miscellaneous abnormalities, as

  - in alcoholism;
  - after cardiopulmonary bypass;
  - in uraemia;
  - due to drugs.

Many **drugs** adversely affect platelet function. However, few do so in a manner quantitative enough to cause clinical bleeding, unless there is some other concomitant haemostatic impairment.

Of the drugs causing quantitatively significant platelet dysfunction, aspirin is the archetypal agent. Like all NSAIDs, it impairs platelet aggregation by inhibiting cyclo-oxygenase and decreasing thromboxane A_2 (TXA_2).

Other drugs which cause clinically significant defects include:

- beta-lactam antibiotics

  - classically carbenicillin, but also other members of this family to a lesser extent;

- dextran 70;
- ticlopidine and clopidrogel;
- selective serotonin reuptake inhibitors (SSRIs).

Many agents can impair platelet function in a minor way, including especially:

- anaesthetics agents;
- antihistamines;
- beta blockers;
- calcium channel blockers;
- clofibrate;
- nitrates;
- psychotropic agents;
- radiographic contrast media.

Certain foods can produce similar effects, including:

- garlic;
- ginger;
- onions;
- several spices.

Treatment of clinical bleeding due to a platelet function defect is with **platelet concentrates** *and/or* **DDAVP** *(see Desmopressin).*

Bibliography

Deykin D 1983 Uremic bleeding. Kidney Int 24: 698.

Ferrara JLM 1995 The febrile platelet transfusion reaction: a cytokine shower. Transfusion 35: 89.

George JN, Shattil SJ 1991 The clinical importance of acquired abnormalities of platelet function. N Engl J Med 324: 27.

Sattler FR, Weitekamp MR, Ballard JO 1986 Potential for bleeding with the new beta-lactam antibiotics. Ann Intern Med 105: 924.

Schafer AI 1984 Bleeding and thrombosis in the myeloproliferative disorders. Blood 64: 1.

Yang Z, Stulz P, von Segesser L et al 1991 Different interactions of platelets with arterial and venous coronary bypass vessels. Lancet 337: 939.

Pleural cavity

Pleural disorders include:

1. pneumothorax (see below);

2. pleurisy (see below) due to underlying disease (infection, inflammation, pulmonary embolism, neoplasm, trauma);

3. pleural effusion (see below);

4. plaques, thickening and calcification following prior pleural disease, (see Asbestos);

5. tumours – mesothelioma (either localized, (i.e. fibroma) or diffuse, (i.e. malignant)).

Pneumothorax refers to the presence of air within the pleural cavity. This process may be:

- spontaneous, or
- traumatic (including iatrogenic).

Either type may be under 'tension'.

Spontaneous pneumothorax:

- can arise in otherwise healthy subjects (primary pneumothorax); or

- can occur as a complication of another lung disorder (secondary pneumothorax).

Primary pneumothorax occurs most commonly in young tall thin males who are otherwise healthy, though they are usually smokers.

This is thought to be due to the greater apical distending forces operating in association with elastic recoil (which declines with age) and the pleural pressure gradient which is proportional to vertical lung height. There is probably an inherent weakness in the subpleural apical tissue, such as a small bleb, presumably due to a congenital bronchial tree anomaly.

Rarely, primary pneumothorax may be catamenial (i.e. menses-related).

The overall incidence of primary pneumothorax in the population generally is low (about 4 per 10 000 patient-years).

Secondary pneumothorax occurs with:

- diffuse disease processes

  - such as airways obstruction, bullae, interstitial lung disease, Marfan's syndrome,

- focal disease processes,

  - such as carcinoma, infarction, necrotizing pneumonia, rheumatoid nodule, endometriosis, tuberculosis (commonly in the past), *Pneumocystis carinii* pneumonia (more commonly nowadays), and acute lobar collapse (causing pneumothorax ex vacuo).

Traumatic pneumothorax may be:

- **open**

  - as after a penetrating chest wall injury;

- **closed**

  - as after closed chest wall injury, pulmonary barotrauma, transbronchial lung biopsy or central venous catheterization.

The physical signs of pneumothorax may be quite subtle, unless the pneumothorax is large or under tension, when there may be:

- compression of the ipsilateral lung;
- displacement of the mediastinum;
- distortion of the contralateral lung;
- circulatory embarrassment.

A chest X-ray is essential to confirm the presence of a pneumothorax and to assess its size and likely cause.

Treatment of a pneumothorax depends on its size and cause.

- *A small spontaneous pneumothorax (up to 25% reduction of lung volume) may be managed conservatively, unless the patient is on mechanical ventilation, in which case as for larger pneumothoraces an intercostal catheter is required. Resolution of a small pneumothorax normally requires 5–7 days, but this can be substantially hastened by administering oxygen which promotes reabsorption by exaggerating the diffusion gradient for nitrogen between the blood and intrathoracic gas.*
- *A moderate spontaneous pneumothorax may be successfully treated by simple aspiration in many cases, again unless the patient is on mechanical ventilation.*
- *Traumatic pneumothorax is best treated with insertion of an intercostal catheter and underwater seal, since in addition there is often blood in the pleural cavity (haemopneumothorax).*
- *Pleurodesis is usually performed for recurrent pneumothorax, and thoracotomy may be required for a persisting bronchopleural fistula.*

There is a risk of ipsilateral recurrence of spontaneous pneumothorax of about 25% within 2 y. Review of patients with apparently primary spontaneous pneumothorax is essential to exclude underlying pathology which may require treatment.

Pleurisy or inflammation of the parietal pleura is always due to underlying pulmonary disease. It is associated with chest pain which is often severe, and with a pleural friction rub on auscultation. Dry or fibrinous pleurisy may be followed later by pleural effusion, in which case the friction rub disappears because of separation of the parietal and visceral pleura.

Pleural effusion may be:

- either a transudate or exudate
  - i.e. less than or greater than 30 g/L protein, respectively;
  - either may be called a hydrothorax;

- contain
  - blood (haemothorax) (see below);
  - pus (empyema – see Cavitation);
  - chyle (chylothorax) (see below).

An effusion contains at least 500 mL before it can be detected clinically and 100–300 mL before it is apparent radiologically. The pleural effusion may lie free in the pleural space or be loculated either in the general space or into lobular or subpulmonary spaces.

The chief investigation of pleural effusion is pleural aspiration (with or without pleural biopsy). The fluid is examined for:

1. **Macroscopic appearance**

- straw-coloured
  - transudate, exudate;

- purulent
  - empyema or pyothorax;
  - >50 000 WBCs/mL gives appearance of purulence;

- blood-stained
  - haemothorax;
  - >1 mL of blood/L gives RBC count >5000/mL and a serous appearance;
  - haematocrit >50% that of peripheral blood indicates frank bleeding;

- milky
  - chylothorax;
  - chyliform rarely in chronic exudates.

2. **Biochemistry**

- protein
  - <30 g/L indicates transudate;
  - >30 g/L indicates exudate;

- glucose
  - N >50% plasma level;
  - decreased in tuberculosis, malignancy, rheumatoid disease;
  - postpneumonic empyema;

- LDH
  - increased in inflammation;

- cholesterol
  - increased in exudates or lymphatic obstruction;

- amylase
  - increased in pancreatic disease;

- pH
  - low (<7.20) in complicated parapneumonic effusions.

3. **Cytology**

4. **Microbiology**

The chief causes of the different types of pleural effusion are

---

1. **Transudate**
- congestive cardiac failure
  - either bilateral or right-sided,

- constrictive pericarditis,
- hypoproteinaemia
  - cirrhosis,
  - nephrotic syndrome,
  - critical illness,

- Meig's syndrome
  - from ovarian carcinoma,

- polyserositis,
- peritoneal dialysis,
- superior vena cava obstruction,
- myxoedema.

2. Exudate

- bacterial pneumonia

  – parapneumonic sympathetic effusion,

- pulmonary infarction,
- malignancy

  – metastases, especially from cancers of lung, breast, stomach, ovary,
  – primary lung cancer,
  – mesothelioma,

- tuberculosis,
- subphrenic abscess,
- pancreatitis,
- oesophageal perforation,
- collagen-vascular disease,
- lymphoma,
- uraemia,
- ascites

  – mostly gives right-sided effusions.

3. Empyema

- bacterial pneumonia,
- subphrenic abscess,
- penetrating injury,
- septic embolism,
- haematogenous spread.

4. Haemothorax

- trauma

  – including invasive procedures,

- malignancy,
- pulmonary infarction,
- leukaemia,
- tuberculosis,
- pancreatitis,
- oesophageal perforation,
- pulmonary arteriovenous malformation or fistula,
- 'bloody tap'.

5. Chylothorax

- malignancy

  – especially lymphoma,

- trauma,
- surgery,
- left subclavian vein thrombosis,
- lymphangiomyomatosis,
- lymphangiectasia,
- mediastinitis.

Bibliography

Alfageme I, Munoz F, Pena N et al 1993 Empyema of the thorax in adults: etiology, microbiologic findings, and management. Chest 103: 839.

Andrivet P, Djedaini K, Teboul JL et al 1995 Spontaneous pneumothorax: comparison of thoracic drainage vs immediate or delayed needle aspiration. Chest 108: 335.

Bartter T, Santarelli R, Akers SM et al 1994 The evaluation of pleural effusion. Chest 106: 1209.

Baumann MH, Strange C 1997 Treatment of spontaneous pneumothorax. A more aggressive approach? Chest 112: 789.

Baumann MH, Strange C 1997 The clinician's perspective on pneumothorax management. Chest 112: 822.

Belani CP (ed) 1998 International symposium on thoracic malignancies. Chest 113 (suppl): 1S.

Cerfolio RJ, Allen MS, Deschamps C et al 1996 Postoperative chylothorax. J Thor Cardiovasc Surg 112: 1361.

Gunnels J 1978 Perplexing pleural effusions. Chest 74: 390.

Jamal S, Maurer JR 1994 Pulmonary disease and the menstrual cycle. Pulmonary Perspectives 11(3): 3.

Joseph J, Sahn SA 1996 Thoracic endometriosis syndrome: new observations from an analysis of 110 cases. Am J Med 100: 164.

Light RW 1993 Management of spontaneous pneumothorax. Am Rev Respir Dis 148: 245.

Lynch TJ 1993 Management of malignant pleural effusions. Chest 103 (suppl): S385.

Martinez FJ, Villanueva AG, Pickering R et al 1992 Spontaneous hemothorax. Medicine 71: 354.

Muller NL 1993 Imaging of the pleura. Radiology 186: 297.

Romero S, Candela A, Martin C et al 1993
Evaluation of different criteria for the separation
of pleural transudates from exudates. Chest 104:
399.

Sahn SA 1988 The pleura. Am Rev Respir Dis 138:
184.

Sahn SA 1993 Management of complicated
parapneumonic effusions. Am Rev Respir Dis
148: 813.

Shiel WC, Prete PE 1984 Pleuropulmonary
manifestations of rheumatoid arthritis. Semin
Arthritis Rheum 13: 235.

Taylor JR, Ryu J, Colby TV et al 1990
Lymphangioleiomyomatosis. N Engl J Med 323:
1254.

Valentine VG, Raffin TA 1992 The management of
chylothorax. Chest 102: 586.

Walker-Renard PB, Vaughan LM, Sahn SA 1994
Chemical pleurodesis for malignant pleural
effusions. Ann Intern Med 120: 56.

Watt AG 1978 Spontaneous pneumothorax. Med J
Aust 1: 186.

Woodring JH, Baker MD, Stark P 1996
Pneumothorax ex vacuo. Chest 110: 1102.

Plumbism (see Lead)

Plummer–Vinson syndrome (see
Dysphagia and Anaemia)

Pneumatosis coli

Pneumatosis coli describes the uncommon
condition of gas-filled cysts within the bowel
wall. The cysts can occupy the submucosa
and subserosa, and they may affect both the
small and large intestine. Although the
aetiology is unknown, there is an association
with chronic airways obstruction. The
condition is usually asymptomatic and
discovered only incidentally on abdominal X-
ray. Occasionally, it may be considered
responsible for either diarrhoea or
obstruction.

Treatment with **hyperbaric oxygen** *causes the cysts
and any associated symptoms to disappear.*

Pneumoconiosis (see Occupational lung
diseases)

Pneumomediastinum (see Barotrauma)

Pneumonia, exotic (see Exotic
pneumonia)

Pneumonia in pregnancy

Pneumonia in pregnancy presents a special
problem, because it is the commonest serious
non-obstetric infection in the pregnant patient
and because it is the third most frequent cause
of indirect maternal death. It can also have a
significant effect on fetal well-being.

Although the relative incidence of specific
pathogens responsible for pneumonia in
pregnancy is the same as in the non-pregnant
patient, the decreased immune status of
pregnancy renders such infections generally
more serious. This particularly applies to viral,
fungal and mycobacterial infections, because the
chief alteration in maternal defence is in cell-
mediated immunity due to the changed
hormonal environment. These changes are
compounded by secondary anatomical
disadvantages in the respiratory system,
especially a raised diaphragm, decreased
functional residual capacity and reduced ability
to clear tracheobronchial secretions.

Pneumonia in pregnancy may be:

- community-acquired bacterial or atypical;
- complicating influenza (superinfection,
  especially due to *S. aureus*);
- nosocomial (usually Gram-negative);
- aspiration (polymicrobial anaerobic and
  Gram-negative).

*The antibiotics which are indicated in pneumonia and
which are safe in pregnancy comprise chiefly the*
penicillins *and* **cephalosporins***.*

- *A* **macrolide** *(but not erythromycin estolate) is
  indicated for atypical pathogens.*

- *Aminoglycosides* and *vancomycin* *should be used only in very severe infections, because of the risk they pose of fetal ototoxicity and nephrotoxicity.*

Bibliography

Garland SM, O'Reilly MA 1995 The risks and benefits of antimicrobial therapy in pregnancy. Drug Safety 13: 188.

Goodrum LA 1997 Pneumonia in pregnancy. Semin Perinatology 21: 276.

Rigby FB, Pastorek JG 1996 Pneumonia during pregnancy. Clin Obstet Gynecol 39: 107.

Riley L 1997 Pneumonia and tuberculosis in pregnancy. Infect Dis Clin North Am 11: 119.

Pneumothorax (see Barotrauma and Pleural cavity)

Poisoning

Chemical poisoning due to drug overdosage is a very commonly encountered problem in Intensive Care and its management principles are well known. Some uncommon drug poisonings (e.g. amphetamines) are considered in this book (see Drugs).

Many other chemical agents, generally of a non-therapeutic nature, may cause uncommon forms of poisoning following ingestion or other exposure (e.g. cyanide, warfare agents), and these are also discussed (see Chemical poisoning).

Food poisoning (q.v.) is considered separately.

Bibliography

Camporesi EM 1990 Use of hyperbaric oxygen in critical care. In: Lumb PD, Shoemaker WC (eds) Critical Care: State of the Art, Chapter 10. Fullerton: Society of Critical Care Medicine. p 219.

Davis JC 1984 Hyperbaric medicine. In: Shoemaker WC (ed) Critical Care: State of the Art. Fullerton: Society of Critical Care Medicine. p E1.

Haddad LM, Shannon MW, Winchester JF (eds) 1997 Clinical Management of Poisoning and Drug Overdose. 3rd edition. Philadelphia: WB Saunders.

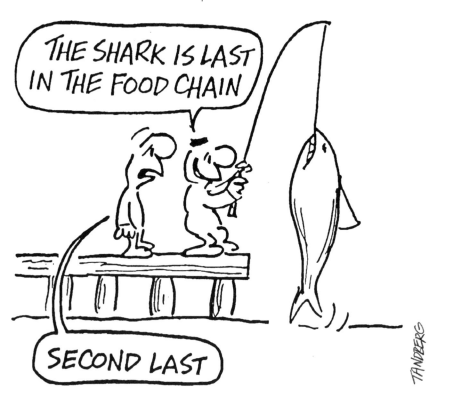

Olson KR (ed) 1998 Poisoning and Drug Overdose. 3rd edition. Norwalk: Appleton & Lange.

Trujillo MH, Guerrero J, Fragachan C et al 1998 Pharmacologic antidotes in critical care medicine: a practical guide for drug administration. Crit Care Med 26: 377.

Poliomyelitis

Poliomyelitis has become rare in developed countries since the development of a successful vaccine in 1955. In developed countries, the occasional reported illness is most likely caused by mutation towards a virulent strain in a relative or recipient.

Poliomyelitis is asymptomatic in 95% of cases. In the remainder, the features are usually similar to mild influenza and gastroenteritis.

It occasionally produces aseptic meningitis and most importantly paralysis from destruction of motor neurones in the spinal cord and brainstem. Paralysis thus occurs of the lower limbs and if severe of the respiratory muscles, with inadequate airway protection and respiratory failure. Residual muscle weakness and wasting are usual.

Treatment is **supportive***.*

There is an ambitious WHO plan for the global eradication of poliomyelitis within the next few years, although the disease is still endemic in at least 50 countries.

Bibliography
Satcher D 1999 Polio eradication by the year 2000. JAMA 281: 221.

Polyarteritis nodosa

Polyarteritis nodosa (PAN) is a multi-system disease with inflammation and necrosis of small and medium arteries. The cause is unknown, but it can sometimes be associated with:

- hepatitis B antigenaemia;
- HIV infection;
- rheumatoid arthritis;
- amphetamine abuse;
- familial Mediterranean fever.

The condition is rare, with a prevalence of 1 in 100000 of the population.

Clinical manifestations are seen most commonly in middle-aged men.

- There is fever, malaise, anorexia, weight loss, weakness, myalgia, arthralgia and subcutaneous nodules.
- There may also be hypertension, acute myocardial infarction, asthma, rash, fits, glomerulonephritis and mononeuritis mutiplex (asymmetrical peripheral neuropathy).
- Renal involvement occurs in 75% of patients and may comprise either glomerulonephritis or vasculitis, with haematuria, proteinuria and uraemia.
- Mesenteric arteritis may cause bowel ischaemia and an abdominal crisis.
- Complications may include aneurysm formation.

Investigations show anaemia, leukocytosis, eosinophilia and raised ESR. Definitive diagnosis is made from histological examination of biopsy material from an involved site, especially muscle, though histology while specific is not very sensitive. Visceral angiography may show microaneurysms and segmental arterial narrowing.

Treatment is that of any underlying disease, together with removal of any identifiable antigen. Otherwise, **corticosteroids** *and sometimes* **cyclophosphamide** *are used.*

Bibliography
Albert DA, Rimon D, Silverstein MD 1988 The diagnosis of poyarteritis nodosa. Arthritis Rheum 31: 1117.

Polycystic kidney disease (see Renal cystic disease)

Polycystic ovary syndrome (see

Amenorrhoea and Hirsutism)

Polycythaemia

Polycythaemia refers to an increased circulating red cell mass, as opposed to erythrocytosis (q.v.), which is an increased red blood cell count without an increased mass.

Relative polycythaemia occurs when there is a decreased plasma volume, as in dehydration, but also in phaeochromocytoma and perhaps in stress. This group also includes **pseudopolycythaemia** (Gaisbock's syndrome), although its mechanism is unknown.

Absolute polycythaemia may be due to:

- hypoxia;
- increased erythropoietin without hypoxia;
- polycythaemia vera.

Hypoxia occurs in:

- cardiopulmonary disease;
- haemoglobinopathy;
- altitude.

In these settings, if the PaO_2 is <60 mmHg (SaO_2 <90%), erythropoietin is appropriately stimulated.

Increased erythropoietin without hypoxia occurs in erythropoietin-secreting tumours. These are usually:

- renal;
- adrenal;
- hepatic;
- ovarian;
- cerebellar.

Polycythaemia vera is an autonomous increase in red cell mass associated with decreased erythropoietin. It is a myeloproliferative disorder, in which the initial clonal change arises in a pluripotent stem cell, so that there are abnormal markers in granulocytic as well as erythroid precursors. However, the red cell series predominates, probably because of inhibition of apoptosis rather than increased sensitivity to erythropoietin.

Clinical features are usually seen in older patients, in whom there is hepatosplenomegaly, ischaemic disease, and typically pruritus, especially after bathing.

Increased viscosity gives rise to thromboembolism, which may be unusual or multiple, and may include the Budd–Chiari syndrome (q.v.).

Investigations show an increased red blood cell mass (unless there is concomitant bleeding) in the absence of hypoxia, and leukocytosis and thrombocytosis.

Treatment is with **venesection** *to a haematocrit of 0.40–0.45 or with* **radiotherapy**.

- **Radiophosphorous** *is used if the patient is refractory to venesection.*
- *Cytotoxic therapy causes a significantly increased risk of the development of leukaemia.*

The prognosis without treatment is a 50% mortality within 1.5 years. This is increased to 3.5 years with successful venesections and 12.5 years following radiotherapy.

The laboratory findings of polycythaemia vera in the absence of clinical features is sometimes referred to as '**primary erythrocytosis**' and is probably a forme fruste of polycythaemia vera.

Bibliography

Berlin NI 1986 Polycythemia vera: an update. Semin Hematol 23: 131.

Challoner T, Briggs C, Rampling MW et al 1986 A study of the haematological and haemorrheological consequences of venesection. Br J Haematol 62: 671.

Editorial 1987 Pseudopolycythaemia. Lancet 2: 603.

Gareau R, Audran M, Barnes R et al 1996 Erthropoietin abuse in athletes. Nature 380: 113.

Golde DW, Hocking WG, Koeffler HP et al 1981 Polycythemia: mechanisms and management. Ann Intern Med 95: 71.

P

Gruppo Italiano Studio Policitemia 1995
Polycthaemia vera. Ann Intern Med 123: 656.
Hinshelwood S, Bench AJ, Green AR 1997
Pathogenesis of polycythaemia vera. Blood Rev
11: 224.
Krantz SB 1991 Erythropoietin. Blood 77: 419.
Schafer AI 1984 Bleeding and thrombosis in
myeloproliferative disorders. Blood 64: 1.
Watts EJ, Lewis SM 1983 Spurious polycythaemia.
Scand J Haematol 31: 241.

Polymyalgia rheumatica (see also

Arteritis)

Polymyalgia rheumatica (PMR) is a clinical
syndrome of profound proximal limb girdle
pain and stiffness, usually seen in older
patients.

> Polymyalgia rheumatica is at one end of a
> spectrum, with giant cell arteritis (most
> commonly temporal arteritis) at the other
> and with overlap in some patients.

Not uncommonly, rheumatoid arthritis may
present with a clinical picture of PMR, with
overt peripheral synovitis becoming apparent
only subsequently.

Clinical manifestations may include fever,
fatigue, weight loss and depression, as well as
the proximal muscle symptoms. The onset is
usually acute but may sometimes be insidious.

Investigations show a markedly increased ESR,
often with anaemia, increased alkaline
phosphatase, normal CK and increased
fibrinogen.

Treatment with **corticosteroids** *(usually 15 mg/day
of prednisolone) gives a dramatic response within
days. Higher doses are needed initially for temporal
arteritis. The dose should usually be tapered to a low
dose for up to 2 y before attempting withdrawal.*

Bibliography

Hamilton CR, Shelley WM, Tumulty PA 1971
Giant cell arteritis: including temporal arteritis and
polymyalgia rheumatica. Medicine 50: 1.
Hunder GG, Bloch DA, Michel BA et al 1990 The
American College of Rheumatology 1990 criteria
for the classification of giant cell arteritis. Arthritis
Rheum 33: 1122.
Zilko PJ 1996 Polymyalgia rheumatica and giant cell
arteritis. Med J Aust 165: 438.

Polymyositis/dermatomyositis

Polymyositis is an uncommon but often serious
condition affecting skeletal muscles. When
associated with skin eruptions, it is referred to as
dermatomyositis.

Although its cause is unknown, it may
sometimes be associated with:

- malignancy (as a paraneoplastic phenomenon
  – q.v.);
- other rheumatic diseases (especially SLE –
  q.v., and scleroderma – q.v.).

The pathogenesis is presumably immunological,
and autoantibodies of various types may be
identified in most patients. However, such
antibodies are probably markers rather than
causes of disease, since they are not usually
directed to muscle components, and the muscle
injury is more likely to be cell-mediated, since
lymphocytes may produce muscle cell
cytotoxin.

> Clinical features are dominated by proximal
> muscle weakness (i.e. shoulder and pelvic
> girdles). In severe cases, distal muscles and
> even the pharynx and diaphragm may be
> involved, with dysphagia, aspiration and
> respiratory failure.

Multi-organ involvement may be seen.

- **Skin**

  - A dark-red eruption is typical, particularly
    on the face, neck, chest and hands.
  - The eyelids may be discoloured and
    oedematous (heliotrope rash).
  - There may be generalized cutaneous
    vasculitis.

- **Lungs**

  – In about 50% of cases, there is either interstitial fibrosis or associated pneumonia.

- **Heart**

  – Arrhythmias and conduction defects may be seen.
  – Myocarditis is now recognized to be present in most patients.

- **Carcinoma**

  – This may be apparent if the polymyositis is a paraneoplastic phenomenon.

Investigations show increased muscle enzymes, especially CK, the most specific muscle enzyme, and particularly the CK-MM isoenzyme. An elevated CK-MB is not necessarily indicative of acute myocardial infarction in this setting, as this isoenzyme is also produced in regenerating skeletal muscle. The AST and LDH are also elevated. The EMG shows characteristic changes of asynchronous muscle fibre contraction. Biopsy shows degeneration and fragmentation of muscle fibres with patchy inflammation.

Diagnosis is made on the basis of the clinical features, together with the elevated muscle enzymes and typical biopsy and perhaps EMG. Imaging with MRI may be useful. Other causes of myopathy (q.v.) should be excluded.

A particularly difficult differential diagnosis is **inclusion body myositis**, suggested by a poor therapeutic response and confirmed by biopsy.

*Treatment is with **corticosteroids**, the dose depending on the severity of the disease. Although most patients improve with corticosteroids, the response is often partial. Following a satisfactory clinical response and normalization of muscle enzymes, the dosage may be tapered. If the response to corticosteroids is inadequate or the dose required for maintenance is unacceptably high, other modalities may be required, including cytotoxic agents (azathioprine or methotrexate), cyclosporin, high-dose immune globulin or plasmapheresis.*

The course of the disease is very variable, ranging from fulminant over a few days to indolent over many years. Typically, there is gradual progression over weeks to months. The mortality is 15–20% at 5 y and is worse in older patients or with associated cardiac, pulmonary or malignant processes. Occasionally there is spontaneous improvement, and sometimes complete and permanent remission may occur with therapy.

Bibliography
Dalakas MC 1991 Polymyositis, dermatomyositis, and inclusion-body myositis. N Engl J Med 325: 1487.
Miller FW 1994 Classification and prognosis of inflammatory muscle disease. Rheum Dis Clin North Am 20: 811.
Sigurgeirsson B, Lindelof B, Edhag O et al 1992. Risk of cancer in patients with dermatomyositis or polymyositis. N Engl J Med 326: 363.
Tazelaar HD, Viggiano RW, Pickersgill J et al 1990 Interstitial lung disease in polymyositis and dermatomyositis: clinical features and prognosis as correlated with histologic findings. Am Rev Resp Dis 141: 727.

Polyneuritis (see Neuropathy)

Polyneuropathy (see Neuropathy)

Porphyria

The porphyrias comprise a group of six mostly inherited diseases,of abnormal porphyrin metabolism. Porphyrin synthesis produces the iron-containing moiety, **haem**, which is the chief component in haemoglobin, cytochromes and other oxidative enzymes.

The enzymic steps from the initial components, glycine and succinyl-CoA, to the eventual production of haem give rise to ring structures via progressive deamination, decarboxylation, oxidation and finally iron chelation. These steps clearly provide multiple sites for enzymic defects, and indeed an abnormality at each of the six steps after the initial production of porphobilinogen causes a distinct disease.

The major sites of haem production are the liver and bone marrow, and thus the sites of the defects in porphyrias are either hepatic (the four most common forms) or erythropoietic (one rare form) or both (one form). Most porphyrias are inherited disorders.

Porphyrias were among the first inborn errors of metabolism to be described, because of their familial pattern, their characteristic clinical features and their obvious chemical markers in the urine (since porphyrins fluoresce under ultraviolet light).

The typical clinical course is one of acute attacks separated by long latent periods. This fluctuating course is explained by the fact that the enzyme defects affect non-rate-limiting steps, whereas the chief endogenous or exogenous stimuli for acute attacks induce the normally rate-limiting initial step controlled by the enzyme, δ-amino laevulinic acid (ALA) synthetase. Thus, precursor production now overwhelms the defective step, and intermediate products spill into the circulation and then into the urine.

Other diseases are also associated with acquired abnormalities of porphyrin metabolism, namely chronic liver disease, haemolysis, malignancy and especially lead poisoning.

1. **Acute intermittent porphyria** (AIP) is an autosomal dominant disease due to deficiency of porphobilinogen (PBG) deaminase to about 50% of normal levels. It is thus due to an abnormality at the first of the six steps from porphobilinogen to haem.

More than 100 different mutations have been described as affecting PBG deaminase in this way. However, 80–90% of those with genetic abnormalities have only latent disease, since many mutations are expressed mildly, and nearly half of those with overt biochemical defects are asymptomatic.

AIP comprises about 5% of porphyrias. Most patients are female.

Like the other hepatic porphyrias, AIP is characterized by the five 'Ps', namely

i.   onset after **P**uberty,
ii. **P**ain, especially abdominal,
iii. **P**olyneuropathy,
iv. **P**hotosensitivity,
v.   **P**sychiatric features.

In over 90% of symptomatic patients, attacks have occurred before the age of 40 years. They are precipitated by the four 'Ms', namely

i. **M**edicines

- especially alcohol, barbiturates, carbamazepine, chloramphenicol, chlordiazepoxide, ergot, griseofulvin, methyldopa, oestrogens, phenytoin, sulfonamides, tolbutamide.
- Fortunately, many drugs are safe, including analgesics, beta blockers, benzodiazepines, chlorpromazine, corticosteroids, penicillin, warfarin.

ii. **M**edical illnesses

- especially infections

iii. **M**alnutrition

- especially carbohydrate deprivation,

iv. **M**enstruation.

- More than half the attacks are precipitated by drugs (usually barbiturates, oral contraceptives, phenytoin, sulfonamides, though many others have varying degrees of reported porphyrinogenicity), followed by menstruation or pregnancy (13%), infections (10%), alcohol (3%), starvation (3%), while in about 15% no precipitating factor can be defined.
- Abdominal pain and tenderness are universal.
- The urine is dark (since PBG in urine polymerizes to form porphobilin, so that the urine becomes dark red on standing).
- Peripheral neuropathy, more motor than sensory, is found in 75% of patients, of whom 15% develop respiratory paralysis.

- About half the patients show neuropsychiatric changes of behaviour and/or mood, often with cranial nerve involvement and sometimes with fits.
- Fever, tachycardia and labile hypertension are common.

Investigations show increased urinary δ-ALA and PBG in all patients, even in remission. Urinary uroporphyrin (>40 nmol/day) and faecal coproporphyrin are increased in all cases acutely. Other investigations show leukocytosis, hyponatraemia, hypochloraemia, hypovolaemia, abnormal EEG and EMG, sometimes and abnormal CSF, and dilated bowel loops on abdominal X-ray.

The differential diagnosis includes in particular any cause of acute abdominal pain.

*Treatment is **symptomatic** with analgesics.*

- ***Glucose*** *in the form of 10% dextrose 200 mL/h is recommended, though added insulin may be required.*
- *Tachycardia and hypotension respond to **beta blockers**.*
- *Fits may be controlled with **gabapentin**.*
- *If respiratory paralysis occurs, **ventilatory support** is required, but even then the reported mortality is up to 50%.*
- *Fluids, electrolytes and nutritional support are required.*
- *Specific treatment in the form of **haematin**, the ferric form of haem (200 mg iv over 20 min bd), provides improvement within a few days but can give rise to disseminated intravascular coagulation.*

The prognosis is probably better than traditionally reported, since modern screening now shows that many patients are asymptomatic, and prophylactic avoidance of precipitating factors is effective. Family screening is recommended.

2. **Variegate porphyria** (porphyria variegata, PV) is due to a decreased protoporphyrinogen oxidase. It is thus due to an abnormality at the fifth of the six steps from porphobilinogen to haem. It is inherited and comprises about 5% of porphyrias.

It is associated with solar skin lesions, as there is photosensitivity, even indoors or under transparent sunscreens, because long-wavelength ultraviolet light penetrates transparent media. There is associated skin fragility and also neuropathic lesions, and blisters, ulcers and scars of various stages are seen.

Acute, systemic attacks can occur, similar to those in acute intermittent porphyria. The two conditions are distinguished by the demonstration of the appropriate porphyrins, usually in faeces, since the defective enzyme itself is not readily assayed.

Treatment is the same as for acute intermittent porphyria.

3. **Hereditary coproporphyria** (HC) is the least common hepatic porphyria (2% of porphyrias) and is due to a deficiency of coproporphyrinogen oxidase. It is thus due to an abnormality at the fourth of the six steps from porphobilinogen to haem.

It is clinically indistinguishable from variegate porphyria and thus overlaps acute intermittent porphyria.

Treatment principles are therefore similar.

4. **Porphyria cutanea tarda** (PCT) is the most common porphyria (80% of porphyrias) and is due to a deficiency of uroporphyrinogen decarboxylase. It is thus due to an abnormality at the third of the six steps from porphobilinogen to haem. Unlike the other porphyrias, most cases (up to 90%) are not familial.

The majority (75%) of affected cases are men, and the peak age of onset is in the 50s. More than half the cases are precipitated by alcohol and the rest by either oestrogens or liver disease, in which case there are abnormal liver function tests and histology. The condition can thus be associated with hepatitis, biliary disease or hepatoma.

All patients show photosensitivity, with vesiculation, hyperpigmentation, hypertrichosis and skin fragility. In 50% of cases, the urine becomes dark on standing.

Investigations show an increased urinary uroporphyrin (>40 nmol/day) and increased total porphyrins in urine and in plasma. Iron overload is seen in 75% of cases and may require venesection or even desferrioxamine (see Haemochromatosis).

*Treatment measures include **avoidance** of sun, alcohol, iron and oestrogens.*

- **Beta–carotene** *may be useful.*
- **Iron depletion therapy** *is required in most patients (see Haemochromatosis).*

5. **(Erythropoietic) Protoporphyria** (EPP) is due to a deficiency of ferrochetalase. It is thus due to an abnormality at the last of the six steps from porphobilinogen to haem. The deficient enzyme occurs in erythrocytes, as well as in liver cells. It is inherited and comprises about 8% of porphyrias.

The chief clinical feature is photosensitivity.

*It may be treated with **beta–carotene**.*

6. **Congenital erythropoietic porphyria** is a very rare autosomal recessive condition with a deficiency of uroporphyrinogen cosynthetase. It is thus due to an abnormality at the second of the six steps from porphobilinogen to haem. The deficient enzyme occurs only in the erythrocyte series.

It is associated with photosensitivity, haemolysis, dark urine and red teeth.

*It has been successfully treated with **bone marrow transplantation**.*

Bibliography

Brodie MJ, Moore MR, Thompson GG et al 1977 Pregnancy and the acute porphyrias. Br J Obstet Gynaec 84: 726.

Grandchamp B 1998 Acute intermittent porphyria. Semin Liver Dis 18: 17.

Kauppinen R, Mustajoki P 1992 Prognosis of acute porphyria: occurrence of acute attacks, precipitating factors, and associated diseases. Medicine 71: 1.

Lamon JM, Bennett M, Frykholm BC et al 1978 Prevention of acute porphyric attacks by intravenous haematin. Lancet 2: 492.

Moore MR 1993 Biochemistry of porphyria. Int J Biochem 25: 1353.

Mustajoki P, Nordman Y 1993 Early administration of heme arginate for acute porphyric attacks. Arch Intern Med 153: 2004.

Yeung Laiwah AC, Moore MR, Goldberg A 1987 Pathogenesis of acute porphyria. Quart J Med 63: 377.

Post-transfusion purpura (see Thrombocytopenia)

Pre-eclampsia

Pre-eclampsia (toxaemia of pregnancy, gestosis in Eastern Europe) occurs in 5–10% of all pregnancies, most commonly in the third trimester of the first pregnancy. It occurs earlier, even in the first trimester, in the presence of hydatidiform mole or underlying renal disease.

The aetiology remains unknown but clearly requires the presence of the trophoblast, as the condition is unique to pregnancy. It is associated with uteroplacental ischaemia, which in turn is associated with structural abnormalities of the spiral arteries, abnormalities of prostaglandin metabolism, increased platelet responsiveness, generalized increase in pressor responsiveness and endothelial cell swelling in the glomeruli. Its pathogenesis may be immunological and perhaps an abnormal response to feto–placental tissue.

Pre-eclampsia consists of the gradual onset of:

- hypertension (to >140/90 mmHg);
- oedema;
- proteinuria (often to >3.5 g/day, i.e. the nephrotic range, but with a normal renal sediment and normal renal function).

The progression from pre-eclampsia to eclampsia is indicated by convulsions and occurs in about 1 in 200 cases. Even in the absence of convulsions (eclampsia), severe pre-eclampsia is associated with neurological features of headache, visual disturbance and increased reflexes. The disparity in the responses of eclamptic and epileptic seizures to benzodiazepines and phenytoin suggests that their mechanism of production is different.

There may be upper abdominal tenderness due to liver distension. Sometimes, the HELLP syndrome (q.v.) may occur, and indeed about 10% of more severe cases suffer this complication.

> In 20–30% of cases of eclampsia, the onset is post-partum and any ante-partum pre-eclampsia may have been mild. Eclampsia may thus be an unpredictable complication for up to 7 days after delivery.

Since pre-eclampsia does not cause renal impairment, the presence of renal failure indicates another associated complication, such as:

- sepsis;
- abruptio placentae;
- urinary tract obstruction;
- acute fatty liver;
- haemolytic–uraemic syndrome (especially post-partum);
- hypovolaemia (due either to hyperemesis or to diabetes insipidus, the latter sometimes seen from excess placental metabolism of vasopressin by vasopressinase).

The differential diagnosis is underlying hypertension or renal disease.

*Treatment is by **delivery** if the mother is stable and fetal maturity is satisfactory.*

- ***Hypertension** may be treated satisfactorily with beta-blockers, methyldopa, hydralazine, or probably calcium channel inhibitors, but ACE inhibitors should be avoided because of increased fetal morbidity and because of possible hypovolaemia.*
- *Hypovolaemia should be treated, and cardiac filling pressures may need to be monitored.*

- ***Magnesium sulfate** is the agent of choice for the prevention and treatment of convulsions (i.e. eclampsia). To achieve a 'therapeutic serum magnesium level' of 2–4 mmol/L, 20 mmol (0.5 g) of magnesium (i. e. 5 g of magnesium sulfate) should be given, as 10 mL iv of 50% magnesium sulfate in 100 mL of 5% dextrose over 20 min. This should be followed by a continuous iv infusion of 5–10 mmol/h for 24 h to maintain a magnesium level which is effective but not toxic. If seizures recur, 50% of the initial loading dose is repeated. Toxicity is monitored by assessment of tendon reflexes for hyporeflexia and by measurement of the serum magnesium level (see Magnesium).*
- *Effective prophylaxis in high-risk patients may be achieved with low-dose **aspirin**.*

The maternal prognosis is good, and there is no increased incidence of subsequent hypertension or renal disease. If the disease has progressed to frank eclampsia, there is a risk of maternal mortality from cerebral haemorrhage. There is an increased fetal risk.

There is a low likelihood of recurrence, unless:

- the condition is severe;
- it has occurred in a multigravida;
- there is a different partner for a subsequent pregnancy;
- there is underlying renal disease.

Bibliography

Arbogast BW, Taylor RN 1997 Molecular Mechanisms of Pre-eclampsia. Berlin: Springer-Verlag.

Bucher HC, Guyatt GH, Cook RJ et al 1996 Effect of calcium supplementation on pregnancy-induced hypertension and preeclampsia. A meta-analysis of randomised controlled trials. JAMA 275: 1113.

Chua S, Redman CWG 1991 Are prophylactic anticonvulsants required in severe pre-eclampsia? Lancet 337: 250.

CLASP (Collaborative Low-dose Aspirin Study in Pregnancy) Collaborative Group 1994 CLASP: a randomised trial of low-dose aspirin for the prevention and treatment of pre-eclampsia among 9364 pregnant women. Lancet 343: 619.

Cunningham FG, Grant NF 1989 Prevention of preeclampsia – a reality? N Engl J Med 321: 606.

Davison JM, Shiells EA, Barron WM et al 1989 Changes in the metabolic clearance of vasopressin and plasma vasopressinase throughout human pregnancy. J Clin Invest 83: 1313.

Douglas KA, Redman CWG 1994 Eclampsia in the United Kingdom. Br Med J 309: 1395.

Durr JA, Hoggard JG, Hunt JM et al 1987 Diabetes insipidus in pregnancy associated with abnormally high circulating vasopressinase activity. N Engl J Med 316: 1070.

Editorial 1989 Are ACE inhibitors safe in pregnancy? Lancet 2: 482.

Gant NF, Worley RJ, Everett RB et al 1980 Control of vascular responsiveness during human pregnancy. Kidney Int 18: 253.

Ihle BU, Long P, Oats J 1987 Early onset pre-eclampsia: recognition of underlying renal disease. Br Med J 294: 79.

Lucas MJ, Leveno KJ, Cunningham FG 1995 A comparison of magnesium sulfate with phenytoin for the prevention of eclampsia. N Engl J Med 333: 201.

Martin JN, Files FC, Blake PG 1990 Plasma exchange for preeclampsia: I. Postpartum use for persistently severe preeclampsia with HELLP syndrome. Am J Obstet Gynecol 162: 126.

Need JA 1975 Pre-eclampsia in pregnancies by different fathers: immunological studies. Br Med J 1: 548.

Perry KG, Martin JN 1992 Abnormal hemostasis and coagulopathy in preeclampsia and eclampsia. Clin Obstet Gynecol 35: 338.

Redman C 1990 Platelets and the beginnings of preeclampsia. N Engl J Med 323: 478.

Redman CWG, Roberts JM 1993 Management of pre-eclampsia. Lancet 341: 1451.

Roberts J, Taylor R, Goldfen A 1991 Clinical and biochemical evidence of endothelial cell dysfunction in pregnancy syndrome eclampsia. Am J Hypertens 4: 700.

Sibai BM, El-Nazer A, Gonzalez-Ruiz A 1986 Severe preeclampsia in young primigravid women: subsequent pregnancy outcome and remote prognosis. Am J Obstet Gynecol 155: 1011.

The Eclampsia Trial Collaborative Group 1995 Which anticonvulsant for women with eclampsia? Evidence from the Collaborative Eclampsia Trial. Lancet 345: 1455.

Williams DJ, de Swiet M 1997 The pathophysiology of pre-eclampsia. Intens Care Med 23: 620.

Pregnancy

A number of either general or specific problems related to pregnancy have relevance to Intensive Care. The general problems are discussed below and include:

- miscarriage (abortion);
- drugs;
- systemic disorders;
- teratogenicity;
- trophoblastic neoplasia;
- post-partum problems.

Specific problems of importance are discussed separately, namely:

- acute fatty liver of pregnancy (q.v.);
- HELLP syndrome (q.v.);
- pneumonia in pregnancy (q.v.);
- pre-eclampsia (q.v.);
- trauma in pregnancy (q.v.).

Maternal deaths are defined by the WHO as deaths 'during pregnancy, childbirth or in the 42 days of the puerperium, irrespective of the duration and site of the pregnancy, from any cause related to or aggravated by the pregnancy or its management'. Such deaths may be:

- direct (i.e. due to a complication of the pregnancy itself); or
- indirect (i.e. due to some other disease but possibly aggravated by pregnancy).

Deaths during pregnancy may also be incidental to that state (e.g. from trauma, suicide, cancer). Total maternal mortality in Victoria is recorded from all three causes and over the last decade has averaged about 0.1 per 1000 births.

By contrast, the total perinatal mortality was 6.9 per 1000 births (or 4.3 per 1000 births using the more restricted WHO recommendations for international comparison), of which about two thirds of the deaths are stillbirths (i.e. at least 500 g or over 22 weeks gestation) and one third neonatal (i.e. at least 500 g or over 22 weeks gestation, and within 28 days of birth). The infant death rate (i.e. total mortality of liveborn babies up to one year) was 3.8 per 1000 live births. This low figure has been particularly contributed to by the progressive decline in Sudden Infant Death Syndrome (SIDS, cot death) over the past decade from about 30% to 10% of infant deaths.

1. The **risk of miscarriage (abortion)** is increased:

- in the antiphospholipid syndrome (APS) (q.v.);
- in systemic infection (especially brucellosis, toxoplasmosis, typhoid);
- with misoprostol (a synthetic PGE_1 analogue used for NSAID-induced peptic ulceration).

More than half of all cases of recurrent miscarriage can be related to a procoagulant abnormality, which then leads to placental vascular occlusion via thrombosis and infarction. The antiphospholipid syndrome is responsible for two thirds of these abnormalities. Virtually all patients with a procoagulant abnormality can subsequently proceed to term with treatment, usually with aspirin before conception and with aspirin and heparin from conception to delivery.

The **complications of miscarriage** are numerous, the most important acute ones being infective, namely:

- acute pelvic inflammatory disease;
- clostridial or Gram-negative anaerobic infections;
- *Mycoplasma hominis* infection (which may also occur post-partum) giving a mild, self-limited, febrile illness.

2. **Drugs** may cause fetal and sometimes maternal problems.

- Antibiotics

  - erythromycin estolate, quinolones, tetracycline and trimethoprim are contraindicated in pregnancy;
  - aminoglycosides, chloramphenicol, metronidazole and sulfonamides are also best avoided;
  - penicillin and cephalosporins are safe.

- Analgesics and sedatives

  - codeine and paracetamol are safe,
  - narcotics are safe except near term,

  - benzodiazepines and barbiturates are not recommended for long-term use,
  - aspirin should be used only for specifically defined indications, e.g. pre-eclampsia.

- Anaesthetics

  - muscle relaxants are safe,
  - nitrous oxide is safe in late pregnancy,
  - local anaesthetics should be used with caution in late pregnancy.

3. Common **systemic disorders**, such as the antiphospholipid syndrome, cardiac disease, cholestasis, collagen-vascular diseases, diabetes, epilepsy, folic acid deficiency, hypertension, infectious diseases (e.g. listeriosis, toxoplasmosis), renal disease, thromboembolism, and thyroid disease, all present additional problems during pregnancy.

Pulmonary oedema in pregnancy may be:

- cardiogenic;
- associated with pre-eclampsia;
- tocolytic-induced (i.e. a complication of β-agonist therapy).

Pneumonia in pregnancy (q.v.) and trauma in pregnancy (q.v.) present particular problems and are discussed separately.

4. Some occupational and environmental exposures are **teratogenic**.

5. **Neoplasia** may arise in the gestational trophoblast. Such neoplasia includes:

- hydatidiform mole, which can be partial, complete or invasive;
- choriocarcinoma, the most invasive form. Choriocarcinoma usually arises from a molar pregnancy, but it can also occur after spontaneous abortion (1:5000 cases), ectopic pregnancy (1:15000 cases) or full-term pregnancy (1:150000 cases).

A molar pregnancy should be considered if there is excessive uterine enlargement, pre-eclampsia, hyperemesis or abnormal vaginal bleeding. The hCG level is markedly elevated, associated hyperthyroidism is sometimes seen, and occasionally trophoblastic lung emboli may occur. In choriocarcinoma, metastases occur particularly to the lung and later to the brain and liver.

*Treatment with combination **chemotherapy** carries a very high cure rate, even for advanced metastatic disease (85% in such cases).*

6. **Post-partum problems** are similar to the systemic problems encountered during pregnancy and listed above, but they can especially include thromboembolism and hypertension.

Additional problems at this time may include:

- endocrine abnormalities (e.g. pituitary infarction);
- cardiomyopathy;
- streptococcal infection;
- depression.

Bibliography

Arnout J, Spitz B, Wittevrongel C et al 1994 High-dose intravenous immunoglobulin treatment of a pregnant patient with an antiphospholipid syndrome. Thromb Haemost 71: 741.

Australian Drug Evaluation Committee 1999 Prescribing Medicines in Pregnancy. 4th edition. Canberra: Australian Government Printing Service.

Australian Society for the Study of Hypertension in Pregnancy 1993 Management of hypertension in pregnancy: consensus statement. Med J Aust 158: 700.

Barron WM 1984 The pregnant surgical patient: medical evaluation and management. Ann Intern Med 101: 683.

Battino D, Granata T, Binelli S et al 1992 Intrauterine growth in the offspring of epileptic mothers. Acta Neurol Scand 86: 555.

Beischer NA (chairman) 1998 Annual Report for the Year 1997. Melbourne: Consultative Council on Obstetric and Paediatric Mortality and Morbidity.

Beeley L 1981 Adverse effects of drugs in later pregnancy. Clin Obstet Gynaecol 24: 275.

Bick RL 2000 Recurrent miscarriage syndrome due to blood coagulation protein/platelet defects: prevalence, treatment and outcome results. Clin Appl Thromb Hemost 6: 115.

Branch DW, Scott JR, Kochenour NK et al 1985 Obstetric complications associated with the lupus anticoagulant. N Engl J Med 313: 1322.

Briggs GG, Freeman RL, Yaffe SJ (eds) 1990 Drugs in Pregnancy and Lactation. 3rd edition. Baltimore: Williams & Wilkins.

Brodie MJ, Moore MR, Thompson GG et al 1977 Pregnancy and the acute porphyrias. Br J Obstet Gynaec 84: 726.

Brown MA, Buddle ML 1996 Hypertension in pregnancy: maternal and foetal outcomes according to laboratory and clinical features. Med J Aust 165: 360.

Brown M, Whitworth J 1992 The kidney in hypertensive pregnancies – victim and villain. Am J Kidney Dis 20: 427.

Burrow GN 1985 The management of thyrotoxicosis in pregnancy. N Engl J Med 313: 562.

Cope I 1991 Medicines in pregnancy. Med J Aust 155: 214.

Cowchock FS, Reece EA, Balaban D et al 1992 Repeated fetal losses associated with antiphospholipid antibodies. Am J Obstet Gynecol 166: 1318.

Dansky LV, Rosenblatt DS, Andermann E 1992 Mechanisms of teratogenesis: folic acid and antiepileptic therapy. Neurology 42 (suppl 5): 32.

Editorial 1989 Are ACE inhibitors safe in pregnancy? Lancet 2: 482.

Fildes J, Reed L, Jones N et al 1992 Trauma: the leading cause of maternal death. J Trauma 32: 643.

Ginsberg JS, Hirsh J 1992 Use of antithrombotic agents during pregnancy. Chest 102 (suppl 4): 385S.

Ginsberg JS, Brill-Edwards P, Johnston M et al 1992 Relationship of antiphospholipid antibodies to pregnancy loss in patients with systemic lupus erythematosus. Blood 80: 975.

Greer IA 1999 Thrombosis in pregnancy: maternal and foetal issues. Lancet 353: 1258.

Grunfeld J-P, Pertuiset N 1987 Acute renal failure in pregnancy. Am J Kidney Dis 9: 359.

Hanly JG, Gladman DD, Rose TH et al 1988 Lupus pregnancy: a prospective study of placental changes. Arthritis Rheum 31: 358.

Hayslett JP 1985 Postpartum renal failure. N Engl J Med 312: 1556.

Hiilesmaa VK 1992 Pregnancy and birth in women with epilepsy. Neurology 42 (suppl 5): 8.

Homans DC 1985 Peripartum cardiomyopathy. N Engl J Med 312: 1432.

Horowitz MD, Gomez GA, Santiesteban R et al 1985 Acute appendicitis during pregnancy. Arch Surg 120: 1362.

Imperiale TF, Petrulis AS 1991 A meta-analysis of low-dose aspirin for the prevention of pregnancy-induced hypertensive disease. JAMA 266: 237.

Johns KR, Morand EF, Littlejohn GO 1998 Pregnancy outcome in systemic lupus erythematosus. Aust NZ J Med 28: 18.

Johnson MJ 1997 Obstetric complications and rheumatic disease. Rheum Dis Clin North Am 23: 169.

Jones WB, Lewis JL 1988 Integration of surgery and other techniques in the management of trophoblastic malignancy. Obstet Gynecol Clin North Am 15: 565.

Kjellberg U, Andersson N-E, Rosen S et al 1999 APC resistance and other haemostatic variables during pregnancy and puerperium. Thromb Haemost 81: 527.

Koch S, Losche G, Jager-Roman E et al 1992 Major and minor birth malformations and antiepileptic drugs. Neurol 42 (suppl 5): 83.

Koshy M, Burd L 1991 Management of pregnancy in sickle cell anemia. Hematol Oncol Clin North Am 5: 585.

Lapinsky SE 1996 Respiratory care of the critically ill pregnant patient. Curr Opinion Crit Care 3: 1.

Laskin CA, Bombardier C, Hannah ME 1997 Prednisolone and aspirin in women with autoantibodies and unexplained recurrent fetal loss. N Engl J Med 337: 148.

Ledger WJ 1977 Antibiotics in pregnancy. Clin Obstet Gynaecol 20: 411.

Lemire RJ 1988 Neural tube defects. JAMA 259: 558.

Leung AS, Millar LK, Koonings PP et al 1993 Perinatal outcome in hypothyroid pregnancies. Obstet Gynecol 81: 349.

Lim V, Katz A, Lindheimer M 1976 Acid–base regulation in pregnancy. Am J Physiol 231: 1764.

Lindheimer MD, Katz AI 1985 Hypertension in pregnancy. N Engl J Med 313: 675.

Lockshin MD 1985 Lupus pregnancy. Clin Rheum Dis 11: 611.

McDonald CF, Burdon JGW 1996 Asthma in pregnancy and lactation: a position paper for the Thoracic Society of Australia and New Zealand. Med J Aust 165: 485.

McPartin J, Halligan A, Scott JM et al 1993 Accelerated folate breakdown in pregnancy. Lancet 341: 148.

Oakley CM 1995 Anticoagulants in pregnancy. Br Heart J 74: 107.

Persellin RH 1977 The effect of pregnancy on rheumatoid arthritis. Bull Rheum Dis 27: 922.

Pisani RJ, Rosenow EC 1989 Pulmonary edema associated with tocolytic therapy. Ann Intern Med 110: 714.

Rizk NW, Kalassian KG, Gilligan T et al 1996 Obstetric complications in pulmonary and critical care medicine. Chest 110: 791.

Rubin PC 1981 Beta-blockers in pregnancy. N Engl J Med 305: 1323.

Schrier RW 1988 Pathogenesis of sodium and water retention in high-output and low-output cardiac failure, nephrotic syndrome, cirrhosis, and pregnancy. N Engl J Med 319: 1065, 1127.

Stirrat GM 1990 Recurrent miscarriage. Lancet 336: 673.

Wald NJ, Bower C 1994 Folic acid, pernicious anaemia, and prevention of neural tube defects. Lancet 343: 307.

Yerby MS 1991 Pregnancy and epilepsy. Epilepsia 32 (suppl 6): S51.

Yerby M, Koepsell T, Darling J 1985 Pregnancy complications and outcomes in a cohort of women with epilepsy. Epilepsia 26: 631.

Yerby MS, Friel PN, McCormick K 1992 Antiepileptic drug disposition during pregnancy. Neurology 42 (suppl 5): 12.

Yerby MS, Leavitt A, Erickson DM et al 1992 Antiepileptics and the development of congenital anomalies. Neurology 42 (suppl 5): 132.

Priapism

Priapism refers to painful and prolonged erection of the penis. It is an uncommon complication of:

- sickle cell anaemia;
- spinal cord lesions;
- polycythaemia vera;
- rarely other thrombotic disorders.

It is sometimes seen as a complication of local therapy for impotence, while priapism itself may in turn lead to impotence. It has occasionally been reported as a side-effect of the non-tricyclic antidepressant agent, trazodone.

Procalcitonin (see Calcitonin)

Proctitis (see Anorectal infections)

Progressive multifocal leukoencephalopathy (see

Demyelinating diseases)

Protein C

Protein C is an important natural inhibitor of coagulation. It is a vitamin K dependent factor and is a serine protease, like most coagulation factors.

Protein C is activated when thrombin couples with thrombomodulin on the endothelial cell surface. It then combines with membrane-bound protein S to form an active complex. This complex antagonizes the large activated cofactors, Va and VIIIa, as they assist the activation of II to IIa and X toXa, respectively.

Protein C has a molecular weight of 62 kD, plasma concentration of 4mg/L (0.0645 μM) and half life of about 12 h.

Protein C deficiency is implicated in the rare warfarin–induced skin necrosis (q.v.). This is because Protein C (and probably protein S) have shorter half-lives than the four vitamin K-dependent coagulation factors (factors II, VII, IX & X) and the initial effect of warfarin, especially in higher dose, must therefore be transiently thrombotic (i.e. the anticoagulant factors are decreased before the coagulation factors). Similarly, in vitamin K deficiency, the administration of vitamin K must result in a transiently haemorrhagic state (i.e. the anticoagulant factors are increased before the coagulation factors).

Protein C deficiency may be either congenital or acquired and leads to a hypercoagulable state.

Congenital protein C deficiency is lethal (with purpura fulminans) in early life if it is homozygous, but heterozygotes are common (1 in 250 of the population). In these subjects, protein C levels overlap the low normal range, and thromboses can occur even with levels of about 50% of normal. Venous and arterial thromboses may occur, and these are sometimes unusual in affecting e.g. cerebral or splenic vessels.

*Treatment is normally with life-long **warfarin**.*

Acquired protein C deficiency occurs in:

- vitamin K deficiency (q.v.);
- liver disease;
- disseminated intravascular coagulation.

Activated protein C resistance is a recently recognized familial thrombophilia, with a Caucasian population incidence of about 5%. It has been found to be the major risk factor for venous thrombosis, being demonstrated in 20–50% of such patients (the higher incidence being found in patients with a family history of thromboembolism).

The phenomenon is due to a point mutation with a single-base substitution of adenine for guanine in the Factor V gene. In the resultant Factor V molecule (Factor V Leiden) an arg at amino acid 506 is replaced by a glu at the cleavage site for protein C, thus rendering Factor Va resistant to inactivation by activated protein C (APC).

Heterozygous subjects have a thrombotic risk which is similar to that seen in heterozygous protein C or protein S deficiency and which increases with age, malignancy and oral contraceptives. APC resistance may also predispose to arterial thrombosis.

Treatment principles are the same as those previously established for protein C or S deficiency (q.v.).

Protein C levels have been found to be low in sepsis and to be correlated with outcome. Protein C replacement was reported to be of benefit in the treatment of small numbers of patients with this condition, and the initial results of a recent large multicentre randomized controlled study using recombinant human activated protein C (drotrecogin alfa) are promising.

Bibliography
Bernard GR, Vincent J-L, Laterre P-F et al 2001
    Efficacy and safety of recombinant human

activated protein C for severe sepsis. N Engl J Med 344: 699.

Bertina RM, Koeleman RPC, Koster T et al 1994 Mutation in blood coagulation factor V associated with resistance to activated protein C. Nature 369: 64.

Dowd P, Ham S-W, Naganathan S et al 1995 The mechanism of action of vitamin K. Annu Rev Nutr 15: 419.

Esmon C 2000 The protein C pathway. Crit Care Med 28: 556.

Esmon CT, Johnson AE, Esmon NL et al 1991 Initiation of the protein C pathway. Ann NY Acad Sci 614: 30.

Hillarp A, Dahlback B 1997 Activated protein C resistance. Vessels 3: 4.

Koster T, Rosendaal FR, de Ronde H, Briet E, Vandenbroucke JP, Bertina RM 1993 Venous thrombosis due to poor anticoagulant response to activated protein C. Lancet 342: 1503.

Matsuzaka T, Tanaka H, Fukuda M et al 1993 Relationship between vitamin K dependent coagulation factors and anticoagulants (protein C and protein S) in neonatal vitamin K deficiency. Arch Dis Child 68: 297.

Papinger I, Kyrle PA, Heistinger M et al 1994 The risk of thromboembolism in asymptomatic patients with protein C and protein S deficiency. Thromb Haemost 71: 441.

Rose VL, Kwaan HC, Williamson K et al 1986 Protein C antigen deficiency and warfarin necrosis. Am J Clin Pathol 86: 653.

Shearer MJ 1995 Vitamin K. Lancet 345: 229.

Smith OP, White B, Vaughan D et al 1997 Use of protein C concentrate, heparin, and haemodiafiltration in meningococcus-induced purpura fulminans. Lancet 350: 1590.

Svensson PJ, Dahlback B 1994 Resistance to activated protein C as a basis for venous thrombosis. N Engl J Med 330: 517.

Zoller B, Hillarp A, Dahlback B 1997 Activated protein C resistance: Clinical implications. Clin Appl Thromb Hemost 3: 25.

Protein S

Protein S is, like protein C, also vitamin K dependent. It is a cofactor for protein C. It has a molecular weight of 69 kD and plasma concentration of 25 mg/L (10 mg/L free, 0.1449 μM), but its half-life is uncertain.

Protein S provides one of the links between the processes of inflammation and thrombosis. Thus, circulating protein S is bound to the C4b component of complement (an acute phase reactant) and is thereby inhibited. In addition, IL-1 decreases thrombomodulin on endothelial cells by two thirds, so that the protein C–protein S complex functions at only about 10% of its normal capacity in this setting.

Like protein C deficiency, protein S deficiency may be either congenital or acquired (e.g. in pregnancy and in the nephrotic syndrome) and is a cause of a thrombotic tendency. Such thromboses can affect cerebral, mesenteric, renal and other veins.

*Treatment is with life-long **warfarin**.*

Bibliography

Dowd P, Ham S-W, Naganathan S et al 1995 The mechanism of action of vitamin K. Annu Rev Nutr 15: 419.

Engesser L, Broekmans AW, Briet E et al 1987 Hereditary protein S deficiency: clinical manifestations. Ann Intern Med 106: 677.

Matsuzaka T, Tanaka H, Fukuda M et al 1993 Relationship between vitamin K dependent coagulation factors and anticoagulants (protein C and protein S) in neonatal vitamin K deficiency. Arch Dis Child 68: 297.

Papinger I, Kyrle PA, Heistinger M et al 1994 The risk of thromboembolism in asymptomatic patients with protein C and protein S deficiency. Thromb Haemost 71: 441.

Rose VL, Kwaan HC, Williamson K et al 1986 Protein C antigen deficiency and warfarin necrosis. Am J Clin Pathol 86: 653.

Shearer MJ 1995 Vitamin K. Lancet 345: 229.

Proteinuria

Proteinuria, like haematuria, is a common abnormality detected on urinalysis.

Proteinuria is defined as >150 mg/day. It should be remembered that:

- 150 mg of protein in this setting contains <20 mg of albumin;

- the dipstick test has a threshold of detection of 2–3-fold higher than this;
- the dipstick test does not detect non-albumin protein.

Proteinuria is:

- mild if <1 g/day;
- severe if >3 g/day.

Proteinuria is clinically important if it is persistent and not solely orthostatic. It may be due to:

1. **Glomerular disease**

In this case, the protein is chiefly albumin.

2. **Tubulointerstitial disease** (including reflux nephropathy)

In this case, the protein is chiefly beta$_2$-microglobulin (q.v.).

Proteinuria comprising mainly low molecular weight material is also seen when there is greatly increased production of such species, e.g. light chains in multiple myeloma (q.v.).

3. **'Overflow'**

This occurs in multiple myeloma, acute leukaemia or following heavy exercise. In these cases, both high-molecular-weight (albumin) and low-molecular-weight (beta$_2$-microglobulin) fractions are excreted.

A similar phenomenon occurs with increased glomerular permeability, as in infection, cardiac failure or following exertion.

Appropriate investigations of proteinuria include examination of urine, renal biopsy and ultrasound examination.

Bibliography
Robinson RR 1980 Isolated proteinuria in asymptomatic patients. Kidney Int 18: 395.

Prussian blue (see Thallium)

Pseudogout (see Gout)

Pseudohyperkalaemia

Pseudohyperkalaemia is not a clinical problem but solely an in vitro phenomenon.

> It is best known as a consequence of in vitro haemolysis, but it also occurs in the presence of marked leukocytosis ($>100 \times 10^9$/L) or thrombocytosis ($>1000 \times 10^9$/L).
>
> Hyperkalaemia in these circumstances should always raise some suspicion as to its correctness. Sometimes, of course, the hyperkalaemia is correct, though unexpected and transient.

Bibliography
Greenberg S, Reiser IW, Chou SY et al 1993 Trimethoprim-sulfamethoxazole induces reversible hyperkalemia. Ann Intern Med 119: 291.

Pseudohyponatraemia (see also Syndrome of inappropriate antidiuretic hormone and Central pontine myelinolysis)

Pseudohyponatraemia refers to a decreased plasma sodium in the presence of a normal or increased plasma osmolality. It may be referred to as isotonic hyponatraemia.

True hyponatraemia is always associated with hypo-osmolality.

Pseudohyponatraemia is due to the presence of other active osmols in plasma, which therefore cause water to move from the intracellular space to the extracellular space and thus dilute the plasma sodium. It therefore occurs in the presence of high concentrations of glucose or mannitol. As a rule of thumb, an increased plasma glucose of 3.5–5 mmol/L decreases the plasma sodium by 1 mmol/L.

Increased concentrations of lipids and proteins can cause up to one third decrease in plasma sodium, because there is less water per litre of plasma, and the phenomenon is thus a measurement artifact.

Glycine irrigation solution, as sometimes used in urology, gives isosmotic dilution of plasma sodium, which can fall as low as 100 mmol/L. Consequent symptoms such as fits are due to glycine toxicity as well as to hyponatraemia.

The diagnosis of pseudohyponatraemia is important, because it is the underlying disease and not the low plasma sodium which requires treatment. When the plasma osmolality is measured in such circumstances, it is important to subtract any contribution from a raised urea, as in renal failure, to provide an estimate of the true osmolality.

Bibliography

Bonventre JV, Leaf A 1982 Sodium homeostasis: steady states without a set point. Kidney Int 21: 880.

Dixon B, Ernest D 1996 Hyponatraemia in the transurethral resection of prostate syndrome. Anaes Intens Care 24: 102.

Weinberg LS 1989 Pseudohyponatremia: a reappraisal. Am J Med 86: 315.

Pseudohypoparathyroidism (see Hypoparathyroidism)

Pseudomembranous colitis (see Colitis)

Pseudo-obstruction of the colon

Pseudo-obstruction of the colon (Ogilvie syndrome) is a relatively common acute complication of a number of conditions in sick hospitalized patients, including surgery, trauma, sepsis, diabetes, neurological disorders, scleroderma, amyloid, and of course drugs which inhibit gastrointestinal motility. As its name suggests, there is no mechanical obstruction, though the pathogenesis is uncertain.

Colonic dilatation is evidenced by a caecal diameter at least 10 cm shown radiologically. Although the condition tends to resolve with conservative treatment, it is a serious condition,

because it can sometimes cause perforation and thus peritonitis and even death.

*Treatment is chiefly of the underlying condition. If this fails, early **colonoscopic decompression** is recommended, though this procedure can be both difficult and hazardous in some patients.*

*Recently, the anticholinesterase **neostigmine** (2 mg iv over 3–5 min) has been shown to be rapidly effective, with decompression in less than 30 min. This agent should be given only in the Intensive Care Unit, because significant muscarinic effects including bradycardia (requiring atropine) may occur, as well as abdominal pain. Needless to say, subtle as well as overt mechanical bowel obstruction (e.g. volvulus) must be excluded before this cholinergic agent can be safely given.*

Bibliography

Ponec RJ, Saunders MD, Kimmey MB 1999 Neostigmine for the treatment of acute colonic pseudo-obstruction. N Engl J Med 341: 137.

Pseudo primary aldosteronism

(see Conn's syndrome)

Psoriasis

Psoriasis is a chronic papulosquamous disease, with a population incidence of 0.5–3%. Its aetiology is unknown, but both hereditary and environmental factors may be involved. There is a 3-fold increased incidence in smokers, and the condition is worse in alcoholics.

The Auspitz sign refers to small bleeding points following scraping of the lesion's scales and is diagnostically helpful. The Kobner response refers to the production of a new lesion following local trauma at an uninvolved site, though this phenomenon is not specific for psoriasis. Scratching thus can aggravate the condition.

The individual lesions tend to coalesce to form plaques which can become extensive, especially on the elbows, knees, lower back and scalp.

Even the palms, soles and genitals may be involved, and the nails become pitted. The lesions can last for many years unless treated. Discomfort and pruritus occur in 60% of cases.

Local treatment includes dithranol, phototherapy, steroids and tar.

- *Systemic therapy chiefly includes methotrexate, etretinate (related to isotretinoin) and probably cyclosporin, though many other agents have also been used with some benefit.*
- *Drugs including antimalarials, beta blockers, indomethacin and lithium may adversely affect psoriasis and should be avoided if possible.*

The prognosis is very variable and the condition can fluctuate greatly spontaneously.

Variants of psoriasis include:

- **Erythroderma** (see Exfoliative dermatitis);
- **Guttate psoriasis**, occurring especially after upper respiratory tract infection, because infecting organisms can act as superantigens and boost the immune response, causing guttate flares;
- **Seborrhoeic psoriasis**, also included in the spectrum of seborrhoeic dermatitis (see Dermatitis);
- **Psoriasis associated with arthritis** and overlapping with Reiter's syndrome (q.v.);
- **Pustular psoriasis**, either generalized (in 80% of cases and associated with hypocalcaemia) or localized (usually to the palms and soles). The lesions appear infected but in fact are not.

Bibliography

Calvert HT, Smith MA, Wells RS 1963 Psoriasis and the nails. Br J Dermatol 75: 415.

Farber EM, Nall ML 1974 The natural history of psoriasis in 5,600 patients. Dermatologica 148: 1.

Farber EM, Nall ML 1992 An appraisal of measures to prevent and control psoriasis. J Am Acad Dermatol 26: 736.

Fox BJ, Odom RB 1985 Papulosquamous diseases: a review. J Am Acad Dermatol 12: 597.

Ingram JT 1958 Pustular psoriasis. Arch Dermatol 77: 314.

Lebwohl M 2000 Advances in psoriasis therapy. Dermatol Clin 18: 13.

Whyte HJ, Baughman RD 1964 Acute guttate psoriasis and streptococcal infection. Arch Dermatol 89: 350.

Ptosis

Ptosis, or drooping eyelid, may be unilateral or bilateral.

- If **unilateral**, it is due to:
  - III nerve lesion;
  - Horner's syndrome (q.v.).
- If **bilateral**, it is either associated with:
  - ophthalmoplegia (q.v.);
  - generalized muscle disorder (see Myopathy).

Pulmonary alveolar proteinosis

Pulmonary alveolar proteinosis (PAP) is a disease of unknown cause and indeed with no known precipitating factor.

There is an accumulation in the alveoli of glycoprotein and lipid material resembling surfactant. It may therefore be a condition of abnormal surfactant production or clearance. It is of interest that GM-CSF 'knockout' mice develop a strikingly similar condition.

Microscopically, this material is amorphous and eosinophilic, with a characteristic positive reaction to periodic acid–Schiff (PAS) reagent. On electron microscopy, there are lamellar bodies similar to those seen in alveolar type II cells. Inflammation is usually minimal, and the lung structure remains intact.

Clinical features comprise cough and dyspnoea, through some patients are asymptomatic. Chest signs are minimal. While occasionally it may cause respiratory failure, most patients are not seriously ill.

The chest X-ray shows a bilateral, butterfly-shaped, pulmonary infiltrate resembling pulmonary oedema but without cardiomegaly, pulmonary vascular congestion, Kerley B lines or pleural effusion. The disease is thus one of the uncommon causes of this common X-ray picture in seriously ill patients.

> The diagnosis is made by the demonstration in turbid fluid obtained by bronchoalveolar lavage of abundant PAS-positive material.
>
> - Since secondary infection may occur, particularly with mycobacteria, nocardia or fungi, the lavage fluid should always be cultured for these micro-organisms.
> - PAS-positive material and a somewhat similar chest X-ray may be found in pneumonia due to *P. carinii*. Thus, the presence of this micro-organism should always be sought in such cases.

Treatment is indicated only if dyspnoea is significant or if the disease fails to remit spontaneously as it does in most cases within a few months.

- *Therapy consists of unilateral **lung lavage**, using a double-lumen endotracheal tube to isolate the contralateral lung from the procedure. The other lung is similarly treated on a subsequent occasion. Corticosteroids are contraindicated.*
- ***GM-CSF** therapy has recently been reported to be dramatically helpful in some patients.*

Bibliography

Claypool WD, Rogers RM, Matuschak GM 1984 Update on the clinical diagnosis, management, and pathogenesis of pulmonary alveolar proteinosis (phospholipidosis). Chest 85: 550.

Goldstein LS, Kavuru MS, Curtis-McCarthy P et al 1998 Pulmonary alveolar proteinosis: clinical features and outcome. Chest 114: 1357.

Pulmonary hypertension

Pulmonary hypertension is a common association of many lung diseases. It also follows a number of non-pulmonary disorders, especially those of a cardiac nature.

> Pulmonary hypertension is defined as an increase in the pulmonary artery pressure (PAP) above 30/15 mmHg (mean PAP >20–25 mmHg).

Cor pulmonale refers to right ventricular hypertrophy and/or dilatation secondary to pulmonary disease and in response to pulmonary hypertension. There may or may not be overt right ventricular failure. The development of right ventricular hypertrophy implies that the process is chronic. Right ventricular dilatation, however, may be acute.

> There are three groups of causes of pulmonary hypertension.
>
> ### 1. **Increased left atrial pressure**
>
> This is due to left heart failure and causes passive pulmonary hypertensio. Since the pulmonary venous pressure is increased, pulmonary oedema eventually occurs.
>
> ### 2. **Increased pulmonary blood flow**
>
> This is due to left-to-right shunt and causes hyperkinetic pulmonary hypertension
>
> ### 3. **Increased pulmonary vascular resistance**
>
> This may be due to:
>
> - vascular constriction, usually caused by hypoxia;
> - vascular obliteration, usually caused by diffuse parenchymal damage, sometime by vasculitis or rarely by veno-occlusive disease;
> - vascular obstruction, usually caused by pulmonary embolism.

Regardless of the initial cause, secondary structural changes eventually occur in the pulmonary arteries. In addition, plexiform (or microaneurysmal) lesions, microvascular thromboses or reactive vasoconstriction occur in some patients. These complications further exacerbate the hypertension.

Chronic airways obstruction, particularly chronic bronchitis, is the main cause of pulmonary hypertension due to parenchymal lung disease. Other causes include diffuse interstitial lung disease, bronchiectasis, kyphoscoliosis, vasculitis, primary pulmonary hypertension and pulmonary veno-occlusive disease. However, any lung disease if sufficiently severe and widespread can cause pulmonary hypertension. Rare causes include tumour or talc embolization, HIV infection, amyloidosis, and familial capillary haemangiomatosis. There may also be an association with portal hypertension and chronic liver disease in some patients. Clusters of cases have been reported following the ingestion of denatured rapeseed oil or appetite suppressants (initially aminorex and subsequently fenfluramines, which have therefore been recently withdrawn from the market). Indeed, recent surveillance has suggested that anorexigens may not only cause primary pulmonary hypertension but also contribute to the secondary pulmonary hypertension associated with other underlying diseases.

The clinical features include symptoms due to low cardiac output, such as fatigue, dyspnoea and angina.

Physical examination shows a prominent 'a' wave of the jugular venous pulse, right ventricular hypertrophy, loud pulmonary component with narrowed split of the second sound, and right heart gallop. In advanced cases, systolic ejection click and pulmonary diastolic and tricuspid pansystolic murmurs may be heard.

There may be evidence of overt right ventricular failure, with increased jugular venous pressure, hepatomegaly and peripheral oedema.

The investigation of patients with pulmonary hypertension requires chest X-ray, ECG, echocardiography and appropriate lung function tests. In addition, right heart catheterization will confirm the presence of pulmonary hypertension, indicate the left atrial pressure (indirectly by the pulmonary artery wedge pressure), demonstrate the presence of left-to-right shunt by right heart blood gas sampling, permit calculation of pulmonary vascular resistance and allow pulmonary angiography.

The treatment of pulmonary hypertension and cor pulmonale is that of the underlying condition.

- *Diuretics and especially digitalis should be used with considerable caution.*
- *In cases with significant arterial hypoxaemia, long-term oxygen therapy is helpful.*

Primary pulmonary hypertension (PPH) is an uncommon condition of unknown aetiology primarily affecting young women. Some cases are familial. Its prevalence is about 1000 per million population and its incidence about 1 per million population per year. Its distinction from chronic, recurrent, pulmonary thromboembolism is not always possible.

The chief symptoms are fatigue, dyspnoea (of unknown mechanism) and syncope on exertion, and sometimes chest pain. Physical signs of cor pulmonale are usually marked. Often there is peripheral vasoconstriction (including Raynaud's phenomenon) and cyanosis.

The median age of diagnosis is 36 years and the average survival is only about 3 y from the onset of symptoms.

Treatment includes avoidance of systemic vasodilators and of pregnancy.

- *Long-term **anticoagulation** is usually recommended, because the distinction from pulmonary embolism is not always possible and because supervening pulmonary artery thrombosis may occur.*
- *Pulmonary **vasodilator** therapy is tempting, but in fact most available pulmonary vasodilators are also systemic vasodilators. Thus, even if the pulmonary vascular resistance is decreased, cardiac output may be increased, so that the pulmonary artery pressure may be unchanged or even increased, while there may be systemic*

hypotension. *Assessment of such agents therefore requires complex haemodynamic monitoring in an Intensive Care setting. If a favourable acute vasodilator response is obtained, high-dose calcium channel blockers (e.g. nifedipine 240 mg/day) may be used. A suitable pulmonary vascular response may perhaps be best assessed following prostacyclin (epoprostenol) infusion or aerosol. Inhaled nitric oxide gives a similar though transient effect. The continuous intravenous infusion of prostacyclin for 12 weeks has recently been reported to improve symptoms, haemodynamics and survival, and long-term treatment is now commonly recommended though there is wide variation in the regimens used.*

- *Single lung or heart–lung **transplantation** has been reported to be relatively effective.*

Bibliography

Auger WR, Channick RN, Kerr KM et al 1999 Evaluation of patients with suspected chronic thromboembolic pulmonary hypertension. Semin Thorac Cardiovasc Surg 11: 179.

Barst RJ, Rubin LJ, Long WA et al 1996 A comparison of continuous intravenous epoprostenol (prostacyclin) with conventional therapy for primary pulmonary hypertension. N Engl J Med 334: 296.

Dantzker DR, Grant BJB 1983 Pulmonary hypertension. In: Shoemaker WC, Thompson WL (eds) Critical Care: State of the Art. Fullerton: Society of Critical Care Medicine. p F1.

Fishman AP 1999 Aminorex to fen/phen: an epidemic foretold. Circulation 99: 156.

Gaine SP, Rubin LJ 1998 Primary pulmonary hypertension. Lancet 352: 719.

Libby DM, Briscoe WA, Boyce B et al 1982 Acute respiratory failure in scoliosis or kyphosis: prolonged survival and treatment. Am J Med 73: 532.

McGregor M, Sniderman A 1985 On pulmonary vascular resistance: the need for more precise definition. Am J Cardiol 55: 217.

Palevsky HI, Fishman AP 1991 The management of primary pulmonary hypertension. JAMA 265: 1014.

Pepke-Zaba J, Higenbottam TW, Dinh-Xuan AT et al 1991 Inhaled nitric oxide as a cause of selective pulmonary vasodilatation in pulmonary hypertension. Lancet 338: 1173.

Rich S 1988 Primary pulmonary hypertension. Prog Cardiovasc Dis 31: 205.

Rich S, Rubin L, Walker AM et al 2000 Anorexigens and pulmonary hypertension in the United States. Chest 117: 870.

Roberts WC 1986 A simple histologic classification of pulmonary arterial hypertension. Am J Cardiol 58: 385.

Rubin LJ 1997 Primary pulmonary hypertension. N Engl J Med 336: 111.

Rubin LJ (ed) 1998 Brenot memorial symposium on the pathogenesis of primary pulmonary hypertension. Chest 114: no.3 Suppl.

Shure D 1996 Primary pulmonary hypertension – good news and bad. Pulmonary Perspectives 13(3): 6.

Versprille A 1984 Pulmonary vascular resistance: a meaningless variable. Intens Care Med 10: 51.

Walmrath D, Schneider T, Pilch J et al 1995 Effects of aerosolized prostacyclin in severe pneumonia. Am J Resp Crit Care Med 151: 724.

Pulmonary infiltrates

The chief causes of a diffuse **pulmonary infiltrate** are:

1. pneumonia;

2. interstitial lung disease

   – sarcoidosis;
   – diffuse fibrosing alveolitis;
   – other interstitial lung disease;
   – collagen–vascular disease;
   – PIE;

3. malignancy

   – lymphoma;
   – metastases;
   – lymphangitis carcinomatosa;
   – alveolar cell carcinoma;

4. pulmonary oedema;

5. acute (adult) respiratory distress syndrome;

6. pneumoconiosis;

7. hypersensitivity pneumonitis;

8. aspiration pneumonitis;

9. drug reaction (see Drugs and the lung);

10. Wegener's granulomatosis;

11. Goodpasture's syndrome;

12. military tuberculosis;

13. radiation pneumonitis;

14. uraemia.

Most of these conditions are separately considered elsewhere in this book.

Bibliography

Crystal RG, Bitterman PB, Rennard SI et al 1984 Interstitial lung diseases of unknown cause. N Engl J Med 310: 154, 235.

Muller NL, Miller RR 1990 Computed tomography of chronic diffuse infiltrative lung disease. Am Rev Respir Dis 142: 1440.

Pulmonary infiltration with eosinophilia (see Eosinophilia and lung infiltration)

Pulmonary nodules

Pulmonary nodules may be:

- small and single (a 'coin' lesion);
- large (>6 cm diameter) and single;
- multiple.

The diagnosis cannot usually be made from the clinical features, since most patients are asymptomatic. It frequently requires comparison with previous films (if available), tomography, CT scanning (with percutaneous needle biopsy/aspiration), bronchoscopy, and sometimes thoracotomy and resection.

The chief causes of a **small and single pulmonary nodule** are:

1. carcinoma

   – usually primary and especially adenocarcinoma;

2. infection

   – granuloma, especially tuberculous or fungal;

3. hamartoma;

4. arteriovenous malformation;

5. bronchogenic cyst

   – for which there may be a clue from 'popcorn' calcification.

The chief causes of a **large and single pulmonary nodule** are:

1. neoplasm

   – usually primary, and especially large cell carcinoma or alveolar cell carcinoma;
   – sometimes lymphoma;

2. infection

   – bacterial pneumonia, fungal infection;

3. sequestration;

4. bronchogenic cyst.

The chief causes of **multiple pulmonary nodules** are:

1. neoplasm

   – usually metastases;
   – sometimes in women 'benign metastasizing' uterine leiomyoma;

2. infection

   – septic emboli, especially in *S. aureus* infection;
   – granulomas, as in fungal or nocardial infection, or in melioidosis or paragonimiasis;

3. arteriovenous malformations;

4. Wegener's granulomatosis;

5. rheumatoid lung;

6. sarcoidosis;

7. amyloid.

Bibliography

Dines DE, Arms RA, Bernatz PE et al 1974 Pulmonary arteriovenous fistulas. Mayo Clin Proc 48: 460.

Faughnan ME, Lui YW, Wirth JA et al 2000 Diffuse pulmonary arteriovenous malformations: characteristics and prognosis. Chest 117: 31.

Lillington GA 1993 Management of the solitary pulmonary nodule. Hosp Pract 28: 41.

Savic B, Birtel FJ, Tholen W et al 1979 Lung sequestration. Thorax 34: 96.

Steele JD 1963 The solitary pulmonary nodule. J Thorac Cardiovasc Surg 46: 21.

Terry PB, Barth KH, Kaufman SL et al 1980 Balloon embolization for the treatment of pulmonary arteriovenous fistulas. N Engl J Med 302: 1189.

White RJ, Lynch-Nyhan A, Terry P et al 1988 Pulmonary arteriovenous malformation: techniques and long-term outcome of embolotherapy. Radiology 169: 663.

Pulmonary oedema (see Acute pulmonary oedema)

Pulmonary veno-occlusive disease

Pulmonary veno-occlusive disease may be seen in a number of settings. In primary pulmonary hypertension (PPH), about 5% of patients have involvement predominantly affecting the pulmonary veins instead of the arteries, with intimal proliferation, thrombosis, obliteration and fibrosis. In these cases, it appears to be an uncommon variant of PPH. Sometimes, the condition may be seen in association with mediastinal fibrosis (see Mediastinum). It has also been reported in collagen-vascular diseases, and after radiation, cancer chemotherapy and bone marrow transplantation.

The chest X-ray shows pulmonary congestion, and the lung scan shows patchy abnormality. Although the pulmonary artery wedge pressure is often increased, it underestimates the true pulmonary capillary or filtration pressure, because in this condition the capillary pressure is much greater than the venous pressure. Lung function tests show marked impairment of gas transfer. Lung biopsy shows intimal fibrosis and eventual arterialization, particularly of the smaller pulmonary veins.

Medical treatment is ineffective. Vasodilator drugs are not usually of value and may paradoxically exacerbate acute pulmonary oedema or even death.

Lung transplantation *is the only potentially curative treatment.*

Bibliography

Heath D, Segal N, Bishop J 1966 Pulmonary veno-occlusive disease. Circulation 34: 242.

Holcomb BW, Loyd JE, Ely EW et al 2000 Pulmonary veno-occlusive disease. Chest 118: 1671.

Palevsky HI, Pietra GG, Fishman AP 1990 Pulmonary veno-occlusive disease and its response to vasodilator agents. Am Rev Respir Dis 142: 426.

Palmer SM, Robinson LJ, Wand A et al 1998 Massive pulmonary edema and death after prostacyclin infusion in a patient with pulmonary veno-occlusive disease. Chest 113: 237.

Purpura

Purpura refers to skin and mucous membrane bleeding, with lesions that range from as small as petechiae to as large as ecchymoses.

> Purpura is caused by:
> - thrombocytopaenia (q.v.);
> - platelet function disorders (q.v.);
> - increased microvascular permeability (i.e. vascular purpura).

Increased microvascular permeability may be due to:

- endothelial cell damage;
- damage to supporting structures;
- miscellaneous conditions.

P

Endothelial cell damage may be:

- toxic, from

  - infections, especially Gram-negative or rickettsial;
  - snake venom;

- embolic, due to

  - sepsis;
  - disseminated intravascular coagulation;
  - thrombotic thrombocytopenic purpura (q.v.);
  - subacute bacterial endocarditis (see Endocarditis);
  - cholesterol;
  - fat;

- leukocytoclastic (see Vasculitis), due to immune-mediated neutrophil aggregation, as

  - in Henoch–Schonlein (or Schonlein–Henoch) purpura;
  - in collagen-vascular disease;
  - in hepatitis B infection;
  - with some drugs (e.g. sulfonamides).

Damage to supporting structures occurs with:

- scurvy (q.v.);
- corticosteroids;
- senile purpura;
- hereditary haemorrhagic telangiectasia (q.v.);
- amyloid (see Multiple Myeloma);
- hereditary connective tissue disorders

  - Ehlers–Danlos syndrome, Marfan's syndrome (q.v.), pseudoxanthoma elasticum.

Miscellaneous conditions primarily include **auto-erythrocyte purpura**. This is an unusual and uncommon condition in middle-aged women. It is manifest as large painful subcutaneous haematomas. Its name derives from its reproduction by subcutaneous injection of the patient's own red blood cells.

Treatment is ineffective.

Bibliography

Cameron JS 1984 Henoch–Schonlein purpura: clinical presentation. Contrib Nephrol 40: 246.

Pyoderma gangrenosum

Pyoderma gangrenosum is a non-infective and probably immunological condition in which purple, non-crepitant, somewhat painful nodules develop usually on the limbs or lower body. The lesions vesiculate, coalesce and ulcerate, leaving a ragged and undermined edge. They can become large and are often multiple. There is no systemic toxicity.

The course is very variable from acute to chronic. The condition is most commonly associated with serious underlying systemic disease, such as a myeloproliferative disorder, rheumatoid arthritis, chronic active hepatitis, gastrointestinal malignancy, or especially inflammatory bowel disease.

The chief differential diagnosis is infectious gangrenous cellulitis (see Gangrene).

Treatment is local, though systemic **corticosteriods** *may be required.*

- *In resistant cases,* **immunosuppression** *with cyclophosphamide, cyclosporin, thalidomide or recently tacrolims (a macrolide antibiotic with an action similar to that of cyclosporin) is indicated.*
- **Dapsone** *and* **hyperbaric oxygen** *have been reported to be helpful in some cases.*

Bibliography

Hecker MS, Lebwohl MG 1998 Recalcitrant pyoderma gangrenosum: treatment with thalidomide. J Am Acad Dermatol 38: 490
Newell LM, Malkinson FD 1982 Pyoderma gangrenosum. Arch Dermatol 118: 769.
Schwaegerle SM, Bergfeld WF, Senitzer D et al 1988 Pyoderma gangrenosum: A review. J Am Acad Dermatol 18: 559

Pyrexia

It is well known that normal body temperature is defended within very narrow limits, with an additional circadian range from about 36.1C in the morning to 37.4°C in the evening.

Heat is produced by metabolic processes, particularly by the liver and heart at rest and by skeletal muscles on exercise. Skeletal muscle can generate large amounts of energy and the body is only about 25% efficient in translating metabolic energy to external work, the rest being converted to heat.

Heat is lost from the skin (90%) and lungs (10%), two thirds by radiation and one third by evaporation, though the latter component increases with increased environmental temperature and on exercise, when sweating which may reach up to 2 L/h becomes the body's main method of achieving external heat loss. Normally, this external heat loss is very efficient, so that even a prolonged increase in metabolic rate of 15-fold or more for two hours or more, as in elite marathoners, raises the body temperature to only 38–40°C (whereas without such heat loss, the temperature would increase by 1°C each 5 min).

The temperature control centre resides in the pre-optic nucleus in the anterior hypothalamus, from where it stimulates the autonomic nervous system to produce either vasodilatation and sweating to increase heat loss of vasoconstriction and shivering to decrease heat loss.

Increased body temperature is referred to as **pyrexia**. Pyrexia may take one or two forms, namely:

- **hyperthermia**
  - i.e. failure of heat control, so that heat production exceeds heat loss;
- **fever**
  - i.e. an increased set-point, so that heat control achieves an increased temperature

Hyperthermia can be caused by:

- increased heat production;

- decreased heat loss;
- hypothalamic disease.

In practice, hyperthermia is usually associated with exercise (in which heat production can increase 20-fold), particularly in association with dehydration or adverse environmental conditions (see Heat stroke).

However, some disease states also produce hyperthermia rather than fever, often with very high body temperatures (e.g. >41°C). These diseases include:

- malignant hyperthermia;
- neuroleptic malignant syndrome;
- salicylate poisoning;
- thyroid storm;
- phaeochromocytoma;
- hypothalamic disease
  - due to encephalitis, cerebrovascular disease, neurotrauma, neoplasia, sarcoidosis, drugs.

The clinical distinction between hyperthermia and fever cannot be made on the basis of temperature level and can be particularly difficult in endocrine or hypothalamic disease. Recurrent pyrexia makes fever more likely than hyperthermia.

The treatment for hyperthermia is that of the underlying disease, with specific therapy if possible. In addition, systemic measures are important, including physical cooling and circulatory support.

Fever, unlike hyperthermia, is always due to disease. It has been known since antiquity to be one of the cardinal signs of significant disease.

Fever arises from the production, especially by mononuclear phagocytes, of cytokines which are acute inflammatory mediators. These include especially IL-1 and TNF but also IL–6 and IFNγ. The cytokine, interleukin-1 receptor antagonist (IL-1ra), opposes the inflammatory response.

IL–1 in particular is a pyrogen, in which role it acts as a hormone rather than a cytokine. Thus, it is distributed by the circulation and acts on receptors remote from the original site of inflammation and cytokine production. Following binding to cell membrane receptors in the hypothalamus, IL-1 activates phospholipase to release from membrane phospholipids the family of arachidonic acid metabolites and in particular prostaglandins (especially of the E series). These substances increase the temperature set-point in the hypothalamus and activate the heat control mechanisms accordingly. It is because of the central role of prostaglandins in this pathway that aspirin is so effective in fever.

Several other cytokines are also pyrogenic, including TNF (which is indirect and acts via stimulating IL-1) and IL-6 and IFNγ (which are direct). As is well known, the 'pro-inflammatory' cytokines are also immunostimulatory, with a variety of actions incorporated into the acute phase response. These include stimulation of T and B cells, activation of macrophages, release of other cytokines, stimulation of neutrophil release from the bone marrow, stimulation of neutrophil chemotaxis (thus causing leukocytosis systemically and inflammatory cell infiltration locally), stimulation of production by the liver of acute phase proteins (thus causing an increased ESR), increased procoagulant activity and platelet adhesion, vasodilatation and increased vascular permeability, and subsequently fibroblast proliferation for repair.

The net effect of the endocrine–immune interactions and the consequent inflammatory and related responses is the 'sick everything' syndrome.

This is a pyrexial, euthyroid, diabetogenic and hypogonadal state, whose details are more apparent as laboratory than as clinical findings.

Apart from being a marker of potentially serious illness, the clinical significance of this state remains uncertain.

Fever of unknown origin (FUO) should perhaps more properly be termed pyrexia of unknown origin (PUO). This is because no assumption should be made in advance as to whether the set-point is or is not increased, though in most cases of course the set-point is in fact increased and the condition may rightly be termed fever.

Fever of unknown origin (FUO) has been defined as:

- core body temperature >38.3°C;
- of at least 3 weeks duration;
- excluding major well known infective and postoperative causes; and
- unclarified despite one week of investigations.

This definition immediately excludes the majority of cases of fever, since although one third of hospital patients develop fever (most due to infection), nearly 90% of these have straightforward diagnoses and in most of the rest the fever is short-lived and has no ill-effects.

The causes of FUO have been well documented in published series, and it is worth remembering that in this, as in many situations of diagnostic difficulty, the uncommon manifestations of common diseases are more likely to be encountered than the common manifestations of uncommon diseases.

The causes of FUO have thus been found to be:

- infections (23–36%);
- neoplasms (7–31%);
- collagen-vascular diseases (9–18%);
- other less common specific diseases (18–29%);
- undiagnosed (7–23%).

Infections

1. Systemic

- Brucellosis, leptospirosis, listeriosis, mycosis, psittacosis, toxoplasmosis should be considered.
- Viral infections do not produce fever for >3 weeks, except for CMV, which is especially seen in transplant recipients.
- Endocarditis and tuberculosis should always be specifically excluded.
- Other infections are rare, except in travellers.

2. Local

- A localized collection or abscess should always be sought, especially if there has been local injury, particularly to the abdomen. Subphrenic, intrahepatic or other intra-abdominal collections should be considered in such cases.
- Occult local infection sometimes involves the urinary tract, paranasal sinuses or teeth.

Neoplasms

- Lymphoma.
- Haematological malignancy.
  - In these cases however the usual cause of fever is infection rather than malignancy itself.
  - If the latter, however, it typically responds to NSAIDs.
- Carcinoma of the kidney.
- Phaeochromocytoma.
- Extensive metastatic disease.

Collagen-vascular diseases

- Especially SLE.
- In the elderly, polymyalgia rheumatica and temporal arteritis should be considered.
- Associated arthralgia and high ESR are useful clues to this category of illness.

Other less common specific diseases

- Alcoholic hepatitis.
- CNS lesions,
  - usually associated with coma and known brain damage.
- Drugs
  - particular culprits are beta-lactam antibiotics, isoniazid, hydralazine, methyldopa, phenytoin, sulfonamides.
  - The presence of a rash and/or eosinophilia may provide a useful clue.
  - In addition, the responsible drug has usually been administered only recently, except that both methyldopa and phenytoin can produce late-presenting fever.
- Factitious.
- **Familial Mediterranean fever** (FMF). This condition presents with attacks of abdominal pain and polyserositis, as well as fever and leukocytosis, but the patient is well between attacks. The patient is usually an Arab, Armenian or Sephardic Jew.

There is an increased incidence of amyloidosis with nephrotic syndrome and of polyarteritis nodosa.

The differential diagnosis is wide and includes diabetic ketoacidosis, acute porphyria, SLE, lead colic, tabetic crisis, and perhaps common intrathoracic conditions, such as AMI or pneumonia.

- Granulomatous diseases, especially sarcoidosis.
- Inflammatory bowel disease.
- Pulmonary thromboembolism
  - though fever prolonged for >1 week is uncommon.
- Whipple's disease.

The height and pattern of fever are not usually diagnostically helpful. Diagnosis requires detailed history and clinical examination and appropriate investigations (particularly microbiological, imaging and histological) to cover the conditions listed above. Occasionally, diagnosis made be assisted by antibiotics or corticosteroids in a therapeutic trial.

Fever in the Intensive Care Unit may also be considered as core temperature 38.3°C (SCCM definition). For practical purposes, temperature elevations less than this do not usually warrant complex investigation in themselves. Most cases of fever in ICU are caused by obvious infections,

- particularly

  – nosocomial pneumonia
  – line-related sepsis
  – abdominal sepsis,
  – wound infection,

- sometimes

  – sinusitis
  – urinary tract infection
  – *C. difficile* colitis

Some cases of fever in ICU are due to non-infectious causes and can be frustrating to clarify. While most such causes usually produce only minor elevations of temperature, sometimes they may produce genuine fever. These conditions include:

- pancreatitis;
- acalculous cholecystitis;
- gut ischaemia;
- gut bleeding;
- thromboembolism;
- drug fever;
- transfusion;
- myocardial infarction;
- cerebral haemorrhage;
- haematoma;
- phlebitis.

While the hazards of pyrexia are well known, the possible benefits of fever remain controversial.

The **adverse consequences of pyrexia** include:

- catabolic state;
- hyperdynamic circulation;
- delirium;
- convulsions (usually in children);
- cellular damage if the temperature is extreme (i.e. >41°C), though usually such damage may be primarily attributable to the underlying disease.

The **beneficial consequences of fever** have not been established in humans, although cytokine release appears to have evolved over hundreds of millions of years, so that in many species it presumably enhances host defence. Certainly, fever benefits some infected poikilotherms and even mammals.

However, fever is not helpful in humans, since although some infecting organisms are heat sensitive the body temperatures achieved during fever are not high enough to take advantage of this potential microbial weakness. Similarly,

- fever therapy as used in the past was not helpful in infections, though it was not harmful, and
- antipyretic medication is not harmful, though it is not helpful except symptomatically.

More recently, whole body hyperthermia has been used in some oncology centres as part of a range of cancer treatment modalities.

Treatment of fever is that of the underlying disease, together with symptomatic measures (aspirin or paracetamol) and general support. Since the temperature set-point is increased, physical cooling can be distressing, though it may be considered useful (as in hyperthermia) if the temperature is particularly high (i.e. >40–41°C), especially at extremes of age and in cardiovascular disease.

Bibliography

Adaun RP, Fauci AS, Dale DC et al 1979 Factitious fever and self-induced infection. Ann Intern Med 90: 230

Bernheim HA, Block LH, Atkins E 1979 Fever: pathogenesis, pathophysiology, and purpose. Ann Intern Med 91: 261

Blumenthal I 1997 Fever – concepts old and new. J R Soc Med 90: 391.

Dinarello CA, Cannon JG, Wolff SM 1988 New concepts on the pathogenesis of fever. Rev Infect Dis 10: 168.

Editorial 1980 Familial Mediterranean fever. Br Med J 281: 2.

Eliakim M, Levy M, Ehrenfeld M 1981 Recurrent Polyserositis (Familial Mediterranean Fever, Periodic Disease). Amsterdam: Elsevier.

Jacoby GA, Swartz MN 1973 Fever of undetermined origin N Engl J Med 289: 1407.

Kluger MJ, Ringler DH, Anver MR 1975 Fever and survival. Science 188: 166.

Knockaert DC, Vanneste LJ, Vanneste SB et al 1992 Fever of unknown origin in the 1980s. Arch Intern Med 152: 51.

Mackowiak PA 1994 Fever: blessing or curse? A unifying hypothesis. Ann Intern Med 120: 1037.

Mackowiak PA 1998 Concepts of fever. Arch Intern Med 158: 1870.

Mackowiak PA, LeMaistre CF 1987 Drug fever: a critical appraisal of conventional concepts. Ann Intern Med 106: 728.

Marik PE 2000 Fever in the ICU. Chest 117: 855.

Musher DM, Fainstein V, Young EJ 1979 Fever patterns: their lack of clinical significance. Arch Intern Med 139: 1225.

Nimmo SM, Kennedy BW, Tullet WM et al 1993 Drug-induced hyperthermia. Anaesthesia 48: 892.

O'Grady NP, Barie PS, Bartlett J et al 1998 Practice guidelines for evaluating new fever in critically ill adult patients. Crit Care Med 26: 392.

Olson KR, Benowitz NL 1984 Environmental and drug-induced hyperthermia: pathophysiology, recognition and management. Emerg Med Clin North Am 2: 459.

Petersdorf RG, Beeson PB 1961 Fever of unexplained origin. Medicine 40: 1.

Roberts NJ 1991 Impact of temperature elevation on immunologic defenses. Rev Infect Dis 13: 462.

Robins HI, Longo W 1999 Whole body hyperthermia. Intens Care Med 25: 898.

Rosenberg J, Pentel P, Pond S et al 1986 Hyperthermia associated with drug intoxication. Crit Care Med 14: 964.

Saper CB, Breeder CD 1994 The neurologic basis of fever. N Engl J Med 330: 1880.

Shann F 1995 Antipyretics in severe sepsis. Lancet 345: 338.

Simon HB 1993 Hyperthermia. N Engl J Med 329: 483.

Simon HB, Daniels GH 1979 Hormonal hyperthermia: endocrinologic causes of fever. Am J Med 66: 257.

Sohar E, Gafni J, Heller H 1967 Familial Mediterranean fever. Am J Med 43: 227.

Swartz MN, Simon HB 1992 Pathophysiology of fever and fever of undetermined origin. Sci Am Med section 7, chapter XXIV: 1.

Pyroglutamic acid (see Lactic acidosis)

Q fever (see Rickettsial diseases)

Rabies

Rabies is a dramatic example of one of many viral **zoonoses** in animals which may be incidentally transmitted to humans, where an entirely different disease is produced from that seen in the original reservoir. Contact may be direct or via a vector.

Most such animal viruses rarely spread to humans. The best known examples apart from rabies are:

- dengue;
- haemorrhagic fevers (including possibly Ebola fever);
- yellow fever;
- equine morbillivirus (first described in 1994 in Australia, and now called Hendra virus);
- lyssavirus of fruit bat origin (first described in 1996 in Australia, called Australian bat lyssavirus (ABL), and closely related to classic rabies virus).

Some human viruses on the other hand may be transmitted to animals, such as:

- hepatitis;
- measles;
- poliomyelitis;
- avian influenza.

Rabies is found in many carnivores in most countries (except Australia, United Kingdom and Hawaii). Dogs are the main source of infection in humans. The disease is particularly prevalent in Asia, Africa, and Central and South America.

Usually, direct inoculation occurs from infected salvia following a bite.

- The virus replicates in adjacent muscle cells and then passes via the nerves to the CNS.
- There is an incubation period of about 30 days (though 12 days to >4 y have been reported).
- Clinical features comprise local pain and numbness and systemic features of irritability,

apprehension, dyspnoea, nausea and diarrhoea.

- Hydrophobia occurs in some patients and is characteristic.
- Subsequently, excitation occurs with hyperventilation, seizures and disorientation.
- Finally, paralysis occurs, even involving autonomically innervated structures, and death follows from cardiorespiratory failure.

The diagnosis requires a careful history, especially of travel. It is confirmed by viral isolation and positive serology.

Treatment is with local wound cleaning and general supportive measures.

- *Although no person to person transmission has been reported, **isolation** is usually recommended.*
- *Post-exposure prophylactic **vaccination** is now very effective but is complex and requires consultation with local health authorities. No vaccination however is required if a suspected animal remains healthy after 10 days of observation or if the animal is killed and laboratory tests are negative.*

The condition is always fatal within three weeks of illness in unvaccinated patients.

Bibliography
Fishbein DB, Robinson LE 1993 Rabies (review). N Engl J Med 329: 1632.

Radiation injury

Radiation has dose-related consequences, both local and systemic. In particular, the patient becomes a compromised host with

- loss of integrity of the mucocutaneous surface barrier (especially the gut),
- decreased number and impaired function of circulating neutrophils and lymphocytes,
- impaired function of both circulating and fixed mononuclear phagocytes.

In radiotherapy, either subatomic particle radiation or electromagnetic radiation (megavoltage X-ray or gamma-rays from radioactive isotopes) may be used. Both modalities deliver photons to the tissues where intracellular structures (e.g. DNA) are ionized in both malignant and normal cells. Some malignant tissues (lymphoma, seminoma) are much more sensitive to radiation than are normal tissues, but unfortunately the converse applies for the gut, kidneys, liver, lungs and nervous system. Radiation injury is an important complication of therapeutic radiation, even though appropriate precautions are taken to minimize the exposure of normal tissues.

> **Acute effects** of radiation include damage to proliferating cells with erythema, desquamation, nausea, oesophagitis and bone marrow suppression.
>
> **Late effects** of radiation are due to vascular occlusion, tissue necrosis or possibly stem cell damage.

Carcinogenic influences in the environment, including radiation, can affect almost all organs by activation of cellular oncogenes. The tumours which may result include especially leukaemia but also carcinoma of the skin, thyroid and breast, bone and soft tissue sarcomas, and brain tumours. Previous radiotherapy for Hodgkin's disease may give rise to such tumours subsequently (as well as to an excess cardiac mortality).

Local effects of radiation can be prominent.

- In the **pelvis**, proctitis and cystitis may result.
- In the **head and neck**, there may be hoarseness, sore and dry mouth and throat, with loss of taste, mucositis, ulcers, fistulae and cutaneous erythema.
- **Neurological** changes of encephalopathy or myelopathy may be produced from local vascular damage.
- Late **pericarditis** may be produced.
- **Radiation pneumonitis** is an acute, primary, vascular reaction, initially with pulmonary vascular congestion and alveolar

oedema, and later with small vessel thrombosis and alveolar epithelial desquamation. It is of variable extent and severity, but it occurs to some degree in all patients having chest irradiation. It may resemble *P. carinii* pneumonia, from which it therefore needs to be distinguished.

Symptoms appear some weeks after radiation and include dry cough and dyspnoea. The overlying skin may show increased pigmentation.

Chest X-ray shows a new pulmonary infiltrate, often typically confined to the area of the radiation port. BAL helps exclude infection or malignancy and may show lymphocytes and dysplastic or damaged alveolar type II cells.

Severe symptoms are probably helped with **corticosteroids**, *and concomitant* **antibiotics** *are usually given because of the likelihood of superinfection.*

- **Radiation fibrosis** is a natural progression of radiation pneumonitis over the succeeding months.

The process is often clinically silent, but dyspnoea can occur and may be progressive and disabling.

Chest X-ray shows infiltration and contraction of the affected part of the lung.

There is no effective treatment.

Bibliography

Gross NJ 1977 Pulmonary effects of radiation injury. Ann Intern Med 86: 81.

Rat bites (see Bites and stings)

Raynaud's phenomenon/disease

Raynaud's phenomenon is a peripheral vasospastic disorder, secondary to organic disease such as SLE or scleroderma which it often precedes.

Raynaud's disease is a primary or idiopathic form of the condition, which in its mildest form occurs in about 25% of young women. It may represent an increased sensitivity to α_2 agonists due to an increased density of receptors in the digital arteries.

Treatment is primarily symptomatic and physical.

- **Calcium channel blockers** *are helpful, though direct vasodilator agents are ineffective.*
- **Captopril** *and* **ketanserin** *are reportedly helpful.*

Bibliography

Coffman JD 1991 Raynaud's phenomenon: an update. Hypertension 17: 593.
Sturgill MG, Seibold JR 1998 Rational use of calcium-channel antagonists in Raynaud's phenomenon. Curr Opin Rheumatol 10: 584.

Reactive arthritis (see Reiter's syndrome)

Reiter's syndrome

Reiter's syndrome comprises the triad of arthritis, urethritis and conjunctivitis. Occasionally, there may be a tetrad, with the additional features of painless ulcers in the mouth or rash on the glans penis (circinate balanitis). The joint involvement is a **reactive arthritis**.

It occurs particularly in young men, in whom it is the commonest inflammatory monoarthropathy or oligoarthropathy, with a prevalence of 3.5 per 100 000. There is a 37-fold increased incidence in subjects with the specific genetic HLA antigen B27, and 70–90% of patients with the condition are B27-positive.

Reiter's syndrome usually follows a specific infection, either epidemic or endemic.

- Epidemic causes are usually dysenteric, especially from salmonella, shigella, campylobacter or *Yersinia enterocolitica*.
- Endemic infections are usually venereal, either from chlamydia or mycoplasma.

Although the pathogenetic mechanisms of the illness are uncertain, there may be cross-reactivity between bacterial antigens and self-antigens.

Clinical features include arthritis, usually asymmetrical and involving the knees, ankles or feet. Achilles tendonitis, plantar fasciitis and tenosynovitis are common. There may be associated sacroiliitis or overlap with ankylosing spondylitis (q.v.). There may sometimes be associated skin lesions, namely keratoderma blennorrhagicum with hyperkeratotic lesions. Conjunctivitis is usual, and there may sometimes be uveitis.

In AIDS, the condition is more severe, though probably not more frequent. This is in contrast to other rheumatic disorders, such as rheumatoid arthritis and SLE, which may improve in the presence of AIDS.

Investigations usually show a raised ESR. Examination of the synovial fluid shows a high complement level, reflecting inflammation (in contrast to rheumatoid arthritis in which the level is low). In chronic disease, there may be IgA antibodies to the trigger organism, consistent with a continuing mucosal infection. The diagnosis is made on the basis of the clinical features and not the laboratory tests.

Treatment is with **NSAIDs,** *to which symptoms of arthritis usually respond.*

- *In occasional severe cases,* **salazopyrine** *or* **methotrexate** *and sometimes* **corticosteroids** *may be required (though some of these agents are contraindicated in HIV-positive cases).*
- *Any predisposing urethritis or bacterial gastroenteritis is treated on its merits.*

The condition is usually self-limited, but sometimes it may progress to produce considerable and prolonged disability.

Bibliography

Amor B 1998 Reiter's syndrome. Rheum Dis Clin North Am 24: 677.

Editorial 1980 Reactive arthritis. Br Med J 281: 311.

Gibofsky A, Zabriskie JB 1995 Rheumatic fever and poststreptococcal reactive arthritis. Curr Opin Rheumatol 7: 299.

Keat A 1999 Reactive arthritis. Adv Exp Med Biol 455: 201.

McEwen C, DiTata D, Lingg C et al 1971 Ankylosing spondylitis and spondylitis accompanying ulcerative colitis, regional enteritis, psoriasis and Reiter's disease. Arthritis Rheum 14: 291.

Winblad S 1975 Arthritis associated with Yersinia enterocolitica infections. Scand J Infect Dis 7: 191.

Relapsing fever

Relapsing fever occurs following infection with one of several species of spirochaete of the genus borrelia, which are transmitted by arthropod vectors (lice or ticks).

- Louse-borne infection often occurs in epidemics and follows natural or man-made disasters. It has thus been associated with typhus and has occurred mainly in Africa, Asia and South America.
- Tick-borne infection is widely distributed and usually arises from exposure to infected rodents.

Both forms of infection are clinically similar.

- Following an incubation period of about 7 days,
  - symptoms comprise high fever with chills, headache, myalgia, prostration, confusion, cough and gastrointestinal complaints,
  - clinical findings include tachycardia, hyperventilation, rash, splenomegaly,
  - sometimes, there is hepatomegaly, lymphadenopathy, disseminated intravascular coagulation.
- After 3–6 days,
  - the febrile illness comes to an abrupt end in a drenching sweat.
- In another 6–10 days,
  - there is a febrile recurrence, but the illness on this occasion is shorter.
  - Sometimes, there may be only one relapse, but often there are many.
  - However, on each occasion the symptom-free interval is longer and the actual relapse is milder and briefer.
  - Resolution occurs because of the production of antibody, but recurrence occurs because of the process of antigen variation.

Spirochaetes are seen on the blood film, except during symptom-free intervals. Borrelia cannot be cultured on artificial media. There is anaemia, thrombocytopenia and disseminated intravascular coagulation, but the white cell count is normal. Liver function tests are abnormal in severe cases.

The differential diagnosis includes:

- bacteraemia;
- infectious mononucleosis;
- malaria;
- salmonellosis;
- leptospirosis;
- spotted fevers.

Treatment is with **tetracycline** *for 10 days, though a single dose of doxycycline 100 mg has been used in epidemics.*

- *Chloramphenicol, penicillin and ceftriaxone are also effective.*
- *Treatment can be associated with the* **Jarisch–Herxheimer reaction** *(q.v.).*

The mortality is usually 2–5%, though it can increase to 40% in epidemics because of concomitant diseases.

Bibliography
Spach D, Liles W, Campbell G et al 1993 Tick-borne diseases in the United States. N Engl J Med 329: 936.

Renal artery occlusion

Renal artery occlusion may be due to:

- emboli;
- thrombi;
- vascular disease.

Emboli arise from:

- cardiac thrombi, due to acute myocardial infarction or atrial arrhythmias. A frequent consequence of embolization of such material is renal artery occlusion, because the kidneys take 20% of the cardiac output.
- athero-emboli (cholesterol emboli). This is usually seen in older patients with extensive atherosclerotic disease who have had a radiological or surgical procedure proximal to the kidneys. An acute increase in plasma creatinine after such procedures is an important clue to this mechanism, though it requires differentiation from contrast-induced renal damage. It may be associated with more peripheral embolization and livedo reticularis (q.v.).
- subacute bacterial endocarditis, tumour or fat. These are uncommon sources of clinically significant renal artery emboli.

Thrombi are usually associated with underlying arterial damage from atheroma or trauma.

Vascular disease is usually associated with abdominal aortic aneurysm.

Renal artery occlusion causes ischaemic damage to the kidney, with a typically wedged-shaped infarct or more general atrophy. The consequences depend on the speed, extent and duration of the process, with irreversible changes often appearing after 2 h of occlusion.

Clinical features typically comprise:

- loin pain and tenderness;
- systemic symptoms of fever and nausea.

Sometimes, the process may be clinically silent. Often in embolic disease there are emboli apparent elsewhere, and the site of embolization is apparent. Hypertension is common. A skin rash may be seen, in the form of livedo reticularis (q.v.).

Investigations show haematuria in one third of cases. The LDH but not the AST is typically elevated. A renal isotope scan is the preferred technique to show either segmental or generalized decrease in renal perfusion.

The diagnosis of renal artery occlusion can be difficult, especially if there is no apparent initiating event and the process is persistent or recurrent.

In severe cases, the differential diagnosis includes acute tubular necrosis.

The urine sediment is sometimes 'active', with haematuria, red blood cell casts and occasionally eosinophils. An eosinophilia may be noted on peripheral blood examination.

Treatment is with **anticoagulation**, *though local thrombolytic therapy has also been reported to be successful.*

Bibliography

Bell SP, Frankel A, Brown EA 1997 Cholesterol emboli syndrome – uncommon or unrecognized? J R Soc Med 90: 543.

Corwin HL, Korbet SM, Schwartz MM 1985 Clinical correlates of eosinophiluria. Arch Intern Med 145: 1097.

Crosby RL, Miller PD, Schrier RW 1986 Traumatic renal artery thrombosis. Am J Med 81: 890.

Lessman RK, Johnson SF, Coburn JW et al 1978 Renal artery embolism. Ann Intern Med 89: 477.

Peat DS, Mathieson PW 1996 Cholesterol emboli may mimic systemic vasculitis. Br Med J 313: 546.

Smith MC, Ghose MK, Henry AR 1981 The clinical spectrum of renal cholesterol embolization. Am J Med 71: 174.

Renal calculous disease (see Nephrolithiasis)

Renal cortical necrosis

Renal cortical necrosis refers to infarction of the entire renal cortex with consequent acute anuric renal failure. The juxtamedullary glomeruli probably survive and are responsible for the partial recovery seen in some patients.

Renal cortical necrosis is:

- traditionally associated with prolonged shock or severe hypovolaemia;
- classically associated with obstetric disasters.

Clinically, there may be loin pain, hypotension and anuria, preceded sometimes by haematuria.

Urinalysis shows casts (as in acute tubular necrosis), and renal function is non-specifically abnormal.

The differential diagnosis includes:

- acute tubular necrosis;
- post-renal obstruction;
- severe glomerulonephritis;
- bilateral vascular occlusion;
- haemolytic–uraemic syndrome (rarely).

An ultrasound examination is required to exclude obstruction, and diagnostic confirmation may require renal biopsy.

*Treatment is **supportive**.*

About one third of patients recover sufficiently to be dialysis-free but with renal function only 15–50% of normal and with proneness to a gradual decline thereafter.

Renal cystic disease

Renal cystic disease comprises a wide variety of conditions.

1. **Simple cysts** are fluid-filled, epithelial-lined structures. They are clinically silent and are found in about 50% of older patients.

2. **Acquired cystic disease** refers to the presence of more than five cysts, accompanied by renal impairment and usually with small scarred kidneys. This process arises in the proximal tubules and occurs in about 50% of patients on long-term dialysis. These cysts can cause haematuria, loin pain and erythrocytosis. They may also become infected or malignant.

3. **Polycystic disease** is a common condition inherited as an autosomal dominant. It is commonly referred to as autosomal dominant polycystic kidney disease (ADPKD) and has a prevalence of at least 1:1000. In 90% of cases, there is an abnormal gene on the short arm of chromosome 16 (ADPKD1 locus). Though the cysts commence in utero as outpouchings of the renal tubule and Bowman's capsule, the condition is clinically silent until adult life. There is interstitial scarring and compression of adjacent normal tissue, giving rise to:

- loin pain;
- hypertension;
- palpable abdominal mass;
- urinary tract infection;
- renal calculi;
- haematuria;
- renal impairment.

The most useful diagnostic imaging is with ultrasound. There may also be:

- cysts elsewhere (especially in the liver, pancreas or spleen);
- cerebral arterial berry aneurysms (and thus subarachnoid haemorrhage);
- mitral valve prolapse;
- colonic diverticula.

4. **Medullary cystic disease** is an autosomal dominant condition of cystic development in the medulla. It presents in young adults with:

- scarred, shrunken kidneys;
- loss of concentrating ability and thus polyuria;
- renal failure.

5. **Medullary sponge kidney** is due to cystic outpouching from the collecting ducts, giving rise to the characteristic flower-spray appearance on intravenous pyelogram. Some cases are familial. The condition presents with:

- haematuria;
- renal calculi;
- occasional tubular effects (e.g. renal tubular acidosis);

but not renal failure.

Bibliography

Amis ES, Cronan JJ, Yoder IC et al 1982 Renal
cysts: curios and caveats. Urol Radiol 4: 199.

Gabow PA 1993 Autosomal dominant polycystic
disease. N Engl J Med 329: 332.

Ishikawa I 1991 Acquired cystic disease: mechanisms
and manifestations. Semin Nephrol 11: 671.

Renal tubular acidosis

Classical renal tubular acidosis (distal RTA
or type 1) is caused by a defect of the distal
tubules preventing H^+ excretion.

Thus,

- the urine cannot be fully acidified,
- the urine pH is always >5.3,
- there is a metabolic acidosis with a normal
  anion gap.

The urinary anion gap is positive.

A similar phenomenon is found in some cases of
diarrhoea, but this should be apparent clinically.
Moreover, the normal negative urinary anion
gap is still seen in such patients with diarrhoea.

H^+ is normally secreted as NH_4^+ from the
alpha-intercalated cell into the lumen of the
collecting tubule under the action of
aldosterone via an ATP-ase pump. The urinary
anion gap is an approximate index of urinary
ammonium, with a negative anion gap
suggesting normal acidification. Potassium is
excreted from the adjacent principal cell also
under aldosterone action to restore
electrochemical neutrality following the active
reabsorption of Na^+ from the lumen. When H^+
is secreted from the cell, bicarbonate remains
and diffuses into the blood in exchange for Cl^-,
also to maintain electrical neutrality. In RTA
only potassium secretion is available to
compensate for sodium reabsorption, so that
hypokalaemia results. Since citrate excretion is
also impaired, the less soluble phosphate appears
in the tubules, and this precipitates with calcium
to give nephrocalcinosis. A similar phenomenon

may occur in chronically alkaline urine from
other causes.

RTA type 1 may be:

- genetic

  - sometimes associated with Marfan's
    syndrome;

- idiopathic;
- associated with

  - drugs (amphotericin, lithium);
  - autoimmune disease;
  - hypocalcaemia;
  - hypergammaglobulinaemia;
  - medullary sponge kidney.

A rare form of RTA may be hyperkalaemic and
associated with:

- urinary tract obstruction;
- renal transplant rejection;
- SLE;
- sickle cell anaemia;
- drugs (amiloride, silver sulfadiazine).

Proximal renal tubular acidosis (proximal
RTA or type 2) is associated with a defect of
proximal tubular reabsorption of bicarbonate.

Thus,

- there is excess sodium bicarbonate in the
  urine,
- the urine pH is >5.3 (when the filtered
  load exceeds the absorptive capacity),
- the plasma bicarbonate is low.

This condition is usually associated with other
proximal tubular defects, for example of
glucose, amino acids, phosphates and uric acid,
so that these substances appear in excess in the
urine, a condition called the Fanconi syndrome
(q.v.).

By contrast, carbonic anhydrase inhibitors
which also increase bicarbonate in the urine do
not cause any of these additional abnormalities.

RTA type 2 may be:

- hereditary
  - as in a variety of metabolic disorders, such as glycogen storage diseases, Wilson's disease, etc.,
- acquired
  - following drugs (cadmium, copper, lead, mercury, outdated tetracycline),
  - associated with multiple myeloma or hyperparathyroidism.

Renal vein thrombosis

Renal vein thrombosis is generally associated with the nephrotic syndrome, but it can also occur in renal carcinoma and thus with normal renal function. The nephrotic syndrome occurs with acute occlusion, but if the thrombosis is gradual, there may be appropriate compensation and the process may be silent.

> While renal vein thrombosis may cause the nephrotic syndrome in association with a thrombophilic state, membraneous nephropathy may also lead to renal vein thrombosis in its own right in about 50% of patients.

Renal vein thrombosis may be bilateral and may be acute enough to cause infarction. Usually it is more gradual and may even be clinically silent, though it can lead to loin pain and haematuria.

Diagnosis is by renal vein Doppler ultrasound examination.

Treatment is with long-term **anticoagulation**.

Bibliography
Cronin RE, Kaehny WD, Miller, PD et al 1976 Renal cell carcinoma: unusual systemic manifestations. Medicine 55: 291.

Llach F 1985 Hypercoagulability, renal vein thrombosis, and other thrombotic complications of the nephrotic syndrome. Kidney Int 28: 429.

Llach F, Papper S, Massry SG 1980 The clinical spectrum of renal vein thrombosis: acute and chronic. Am J Med 69: 819.

Renin–angiotensin–aldosterone

The renin–angiotensin–aldosterone (RAA) system is one of the key mechanisms for salt and water balance and thus for circulatory control.

Renin is a proteolytic enzyme produced by modified smooth muscle cells in the afferent arteriole of the kidney in the juxtaglomerular cells. Its release is regulated by tubular sodium concentration, sensed in the adjacent epithelial cells of the macula densa in the distal convoluted tubule. Renin release is also influenced by adrenergic stimuli.

The substrate for rennin is a circulating α_2-globulin (angiotensinogen) which is produced in the liver. From it, renin cleaves the inactive decapeptide, angiotensin I. Angiotensin I is converted to the octapeptide, angiotensin II, in the lungs by angiotensin-convertin enzyme (see Angiotensin-converting enzyme), and angiotensin II is the main stimulus to the production of aldosterone in the adrenal gland (see Aldosterone). Angiotensin II also activates the adrenergic system and is thus a vasopressor and mild inotrope. These well known effects are mediated via the AT_1 receptors.

In addition to these effects which have been recognized for many decades, it has more recently been appreciated that angiotensin II has a second subtype of receptors, AT_2, which mediate a variety of other less well defined actions. Thus, angiotensin II also increases intracellular Ca^{++} release and cell growth (i.e. it affects gene expression by enhancing protein synthesis in smooth muscle and myocardial cells). Angiotensin II is thus an extracellular messenger, and its mechanism of action is via binding to the specific cell surface receptors, which initiates a complex signalling cascade to release intracellular Ca^{++} and to activate protein kinase C.

Angiotensin II receptor antagonists (ARAs), i.e. losartan, irbesartan and related compounds, target the AT_1 receptor. They thus provide more complete angiotensin blockade than do the ACE inhibitors, because angiotensin can also be formed to some extent via pathways other than renin. Since the angiotensin receptor antagonists do not block the inactivation of bradykinin like the ACE inhibitors do, they were not expected to produce cough or angioedema, but this early promise has not been borne out in practice. On the other hand, the potentiation of bradykinin may be responsible also for some of the beneficial effects of the ACE inhibitors. In addition, the ARAs have been reported to cause occasional hepatotoxicity and to exacerbate hyperglycaemia in some diabetics. In clinical trials, angiotensin receptor antagonists have been found to be as effective as ACE inhibitors in hypertension and more effective in reducing mortality in heart failure.

Since renin release is influenced by sodium concentration, adrenergic stimuli and renal perfusion pressure, it is ideally attuned to controlling blood volume.

Abnormalities of renin secretion include both:

- **overproduction** in

    - renal artery stenosis;
    - the rare Bartter's syndrome, in which there is an increased renal synthesis of PGE_2 and hypokalaemic metabolic alkalosis;

- **deficiency** in

    - renal disease, especially diabetic nephropathy;
    - Conn's syndrome.

Abnormalities of aldosterone production follow the abnormalities of renin secretion, though there are also other causes of dysaldosteronism.

- **Hypoaldosteronism** may be

    - hyporeninaemic,
    - idiopathic.

- **Hyperaldosteronism** may be

    - hyper-reninaemic,
    - primary,
    - secondary to cardiac, hepatic or renal disease.

Bibliography

Curry SC, Arnold-Capell P 1991 Nitroprusside, nitroglycerin, and angiotensin-converting enzyme inhibitors. Crit Care Clin 7: 555.

Melby JC 1991 Diagnosis of hyperaldosteronism. Endocrinol Metab Clin North Am 20: 247.

Oparil S, Haber E 1974 The renin–angiotensin system. N Engl J Med 291: 389 & 446.

Pitt B, Segal R, Martinez FA et al 1997 Randomised trial of losartan versus captopril in patients over 65 with heart failure (Eavaluation of Losartan in the Elderly Study, ELITE). Lancet 349: 747.

Quinn SJ, Williams GH 1988 Regulation of aldosterone secretion. Ann Rev Physiol 50: 409.

Stoll M, Steckelings UM, Paul M et al 1995 The angiotensin AT2-receptor mediates inhibition of cell proliferation in coronary endothelial cells. J Clin Invest 95: 651.

Williams GH 1986 Hyporeninemic hypoaldosteronism. N Engl J Med 314: 1041.

Respiratory burns (see Burns (respiratory complications))

Respiratory diseases

Issues related to the management of major respiratory problems comprise much of the backbone of Intensive Care, particularly problems concerning mechanical ventilation, acute (adult) respiratory distress syndrome and nosocomial pneumonia. While many other respiratory problems are also common, especially asthma, acute pulmonary oedema, community-acquired pneumonia and pulmonary thromboembolism, some may have uncommon causes or differential diagnoses. These uncommon aspects of common conditions, together with the more clearly uncommon conditions themselves, are therefore considered in this book and include:

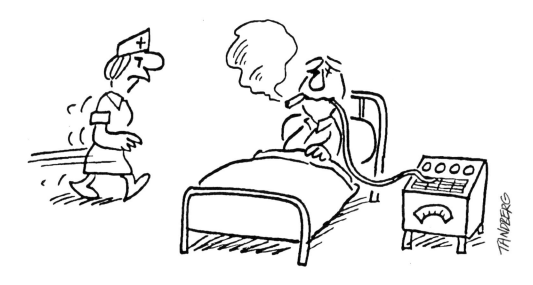

- acute lung irritation;
- acute pulmonary oedema;
- alpha$_1$-antitrypsin deficiency;
- aspiration;
- asthma;
- barotrauma;
- bronchiectasis;
- bronchiolitis obliterans;
- burns;
- cancer;
- cavitation;
- cystic fibrosis;
- diffuse fibrosing alveolitis;
- drowning;
- drugs and the lung;
- eosinophilia and lung infiltration;
- exotic pneumonia;
- Goodpasture's syndrome;
- haemoptysis;
- histiocytosis X;
- hypersensitivity pneumonitis;
- idiopathic pulmonary fibrosis;
- interstitial lung diseases;
- interstitial pneumonitis;
- occupational lung diseases;
- pneumoconiosis;
- pulmonary alveolar proteinosis;
- pulmonary hypertension;
- pulmonary infiltrates;
- pulmonary nodules;
- pulmonary veno-occlusive disease;
- radiation;
- sarcoidosis;
- sleep disorders of breathing;
- systemic diseases and the lung;
- Wegener's granulomatosis.

Non-respiratory thoracic disorders are also considered, in relation to the:

- chest wall;
- diaphragm;
- mediastinum;
- pleural cavity.

Bibliography

Abraham E, Terada L (eds) 1999 Acute lung injury. Chest 116 (suppl 1).

Albertson TE, Walby WF, Derlet RW 1995 Stimulant-induced pulmonary toxicity. Chest 108: 1140.

Bascom R, Bromberg PA, Costa DL et al 1996 Health effects of outdoor pollution. Am J Resp Crit Care Med 153: 3, 477.

Berger AJ, Mitchell RA, Severinghaus JW 1977 Regulation of respiration. N Engl J Med 297: 92, 138, 194.

Cade JF, Pain MCF 1988 Essentials of Respiratory Medicine. Oxford: Blackwell.

Caruana-Montaldo B, Gleeson K, Zwillich CW 2000 The control of breathing in clinical practice. Chest 117: 205.

Craddock PR, Fehr J, Brigham KL et al 1977 Complement and leukocyte-mediated pulmonary dysfunction in hemodialysis. N Engl J Med 296: 769.

Editorial 1989 Polycythaemia due to hypoxaemia: advantage or disadvantage? Lancet 2: 20.

Gardner WN 1996 The pathophysiology of hyperventilation disorders. Chest 109: 516.

Goldstein RA, Rohatgi PK, Bergofsky EH et al 1990 Clinical role of bronchoalveolar lavage in adults with pulmonary disease. Am Rev Respir Dis 142: 481.

Green M 1995 Air pollution and health. Br Med J 311: 401.

Heffner JE, Harley RA, Schabel SI 1990 Pulmonary reactions from illicit substance abuse. Clin Chest Med 11: 151.

Irwin RS (ed) 1998 Managing cough as a defense mechanism and as a symptom: a consensus panel report of the American College of Chest Physicians. Chest 114: no.2 Suppl.

Jamal S, Maurer JR 1994 Pulmonary disease and the menstrual cycle. Pulmonary Perspectives 11(3): 3.

Kopec SE, Irwin RS, Umali-Torres CB et al 1998 The postpneumonectomy state. Chest 114: 1158.

Kryger M, Bode F, Antic R et al 1976 Diagnosis of obstruction of the upper and central airways. Am J Med 61: 85.

Leatherman JW, Davies SF, Hoidal JR 1984 Alveolar hemorrhage syndromes: diffuse microvascular lung hemorrhage in immune and idiopathic disorders. Medicine 63: 343.

Leatherman JW, Mcdonald FM, Niewohner DE 1985 Fluid-containing bullae in the lung. South Med J 78: 708.

McGregor M, Sniderman A 1985 On pulmonary vascular resistance: the need for more precise definition. Am J Cardiol 55: 217.

Parsons PE 1994 Respiratory failure as a result of drugs, overdoses, and poisonings. Clin Chest Med 15: 93.

Ray CS, Sue DY, Bray G et al 1983 Effects of obesity on respiratory function. Am Rev Respir Dis 128: 501.

Savic B, Birtel FJ, Tholen W et al 1979 Lung sequestration. Thorax 34: 96.

Schatz M, Wasserman S, Patterson R 1981 Eosinophils and immunologic lung disease. Med Clin North Am 65: 1055.

Sugarbaker DJ (ed) 1997 Multimodality therapy of chest malignancies – update '96. Chest 112: 181S.

Terry PB, Barth KH, Kaufman SL et al 1980 Balloon embolization for the treatment of pulmonary arteriovenous fistulas. N Engl J Med 302: 1189.

Trulock EP 1997 Lung transplantation. Am J Respir Crit Care Med 155: 789.

Versprille A 1984 Pulmonary vascular resistance: a meaningless variable. Intens Care Med 10: 51.

Walmrath D, Schneider T, Pilch J et al 1995 Effects of aerosolized prostacyclin in severe pneumonia. Am J Resp Crit Care Med 151: 724.

White RJ, Lynch-Nyhan A, Terry P et al. 1988 Pulmonary arteriovenous malformation: techniques and long-term outcome of embolotherapy. Radiology 169: 663.

Winterbauer RH, Belic N, Moores KD 1973 Clinical interpretation of bilateral hilar adenopathy. Ann Intern Med 78: 65.

Wohl MEB, Chernick V 1978 Bronchiolitis Am Rev Respir Dis 118: 759.

Wright BA, Jeffrey PH 1990 Lipoid pneumonia. Semin Respir Infect 5: 314.

Wu T-C, Tashkin DP, Djahed B et al 1988 Pulmonary hazards of smoking marijuana as compared with tobacco. N Engl J Med 318: 347.

Restless legs

Restless legs syndrome is classically a benign idiopathic disorder, though it may also be a precursor to toxic/metabolic neuropathy, especially due to uraemia.

There is aching of the legs, with crawling sensations, especially at night. Symptoms may be present for a long time without any progression.

*Treatment with **carbamazepine, clonazepam** or **levodopa** may give relief.*

Bibliography
O'Keefe ST 1996 Restless legs syndrome: a review. Arch Intern Med 156: 243.

Telstad W, Sorensen O, Larsen S et al 1984 Treatment of the restless legs syndrome with carbamazepine. Br Med J 288: 444.

Reticulocytes

The red blood cell is produced when the late normoblast extrudes its nucleus. For the first four days of its life-span (three days in the bone marrow and one in the peripheral blood), the new red blood cell is termed a reticulocyte, because it contains residual ribosomes which are apparent on supravital stain, since the RNA is precipitated by methylene blue. Following the loss of this residual ribosomal material, the red blood cell becomes mature. When nuclei are extruded from even earlier normoblasts, as in severe anaemia, 'stress reticulocytes' are produced.

The reticulocyte count reflects the vigour of marrow production.

> The absolute reticulocyte count may be calculated as the red blood cell count, multiplied by the percentage of reticulocytes, corrected for the time in the peripheral circulation (normally one day).

Maturation time in the peripheral blood is prolonged in anaemia (e.g. it is two days when the PCV has fallen to 0.25). Since the reticulocyte count is normally 0.5–2.5% of the total red blood cell count, the normal corrected reticulocyte count is $50 \pm 25 \times 10^9$/L.

> - **An increased reticulocyte count**
>   - is seen in increased marrow production.
>   - This occurs in many forms of anaemia.
> - **A decreased reticulocyte count**
>   - is seen in decreased marrow production.
>   - This occurs in renal disease, aplastic anaemia, megaloblastic anaemia, sideroblastic anaemia, thalassaemia and myelofibrosis.

Retinal haemorrhage

Retinal haemorrhage is seen most typically:

- in uncontrolled hypertension;
- with increased local venous pressure, as in cavernous thrombosis.

It may also be seen in:

- some infections
  - such as with CMV or in SBE;

- a number of other settings
  - such as carbon monoxide poisoning, fat embolism and high altitude.

Retrobulbar neuritis

Retrobulbar neuritis is usually due to demyelination (see Demyelinating diseases). It may also be caused by:

- cyanide poisoning (q.v.);
- nicotine
  - tobacco amblyopia, traditionally seen in pipe smokers;
- vitamin B_{12} deficiency (q.v.).

Reye's syndrome

Reye's syndrome is a serious systemic disorder, which follows a viral infection and which involves particularly the brain and liver. Although originally described in children, it is now known also to affect young adults and even sometimes older patients.

Epidemiologically, it has been linked to prior influenza (and probably other viral infections, such as varicella), together with the concomitant use of salicylates. However, its pathogenesis remains unknown. Moreover, its incidence appears to have declined significantly since the 1980s, perhaps partly because of greater avoidance of aspirin and partly because many cases became reclassified as due to other metabolic disorders.

> Clinical features comprise the rapid onset, some days after the viral illness, of
>
> - refractory vomiting,
> - hepatomegaly,
> - fits,
> - drowsiness,
> - eventually coma.

Investigations show abnormal liver function tests, except that the bilirubin usually remains normal. Liver biopsy shows microvesicular steatosis, with minimal inflammation (a similar fatty infiltration occurring in other viscera). The CSF is normal, except that the pressure may be raised.

The diagnosis is generally made clinically, because liver biopsy may be unsafe due to the associated coagulopathy.

Treatment is **supportive** *with clotting factor replacement, mechanical ventilation, lactulose, and measures to decrease intracranial hypertension (including mannitol and/or dexamethasone).*

Prevention includes the use of paracetamol rather than aspirin for young people with acute viral infections and influenza vaccine for those few patients who need to have aspirin.

Bibliography

Atkins JN, Haponik EF 1979 Reye's syndrome in the adult patient. Am J Med 67: 672.
Reye RDK, Morgan G, Baral J 1963 Encephalopathy and fatty degeneration of the viscera: a disease entity in children. Lancet 2: 749.
Sarnaik AP 1999 Reye's syndrome: hold the obituary. Crit Care Med 27: 1674.

Rhabdomyolysis

Rhabdomyolysis refers to the necrosis of muscle tissue. There is consequent release of myoglobin and muscle enzymes into the circulation. The causes of rhabdomyolysis are as follows.

- **Idiopathic**
  - paroxysmal, with muscle pain, tenderness and weakness,
  - usually after exertion and lasting for 2–3 days,
  - sometimes familial, and there may be enzyme defects.
  - There is an increased intracellular Ca^{++} and thus dantrolene may be helpful by inhibiting calcium release from the sarcoplasmic reticulum.

- **Heat stroke**
  - q.v.

- **Malignant hyperthermia**
  - q.v.

- **Neuroleptic malignant syndrome**
  - q.v.

- **Metabolic disorders**
  - hypokalaemia, diabetic ketoacidosis, hyperosmolality.

- **Muscle damage**
  - from ischaemia, severe exertion, status epilepticus, trauma.

- **Polymyositis**
  - q.v.

- **Toxic agents**
  - alcohol, cocaine, drug overdose, lovastatin, snake venom.

- **Viral (and rarely bacterial) infection**
  - especially influenza,
  - also adenovirus, EBV, HSV,
  - occasionally Gram-positive bacteria.

The most important clinical consequence of rhabdomyolysis is acute renal failure from tubular obstruction due to pigment casts. There may also be tubular cell damage and afferent-efferent arterial imbalance, as well as hypovolaemia.

Rhabdomyolysis is thus similar to haemolysis, with myoglobinuria causing problems similar to those from haemoglobinuria, but with some clearly distinguishing features, as indicated in the table below.

Myoglobinuria v haemoglobinuria

	Myoglo-binuria	Haemo-globinuria
Molecular weight	170 kD	69 kD
Plasma colour	normal	dark red
Urine colour	dark red	dark red
Urine dipstick test for blood	positive	positive
Urine red blood cells	negative	negative
Renal damage	yes	yes

Other renal investigations show:

- pigment casts in the urine sediment;
- raised plasma creatinine and urea;
- hyperkalaemia;
- hyperphosphataemia;
- hypercalcaemia;
- very low urine sodium concentration, in contrast to the more normal level in typical acute tubular necrosis.

The plasma CK is also high, as are other muscle enzyme levels.

*Treatment is with **hydration** with iv saline to improve renal perfusion and urine flow. A urine output of 300 mL/h should be obtained, if necessary with mannitol diuresis. The urine pH should be maintained >6.5 until the urine colour has normalized. A positive fluid balance may be expected in the first 6–12 h, because of fluid sequestration in damaged muscle. Because of the likelihood of renal failure, and difficulties with fluid balance, cardiac filling pressures should be monitored.*

*Although **hypocalcaemia** is usual in the early phases due to calcium transit into ischaemic muscle, and although it may be aggravated by alkalinization, hypercalcaemia occurs in 20–30% of cases during the recovery. This may be an unexpected phenomenon and arises from mobilization of calcium from injured muscle. Calcium administration should thus be avoided, even during the early stages of hypocalcaemia.*

Bibliography

Gabow PA, Kaehny WD, Kelleher SP 1982 The spectrum of rhabdomyolysis. Medicine 61: 141.
Knochel JP 1981 Rhabdomyolysis and myoglobinuria. Semin Nephrol 1: 75.
Miller FW 1994 Classification and prognosis of inflammatory muscle disease. Rheum Dis Clin North Am 20: 811.

Rheumatology

Connective tissue and musculoskeletal disorders mostly have no currently identifiable specific aetiology. However, as for other conditions, a classification is useful, though it must necessarily be somewhat arbitrary.

Many rheumatological conditions are very common in the population, including soft tissue rheumatic syndromes, osteoarthritis, post-traumatic damage, rheumatoid arthritis and vasomotor disorders. Thus, while some connective tissue and musculoskeletal conditions may have manifestations severe enough to require Intensive Care admission, more common reasons for Intensive Care in such patients are either comorbidity, because of the chronicity of many of these conditions, or other illness, with the rheumatic disorder being coincidental.

A large variety of rheumatological conditions may therefore be seen in Intensive Care patients, and while not usually primary problems they can give rise to added difficulties of management of pain, immobility, stiffness and concomitant drug needs. The chief such conditions include:

- ankylosing spondylitis;
- arthritis and arthropathies;
- cricoarytenoid arthritis;
- Felty's syndrome;
- gout and pseudogout;
- kyphoscoliosis;
- mixed connective tissue disease;
- myositis;
- polyarteritis nodosa;
- polymyalgia rheumatica;
- polymyositis and dermatomyositis;
- Reiter's syndrome and reactive arthritis;
- rhabdomyolysis;
- scleroderma;
- Sjögren's syndrome;
- spondyloarthritis;
- systemic lupus erythematosus.

Bibliography

Ahern MJ, Smith MD 1997 Rheumatoid arthritis. Med J Aust 166: 156.
Gibofsky A, Zabriskie JB 1995 Rheumatic fever and poststreptococcal reactive arthritis. Curr Opin Rheumatol 7: 299.
Hamerman D 1989 The biology of osteoarthritis. N Engl J Med 320: 1322.
Hruska KA, Teitelbaum SL 1995 Renal osteodystrophy. N Engl J Med 333: 166.
Jowsey J 1977 Metabolic Disease of Bone. Philadelphia: WB Saunders.

Kelley WN, Harris ED, Ruddy S et al (eds) 1997
Textbook of Rheumatology. 5th edition.
Philadelphia: Saunders.

Littlejohn GO 1996 Fibromyalgia syndrome. Med J
Aust 165: 387.

Mandell BF (ed) 1994 Acute Rheumatologic and
Immunological Diseases: Management of the
Critically Ill Patient. New York: Marcell Dekker.

Miller FW 1994 Classification and prognosis of
inflammatory muscle disease. Rheum Dis Clin
North Am 20: 811.

Mills PR, Sturrock RD 1982 Clinical associations
between arthritis and liver disease. Ann Rheum
Dis 41: 295.

Parniapour M, Nordin M, Skovron ML et al 1990
Environmentally induced disorders of the musculoskeletal system. Med Clin North Am 74: 347.

Posen S 1992 Paget's disease: current concepts. Aust
NZ J Surg 62: 17.

Prockop DJ 1992 Mutations in collagen genes as a
cause of connective-tissue diseases. N Engl J Med
326: 540.

Rodan GA 1992 Introduction to bone biology. Bone
13: 53.

Schumacher HR, Klippel JH, Koopman WJ (eds)
1993 Primer on the Rheumatic Diseases. Atlanta:
Arthritis Foundation.

Shiel WC, Prete PE 1984 Pleuropulmonary
manifestations of rheumatoid arthritis. Semin
Arthritis Rheum 13: 235.

Simon LS, Mills JA 1980 Drug therapy: nonsteroidal
antiinflammatory drugs. N Engl J Med 302: 1179,
1237.

Rickettsial diseases

Rickettsial diseases are produced by infection
with members of a genus of small pleomorphic
obligate intracellular parasites which contain
both DNA and RNA and are coccobacillary in
appearance. In general, they have an animal
reservoir and an arthropod vector and are
transmitted to humans only incidentally. They
are taxonomically related to various
proteobacteria, such as legionella.

The organisms multiply at the site of entry and
then disseminate so as to infect endothelial cells
throughout the body. This results in:

- capillary leak syndrome;
- hypovolaemia;
- circulatory failure;
- multi-organ failure.

There are three main groups of rickettsial
diseases, namely:

- the spotted fevers;
- the typhus group;
- Q fever.

In addition, many new rickettsioses have
been identified worldwide in recent years,
including ehrlichiosis and bartonella
infection (cat-scratch disease, trench fever
and bacillary angiomatosis).

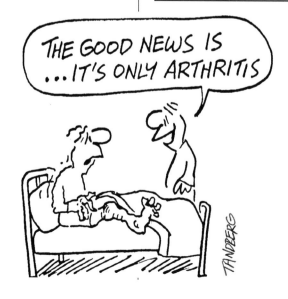

1. **Spotted fevers** are widely distributed, particularly in the Rocky Mountains of the USA, the Mediterranean, Asia and Northern Australia.

A generalized maculopapular rash is accompanied by fever and systemic features.

2. **The typhus group** includes:

- endemic (murine) typhus;
- epidemic (louse-borne) typhus;
- scrub typhus.

Endemic typhus occurs worldwide and is transmitted by rodent fleas. The responsible organism is *R. typhi*. Following an incubation period of 6–14 days, there is fever, an eventual rash and systemic symptoms, especially headache. There may be a pulmonary infiltrate. The illness lasts 10–12 days if untreated.

Epidemic typhus is due to *R. prowazekii* and is transmitted by the body louse, especially in times of war. Following an incubation period of 7 days, there is an abrupt onset of high fever, an eventual rash, severe headache and diffuse vascular lesions. There is often a pulmonary infiltrate and splenomegaly, and if severe, hypotension, confusion, respiratory failure and disseminated intravascular coagulation. Lysis occurs after two weeks without treatment, and mortality is 10–50%, especially in the debilitated. A recrudescence of epidemic typhus may occur many years later and is referred to as Brill–Zinsser disease. The organism has presumably persisted dormant in the reticuloendothelial system prior to reactivation. There is an irregular fever and severe headache but no rash. The illness lasts 7–11 days, following which there is complete recovery.

Scrub typhus is produced by the organism *Orientia tsutsugamushi* (formerly called *R. tsutsugamushi*) and is transmitted by an infected mite, an ectoparasite of small mammals. The condition usually occurs in South East Asia, the Western Pacific or Northern Australia. The bite site may show infection, and there is lymphadenopathy, a high fever and a rash.

3. **Q fever** is caused by the organism, *Coxiella burnetii*, following transmission via milk, faeces or products of conception. The animal reservoir in cattle and sheep is worldwide, and the organism is very infectious, although no person-to-person transmission occurs. It is usually seen in animal workers. The transmission is airborne.

Following an incubation period of about 20 days, there are non-specific initial symptoms followed after 4–5 days by fever, headache, cough, chest pain and primary atypical pneumonia. There is no rash but there is occasionally hepatosplenomegaly. Spontaneous recovery occurs after 1–2 weeks.

Chronic recurrent illness may occur in up to 10% of patients months to years after the acute illness. This can be associated with potentially fatal endocarditis.

The differential diagnosis is difficult, as in the early phases it is similar to many acute febrile illnesses. The history of contact with livestock is important. When pneumonitis appears, the differential diagnosis becomes more confined and includes viral, chlamydial, legionella and mycoplasma infections. In endocarditis, it mimics bacterial infection.

The diagnosis of rickettsial diseases is confirmed serologically.

*The organisms are sensitive to **tetracycline** (0.5 g qid or doxycycline 100 mg bd) or chloramphenicol (0.5 g qid), to either of which antibiotic group a rapid response is seen. Ciprofloxacin is also effective.*

Bibliography

Caron F, Meurice JC, Ingrand P et al 1998 Acute Q fever pneumonia. Chest 114: 808.

Spach D, Liles W, Campbell G et al 1993 Tick-borne diseases in the United States. N Engl J Med 329: 936.

Winkler HH 1990 Rickettsia species. Annu Rev Microbiol 44: 131.

Salicylism (see Aspirin)

Salpingitis

Salpingitis or infection involving the Fallopian tubes commonly also involves the uterus and adjacent structures, and together these infections comprise **acute pelvic inflammatory disease**.

Except when the organisms are directly implanted following abortion, pregnancy or surgery, the pathogens usually have ascended from the vagina. Thus, aerobic and anaerobic faecal flora and cervicovaginal flora (especially bacteroides and anaerobic Gram-negative cocci) are responsible for 50% of infections. Other organisms commonly involved include *N. gonorrhoeae*, *Chlamydia trachomatis*, *Mycoplasma hominis*, *Ureaplasma urealyticum*.

There are both local and systemic features of infection and occasionally extension to produce peritonitis.

Subsequent problems include recurrent abdominal pain, ectopic pregnancy and infertility.

The differential diagnosis can sometimes be difficult and includes:

- appendicitis;
- mesenteric adenitis;
- endometriosis;
- ruptured ovarian cyst;
- ovarian tumour;
- ectopic pregnancy.

In 25% of cases presenting with a putative diagnosis of salpingitis, no definitive diagnosis is made even at laparoscopy.

*Treatment is with **antibiotics**, preferably tetracycline (doxycycline) and a cephalosporin (cefoxitin). Recently, quinolones have also been shown to be effective. If severe, gentamicin plus metronidazole or even imipenem may be indicated. In either event, doxycycline should also be given for up to two weeks to cover chlamydia. If poor compliance with such a regimen is anticipated, a single dose of azithromycin*

1 g is a cost-effective alternative. Failure of antibiotic therapy indicates the likelihood of an abscess, which needs to be identified by imaging (usually CT) and drained.

Bibliography

Peterson HB, Walker CK, Kahn JG et al 1991 Pelvic inflammatory disease: key treatment issues and options. JAMA 266: 2605.

Rice PA, Schachter J 1991 Pathogenesis of pelvic inflammatory disease: what are the questions? JAMA 265: 2587.

Webster DP, Schneider CN, Cheche S et al 1993 Differentiating acute appendicitis from pelvic inflammatory disease in women of child-bearing age. Am J Emerg Med 11: 569.

Sarcoidosis

Sarcoidosis is a multisystem disease characterized by non-caseating granulomas. It is found worldwide, but there is great regional variation in incidence. In general, it is more common in temperate than in tropical climates. Occasional familial clustering is seen, perhaps indicating some genetic predisposition.

The aetiology is most likely to be one or more, as yet unidentified, transmissible agents. Although it has been linked with a number of infections, none of these associations have stood up to close scrutiny, except perhaps for reports of its occurrence after yersinia infections. In turn, sarcoidosis may predispose to listeria or cryptococcal infection. Moreover, many conditions both infectious (e.g. histoplasmosis, non-caseating tuberculosis) and non-infectious (e.g. berylliosis) may also produce granulomas similar to those seen in sarcoidosis.

It is a relatively common condition, especially in young adults, with a prevalence generally from 5–20 per 100 000 population.

Although the clinical features are protean, the chief manifestations are pulmonary, with over 95% of patients having an abnormal chest X-ray. Physical examination of the chest is frequently normal, but crackles and wheezes are sometimes noted. Respiratory symptoms correlate much better with functional or pathological changes than with radiological changes, the latter often being either considerably greater or less than the symptoms would suggest.

> Clinical staging is based on the lung involvement, though there is no necessary progression or retrogression serially through the individual stages.
>
> - **Stage I** (50% of cases)
>
> This consists of bilateral hilar lymphadenopathy which is usually asymptomatic. There are however systemic features of fever, malaise, weight loss, arthralgia and erythema nodosum. About 10% of these patients have extrapulmonary involvement (especially of CNS, eyes, lacrimal glands). Most cases (75%) resolve after two years, and only 10–15% develop progressive pulmonary disease. An acute onset with erythema nodosum especially heralds a self-limited course and spontaneous resolution.
>
> - **Stage II** (25% of cases)
>
> This involves both bilateral hilar lymphadenopathy and diffuse lung infiltration. In addition to systemic features, there are usually pulmonary symptoms of cough and dyspnoea. Remission occurs in about 50% of patients within two years, but some progress to develop chronic disease.
>
> - **Stage III** (15% of cases)
>
> This refers to diffuse lung infiltration without hilar lymphadenopathy. Respiratory symptoms are usual, though these are much less striking than the chest X-ray would predict. Although most patients at this stage have progressed through the previous stages, about 10% of cases in fact present at this stage. Remission still occurs in about one third of patients by two years, though progression to relentless progressive chronic pulmonary fibrosis is common, especially in

patients with an insidious onset. Extrapulmonary involvement is frequent.

> - **Stage 0** (the remaining 10% of cases)
>
> This term is sometimes applied to those who have normal chest X-rays.

Uncommon intrathoracic manifestations include the following.

- **Pleural effusion** or pleural thickening, seen in 1–4% of cases. The effusion is usually small, and there is a high lymphocyte count in the pleural fluid.
- **Lung nodules**, often large (i.e. 2–10 cm diameter) and needing to be distinguished from tuberculosis, mycetoma or carcinoma.
- **Cavitation**, rarely.
- **Calcification of nodes**, seen in 5% of cases as a late phenomenon.
- **Atelectasis**, due to endobronchial involvement and with associated wheeze.
- **Respiratory failure**, due to extensive consolidation.
- An unusual variant is **necrotizing sarcoid granulomatosis with pulmonary arteritis**.

Extrapulmonary manifestations are numerous and varied, and they may be apparent in virtually any organ system.

- **Skin**. Erythema nodosum is seen in 90% of patients with stage I disease. Sometimes, there may be skin granulomas, nodules or lupus pernio (usually in stage III disease).
- **Eyes** are involved in 25% of patients. Typically, there is uveitis with painless photophobia and lacrimation. Classically but uncommonly, there may be uveoparotid fever (with associated salivary gland enlargement, systemic symptoms, meningitis and cranial nerve palsies) or chorioretinitis (with blurred vision). Keratoconjunctivitis sicca may occur.
- **Neurological changes** are seen in <5% of patients. They may involve either the central nervous system (encephalopathy, hypothalamic lesions, granulomas, cranial

nerve palsies, fits, chronic meningitis in which the CSF shows increased protein and lymphocytes) or peripheral nervous system (with peripheral neuropathy of a sensory and/or motor form).

- **Liver** and **spleen** may contain granulomas, occasionally there may be overt enlargement or dysfunction, and associated lymphadenopathy may be seen.
- **Musculoskeletal system** is involved in 1–10% of patients, with arthritis, swelling and cystic lesions in the bones of the digits.
- **Endocrine changes** comprise hypercalcaemia and especially hypercalcuria, and occasionally pituitary dysfunction, especially with diabetes insipidus.
- **Heart**, with granulomas causing failure, arrhythmias and pericardial disease, though in fact most cardiac involvement is occult.
- **Upper respiratory tract**, with nasal granulomatous involvement simulating rhinitis or supraglottic laryngeal plaque involvement causing hoarseness.
- **Renal**, with tubulointerstitial nephritis, associated with either interstitial infiltration, granulomas or nephrocalcinosis. There is sterile pyuria, mild proteinuria and defects of concentration and acidification and thus tubular function. Renal involvement is however usually asymptomatic, and like the cardiac involvement it is generally found only at autopsy.

The diagnosis is established most securely when clinicoradiographic findings are supported by histological evidence of widespread noncaseating epithelioid-cell granulomas in more than one organ. Although often only lung material obtained by transbronchial lung biopsy is available for examination, additional biopsy of lymph node, Kveim nodule (formerly) or other tissue greatly assists diagnosis.

Bronchoalveolar lavage fluid shows lymphocytosis, though this is non-specific.

Chest X-ray shows that the diffuse lung involvement may be miliary, nodular or reticular. Confluent infiltrates may occur and are sometimes massive. Chest radiography is always essential, as clinically silent pulmonary involvement is usual, even if the presentation is extrapulmonary.

Lung function tests may show decreased ventilatory capacity, usually restrictive but occasionally obstructive in pattern, hypoxaemia and hypocapnia, decreased lung volumes, decreased compliance and decreased gas transfer. The latter is probably the most sensitive functional test and the best for serial follow-up. Although these functional changes correlate quite well with pathological changes, they are not helpful prognostically.

There is depressed cell-mediated immunity (i.e. anergy, with a negative Mantoux test) but often enhanced humoral or B-lymphocyte activity (with raised or abnormal immunoglobulins).

A positive Kveim test has been obtained in about 80% of cases, though this test is no longer performed.

Microbiological examination of sputum should exclude acid-fast bacilli.

Hypercalcaemia and especially hypercalcuria may be demonstrated.

The serum angiotensin converting enzyme (ACE) level is increased in most patients with acute disease. However, this finding is non-specific, importantly being also seen in miliary tuberculosis, as well as in pneumoconiosis, biliary cirrhosis and leprosy.

The chief differential diagnosis is:

- tuberculosis;
- lymphoma;
- metastatic carcinoma;
- amyloid.

Treatment is not required in many patients, because the disability is mild and remission is usual, but **corticosteroids** *are indicated in symptomatic disease. Corticosteroids both relieve symptoms and suppress inflammation and granuloma formation. They thus suppress the manifestations of acute sarcoidosis, but* *whether they alter the long-term outcome remains unproven. Most clinicians, however, would use corticosteroids in Stage II or III disease with dyspnoea and abnormal lung function and in serious extrapulmonary disease. Low doses are usually effective, and treatment can often be ceased after one year.*

- *No benefit has been found from the addition of cyclosporin to corticosteroids.*
- *There is some trial evidence to suggest that prolonged treatment with **chloroquine** may be helpful in some patients.*

The prognosis is usually good, because about 75% of patients with stage I disease undergo a complete remission within two years. In about 10% of patients, progression to fibrosis occurs. In individual patients, the course and prognosis may correlate with the mode of onset, as indicated above. Severe chronic extrapulmonary lesions are usually associated with pulmonary fibrosis. The overall mortality is less than 5% and is most commonly due to respiratory failure secondary to severe pulmonary fibrosis.

Bibliography

British Thoracic Society Sarcoidosis Study 1996 Effects of long term corticosteroid treatment. Thorax 51: 238.

Newman LS, Rose CS, Maier LA 1997 Sarcoidosis. N Engl J Med 336: 1224.

Selroos O, Astra Draco AB 1996 Glucocorticosteroids and pulmonary sarcoidosis. Thorax 51: 229.

Thomas PD, Hunninghake GW 1987 Current concepts of the pathogenesis of sarcoidosis. Am Rev Respir Dis 135: 747.

Winterbauer RH, Belic N, Moores KD 1973 Clinical interpretation of bilateral hilar adenopathy. Ann Intern Med 78: 65.

Wyser CP, van Schalkwyk EM, Alheit B et al 1997 Treatment of progressive pulmonary sarcoidosis with cyclosporin A. Am J Respir Crit Care Med 156: 1371.

Scalded skin syndrome (see

Exfoliative dermatitis)

Scarlet fever

Scarlet fever is usually produced by the Group A beta-haemolytic streptococcus, S. pyogenes. This organism produces the type A erythrogenic toxin which causes extensive capillary damage. Although scarlet fever declined in incidence and severity following the introduction of penicillin, there has been a recent re-emergence of the condition.

> The original site of streptococcal infection can be skin and soft tissue, e.g. cellulitis or necrotizing fasciitis, rather than an upper respiratory tract infection. Usually, there is associated bacteraemia.

Following a fever and sore throat, there is a fine, red, sandpaper-like rash within 1–5 days. Although the rash includes the oral cavity, it typically tends to spare the perioral region. There is nausea and even severe prostration. When the rash fades, desquamation accompanies the healing process.

Complicating features, often in the absence of a rash, include:

- ARDS;
- renal failure;
- a toxic-shock syndrome resembling that caused by staphylococci (see Toxic-shock syndrome). In this setting, the mortality is 30% despite high-dose penicillin and Intensive Care.

Schistosomiasis

Schistosomiasis arises from infection with a trematode, one of the major groups of helminthic parasites.

Helminths are multicellular organisms with complex extra-human life-cycles and include **trematodes** (flukes), **nematodes** (roundworms) and **cestodes** (tapeworms).

The three major species of fluke are *S. mansoni*, *S. japonicum* and *S. haematobium*. They are mostly found in Africa, Asia, and Central and South America. Because of the absence of an intermediate host, they are not found in developed countries, though infection may be seen in travellers.

Following passage of the eggs in human faeces into water, the hatchlings become free-swimming miracidia which enter the fresh water snail, the immediate host. These release free-swimming cercaria, which penetrate human skin and become schistosomula, which in turn circulate in the blood and mature and mate in portal vessels. These then lodge in blood vessels in different parts of the body, where they shed eggs, which are excreted or transported elsewhere. In particular, *S. mansoni* lodges in the colon, *S. japonicum* in the entire intestine and *S. haematobium* in the bladder.

There are three stages of clinical disease.

- **First stage**

There is dermatitis at the site of penetration of the parasite into the skin.

- **Second stage**

About 4–8 weeks later, if the original infestation has been heavy, acute disease now occurs (Katayama fever). There is fever, malaise, myalgia, urticarial rash, cough, hepatosplenomegaly and eosinophilia.

- **Third stage**

The eggs are now found in the liver, gut and bladder. This gives rise to fever, malaise, diarrhoea, haematuria, hepatosplenomegaly and later portal hypertension. Liver failure does not occur because the hepatic parenchyma is spared. Embolization to the lungs may cause pulmonary hypertension and to the brain may cause focal CNS signs. The diagnosis is made following demonstration of the eggs in faeces or urine.

*Treatment is with **praziquantel** (40–60 mg/kg as a single dose). This drug is very effective and has few side-effects.*

Bibliography

Hiatt RA, Sotomayor ZR, Sanchez G et al 1979 Factors in the pathogenesis of acute *Schistosomiasis mansoni*. J Infect Dis 139: 659.

Schonlein–Henoch purpura (see Purpura)

Scleroderma

Scleroderma (systemic sclerosis) is a generalized disorder of connective tissue of unknown aetiology. It is characterized by degenerative and inflammatory changes that lead to intense fibrosis, particularly in the skin. Possible fetal microchimerism with a consequent form of graft-versus-host disease has been reported as an interesting pathogenetic mechanism in some cases of scleroderma in women.

This process may be extensive and involve many other organs, especially lungs and kidneys, but sometimes it may be localized to skin and subcutaneous tissue and even comprise a single linear lesion. Pathogenetically, the fibrous proliferation comprises quantitatively but not qualitatively abnormal collagen. There is an associated vasculopathy involving small arteries.

Clinical manifestations of scleroderma can be widespread, with multi-organ involvement.

- **Skin**

  - There is early thickening and later atrophy.
  - There is loss of pliability, mobility and appendages, especially on the hands (sclerodactyly) and face.
  - There is often associated telangiectasia.
  - The involvement of cutaneous vessels may give Raynaud's phenomenon.
  - Sometimes, there is subcutaneous calcinosis.

- **Musculoskeletal**

  - There is polyarthralgia and sometimes polyarthritis, and tenosynovitis.

- Acral osteolysis with loss of terminal bone and soft tissue from the digits is seen.
- There can be flexion contractures and myopathy.

- **Gastrointestinal tract**

  - There is dilatation and impaired contractility of the oesophagus.
  - This process may also involve the intestine, and sometimes there may be pneumatosis intestinalis.
  - Some patients have associated Sjögren's syndrome (q.v.).

- **Lungs**

  - There may be diffuse interstitial fibrosis and pulmonary hypertension.

- **Heart**

  - Cardiomyopathy, arrhythmias, conduction defects, cardiac failure may occur.

- **Kidneys**

  - Malignant hypertension (renal crisis) can be produced.

- **Nerves**

  - Trigeminal neuralgia and other cranial neuropathies may be seen rarely.

Investigations show a positive ANA test in most patients, and diffuse hypergammaglobinaemia may be present. A specific antibody is demonstrable to the enzyme, topoisomerase I (Scl–70).

*Treatment is **symptomatic** and depends on the extent of involvement and the speed of progression. Symptoms should be managed on their individual merits.*

***Corticosteroids** and **cyclophosphamide** arrest the progress of pulmonary fibrosis, and **ACE inhibitors** are recommended in renal crisis.*

The prognosis depends on the extent and type of involvement. Renal crisis used to be fatal, but patients now often survive with aggressive antihypertensive therapy, and pulmonary involvement is now the chief cause of death. The mortality is very variable, though the average is 50% at 5 y in diffuse disease and 35% at 10 y overall. Although the condition only occasionally remits, its progress is usually slow, especially after the first two to five years. Localized disease itself does not adversely affect life expectancy.

Variants of scleroderma include the following.

- **Overlap syndromes**

  - mixed connective tissue disease (q.v.).

- **Limited cutaneous scleroderma**

  - CREST syndrome, namely calcinosis, Raynaud's phenomenon, oesophageal immobility, sclerodactyly, telangiectasia.
  - This variant of scleroderma is a milder form with limited skin involvement, less organ damage (except for biliary cirrhosis) and less progression.
  - However, some patients develop severe pulmonary hypertension late in the course of this illness.
  - An anti-centromere antibody is usually demonstrable.

Bibliography

Donohoe J 1992 Scleroderma and the kidney. Kidney 41: 462.

Evans PC, Lambert N, Maloney S et al 1999 Long-term fetal microchimerism in peripheral blood mononuclear cell subsets in healthy women and women with scleroderma. Blood 93: 2033.

Rasaratnam I, Ryan PFJ 1997 Systemic sclerosis and the inflammatory myopathies. Med J Aust 166: 322.

Silver RM, Miller KS, Kinsella MB et al 1990 Evaluation and management of scleroderma lung disease using bronchoalveolar lavage. Am J Med 88: 470.

Scombroid

Scombroid poisoning is the commonest seafood poisoning worldwide. Enteric marine flora can degrade histidine, present in high concentration in the dark meat of many fish, to form histamine, the likely toxin in this condition. This process arises when caught fish are not cooled, and it can occur within even a few hours at room temperature. Once formed, the toxin is not destroyed by subsequent freezing or by smoking.

The victim may note that the fish tasted metallic or peppery. The onset of symptoms is rapid with headache, flush, pruritus, gastrointestinal symptoms and occasionally bronchospasm. It is not an allergic process.

The administration of **antihistamines**, *including H2 antagonists, is recommended for symptomatic relief.*

The condition is non-fatal and self-limited.

Bibliography
Morrow JD, Margolies GR, Rowland J et al 1991 Evidence that histamine is the causative toxin of scombroid-fish poisoning. N. Engl J Med 324: 716.

Scorpion stings (see Bites and stings)

Scurvy

Scurvy is due to vitamin C deficiency and is the oldest known nutritional disorder of man. It was well described during the Crusades and later it afflicted sailors. It was recognized in 1753 as dietary in origin.

Since vitamin C is required for the synthesis of collagen, patients with scurvy have deficient supporting structures for small vessels. There is thus microvascular bleeding (especially of the gums), commonly with vascular purpura and sometimes with deep haematomas. There are also abnormalities of the hair shafts and of keratinization.

Scurvy is commonly associated with other vitamin deficiencies and with malnutrition.

Treatment is with **vitamin C** *1 g daily.*

Bibliography
Wallerstein RO, Wallerstein RO Jr 1976 Scurvy. Semin Hematol 13: 211.

Selenium

Selenium (Se, atomic number 34, atomic weight 79) was discovered in 1818 and is related chemically and physically to sulfur, being intermediate between metals and non-metals. It is widely distributed in nature in small quantities, and it is ingested in grains, meats and seafood.

In the body, where it is present in a total amount of 10–20 mg, it is an essential trace element and acts as an anti-oxidant. Over the last decade, it has become apparent that, like iodine, selenium is required for normal thyroid metabolism (see Euthyroid sick syndrome).

Selenium deficiency has been reported to be associated with cardiomyopathy, myositis and osteoarthropathy. More recently, it has been appreciated that low selenium levels may occur in sepsis and trauma and are then associated with increased morbidity and mortality.

The normal plasma level is 0.8–1.2 μmol/L. The daily requirement is 30–80 μg orally and the recommended iv dose is 0.4–1.5 μmol/day.

Bibliography
Berger MM, Cavadini C, Chiolero R et al 1996 Copper, selenium and zinc status and balances after major trauma. J Trauma 40: 103

Diplock AT, Chaudhry FA 1988 The relationship of selenium biochemistry to selenium-responsive disease in man. In: Prasad AS (ed) Essential and Toxic Trace Elements in Human Health and Disease. New York: Liss. p 211.

Forceville X 2001 Selenium and the 'free' electron. Intens Care Med 27: 16.

Levander OA, Burk RF 1986 ASPEN research workshop on selenium in clinical nutrition. JPEN 10: 545.

Rayman MP 2000 The importance of selenium to human health. Lancet 356: 233.

Serotonin syndrome (see Amphetamines)

Serpins (see Alpha$_1$-antitrypsin deficiency)

Serum sickness (see Immune complex disease)

Sheehan's syndrome (see Pituitary)

Short bowel syndrome

The short bowel syndrome occurs following extensive surgical removal of the small intestine usually for ischaemia or malignancy, though sometimes it may follow irradiation.

Malabsorption (q.v.) results, especially when the ileum is lost, because although the ileum can compensate for the loss of the jejunum, vice versa does not apply, especially for specialized absorption sites within the ileum for vitamin B$_{12}$ and bile salts.

The predominant clinical feature is profuse diarrhoea. This occurs because of the increased osmotic load, especially of carbohydrates. Steatorrhoea, weight loss, and vitamin or mineral deficiencies, may occur.

Treatment is with dietary control (i.e. small, frequent and readily absorbed meals), vitamin and mineral supplementation, and anti-diarrhoeal medication.

Shy–Drager disease (see Sweating)

Sickle cell anaemia (see Haemoglobin disorders)

Sideroblastic anaemia

Sideroblastic anaemia refers to a diverse group of conditions associated with ineffective erythropoiesis and thus anaemia. The name derives from the presence in peripheral blood of normoblasts with iron-encrusted mitochondria, the so-called ringed sideroblasts. The peripheral blood film shows hypochromic, distorted red blood cells, but the iron binding capacity is saturated.

The following types may be found.

1. Hereditary benign sideroblastic anaemia

This can occur as either a sex-linked or autosomally inherited condition.

2. Acquired benign sideroblastic anaemia

This is seen in:

- alcoholism;
- lead poisoning;
- pyridoxine deficiency;
- after anti-tuberculous drugs, such as isoniazid.

3. Acquired malignant sideroblastic anaemia

This is a myelodysplastic disorder, accompanied by neutropenia and thrombocytopenia. It may evolve into a myeloproliferative disorder or acute myeloid leukaemia.

Bibliography
Doll DC, List AF 1992 Myelodysplastic syndromes. Semin Oncol 19: 1.
Jacobs A 1986 Primary acquired sideroblastic anaemia. Br J Haematol 64: 415.

Situs inversus

Situs inversus refers to left–right reversal of the normal asymmetrical position of the body's internal organs. If this process involves just the heart, it is of course called isolated dextrocardia.

Situs inversus is characteristic of **Kartagener's syndrome**, described in 1933 as accompanied by bronchiectasis (q.v.). Subsequently, the association of chronic sinusitis was recognized, and 40 y later the further link was made with male infertility associated with live but immotile sperm.

The condition is inherited as an autosomal recessive, involving the absence of ATPase-containing dynein arms of outer microtubular doublets. This is part of the microtubular machinery required for motility in sperm tails and respiratory cilia. Immotile cilia thus lead to respiratory infection, and immotile sperm lead to infertility. Fertility is also decreased in women, because the oviducts and fimbriae are ciliated. Kartagener's syndrome has thus been renamed '**Immotile cilia syndrome**'.

Other abnormalities of disturbed microtubular configurations have more recently also been described. These give rise to motility disturbances (including incoordination instead of immotility) and are thus more generally referred to as primary ciliary dyskinesia.

The clinical features primarily comprise upper respiratory tract and lower respiratory tract infections commencing in childhood. There is thus:

- chronic sinusitis;
- secretory otitis media;
- retained tracheobronchial secretions with chronic productive cough;
- bacterial superinfection;
- ultimately bronchiectasis.

The pattern of disability is similar to that seen in cystic fibrosis, except that it is milder and without the serious sequelae of pneumonia, cor pulmonale and severe airways obstruction. Also in contrast to cystic fibrosis, the micro-organisms involved are chiefly haemophilus, neisseria and streptococci rather than pseudomonas and staphylococci.

Investigations apart from respiratory assessment include examination of the cilia in vitro or their clearance ability in vivo.

Bibliography

Afzelius BA 1976 A human syndrome caused by immotile cilia. Science 193: 317.

Mygind N, Nielsen MH, Pedersen M 1983 Kartagener's syndrome and abnormal cilia. Eur J Respir Dis 64 (suppl 127): 1.

Sjögren's Syndrome

Sjögren's syndrome is a chronic inflammatory condition involving the exocrine glands. It may be associated other autoimmune diseases, especially rheumatoid arthritis, but also SLE and scleroderma.

Since the changes can be subtle, its total incidence is uncertain, but its prevalence may be up to 1 in 100 of the population.

The pathology comprises inflammatory cellular infiltrate of glandular tissue with associated acinar atrophy.

Clinical manifestations are dominated by the **sicca syndrome**.

- This comprises dry eyes and mouth, because the lacrimal and salivary glands are affected.
- Sometimes, the respiratory tract is also dry, with hoarseness, bronchitis and pneumonia.
- The skin and genital mucous membranes may be similarly affected.

There may be associated myositis, neuropathy and thyroiditis. Sometimes, there is concomitant biliary cirrhosis, cryoglobulinaemia, drug hypersensitivity, pancreatitis, renal tubular acidosis or chronic hepatitis C infection. Neuropsychiatric abnormalities may be seen.

Investigations show decreased tear production, which can be conveniently assessed by the Schirmer filter paper test. There is filamentous keratitis on slit-lamp examination and conjunctival staining with Rose Bengal dye. There is decreased salivary flow (e.g. <0.5

mL/min from the parotid duct after lemon juice). Sialography or biopsy may be useful. The ESR and IgG are increased. Rheumatoid factor is positive in most patients, antinuclear antibodies are often present in high titre with a speckled pattern, and antibodies to Ro(SS-A) and La(SS-B) are present in about 60% of patients. There is some genetic predisposition, with primary Sjögren's syndrome associated with HLA B8, DR3.

An unusual complication is lymphoid proliferation to produce either

- **pseudolymphoma**, if the proliferation is pleomorphic, or even
- non-Hodgkin's lymphoma.

*Treatment is usually **symptomatic** with oral fluids and artificial tears.*

Low-dose corticosteroids or hydroxychloroquine are occasionally indicated and sometimes immunosuppression if severe manifestations are present.

Skin necrosis (see also Gangrene)

Warfarin-induced skin necrosis is a rare complication of coumarin therapy, usually seen within the first 10 days of treatment in protein C deficient patients. Red haemorrhagic bullae, which become necrotic and then scar, occur particularly on the breasts, thighs and buttocks of women and on the penis of men.

Heparin-induced skin necrosis is also rare and is similar to that seen after warfarin. It is presumed to be due to immune-mediated platelet aggregation.

Skin signs of internal malignant disease (see Paraneoplastic syndromes)

Sleep disorders of breathing (see also Melatonin)

Disordered breathing comprises:

- periodic and other abnormalities of breathing pattern;
- primary alveolar hypoventilation;
- the sleep apnoea syndromes.

The first two groups of disorders are also more marked during sleep and are thus considered here.

1. **Periodic breathing** is best known in the form of Cheyne–Stokes respiration, in which cycles occur of gradually increasing tidal volume followed by decreasing tidal volume and then transient apnoea, when the cycle is repeated.

It is best explained by a lag in the normal control loop of ventilation. It is thus an expected feature of advanced cardiac disease with a prolonged circulation time. It is also seen in patients with central nervous system lesions involving the deep structures in the cerebral hemispheres and basal ganglia, as in ischaemia or encephalopathy. For uncertain reasons, it may be seen during haemodialysis, in chronic pulmonary disease and in some normal subjects, e.g. at altitude.

Other related abnormal breathing patterns include:

- random, ataxic or Biot's breathing

  - due to medullary, pontine or cerebellar lesions (usually haemorrhage or trauma);
  - in these cases, apnoea is readily produced by sedatives or narcotics;

- apneustic breathing

  - due to lower pontine lesions and characterized by an end-inspiratory pause.

2. **Primary alveolar hypoventilation** is usually due to a brainstem lesion, commonly vascular or inflammatory. There is:

- hypoxaemia;
- hypercapnia;
- grossly impaired ventilatory response to carbon dioxide, hypoxia and exercise;
- normal pulmonary function;
- normal neuromuscular function;
- normal chest wall;
- normal blood gases on voluntary hyperventilation.

Clinical features include headache, lethargy and somnolence but not dyspnoea. There is cyanosis, polycythaemia and cor pulmonale.

The extreme of the condition has been picturesquely called **'Ondine's curse'**.

When associated with obesity and often also obstructive sleep apnoea, it is sometimes referred to as the **'Pickwickian syndrome'**.

---

3. **Sleep apnoea syndromes** comprise those impairments of breathing, either hypoventilation or frank apnoea, that occur chiefly or solely during sleep. **Obstructive sleep apnoea** (OSA) is the severe end and chronic snoring is the mild end of the spectrum of conditions referred to as sleep disordered breathing (SDB) due to increased upper airway resistance.

The sleep apnoea syndromes are most commonly due to upper airway obstruction, though the cause may be sometimes either central or a combination of both mechanisms. Although most patients are overweight middle-aged men, the condition is in fact widespread and may affect 2–5% of the population to some degree.

It may also occur as a new phenomenon in patients discharged from intensive care after prolonged mechanical ventilation.

Clinical features are dominated by:

- somnolence during the daytime

  – due to nocturnal sleep fragmentation;

- snoring, restlessness and apnoeic episodes during the night

  – observed by bed partners;

- the longer-term consequences of repeated asphyxia

  – polycythaemia, hypercapnia, cor pulmonale, intellectual deterioration, sexual dysfunction, headache;

- cardiovascular consequences

  – arrhythmias, hypertension, an increased incidence of acute myocardial infarction and stroke.

Pathogenetic mechanisms, generally worse during REM-sleep in most patients, include relaxation of the muscles of the upper airway during sleep (a process exacerbated by alcohol or sedative drugs), decreased ventilatory response to carbon dioxide during sleep, or pathological abnormalities of the upper airway, chest wall or neuromuscular function. Sedative drugs impair the arousal response to obstruction, hypoxaemia and hypercapnia, and thus prolong the apnoeic episodes.

The diagnosis is suggested by clinical suspicion based on the constellation of features described above, but it should be confirmed by formal polysomnography in a sleep laboratory. Such studies show that sleep disruption with apnoea and arousal may occur up to 60 times or more per hour.

Treatment options include:

- *cessation of alcohol and sedatives;*
- *weight control;*
- *attention to any local pathology (e.g. tonsillar hypertrophy);*
- *avoidance of androgens;*
- *use of drugs, such as medroxyprogesterone (a respiratory stimulant) or protryptyline (to decrease REM-sleep), which may sometimes be helpful;*
- *low-flow oxygen if hypoxaemia is the dominant consequence;*
- **nasal CPAP**, *the most dramatically effective measure, even in non-obstructive cases;*
- *other mechanical aids, but those available are generally poorly effective;*
- *nasal positive pressure ventilation in severe cases;*
- *attention to non-obstructive causes;*
- *surgery, which is occasionally indicated, usually tracheostomy but sometimes uvulopalatopharyngoplasty (UPPP), though the results are often disappointing and there is an absence of good trial data.*

Bibliography

Aldrich MS 1992 Narcolepsy. Neurology 42 (suppl): 34.

Burwell CS, Robin ED, Whaley RD et al 1956 Extreme obesity associated with alveolar hypoventilation: a Pickwickian syndrome. Am J Med 21: 811.

Canto RG, Zwillich CW 1993 Central sleep apnea. Pulmonary Perspectives 10(3): 4.

Chan CS, Grunstein RR, Bye PT et al 1989 Obstructive sleep apnea with severe chronic airflow limitation. Am Rev Respir Dis 140: 1274.

Cherniack NS, Longobardo GS 1973 Cheyne–Stokes breathing: instability in physiologic control. N Engl J Med 288: 952.

Chishti A, Batchelor AM, Bullock RE et al 2000 Sleep-related breathing disorders following discharge from intensive care. Intens Care Med 26: 426.

Exar EN, Collop NA 1999 The upper airway resistance syndrome. Chest 115: 1127.

Fishman AP, Goldring RM, Turino GM 1966 General alveolar hypoventilation: a syndrome of respiratory and cardiac failure in patients with normal lungs. Q J Med 35: 261.

Hudgel DW, Thanakitcharu S 1998 Pharmacologic treatment of sleep-disordered breathing. Am J Respir Crit Care Med 158: 691.

Ingbar DH, Gee JBL 1985 Pathophysiology and treatment of sleep apnea. Annu Rev Med 36: 369.

Kales A, Vela-Bueno A, Kales JD 1987 Sleep disorders: sleep apnea and narcolepsy. Ann Intern Med 106: 434.

Krachman SL, D'Alonzo GE, Griner JG 1995 Sleep in the intensive care unit. Chest 107: 1713.

McNicholas WT 1999 Sleep apnoea and driving risk. Eur Respir J 13: 1225.

Naughton M, Pierce R 2000 Snoring, Sleep Apnoea and Other Sleep Problems. 2nd edition. Spring Hill: Australian Lung Foundation.

Neill AM, McEvoy RD 1997 Obstructive sleep apnoea and other sleep breathing disorders. Med J Aust 167: 376.

O'Keefe ST 1996 Restless legs syndrome: a review. Arch Intern Med 156: 243.

Pack AI 1994 Obstructive sleep apnea. Adv Intern Med 39: 517.

Powell NB, Riley RW, Robinson A 1998 Surgical management of obstructive sleep apnea syndrome. Clin Chest Med 19: 77.

Ray CS, Sue DY, Bray G et al 1983 Effects of obesity on respiratory function. Am Rev Respir Dis 128: 501.

Riley RW, Powell NB 1990 Maxillofacial surgery and obstructive sleep apnea syndrome. Otolaryngol Clin North Am 23: 809.

Saunders NA, Sullivan CE (eds) 1984 Sleep and Breathing. Lung Biology in Health and Disease, Vol 21. New York: Marcel Dekker.

Severinghaus JW, Mitchell RA 1962 Ondine's curse – failure of respiratory center automaticity while awake. Clin Res 10: 122.

Strohl KP, Redline S 1986 Nasal CPAP therapy, upper airway muscle activation, and obstructive sleep apnea. Am Rev Respir Dis 134: 555.

Strollo PJ, Rogers RM 1996 Obstructive sleep apnea. N Engl J Med 334: 99.

Sullivan CE, Issa FG, Berthon-Jones M et al 1981 Reversal of obstructive sleep apnoea by continuous positive airway pressure applied through the nares. Lancet 1: 862.

Young T, Palta M, Dempsey J et al 1993 The occurrence of sleep-disordered breathing among middle-aged adults. N Engl J Med 328: 1230.

Worsnop C, Pierce R, McEvoy RD 1998 Obstructive sleep apnoea. Aust NZ J Med 28: 421.

341

Smoke inhalation (see Burns, respiratory complications)

Snake bites (see Bites and stings)

Sodium nitroprusside (see Cyanide)

Somatomedin C (see Acromegaly)

Somatostatin (see Acromegaly, Ectopic hormone production and Octreotide)

Spider bites (see Bites and stings)

Splenomegaly (see also Hypersplenism)

Splenomegaly may be caused by:

- **congestion**, due to

  - portal or splenic vein obstruction,
  - hepatic cirrhosis,
  - cardiac failure,

- **infectious disease**s, either

  - generalized (such as malaria or infectious mononucleosis),
  - granulomatous and local (e.g. tuberculosis),

- **connective tissue disorders**, such as

  - collagen-vascular diseases,
  - vasculitis,

- **infiltrations**, such as

  - sarcoidosis,
  - amyloid,
  - lipoidosis,

- **neoplasia**, particularly

  - lymphoma,
  - myeloproliferative disorders,

- **haemolytic diseases**.

Bibliography

Bohnsack JF, Brown EJ 1986 The role of the spleen in resistance to infection. Annu Rev Med 37: 49.
Rose WF 1987 The spleen as a filter. N Engl J Med 317: 704.

Spondyloarthritis

Spondyloarthritis refers to combined sacroiliitis and peripheral arthropathy. Although the chief such condition is **ankylosing spondylitis** (q.v.), other diseases may cause a similar condition and indeed there may be considerable overlap between them. Sometimes, the specific type is difficult to characterize and the term undifferentiated spondyloarthritis is used. They are associated with the major histocompatibility complex class I molecule, the human leukocyte antigen HLA-B27. There is a probable bacterial pathogenesis, most obviously found in reactive arthritis.

The other causes of spondyloarthritis include:

- **enteropathic** spondyloarthritis,

  - associated with Crohn's disease or ulcerative colitis,

- **psoriatic** spondyloarthritis,
- **Reiter's syndrome**,

  - q.v.,

- **reactive arthritis**,

  - occurring after various infections, but without direct microbial joint invasion (see Arthritis),
  - best regarded as a limited form of Reiter's syndrome (q.v.),

- possibly **Behçet's syndrome** (q.v.),
- possibly **Whipple's disease** (q.v.).

Bibliography

Kahn MA (ed) 1994 Spondyloarthropathies. Curr Opin Rheumatol 6: 351.
McEwen C, DiTata D, Lingg C et al 1971 Ankylosing spondylitis and spondylitis accompanying ulcerative colitis, regional enteritis, psoriasis and Reiter's disease. Arthritis Rheum 14: 291.
Reveille JD 1998 HLA-B27 and the seronegative spondyloarthropathies. Am J Med Sci 316: 239.

Spotted fevers (see Rickettsial diseases)

Staphylococcal scalded skin syndrome (see Exfoliative dermatitis)

Stevens–Johnson syndrome (see Erythema multiforme, and Exfoliative dermatitis)

Stings (see Bites and stings)

Stomatitis (see Mouth diseases)

Storage disorders

Storage disorders are due to monocyte/ macrophage defects. These cells normally scavenge cellular debris, a process which involves their lysosomes. Mutations causing enzymatic defects of lysosomal constituents (e.g. hydrolases) thus result in storage abnormalities.

These are classified according to the composition of the retained product and include glycoproteins, mucopolysaccharides, neutral lipids and sphingolipids.

Treatment has generally been with **bone marrow transplantation**, *though for some conditions it is controversial.*

For Gaucher's disease, **alglucerase** *is specific.*

Stridor (see Asthma)

Strychnine

Strychnine is an alkaloid (q.v.) which was discovered in 1818 in the woody vine called St Ignatius' beans in the Philippines (*Strychnos ignatii*). It also occurs in the seeds of the Indian tree, *Strychnos nux-vomica*. It is a very bitter substance and was used formerly as a tonic or cathartic in medicinals. Its common clinical use of the time was parallelled by its frequency in suicide and homicide. Now, however, it is used only as a rodent poison in agriculture, so that human toxicity is rare. The average lethal dose is 100 mg.

It is rapidly absorbed and having a low protein-binding is also rapidly cleared, 80% being metabolized by the liver and 20% excreted unchanged in the urine. The urine thus provides the best sample for clinical measurement.

Neurological toxicity is rapid (within 10–30 min) and dramatic. Since strychnine blocks the inhibitory neurones in the thalamus, brainstem and spinal cord, it produces a hyperexcitable state with powerful spasms and fits and

eventually death from brainstem paralysis. There is facial stiffness, trismus and opisthotonos. Tetanic contraction of the respiratory muscles produces apnoea. A series of fits each followed by exhaustion lasts several hours. Since the patient is awake during these episodes, there is considerable somatic and psychic discomfort. Death occurs primarily from respiratory failure. There may be associated lactic acidosis, rhabdomyolysis and even fractures.

The differential diagnosis includes epilepsy, tetanus and rabies.

Treatment consists of **sedation**, *particularly with a benzodiazepine.*

- *Muscle relaxation and mechanical ventilation is usually required, together with cardiovascular and metabolic support.*
- *Dialysis is not effective.*

If the patient survives for six hours, i.e. the usual period of seizures, total recovery is the rule.

Sturge–Weber syndrome

Sturge–Weber syndrome (encephalo-trigeminal angiomatosis) is a rare neurocutaneous disorder most obviously manifest by a craniofacial naevus, which is a port-wine stain (naevus flammaeus or capillary angioma) of the face. It involves the skin innervated by the first branch of the trigeminal nerve and is due to dilated capillaries in the dermis. Although it is apparent at birth, after puberty the lesion becomes thicker and more nodular, and little regression occurs.

Neurological features include contralateral fits from ipsilateral leptomeningeal and cortical angiomatosis, usually in the parieto-occipital region. There may also be hemiparesis and hemianopia, as well as mental retardation. There is commonly ipsilateral glaucoma.

Treatment is **symptomatic**, *apart possibly from laser therapy for the skin lesion.*

Sucralfate (see Aluminium)

Sweating

Sweating is an important physiological mechanism of temperature control. However, abnormalities are frequent.

Decreased sweating occurs in

- Autonomic nervous system disease.

  - This is usually part of diabetic or alcoholic peripheral neuropathy and is associated with other neurological features, such as hyporeflexia and impotence.
  - Commonly, there is orthostatic hypotension without tachycardia.

- Dehydration.
- Heat stroke.
- **Shy–Drager disease**

  - This was described in 1960 as a condition of autonomic deficiency, associated with neurological degeneration, Parkinsonian features and postural hypotension.
  - It is generally fatal in 7–8 y.

Increased sweating occurs in the following.

- Acromegaly.
- Acute myocardial infarction.
- Anticholinesterase overdose

  - i.e. cholinergic crisis.

- Cardiac tumours.
- Chinese restaurant syndrome.
- Collagen-vascular diseases

  - especially rheumatoid arthritis.

- Drug withdrawal

  - especially from anxiolytic, hypnotic or sedative drugs (colloquially referred to as 'cold turkey').

  - Severe or even life-threatening features can occur within 24–36 h of withdrawal of such drugs, with hyperthermia, fits and coma, as well as sweating.

- Dumping syndrome

  - occurring shortly after a meal.

- Dyshidrosis (or pompholyx)

  - a form of eczematous dermatitis, manifest by recurrent vesicles on the sides of the fingers and on the palms and soles.

- Endocarditis.
- Exercise

  - Sweating is of course the major physiological response to the hyperthermia of exercise.

- Envenomation

  - e.g. spider bite.

- Hot flushes (flashes)

  - which are part of the vasomotor disturbance associated with declining oestrogen levels, particularly at the female menopause.

- Hyperthyroidism.
- Hypoglycaemia.
- Irritable bowel syndrome

  - which is associated with vasomotor instability in many patients.

- Myeloproliferative disorders.
- Phaeochromocytoma.
- Pre-syncope

  - in which there is increased cholinergic stimulation, with pallor, nausea and increased intestinal peristalsis, as well as sweating.

- Needless to the say, increased sweating is one of the accompaniments of fever or hyperthermia (q.v.).

Night sweats are prominent in the following.

- AIDS.
- Chronic myeloid leukaemia.
- Cryptococcosis.
- Eosinophilic pneumonia.
- Fungal infections.
- Hodgkin's disease.
- Melioidosis.
- Paragonimiasis.
- Pulmonary aspergillosis.
- Renal abscess.
- Tuberculosis.

Bibliography
Quinton P 1987 Physiology of sweat secretion. Kidney Int 2 (suppl 21): S102.

Sweet's syndrome (see Paraneoplastic syndromes (dermatoses))

Swimming (see Bathing, Drowning and Diving)

Syndrome of inappropriate antidiuretic hormone

The syndrome of inappropriate antidiuretic hormone (SIADH) secretion occurs in three groups of clinical settings.

1. Increased ADH

Either increased ADH synthesis in the hypothalamus or increased ADH release from the posterior pituitary may be produced by:

- CNS disorders (infection, neoplasia, vascular disease),
- the postoperative state,
- prolonged nausea.

2. Ectopic ADH

This may be produced in a number of tumours,

- particularly carcinoma of the lung,
- also tumours of the gut or thymus,
- neuroblastoma.

3. Increased sensitivity to ADH

This may be produced by a number of drugs, such as:

- carbamazepine,
- chlorpropamide,
- cyclophosphamide.

Of course, vasopressin or oxytocin may also have been administered in their own right.

In SIADH, the osmostat gets reset at a lower level for ADH release, e.g. as low as 275 mOsm/kg. The serum sodium is thus stabilized at a new low level (usually 120–130 mmol/L), despite an abnormally increased urinary sodium concentration and osmolality. This is a relatively stable state, since water restriction gives rise to thirst and thus to further stimulation of ADH, so that the urine becomes more concentrated.

The clinical features are those of hyponatraemia. These are chiefly neurological with headache, malaise, nausea, fits and eventually coma.

The differential diagnosis of SIADH is primarily the other causes of hyponatraemia, in particular:

- volume depletion;
- dilution;
- pseudohyponatraemia.

Adrenal insufficiency should be specifically excluded.

The diagnosis is confirmed by measurements of the plasma and urine sodium concentration and osmolality, as indicated in the table below.

Differential diagnosis of hyponatraemia

Condition	Plasma Na$^+$	Plasma osmo-lality	Urine Na$^+$	Urine osmo-lality
Pseudohypo-natraemia	⇓	⇔	⇔	⇔
Hypovolaemia	⇓	⇓	⇓	⇑
Dilution	⇓	⇓	⇔	⇓
SIADH	⇓	⇓	⇑	⇑

Increased urine Na^+ refers to >20 mmol/L and decreased urine Na^+ refers to <15 mmol/L. Increased urine osmolality refers to >200 mOsm/kg.

In hyponatraemia due to hypovolaemia, if there is associated

- **hypokalaemia and metabolic alkalosis**,

  – hypovolaemia is probably due to vomiting, diuretic therapy or perhaps a villous adenoma,

- **hypokalaemia with metabolic acidosis**,

  – hypovolaemia is probably due to diarrhoea,

- **hyperkalaemia and metabolic acidosis**,

  – hypovolaemia is probably due to adrenal insufficiency.

Treatment is primarily with **water restriction**.

- *Saline may be cautiously administered in severe cases but clearly must be more hypertonic than the urine, so that isotonic saline is generally unsuitable. This is because normal sodium excretion takes less water with it than is administered, so that the plasma sodium falls further.*
- *In persistent cases, an* **ADH antagonist** *may be used, such as a loop diuretic (e.g. frusemide), demethyltetracycline or possibly lithium.*

(see also Central pontine myelinolysis (for further discussion of the treatment of hyponatraemia, including speed of correction and complications).

Bibliography

Berl T 1990 Treating hyponatremia: damned if we do and damned if we don't. Kidney Int 37: 1006.

Robertson GL 1987 Physiology of ADH secretion. Kidney Int 32 (suppl 21): S20.

Rose BD 1986 New approach to disturbances in the plasma sodium concentration. Am J Med 81: 1033.

Sterns RH 1987 Severe symptomatic hyponatremia: treatment and outcome. Ann Intern Med 107: 656.

Vokes TJ, Robertson GL 1988 Disorders of antidiuretic hormone. Endocrinol Metab Clin North Am 17: 281.

Syphilis

Syphilis is a sexually transmitted disease produced by infection with the thin motile spirochaete, *Treponema pallidum*. Humans are its only known host.

There has been a recent recurrence of syphilis, particularly among homosexual men.

Although not culturable in vitro and very labile to heat, cold, drying and soap, a 50% effective inoculum requires only 50–60 organisms. Since most inocula in contacts of even heavily infected cases do not produce the disease, most inocula are therefore presumably very small. Following penetration of mucous membrane or broken skin, there is parasitaemia which lasts 10–60 days.

The **primary lesion** appears as a painless chancre at the site of inoculation after an incubation period of 3–4 weeks. It lasts for 1–6 weeks and then heals. A chancre is highly infective.

A **secondary stage** appears 6 weeks later, with:

- widespread mucocutaneous lesions;
- lymphadenopathy;
- systemic illness.

This resolves after 2–6 weeks. The disease then becomes latent for a variable period up to 20 years or more, during which time there are no symptoms but positive serology.

The **tertiary stage** eventually appears with destructive lesions in the CNS, aorta, bones, skin and elsewhere.

- Neurosyphilis takes the form of meningovascular disease, general paresis, optic atrophy, tabes dorsalis (a motor ataxia accompanied by ptosis), Argyll–Robertson pupils, Charcot's joints, incontinence, visceral crises and lightning pains in the legs.

- The aortic lesions include aortitis and aortic valve incompetence.
- Elsewhere, necrotic granulomas called gummas appear.

The diagnosis is made by dark-field microscopy of infected lesions, which show the parasite, and by serological demonstration of a non-specific antibody directed against the lipoidal antigen produced by the interaction of the parasite with host tissues. Such tests (e.g. VDRL) have a high sensitivity but numerous false-positives. A specific antitreponemal antibody may be demonstrated for confirmation.

*Treatment is with **penicillin** for 7–14 days.*

- *Erythromycin, tetracycline, chloramphenicol and cephalosporins are also effective.*
- *The **Jarisch–Herxheimer** reaction may occur during treatment (q.v.).*

Bibliography
Hook EW, Marra CM 1992 Acquired syphilis. N Engl J Med 326: 1060.

Syringomyelia (see also Neural tube defects)

Syringomyelia refers to local dilatation of the central canal within the cervical and/or thoracic spinal cord. It is usually associated with the Arnold–Chiari malformation (q.v.), but it can follow local injury or be associated with a spinal glioma.

Clinically it causes a myelopathy, with both motor and sensory deficits in one or both arms. The sensory deficit involves especially pain and temperature. There may be neck pain, extending up to the occiput. Occasionally, there is an ipsilateral Horner's syndrome. Eventually, the pyramidal tracts also become involved, with spastic weakness of the lower limbs.

Proximal extension to the medulla gives rise to

syringobulbia, with abnormal signs related to the V, VII, IX, X and XII cranial nerves.

Diagnosis is optimally made by MRI.

*Treatment is with **surgical decompression**.*

Bibliography
Lemire RJ 1988 Neural tube defects. JAMA 259: 558.

Systemic diseases and the lung

Many systemic diseases may have significant pulmonary involvement, either directly or indirectly.

They include:

- collagen-vascular diseases
  - SLE;
  - scleroderma;
  - dermatomyositis;
- rheumatoid arthritis;
- Sjögren's disease;
- polyarteritis nodosa;
- ankylosing spondylitis;
- Stevens–Johnson syndrome;
- obesity;
- neurological disease;
- renal disease
  - uraemia;
  - dialysis problems;
  - disseminated intravascular coagulation;
  - acute glomerulonephritis;
  - collagen-vascular diseases;
  - Goodpasture's syndrome;
  - Wegener's granulomatosis;
  - drug reactions;
  - transplant complications.

Bibliography
Craddock PR, Fehr J, Brigham KL et al 1977 Complement and leukocyte-mediated pulmonary dysfunction in hemodialysis. N Engl J Med 296: 769.

Davies D 1972 Ankylosing spondylitis and lung fibrosis. Q J Med 41: 395.

Marik P, Varon J 1998 The obese patient in the ICU. Chest 113: 492.

Matthay RA, Schwarz MI, Petty TL 1975 Pulmonary manifestations of systemic lupus erythematosus. Medicine 54: 397.

Ray CS, Sue DY, Bray G et al 1983 Effects of obesity on respiratory function. Am Rev Respir Dis 128: 501.

Segal AM, Calabrese LH, Muzaffar A et al 1985 The pulmonary manifestations of systemic lupus erythematosus. Semin Arthritis Rheum 14: 202.

Shiel WC, Prete PE 1984 Pleuropulmonary manifestations of rheumatoid arthritis. Semin Arthritis Rheum 13: 235.

Systemic lupus erythematosus

Systemic lupus erythematosus (SLE) is a chronic multi-system autoimmune disease. Its cause or causes are not yet known.

Pathogenetically, it arises from the loss of immune regulation and tolerance, so that there is an autoimmune reaction to host antigens giving rise to inflammatory damage of vessels and tissues. There is some genetic predisposition, and there may be viral disruption of the suppressor T cell population. Eventually, there is excess B-cell proliferation and circulating immune complexes, with deposits containing DNA, complement and immunoglobulins.

The clinical features are extremely variable and are seen primarily in young women, in whom there is an incidence of 1 in 15 000 per year.

The most common features are rash, fever and arthritis, but there are very many others and indeed the condition can rightly be called protean.

- **Rash** is characteristically manifest as facial erythema, typically of the transient butterfly type, but more commonly it is apparent elsewhere, particularly on the neck and hands. It may be exacerbated by ultraviolet light, and it can be associated with alopecia or mouth ulcers.

- **Fever** is present in many patients, and the differential diagnosis from infection can be difficult.

- **Arthritis** is usually of the non-deforming type and comprises symmetrical polyarthritis with pain, swelling and morning stiffness. Sometimes, it may be indistinguishable from rheumatoid arthritis. There may be associated tendonitis and sometimes avascular necrosis of bone. Arthralgia is common.

- **Heart** involvement is especially manifest by pericarditis. Sometimes, there may be myocarditis or non-infective endocarditis.

- **Kidneys** are commonly involved, as evidenced by haematuria, proteinuria, pyuria and urinary casts. Minor mesangial changes occur in most patients but are asymptomatic. Focal proliferative changes are also common but are benign and reversible. Membranous glomerulonephritis may sometimes occur with consequent nephrotic syndrome, though this too can remit. Diffuse proliferative glomerulonephritis is the most serious renal complication and may lead to renal failure. The renal pathology may vary during the course of the disease.

- **Neurological** involvement occurs in about 50% of patients, although it is often mild. Neuropsychiatric features are common early in the course of the disease. Depression is especially marked, but there may also be organic psychosis or fits. Pyramidal tract or cranial nerve involvement may be seen (especially the latter, with VII nerve and extra-ocular signs). Aseptic meningitis, chorea and peripheral neuropathy may sometimes be seen. Except for cognitive dysfunction, most neurological changes are transient. The CSF is often normal, there are minimal histological changes, and abnormalities noted on MRI in subcortical white matter are reversible.

- **Lungs** are commonly involved, with pleurisy, pleural effusion, diffuse pulmonary infiltrate and propensity to pneumonia. Pulmonary hypertension is sometimes seen. The lungs may also be involved if there is cardiac failure, renal failure or thromboembolism.

- **Antiphospholipid syndrome** (q.v.). This is a hypercoagulable state associated with autoantibodies to phospholipid, the so-called 'lupus anticoagulant' occurring in about 50% of patients with SLE.
- **Myopathy** may be seen (q.v.).
- **Splenomegaly** may occur (q.v.).

Pregnancy can be associated with specific problems in SLE, since pregnancy may sometimes be a cause of SLE exacerbation. Pregnancy-related problems also occur if there is hypertension or antiphospholipid syndrome, and there is an increased incidence of spontaneous abortion, pre-eclampsia and neonatal lupus.

Investigations show anaemia, sometimes of an acute haemolytic nature. There is typically leukopenia and thrombocytopenia. Many autoantibodies can be demonstrated, especially ANA (in >90% of cases), antibodies to many of the antigens in cell nuclei (e.g. to double-stranded DNA in about 70% of cases), and LE cells. Complement levels are usually reduced in active disease. The changes of individual organ involvement may be demonstrated.

Treatment must be individualized, because of the very variable clinical course and the difficulty in evaluating progress.

- *It is usual to recommend avoidance of sun exposure, because 30% of patients are photosensitive and a flare-up involves not just the skin but systemic changes.*
- *Skin manifestations are treated with avoidance of excessive ultraviolet light exposure, topical corticosteroids, and sometimes hydroxychloroquine and low-dose systemic corticosteroids.*
- *Joint manifestations are treated with NSAIDs, hydroxychloroquine and sometimes low-dose corticosteroids.*
- *Problems such as pleurisy or pericarditis may require moderate-dose corticosteroids.*
- *Severe neurological manifestations or diffuse proliferative glomerulonephritis are treated with high-dose corticosteroids. End-stage renal disease is treated with chronic haemodialysis or*

transplantation, after which recurrence of lupus nephritis is fortunately rare.
- *Immunosuppressive therapy (cyclophosphamide, azathioprine) may be used for steroid-sparing or for uncontrolled disease, though they have not been shown to enhance the efficacy of steroids in controlled trials (except for cyclophosphamide iv).*
- *Although corticosteroids may be strikingly helpful symptomatically in a number of situations as described above, it is doubtful whether they alter survival.*
- *Plasmapheresis was found not to be effective in a controlled trial.*

The prognosis is difficult to assess in an individual patient, but it is often good. An average 5 y mortality of 20% is sometimes quoted from referral centres, though the actual rate is greatly dependent on the patient sample studied, with much lower rates applying to the overall population of SLE-affected patients. There is no cure, and while there may be complete remission for several years on the one hand, on the other hand there may be recurrences which can range from mild to severe multi-organ disease. Exacerbations may be precipitated by infection, surgery, some drugs and sometimes pregnancy. The prognosis is worse if there is severe neurological or renal involvement. Death is usually from either infection or renal failure.

Variants include the following.

1. Drug-induced SLE

This is particularly seen after hydralazine and procainamide. It may also follow penicillamine, isoniazid, phenytoin, sometimes phenothiazines and occasionally other drugs.

The risk is about 1% with the high-risk drugs, though about 50% of patients exposed to these drugs develop positive ANA titres and some may have subclinical SLE.

This form of lupus is usually milder and with less renal disease, though sometimes the entire lupus complex may be seen.

Systemic lupus erythematosus

Usually, drug-induced SLE follows the continuous administration of the offending drug for some time (range 3 weeks to 2 years). It is reversible on stopping the drug, though the abnormal laboratory tests may take many months to resolve, unlike the symptoms which usually subside in a few days.

2. Discoid lupus

This comprises skin lesions only and involves the face, scalp, chest and arms. Systemic disease rarely occurs. The serology is negative.

Bibliography

Doherty NE, Siegel RJ 1985 Cardiovascular manifestations of systemic lupus erythematosus. Am Heart J 110: 1257.

Ginsberg JS, Brill-Edwards P, Johnston M et al 1992 Relationship of antiphospholipid antibodies to pregnancy loss in patients with systemic lupus erythematosus. Blood 80: 975.

Johns KR, Morand EF, Littlejohn GO 1998 Pregnancy outcome in systemic lupus erythematosus. Aust NZ J Med 28: 18.

Lee LS, Chase PH 1975 Drug-induced systemic lupus erythematosus. Semin Arthritis Rheum 5: 83.

Matthay RA, Schwarz MI, Petty TL 1975 Pulmonary manifestations of systemic lupus erythematosus. Medicine 54: 397.

Rasaratnam I, Ryan PFJ 1997 Systemic lupus erythematosus. Med J Aust 166: 266.

Segal AM, Calabrese LH, Muzaffar A et al 1985 The pulmonary manifestations of systemic lupus erythematosus. Semin Arthritis Rheum 14: 202.

Steinberg AD 1986 The treatment of lupus nephritis. Kidney Int 30: 769.

Tan EM, Cohen AS, Fries JF et al 1982 The 1982 revised criteria for the classification of systemic lupus erythematosus. Arthritis Rheum 25: 1271.

Takayasu's disease (see Aortic

coarctation and Vasculitis)

Tardive dyskinesia

Tardive dyskinesia describes a syndrome of involuntary facial movements and choreoathetotic movements of the limbs.

It is a severe neurological complication, seen in about 20% of patients on long-term antipsychotic drugs. The best known drugs in this setting are the phenothiazines, but other unrelated compounds may produce similar effects.

> Sometimes, there may be impairment of swallowing, airway control and breathing.

The condition may slowly resolve when the drug is stopped. It is otherwise untreatable.

Temporal arteritis (see Arteritis)

Tetanus (see also Clostridial infections)

Tetanus results from infection with the anaerobic Gram-positive bacillus, *Clostridium tetani*, which is widely distributed in soil and animal (and occasionally human) faeces. Since active immunization is so effective, the disease is most commonly seen in developing countries, where a million deaths per year are produced worldwide due to the fact that the organism is ubiquitous and trauma so frequent. Clinical tetanus does not provide immunity against subsequent episodes.

Inoculated spores germinate at the site of injury and produce a potent neurotoxin (tetanospasmin). This migrates centrally along motor neurone axons to the spinal cord, where it suppresses the inhibition of the reflex arc by internuncial neurones. The reflex antagonist relaxation normally activated during contraction is thus lost, and muscular spasm occurs with a result which depends on the relative strengths of the agonist and antagonist muscle groups involved. Thus, opisthotonos is typical, with upper limb flexion and lower limb extension.

> Most commonly, the organisms penetrate a site of skin injury following trauma. Sometimes, they follow bites, burns, surgery, parenteral narcotic use, delivery or abortion. In 10–20% of cases, there is no identifiable initial lesion.

There is an incubation period of usually more than 2 weeks, but it may range from 1–55 days. The shorter the incubation period, the higher the mortality, which is reportedly 100% if the incubation period is only 1–2 days and about 30% if it is greater than 10 days.

- Trismus (lockjaw) is the first clinical feature noted in over half the patients.
- There is:

  - restlessness;
  - generalized muscle spasm and stiffness;
  - hyper-reflexia (with downgoing plantar reflexes);
  - dysphagia.

- The spasms become progressively violent within 72 h, though there is no loss of consciousness. Tonic seizures follow even minor stimuli and may involve the respiratory muscles, thus potentially giving respiratory arrest.
- There is moderate fever and sympathetic overactivity.
- The illness is severe for the first week, then gradually decreases over several weeks.
- Complications include:

  - respiratory failure;
  - pulmonary aspiration;
  - arrhythmias;
  - fractures of the thoracic vertebrae;
  - pulmonary embolism.

Laboratory results are generally normal, and the organism can be isolated in only 30% of patients.

The differential diagnosis includes:

- strychnine poisoning (q.v.)

  – this is very similar;

- pseudotetanus with trismus

  – this may be caused by phenothiazines and resolves with IV phenytoin;

- spider bite (q.v.);
- trismus from other causes

  – such as jaw infection or encephalopathy;

- hysteria.

*Treatment principles are three-fold, namely to **treat the source**, **neutralize the toxin** and **manage the complications**.*

- *The wound requires debridement and culture.*
- ***Antitoxin**, currently of human origin, is given in a single dose of 3–5000 U im or iv. The wound should be infiltrated with antitoxin also. Antitoxin is not effective for toxin which has already become bound. If human immunoglobulin is not available, equine antitoxin is used in a dose of 100 000 U.*
- *Intensive Care is required with administration of muscle relaxants, sedation, iv fluids and mechanical ventilation. Sedation should be with diazepam, and beta blockers iv are used for arrhythmias. Penicillin is given iv in large doses for one week, but is of limited value in that it affects only the vegetative cells in the wound, though in this way new toxin production is prevented.*

Bibliography

Edsall G 1976 Problems in the immunology and control of tetanus. Med J Aust 2: 216.

Tetrahydroaminoacridine (THA)

(see Anticholinergic agents)

Tetralogy of Fallot

Tetralogy of Fallot is the commonest cyanotic congenital heart disease. It comprises:

- pulmonary stenosis (more commonly infundibular than valvular);
- ventricular septal defect;
- an over-riding dextroposed aorta;
- right ventricular hypertrophy.

There is thus a right-to-left shunt, the degree of which varies with the degree of pulmonary stenosis.

The shunt causes hypoxaemia, cyanosis and secondary polycythaemia. Coagulopathy due to reduced vitamin K–dependent clotting factors and platelet dysfunction give rise to a bleeding tendency, which is especially marked after cardiac surgery.

***Surgical correction** should be performed in childhood (before the age of 5 y). Such surgery nowadays always involves a complete repair.*

In adults who have had an incomplete repair or no surgery, there is an increased risk of:

- infective endocarditis;
- paradoxical embolism, especially of the brain and thus the production of a brain abscess;
- sudden death from arrhythmias.

Bibliography

Nora JJ 1993 Causes of congenital heart disease: old and new modes, mechanisms, and models. Am Heart J 125: 1409.
Wilson NJ, Neutze JM 1993 Adult congenital heart disease: principles and management guidelines. Aust NZ J Med 23: 498, 697

Tetrodotoxin (see Bites and stings (marine invertebrates and marine vetebrates))

Thalassaemia (see Haemoglobin disorders)

Thallium

Thallium (T1, atomic number 81, atomic weight 204, melting point 304°C) is a soft blue-grey metal, malleable like lead but tarnishing in air. It is present in small amounts in lead an zinc ores and was discovered in them in 1861. Neither the metal or its compounds have major commercial application, but since it is a poor conductor of electricity it has found limited industrial use in photoelectric cells and in optics.

However, its toxicity made it popular in insecticides and rodenticides until the 1960s. Following its accidental or deliberate ingestion in humans, there is a classical picture of initial gastroenteritis followed by peripheral neuropathy and later alopecia. The peripheral neuropathy is generally mixed and is manifest particularly by ptosis, retrobulbar neuritis and facial paralysis. A Guillain–Barré-like polyneuritis has also been reported.

> Since thallium ions behaves like potassium, they are secreted into the gut where they may be sequestered by the antidote, **Prussian blue** (potassium ferrihexacyanoferrate), via exchange of potassium for thallium in its molecular lattice.

Prussian blue is given in a dose of 10 g bd orally or by nasogastric or nasoduodenal tube, a tube usually being needed because of associated gastrointestinal stasis. For the same reason, a purgative is generally required to treat the severe constipation which typically occurs. The antidote is continued not only until plasma and urinary levels have declined but more importantly until faecal excretion has ceased. Potassium given intravenously enhances thallium excretion into the gut, but oral potassium is contraindicated since it interferes with the thallium–potassium exchange by the antidote in the gut.

Thermoregulation (see Pyrexia)

Thiamine deficiency (see Beriberi)

Thrombasthenia (see Platelet function disorders)

Thrombocythaemia (see Thrombocytosis)

Thrombocytopenia

Thrombocytopenia refers to a decreased peripheral blood platelet count.

Like deficiencies of the other formed elements, it is due to one or more of the same three mechanisms, namely decreased production, increased removal or sequestration.

The mechanism of platelet production from megakaryocytes has been greatly clarified by the discovery of **thrombopoietin** (TPO) and by its recent cloning and characterization. TPO deficiency may occur in liver disease, since the liver is a major site of its production, and TPO excess may be involved in some states of thrombocytosis. Exogenous TPO is available for clinical trial use in thrombocytopenic conditions.

> The relationship between the platelet count and the risk of bleeding is inexact.
>
> - Thus, there is no single level below which bleeding occurs and above which bleeding does not occur.
> - Nevertheless, a platelet count of 20×10^9/L is commonly regarded as the 'magic number' below which the risk of serious haemorrhage becomes significant.
> - However, a platelet count of at least double this is required for protection against bleeding from invasive procedures (i.e. $40–50 \times 10^9$/L) and double this again (about 100×10^9/L) for haemostatic safety in high-risk procedures, such as neurosurgery.

- In general, one unit of platelet concentrate raises the platelet count by about $10 \times 10^9/L$ per m^2, so that 5–6 units or packs are generally required for haemostasis.
- However, unlike the normal half-life of four days, the half-life of transfused platelets is usually only about 24 h and perhaps as short as only 1 h in severe consumptive disorders.

In addition, a number of other factors both platelet-related and platelet-independent affect bleeding.

- **Platelet-related factors** include platelet size and thus their age and metabolic and functional activity, with larger platelets being younger and more active. In addition, platelet function abnormalities (q.v.) increase the risk of bleeding for any given platelet count.
- **Platelet-independent factors** affecting bleeding include any concomitant haemostatic defect, particularly those of coagulation, as in liver disease, vitamin K deficiency and disseminated intravascular coagulation.

The diagnosis of the cause of thrombocytopenia is assisted by both the associated clinical features and the full blood examination. Platelet kinetics are not feasible as a routine study, though the response to a standard six–unit platelet transfusion gives indirect kinetic information and is thus diagnostically helpful.

The types of thrombocytopenia are:

- decreased production;
- increased removal;
  - either immune or non-immune mediated;
- sequestration.

Deceased production occurs with:

- marrow infiltration;
- aplastic anaemia;
- dysplastic megakaryopoiesis
  - due to alcoholism, or vitamin B$_{12}$ or folic acid deficiency;
- drugs
  - alcohol, gold, sulfonamides, thiazides.

Increased removal may be either immune or non-immune mediated. The two mechanisms are not always clearly separable.

1. **Immune mechanisms** include:

- autoantibodies
  - ITP, lymphoma, SLE;
- drugs (see drug-induced thrombocytopenia below)
  - quinine/quinidine particularly;
  - heparin;
  - possibly diazepam, paracetamol, phenytoin, thiazides;
- infections
  - infectious mononucleosis, malaria;
- **post-transfusion purpura** (PTP).

Post-transfusion purpura is an uncommon condition occurring 2–10 days after the transfusion of any blood products containing platelets.

PTP is considered due to antibody production to the platelet allo-antigen Zwa, a platelet antigen occurring in 90% of the population. Patients with PTP are thus Zwa negative.

The condition is usually seen in middle-aged or elderly women. There tends to be severe thrombocytopenia and clinically significant bleeding.

The chief differential diagnosis is heparin-induced thrombocytopenia, disseminated intravascular coagulation and sepsis.

Treatment with high doses of **corticosteroids** *may be effective.*

- **Plasmapheresis** *may be used in severe and refractory cases.*
- *The best therapy is* **immune globulin** *(IgG 40 g iv over 40 min), followed by 10 units of platelets which are now effective because of reticuloendothelial blockade.*

The condition is reversible within 1–4 months.

2. **Non-immune destruction** occurs because of activation of coagulation, platelet aggregation or endothelial cell damage. It is due to:

- disseminated intravascular coagulation

  - or related conditions, such as haemolytic–uraemic syndrome, thrombotic thrombocytopenic purpura, vasculitis, pre-eclampsia;

- giant haemangioma

  - possibly via disseminated intravascular coagulation;

- Gram-negative septicaemia

  - typically accompanied by DIC if severe;
  - without DIC in milder cases, e.g. platelet count >50×109/L;

- massive transfusion

  - and thus platelet washout.

Sequestration occurs with:

- splenomegaly

  - when the intrasplenic platelet pool may rise from the normal 25% to 50–80%;

- coronary artery bypass grafting

  - when a platelet count $<50 \times 10^9$/L may persist for up to one week or more, especially in the elderly;

- pre-eclampsia and HELLP syndrome (q.v.).

Normal pregnancy is incidentally associated with mild asymptomatic thrombocytopenia in 5–8% of cases.

Thrombocytopenia due to sequestration is usually mild and not clinically significant unless there is concomitant disease. The reason for the failure of the bone marrow to compensate is uncertain.

Drug-induced thrombocytopenia may be difficult to distinguish from ITP, though the history may provide a clue.

Thrombocytopenia due to quinine/quinidine typically develops after about two weeks and is treated with corticosteroids if severe and possibly with immune globulin or plasmapheresis.

Heparin has become recognized as a common cause of thrombocytopenia, which may take one of two forms, sometimes referred to as Types I (mild, early, non-immune) and II (severe, delayed, immune).

1. **Type I**. Mild thrombocytopenia occurs in about 1% of patients given porcine heparin and about 5% of those given bovine heparin.

It becomes apparent within 4–10 days of commencement of unfractionated heparin and is probably non-immune. It may occur even with small doses of heparin.

It is asymptomatic and self-limited, even if heparin is continued.

No treatment or even cessation of heparin is required

2. **Type II**. A more severe form of thrombocytopenia (**heparin-induced thrombocytopenia**, HITS) may sometime be seen, with more profound thrombocytopenia ($<50 \times 10^9$/L), associated with a heparin-dependent IgG antiplatelet antibody.

The antigen recognized is a complex, on a platelet membrane, of heparin's glycosaminoglycans and platelet factor 4 (PF-4, a heparin-binding protein in the platelet's α granule). Antibody binding to this complex causes platelet activation and subsequent platelet removal from the circulation.

There may be in vivo platelet aggregates and endothelial cell damage (because heparin and heparin-like material is bound to the endothelial cell surface) with consequent thromboembolism. While thrombosis is usually venous, it may be arterial or microvascular, and it may affect unusual sites. It can be severe and extensive, and it carries a 20% risk of amputation and a 30% mortality.

Treatment of HITS requires **total cessation of heparin**, *as changing to another animal source or a low molecular weight preparation is mostly ineffective.*

Although some antithrombotic protection may be offered by dextra or aspirin, warfarin is the best therapeutic option. Either the low molecular weight heparinoid, danaparoid, or a member of the hirudin, such as lepirudin, can be specifically useful in the first few days.

Thrombotic thrombocytopenic purpura (TTP) is an uncommon condition, which causes about 1 death per 1 000 000 population per year. It occurs at all ages and is twice as common in women.

TTP was originally described in 1924 by Moschowitz, but it was only in 1982 that its relation to platelet adhesion to damaged endothelial cells via unusually large von Willebrand factor multimers was discovered. The mechanism for this damage was finally elucidated in 1996, when it was found that a metalloprotease is normally responsible for cleaving the large vWF multimers after they are secreted into the plasma by endothelial cells. This vWF-cleaving protease is deficient in TTP, being absent in chronic relapsing TTP and removed by a specific autoantibody in acute TTP. The protease is normal in the seemingly related haemolytic–uraemic syndrome. The protease may now be assayed relatively simply, and this could form the basis of a specific diagnostic test.

TTP is manifest by:

- thrombocytopenia;
- microangiopathic haemolysis;
- generalized symptoms of fever and damage to the brain and kidneys (and sometimes bowel, heart, liver and skin).

It thus has many clinical features in common with haemolytic–uraemic syndrome (q.v.).

There are a number of variants of TTP as yet unclarified as to mechanism, but their predisposing factors include:

- bone marrow transplantation;
- pregnancy;
- the drugs, cyclosporin and ticlopidine;
- HIV infection.

Treatment has not been subjected to formal trials, but **plasmapheresis** *has become the favoured therapy, with daily exchanges for one week in severe cases. Electrolytes, plasma proteins and the platelet count need careful monitoring.*

- **Corticosteroids** *are traditionally used, but former modalities such as aspirin, dipyridamole or vincristine are generally no longer required.*
- *Dextran and prostacyclin have been occasionally used.*
- *In severe and refractory cases,* **splenectomy** *may produce a striking remission.*

Modern treatment has greatly improved the previously rapidly fatal course of this condition, so that survival is now over 70%. However, while many patients remain in complete and long-term remission, about one third relapse during the following 10 y, and 10% of patients develop other serious disease.

Bibliography
Bell WR, Braine HG, Ness PM et al 1991 Improved survival of thrombotic thrombocytopenic purpura hemolytic–uremic syndrome: clinical experience in 108 patients. N Engl J Med 325: 398

Beutler E 1993 Platelet transfusions: the 20, 000/?L trigger. Blood 81: 1411

Bick RL 1997 Heparin-induced thrombocytopenia and paradoxical thromboembolism: Diagnostic and therapeutic dilemmas. Clin Appl Thromb Hemost 3: 63

Chong BH 1995 Heparin-induced thrombocytopenia. Br J Haematol 89: 431.

Chong BH, Ismail F, Cade J et al 1989 Heparin-induced thrombocytopenia: studies with low molecular weight heparinoid, Org 10172. Blood 73: 1592.

Cines DB, Konkle BA, Furlan M 2000 Thrombotic thrombocytopenic purpura: a paradigm shift? Thromb Haemost 84: 528.

Editorial 1991 TTP – desperation, empiricism, progress. N Engl J Med 325: 426.

Farag SS, Savoia H, O'Malley CJ et al 1997 Lack of in vitro cross-reactivity predicts safety of low-molecular weight heparins in heparin-induced thrombocytopenia. Clin Appl Thromb Hemost 3: 58.

Ferrara JLM 1995 The febrile platelet transfusion reaction: a cytokine shower. Transfusion 35: 89.

George JN, El-Harake M, Raskob GE 1994 Chronic idiopathic thrombocytopenic purpura. N Engl J Med 331: 1207.

Greinacher A 1995 Heparin-associated thrombocytopenia. Vessels 1: 17.

Mannucci PM 1999 Thrombotic thrombocytopenic purpura: a simpler diagnosis at last? Thromb Haemost 82: 1380.

Moake JL, Rudy CK, Troll JH et al 1982 Unusually large plasma factor VIII: von Willebrand factor multimers in chronic relapsing thrombotic thrombocytopenic purpura. N Engl J Med 307: 1432.

Mueller-Eckhardt C 1986 Post-transfusion purpura. Br J Haematol 64: 419.

Payne BA, Pierre RV 1984 Pseudothrombocytopenia: a laboratory artifact with potentially serious consequences. Mayo Clin Proc 59: 123.

Tsai HM, Lian ECY 1998 Antibodies to von Willebrand factor-cleaving protease in acute thrombotic thrombocytopenic purpura. N Engl J Med 339: 1585.

Vempaty HT, Zehnder JL 1998 Heparin-induced thrombocytopenia: pathophysiology, laboratory diagnosis and clinical management. Crit Care International Mar–Apr: 8.

Warkentin TE, Levine MN, Hirsh J et al 1995 Heparin-induced thrombocytopenia in patients treated with low-molecular-weight heparin or unfractionated heparin. N Engl J Med 332: 1330.

Warkentin TE, Chong BH, Greinacher A 1998 Heparin-induced thrombocytopenia: towards consensus. Thromb Haemost 79: 1.

Yang Z, Stulz P, von Segesser L et al 1991 Different interactions of platelets with arterial and venous coronary bypass vessels. Lancet 337: 939.

Thrombocytosis/ thrombocythaemia

Thrombocytosis refers to an increased platelet count above 400×10^9/L, and **thrombocythaemia** refers to disease associated with such an increased count.

Thrombocytosis is usually 'reactive' to:

- inflammation;
- trauma;
- neoplasia;
- splenectomy.

The platelets themselves are normal. There are no clinical consequences, even in the presence of a very high count.

> Such high platelet counts can however be a cause of pseudohyperkalaemia.

Thrombocythaemia is an autonomous increase in the peripheral blood platelet count, with megakaryocyte proliferation in the bone marrow. It is usually due to a clonal chronic myeloproliferative disorder, such as chronic myeloid leukaemia, polycythaemia vera, myelofibrosis, and essential thrombocythaemia.

The platelet count is commonly much greater than 1000×10^9/L. Platelet function is commonly abnormal as well.

Life expectancy is relatively unimpaired, but there is an increased incidence of bleeding (about 20%) and/or thromboembolism (about 10%).

Erythromelalgia may be produced and is due to microvascular dysfunction. It is manifest by cyanotic, ischaemic and burning digits.

*Treatment is generally with **aspirin**.*

- **Cytotoxics** *(alkylating agents)*, **radiophosphorus** *(*^{32}*P)*, **hydroxyurea** *or* **interferon** *are used in severe cases. However, alkylating agents, radiophosphorus and recently hydroxyurea have been shown to increase the incidence of leukaemic transformation and are therefore best avoided in younger patients, but the newer agent,* **anagrelide**, *is not mutagenic.*
- **Plateletpheresis** *may be used in emergency cases.*

Bibliography

Anagrelide Study Group 1992 Anagrelide, a therapy for thrombocythemic states. Am J Med 92: 69.

Bentley MA, Taylor KM, Wright SJ 1999 Essential thrombocythaemia. Med J Aust 171: 210.

Kurzrock R, Cohen PR 1991 Erythromelalgia: review of clinical characteristics and pathophysiology. Am J Med 91: 416.

Michiels JJ (ed) 1997 Platelet-dependent vascular complications and bleeding symptoms in essential thrombocythemia and polycythemia vera. Semin Thromb Hemost 23: 333.

Michiels JJ, Abels J, Steketee J et al 1985 Erythromelalgia caused by platelet mediated arteriolar inflammation and thrombosis in thrombocythemia. Ann Intern Med 102: 466.

Tefferi A, Elliott M, Solberg L et al 1997 New drugs in essential thrombocythemia and polycythemia vera. Blood Rev 11: 1.

Thromboembolism (see

Thrombophilia)

Thrombophilia

Thrombophilia refers to a thrombotic tendency, which may be inherited or acquired. The term was coined in 1965 and is a broader term than hypercoagulability, as it includes abnormalities of platelets and fibrinolysis as well as coagulation. It does not however include the other two components of Virchow's triad for thrombosis, namely abnormalities of the vessel wall or of blood flow.

Thrombophilia implies the occurrence of thrombi which are familial, unusual, recurrent or multiple.

Inherited thrombophilia includes:

- activated protein C resistance (Factor V Leiden defect);
- deficiencies (or abnormalities) of

   - antithrombin-III;
   - protein C;
   - protein S;
   - plasminogen;
   - fibrinogen;
   - prothrombin (the recently described mutation, G20210A variant, with G→A nucleotide substitution);
   - low factor XII (46 C→T mutation) has recently been considered paradoxically to be a possible thrombophilic rather than a haemostatic risk (after all, Mr Hageman whose name was originally give to factor XII died of pulmonary embolism);

- hyperhomocystinaemia

   - probably due to a mutant variant (called C677T) of the enzyme, 5, 10-methylenetetrahydrofolate reductase, which causes a relative deficiency of the enzyme responsible for converting homocysteine to methionine;
   - a fasting plasma homocysteine level >18.5mmol/L is significant, possibly via a direct pathogenetic mechanism;
   - possibly ameliorated with folate supplementation;

Interestingly, factor XIII mutation (val34leu) has recently been described as significantly protective against thrombophilia.

Acquired thrombophilia includes:

- antiphospholipid syndrome;
- collagen-vascular disorders;
- malignancy (including chemotherapy);
- nephrotic syndrome;
- myeloproliferative disorders.

Bibliography

Cattaneo M 1999 Hyperhomocysteinemia, atherosclerosis and thrombosis. Thromb Haemost 81: 165.

Dalen JE, Hirsh J, Guyatt GH (eds) 2001 Sixth

ACCP consensus conference on antithrombotic therapy. Chest 119: no. 1 (Suppl).

de Moerloose P, Bounameaux HR, Mannucci PM 1998 Screening tests for thrombophilic patients: which tests, for which patient, by whom, when, and why? Semin Thromb Hemost 24: 321.

den Heijer M, Rosendaal FR, Blom HJ et al 1998 Hyperhomocystinemia and venous thrombosis: a meta-analysis. Thromb Haemost 80: 874.

Franco RF, Reitsma PH, Lourenco D et al 1999 Factor XIII val34leu is a genetic factor involved in the aetiology of venous thrombosis. Thromb Haemost 81: 676.

Khamashta MA, Cuadrado MJ, Mujic F et al 1995 The management of thrombosis in the antiphospholipid-antibody syndrome. N Engl J Med 332: 993.

Lane DA, Mannucci PM, Bauer KA et al 1996 Inherited thrombophilia. Thromb Haemost 76: 651.

Miletich JP, Prescott SM, White R et al 1993 Inherited predisposition to thrombosis. Cell 72: 477.

Prins MH, Hirsh J 1991 A critical review of the evidence supporting a relationship between impaired fibrinolytic activity and venous thromboembolism. Arch Intern Med 151: 1721.

Sacher RA (ed) 1998 Thrombophilia: a forum on diagnosis and management in obstetrics, gynecology and surgery. Semin Thromb Hemost 24: Suppl 1.

Winter M, Gallimore M, Jones DW 1995 Should factor XII assays be included in thrombophilia screening? Lancet 346: 52.

Thrombopoietin (see Thrombocytopenia)

Thrombotic thrombocytopenic purpura (see Thrombocytopenia)

Thyroid function (see Euthyroid sick syndrome, Hyperthyroidism and Hypothyroidism)

Thyroid storm (see Hyperthyroidism)

Ticks (see Bites and stings (insects), Lyme disease and Relapsing fever)

Tinnitus

Tinnitus is the distressing symptom of ringing in the ear(s). It is due to any of the causes of VIII nerve damage (see Neuropathy above), provided the nerve has not been actually destroyed. It is also seen in:

- migraine;
- motion sickness;
- salicylism.

Tongue (see Mouth diseases)

Torulosis (see Cryptococcosis)

Toxic epidermal necrolysis (see Exfoliative dermatitis)

Toxic erythemas (see Erythema multiforme and Exfoliative dermatitis)

Toxic gases and fumes (see Acute lung irritation)

Toxic-shock syndrome

Toxic-shock syndrome (TSS) consists of hypotension, shock and rash following an acute febrile staphylococcal infection.

It was first described in 1978 in children and by 1980 about 1000 cases had been reported, 95% in women and of these by far the majority occurring during menstruation and associated with tampon use. In retrospect, the toxic-shock syndrome may have been the cause of the post-influenzal plague in Athens in 430 BC known as the 'Thucydides syndrome' (although other conditions have also been implicated, e.g. Ebola fever).

The syndrome is due to the staphylococcal toxin, TSST-1, which is secreted following a localized superficial and not necessarily overt staphylococcal infection. One of a considerable variety of local infections may be identified. They may even include deep staphylococcal infections, such as wound infection, abscess, pneumonia, empyema or osteomyelitis. TSST-1 stimulates IL-1 and TNF release, and the entire sequence may be enhanced by impaired host immunity.

Clinical features include:

- high fever;
- scarlatiniform rash with subsequent desquamation, especially on the palms;
- strawberry tongue and sore throat, though without a pharyngeal exudate;
- conjunctival injection;
- vomiting and diarrhoea;
- hypotension and eventually shock.

Multi-organ involvement is demonstrated by:

- myalgia;
- toxic encephalopathy;
- liver dysfunction;
- renal failure;
- thrombocytopenia;
- hypocalcaemia.

The diagnosis is based on the clinical features and the identification of *S. aureus* in culture. The condition is rarely caused by *S. epidermidis*.

The differential diagnosis includes:

- scarlet fever;
- meningococcaemia;
- the Stevens–Johnson syndrome.

Treatment includes **resuscitation, management of the local infection** *and* **systemic antibiotics**. *These should be either a beta-lactamase-resistant penicillin or a cephalosporin.*

- *The potential value of corticosteroids is uncertain.*

The prognosis is good, with recovery in 1–2 weeks and a mortality of only 5%. The incidence has declined and the fatality rate decreased since super-absorbent tampons were withdrawn from the market in 1981. Nowadays, at least 20% of cases bear no relation to menstruation. The condition can be recurrent given appropriate circumstances.

A similar syndrome is produced by some strains of *S. pyogenes* which secrete erythrogenic toxin type A, i.e. the toxin responsible for scarlet fever, though in the **'toxic strep syndrome'** scarlatiniform eruptions are paradoxically absent (see Scarlet fever).

Non-group A streptococcal strains have also been reported recently to cause this condition.

Commonly there is massive soft tissue destruction, but sometimes the preceding streptococcal infection is not severe.

The diagnosis can be particularly difficult, with only flu-like symptoms in some patients and negative blood cultures in 40% of cases.

There has been a preliminary report that the administration of high doses of **C1-esterase inhibitor** *iv may be helpful.*

Bibliography

Cone LA, Woodard DR, Schlievert PM et al 1987 Clinical and bacteriologic observations of a toxic shock-like syndrome due to Streptococcus pyogenes. N Engl J Med 317: 146.

Davis JP, Chesney PJ, Wand PJ et al 1980 Toxic-shock syndrome: epidemiologic features, recurrence, risk factors, and prevention. N Engl J Med 303: 1429.

Fronhoffs S, Luyken J, Steuer K et al 2000 The effect of C1-esterase inhibitor in definite and suspected streptococcal toxic shock syndrome. Intens Care Med 26: 1566.

Kain KC, Schulzer M, Chow AW 1993 Clinical spectrum of nonmenstrual toxic shock syndrome (TSS): comparison with menstrual TSS by multivariate discriminant analysis. Clin Infect Dis 16: 100.

Langmuir AD, Worthen TD, Solomon J et al 1985
The Thucydides syndrome: a new hypothesis for
the cause of the plague of Athens. N Engl J Med
313: 1027.
Stevens DL 1995 Streptococcal toxic-shock
syndrome: spectrum of disease, pathogenesis, and
new concepts in treatment. Emerg Infect Dis 1: 3.
Stevens DL, Tanner MH, Winship J et al 1989
Severe group A streptococcal infections associated
with a toxic shock-like syndrome and scarlet fever
toxin. N Engl J Med 321: 1.

Toxoplasmosis

Toxoplasmosis is caused by infection with the
obligate intracellular protozoan parasite,
Toxoplasma gondii, which has a worldwide
distribution and can infect all mammalian
species.

Human infection usually arises from ingestion
of contaminated raw food or cat faeces, but it
can also arise from transplacental passage, organ
transplantation or blood transfusion. Following
the ingestion of cysts, trophozoites are liberated
in the gut giving rise to parasitaemia and tissue
invasion with eventual cyst formation. Though
quiescent, the cysts remain viable.

- Most infections are clearly asymptomatic,
  since positive serology is found in up to
  50% of populations, even in developed
  countries.
- In adults, there is fever, myalgia, fatigue,
  rash, lymphadenopathy,
  hepatosplenomegaly and atypical
  lymphocytosis.
- The disease is usually mild and subsides
  after several weeks.
- In immunocompromised hosts, a severe
  opportunistic infection may occur with:

  - pneumonitis;
  - myocarditis;
  - meningoencephalitis;
  - a mass lesion.

The diagnosis is made serologically.

The differential diagnosis includes:

- infectious mononucleosis;
- CMV infection;
- lymphoma;
- sarcoidosis.

*Treatment is required if the disease is severe or there is
multisystem involvement. **Pyrimethamine** is used in
a dose of 25–50 mg per day for 4–6 weeks.
Concomitant folinic acid therapy is recommended. It is
usual to add a sulfonamide or clindamycin for cerebral
toxoplasmosis in patients with AIDS.*

Bibliography
Joiner KA, Dubremetz JF 1993 Toxoplasma gondii: a
protozoan for the nineties. Infect Immun 61: 1169.
McCabe R, Remington JS 1988 Toxoplasmosis. N
Engl J Med 318: 313.
Wong S, Remington JS 1994 Toxoplasmosis in
pregnancy. Clin Infect Dis 18: 853.

361

Trace elements

Trace elements are micronutrients or chemical
substances required by living organisms in very
small amounts (each present in the body in an
amount <0.01% of total body weight) and
usually associated with enzyme function.
Confirmation of the essential nature of a
particular trace element requires that its
deficiency is associated with dysfunction and
that its addition prevents or reverses this
dysfunction.

The **essential trace elements** (ETEs) include:

- boron;
- cobalt;
- chromium;
- copper;
- iodine;
- manganese;
- molybdenum;
- selenium;
- zinc;
- possibly nickel;
- possibly silicon;
- possibly vanadium.

Deficiency of any one of these elements gives rise to clinical disease. The major deficiencies are discussed elsewhere in relation to the individual elements.

Recently, there has been new understanding of the requirements for trace elements in critical illness and of their iv dosage in that setting, with particular emphasis on prevention of deficiency. The elements with defined daily dosage for this purpose are listed in the table below.

Trace element requirements

Element	Dosage
Chromium	0.2–0.4
Copper	5–20
Iodine	1.0
Iron	20
Manganese	5
Molybdenum	0.4
Selenium	0.4–1.5
Zinc	50–100

Doses are in μmol/day for iv administration in patients receiving total parenteral nutrition (TPN). They may be conveniently obtained by adding a commercial multi-element preparation (such as 10 mL or 1 ampoule of Additrace from Pharmacia-Upjohn) to the TPN solution. Major minerals such as sodium, potassium, calcium, magnesium and phosphate have to be added separately, as their needs can vary greatly between individual patients.

Bibliography

Berger MM, Cavadini C, Chiolero R et al 1994 Influence of large intakes of trace elements on recovery after major burns. Nutrition 10: 327.

Chandra RK 1992 Effect of vitamin and trace-element supplementation on immune responses and infection in elderly patients. Lancet 340: 1124.

Elia M 1995 Changing concepts of nutrient requirements in disease: implications for artificial nutritional support. Lancet 345: 1279.

Fleming CR 1989 Trace element metabolism in adult patients requiring total parenteral nutrition. Am J Clin Nutr 49: 573.

Mertz W 1981 The essential trace elements. Science 213: 1332.

Prasad AS (ed) 1988 Essential and Toxic Trace Elements in Human Health and Disease. New York: Liss.

Shenkin A 1986 Vitamin and essential trace element recommendations during intravenous therapy: theory and practice. Proc Nutr Soc 45: 383.

Simmer K, Thompson RPH 1990 Trace elements. In: Cohen RD, Lewis B, Alberti KGMM, Denman AM (eds) The Metabolic and Molecular Basis of Acquired Disease. London: Baillere Tindall. p 670.

Supplement 1995 The trace elements: their role and function in nutritional support. Nutrition 2: no.1.

Transverse myelitis (see Demyelinating diseases)

Trauma

The principles of the management of patients with trauma, even those with uncommon aspects of common injuries, are well known in the Intensive Care setting. This book thus considers injuries which themselves are less common, including:

- bites and stings;
- lightning;
- radiation injury;
- respiratory burns;
- trauma in pregnancy;
- water-related accidents.

Bibliography

Barton RN 1985 Trauma and its metabolic products. Br Med Bull 41: 3.

Blaisdell FW, Holcroft JW (eds) 1999 Scientific American Surgery Handbook of Trauma. New York: Scientific American.

Green DR 1988 Trauma and the immune response. Immunol Today 9: 253.

Frayn KN 1986 Hormonal control of metabolism in trauma and sepsis. Clin Endocrinol 24: 577.

Moore EE, Cogbill TH, Malagoni MA et al 1996 Scaling systems for organ specific injuries. Curr Opinion Crit Care 2: 450.

Nelson LD (ed) 1999 New advances in the care of critically injured patients. New Horizons: The Science and Practice of Acute Medicine 7: 1.

Smith RM, Giannoudis PV 1998 Trauma and the immune response. J R Soc Med 91: 417.

Wisner DH 1996 Current priorities in the management of multiple injury. Curr Opinion Crit Care 2: 463.

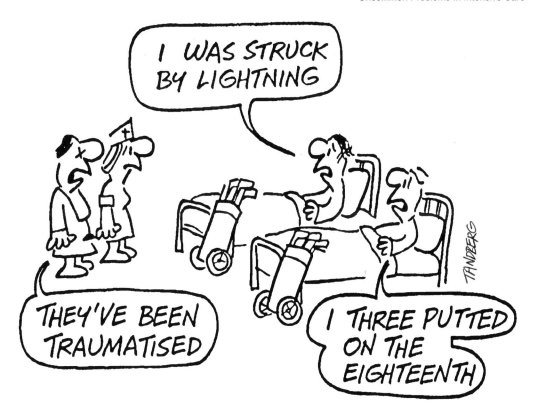

Trauma in pregnancy

Trauma in pregnancy is the commonest cause of maternal death, although only 1 in 20 cases of maternal trauma requires hospitalization. Fetal risk is greater than maternal risk, but in general fetal loss is minimized if maternal health can be maintained.

Trauma during pregnancy may present special problems of assessment and management. This is not just because two patients have to be simultaneously considered, but especially because of the altered abdominal anatomy and general physiology.

While **hypotension** in the pregnant trauma patient may be due to hypovolaemia, it may also be positional. This distinction may be especially difficult, because the blood volume is increased by up to 35% in pregnancy (about 1500 mL at term) and the cardiac output is concomitantly increased, thus masking the usual clinical signs of hypovolaemia. However, putting the patient in the left lateral position will help to differentiate these two causes, because in the supine position inferior caval (or even aortocaval) obstruction can occur. This may reduce the cardiac output by up to 30% and the systolic blood pressure by up to 30 mmHg due to diminished preload.

Early **vascular access** for volume resuscitation is important, because the uterine blood flow is not autoregulated and fetal shock may occur early. Vasopressors are best avoided.

Abdominal examination in pregnancy can be misleading, because the normal anatomical relationships are altered due to stretching of the abdominal wall, relocation of viscera and compartmentalization. Diagnostic peritoneal lavage can be safely performed in any trimester provided it is above the uterus.

Placental abruption (abruptio placentae) occurs in 2–4% of patients with minor injuries and in up to 40% of those with major injuries. It is the major cause of fetal death following maternal trauma. This complication occurs particularly with deceleration forces, and there may therefore be few external signs of injury. It also complicates about 1% of pregnancies in general, particularly when risk factors such as advanced maternal age, smoking or hypertension are present.

Clinical features may include abdominal cramps, uterine tenderness, vaginal bleeding, amniotic fluid leakage (with the resultant vaginal fluid having a pH of 7–7.5), amniotic fluid embolism (q.v.), hypovolaemia (since up to 2 L of blood can accumulate in the uterus), a uterine size which is 'larger than dates', and altered fetal heart rate.

The detection of increased plasma levels of thrombomodulin, a marker of endothelial cell damage, has been reported to have the highest sensitivity of any test for placental abruption.

Cardiotocographic monitoring should be performed for at least 4 h and continued for up to 24 h if any of the clinical features described above are present.

Fetomaternal haemorrhage occurs in 8–30% of cases after trauma. It is detected by the Kleihauer-Betke (KT) acid elution technique on maternal blood. One fetal cell per 1000 maternal cells corresponds to a feto–maternal haemorrhage of 5 mL. All Rh-negative mothers who have a negative indirect Coomb's test and who suffer abdominal trauma during pregnancy should receive Rh immune globulin prophylactically. The dose will depend on the KT test result.

Bibliography
Knudson MM 1996 Acute abdominal injuries during pregnancy. Curr Opinion Crit Care 2: 469.

Magriples U, Chan DW, Bruzek D et al 1999 Thrombomodulin: a new marker for placental abruption. Thromb Haemost 81: 32.
Pearlman MD, Tintinalli JE, Lorenz RP 1990 Blunt trauma during pregnancy. N Engl J Med 323: 1609.
Sorensen VJ, Bivins BA, Obeid FN et al 1990 Management of general surgical emergencies in pregnancy. Am Surg 56: 245.

Trench fever (see Pediculosis and Rickettsial diseases)

Trichlorethylene (see Carbon tetrachloride)

Tropical eosinophilia (see Eosinophilia and lung infiltration)

Tuberculosis

Tuberculosis (TB) is one of the best known chronic infectious diseases. Although in recent decades it had been reduced to a low incidence in developed countries (e.g. <5 notifications per 100 000 population per year), it has remained one of the major causes of death worldwide. Moreover, it has also lately had a resurgence in developed countries, particularly in migrants, indigenous peoples, disadvantaged groups (especially the homeless) and the immunocompromised (especially as a coinfection with HIV). A major conference has emphasized its many different visages and thus the need for adaptable control strategies (Lancet Conference, 1995).

Although treatment principles (standard 6 months chemotherapy with 4-drug combinations) are well established with almost 100% cure rates, perhaps one of the main new challenges is the increasing frequency of multidrug-resistant strains, selected because of inappropriate therapy and evident not only in developing countries. The occurrence of multidrug-resistant tuberculosis (MDR-TB) ranges from <1% of cases of TB in Australia (i.e. about 10 cases per year) to over 13% in India (i.e. about 250000 cases per year). Current agents which may be of use in the treatment of such patients include new fluoroquinolones (e.g. ciprofloxacin), macrolides (e.g. clarithromycin) and rifamycins (e.g. rifabutin), but depressingly no agents are suitable for prophylaxis after contact with isoniazid-resistant strains.

> Clinical staff need to be aware of the risks of hospital-acquired tuberculosis and the need for scrupulous preventative measures, including rapid diagnosis, effective treatment, thorough isolation of infected patients, monitoring of staff, and chemoprophylaxis of close contacts.

Bibliography
Davies PDO, De Cock KM, Leese J et al 1996 Tuberculosis 2000. J R Soc Med 89: 431.
Lancet Conference 1995 The challenge of tuberculosis: statements on global control and prevention. Lancet 346: 809.
Millard FJC 1996 The rising incidence of tuberculosis. J R Soc Med 89: 497.
Ormerod P, Campbell J, Novelli V 1998 Chemotherapy and management of tuberculosis in the United Kingdom: recommendations 1998. Thorax 53: 536.
Snider DE, La Montagne JR 1994 The neglected global tuberculosis problem. J Infect Dis 169: 1189.
Snider DE, Roper WL 1992 The new tuberculosis. N Engl J Med 326: 703.

Tuberous sclerosis

Tuberous sclerosis (Bourneville's disease) is a rare inherited neurocutaneous disorder or phakomatosis. It has a variable hereditary pattern and a prevalence of about 1 per 100000 population.

It is characterized by the triad of facial sebaceous adenoma (butterfly rash over the nose and cheeks), epilepsy and mental retardation. There may also be cafe-au-lait spots. It is one of the uncommon causes of a diffuse pulmonary infiltrate, with an interstitial pattern of extensive fine thin-walled cysts seen on high-resolution CT scanning. There may be associated cardiac, cerebral or renal tumours.

Treatment is **symptomatic**.

Bibliography
Critchley M, Earle C 1932 Tubero-sclerosis and allied conditions. Brain 55: 311.
Lenoir S, Grenier P, Brauner MW et al 1990 Pulmonary lymphangiomyomatosis and tuberous sclerosis: comparison of radiographic and thin-section CT findings. Radiology 175: 329.

Tubulointerstitial diseases

Tubulointerstitial diseases, together with glomerular diseases and vascular diseases, comprise the three main groups of renal disorders. The tubulointerstitial diseases have a large variety of causes and display a considerable spectrum of severity and reversibility and thus clinical features.

> The urine usually shows:
> - haematuria;
> - sterile pyuria;
> - white blood cell casts;
> - proteinuria
>   - the protein is of low molecular weight, i.e. beta$_2$–microglobulin (q.v.),
>   - rather than albumin as in glomerular diseases.
>
> Renal dysfunction shows tubular defects, including:
> - impaired concentration with polyuria and possibly hypovolaemia;
> - hypokalaemia or hyperkalaemia;
> - magnesium loss;

- glycosuria;
- aminoaciduria;
- renal tubular acidosis.

Acute interstitial nephritis is usually an allergic response, especially to drugs. Many drugs (currently more than 50) can be potential causes, but the most common are:

- beta-lactam antibiotics
  - especially with the anti-staphylococcal agents, flucloxacillin and dicloxacillin, and more commonly with the latter (in contrast to hepatic reactions which are more common with the former);
- other antibiotics
  - less commonly;
  - including ciprofloxacin, cotrimoxazole, erythromycin, rifampicin, vancomycin;
- NSAIDs;
- cimetidine;
- diuretics, such as thiazides;
- phenytoin, carbamazepine;
- other drugs
  - allopurinol, methyldopa, propranolol.

It is clinically associated with fever, rash and eosinophilia, which occur on average about two weeks (range 3–42 days) after the drug has been commenced. Oliguria is usual. There is a sterile pyuria, often with eosinophiluria.

This is an important cause of renal dysfunction, because:

- it is third in frequency after pre-renal uraemia and acute tubular necrosis;
- it is reversible if the drug is stopped.

Treatment with **corticosteroids** *is probably not effective, though it is commonly given if recovery is delayed beyond a few days.* **Dialysis** *is required in perhaps one third of cases, occasionally for several weeks.*

Chronic interstitial nephritis may be caused by a large variety of factors. It is a toxic

nephropathy, and some years ago it was commonly called analgesic nephropathy, because in most cases it had been associated with excessive oral analgesic consumption (particularly phenacetin), although the mechanism for this type of damage remains unclear.

The many aetiological factors include:

- drugs most commonly, especially
  - analgesics (not just phenacetin, which was later withdrawn from the market, but also paracetamol/aspirin combinations as well as other NSAIDs);
  - cisplatin;
  - cyclosporin;
  - lithium;
- toxic/metabolic agents
  - cadmium;
  - lead;
  - hypokalaemia;
  - hypercalcaemia;
- physical agents
  - irradiation;
  - obstruction;
  - reflux;
- infection
  - chronic pyelonephritis;
  - systemic infection;
- vascular diseases;
- cystic renal disease;
- transplant rejection;
- systemic diseases
  - SLE;
  - sarcoidosis;
  - dysproteinaemias.

Chronic interstitial nephritis is commonly associated with papillary necrosis. It typically presents as two sequential problems, namely:

- renal dysfunction
  - failure of urinary concentration, acidification and sodium conservation;

- consequent metabolic acidosis and hypovolaemia;

- slowly progressive renal failure

  - sometimes with severe hypertension;
  - eventually with dialysis-dependent end-stage renal disease.

Bibliography

Abraham PA, Keane WF 1984 Glomerular and interstitial disease induced by nonsteroidal anti-inflammatory drugs. Am J Nephrol 4: 1.

Corwin HL, Korbet SM, Schwartz MM 1985 Clinical correlates of eosinophiluria. Arch Intern Med 145: 1097.

Hoitsma AJ, Wetzels JFM, Koene RAP 1991 Drug-induced nephrotoxicity: aetiology, clinical features and management. Drug Safety 6: 131.

Kincaid-Smith P 1980 Analgesic abuse and the kidney. Kidney Int 17: 250.

Linton AL, Clark WF, Driedger AA et al 1980 Acute interstitial nephritis due to drugs. Ann Intern Med 93: 735.

Neilson EG 1989 Pathogenesis and therapy of interstitial nephritis. Kidney Int 35: 1257.

Ronco PM, Flahault A 1994 Drug-induced end-stage renal disease. N Engl J Med 331: 1711.

Tumour lysis syndrome (see Cancer complications.

Typhoid Fever

Typhoid Fever (enteric fever) is caused by the exclusively human pathogen, *Salmonella typhi*. Transmission is via water or food contaminated with human faeces. The disease thus occurs primarily in developing countries, and the rare outbreaks in developed countries usually arise because of food handling by chronic salmonella carriers.

Clinical features comprise:

- fever;
- paradoxical bradycardia;
- headache;
- cough;
- abdominal pain;
- splenomegaly;
- a transient rose-coloured macular rash on the body;
- watery diarrhoea which occurs early with constipation later.

The lymphoid hyperplasia in the terminal ileum may be complicated by haemorrhage or perforation.

Blood cultures are usually positive in the first two weeks, and faecal and urinary cultures become positive during the second and third weeks.

Continued excretion of the organism occurs in up to 3% of patients. Biliary disease predisposes to chronic enteric carriage, and schistosomiasis predisposes to chronic urinary carriage. Chronic carriers are asymptomatic but remain a risk to others.

Treatment traditionally was with **chloramphenicol**, *but* **ampicillin** *and* **cotrimoxazole** *are also effective.*

- *In cases of resistance to these drugs (e.g. in South and South-East Asia), a quinolone or third-generation cephalosporin may be used.*
- *Chronic carriage requires prolonged antibiotic therapy, and* **cholecystectomy** *is generally curative in carriers with biliary disease who do not respond completely to antibiotics.*

Prevention is with public health measures and immunization.

Nontyphoidal salmonellosis is common in developed countries, with the usual sources being inadequately cooked hen's eggs, exotic pets such as turtles and the smoking of contaminated marijuana.

Bibliography

Hornick RB, Greisman SE, Woodward TE et al 1970 Typhoid fever. N Engl J Med 283: 686, 739.

Typhus (see Rickettsial diseases)

U

Ulcerative colitis (see Inflammatory bowel disease)

Ulcers

Ulcers refer to breaches in the skin or mucous membranes. Though common, they may have a large list of causes, some of which are unusual.

Skin ulcers are seen with:

- Anthrax;
- Basal cell carcinoma;
- Blastomycosis;
- Chancroid;
- Chromium poisoning;
- Cryptococcosis;
- Decubitus (pressure);
- Diphtheria;
- Ecthyma;
- Erythema multiforme;
- Felty's syndrome;
- Graft-versus-host disease;
- Granuloma inguinale;
- Histiocytoma;
- Kaposi's sarcoma;
- Ischaemia (including diabetes);
- Leishmaniasis;
- Livedo vasculitis;
- Lymphogranuloma venereum;
- Mucormycosis;
- Mycobacteria (non-tuberculous);
- Mycosis fungoides (cutaneous T-cell lymphoma);
- Pemphigus vulgaris;
- Plague;
- Porphyrias;
- Progressive bacterial synergistic gangrene;
- Pseudomonas;
- Pyoderma gangrenosum;
- Scleroderma;
- Sporotrichosis;
- Squamous cell carcinoma;
- Syphilis;
- Tetanus;
- Tularaemia;

- Venereal inguinal buboes;
- Venous disease;
- Yaws.

Oral ulcers are seen in:

- Aphthous states;
- Behçet's syndrome;
- Bejel;
- Erythema multiforme;
- Graft-versus-host disease;
- Hand-foot-and-mouth disease;
- Herpes simplex virus;
- Leishmaniasis;
- Neutropenia;
- Pemphigus vulgaris, including bullous mucosal pemphigoid;
- Reiter's syndrome;
- Stevens–Johnson syndrome;
- SLE.

Genital ulcers occur in:

- Amoebiasis;
- Behçet's syndrome;
- Chancroid;
- Epstein–Barr virus infection;
- Granuloma inguinale;
- HSV (type 2) infection;
- Lymphogranuloma venereum;
- Reiter's syndrome;
- Syphilis;
- Stevens–Johnson syndrome;
- Trauma.

Bibliography
Antoon JW, Miller RL 1980 Aphthous ulcer – a review of the literature on etiology, pathogenesis, diagnosis, and treatment. JAMA 101: 803.

Urticaria

There are a number of urticarial conditions, but apart from hives they are uncommon.

1. Urticaria thus usually refers to **hives**, which are areas of transient, localized, pruritic oedema, varying in size from 1–20 cm and in number from one to more than 100. They are usually caused by food sensitivity (mostly due to the degranulating chemicals used as colouring and flavouring agents) and aspirin.

The main treatment of hives and indeed of urticaria in general is with **antihistamines** *and if severe with adrenaline and corticosteroids. Photochemotherapy has been used.*

2. **Angioedema** (q.v.).

3. **Physical**, due especially to cold, but also to heat or sun. **Cold urticaria** is produced in some patients by IgE autoantibodies to a cold-dependent skin antigen. It occurs particularly during rewarming and is usually associated with systemic symptoms, such as headache, tachycardia, syncope and wheeze. If severe, it resembles leukocytoclastic vasculitis (see below).

4. **Systemic mastocytosis** produces a similar picture to carcinoid but the main mediator is histamine. There is mast cell accumulation not only in skin (in virtually all cases) but also in non-cutaneous sites, with visceral and bony lesions (in 10–20% of cases). It is probably related to lymphoproliferative disorders or polycythaemia, and there may be associated eosinophilia. In addition to urticaria, there is flushing, headache, fatigue, abdominal pain and diarrhoea, all due to histamine release. In severe cases, hypotension may be produced. These symptoms may be precipitated by alcohol or analgesics.

Treatment is with H_1 and H_2 **antihistamines**, **anticholinergics** *for gastrointestinal symptoms and oral* **cromoglycate**.

5. **Leukocytoclastic vasculitis** is sometimes considered among the urticarial conditions.

- It comprises necrosis of the walls of vessels up to arterioles with extravasation of formed blood elements.
- This usually gives rise to palpable purpura, but some lesions begin as urticaria.
- In addition, chronic lesions tend to become urticarial.

Although it may be idiopathic, it is more usually associated with

- systemic disease (collagen-vascular disease, lymphoma, other malignancy),
- infections (infectious mononucleosis, hepatitis, streptococcal),
- drugs (aspirin, cephalosporins, penicillin, procainamide, thiazides).

369

Bibliography
Denburg JA 1992 Basophil and mast cell lineage in vitro and in vivo. Blood 79: 846.
Dowd PM 1987 Cold-related disorders. Prog Dermatol 21: 1.
Ekenstam E, Callen JP 1984 Cutaneous leukocytoclastic vasculitis. Arch Dermatol 120: 484.
Fine J 1980 Mastocytosis. Int J Dermatol 19: 117.
Gibson LE 1990 Cutaneous vasculitis: approach to diagnosis and systemic associations. Mayo Clin Proc 65: 221.
Lewis RA 1984 Mastocytosis. J Allergy Clin Immunol 74: 755.
Mehregan RD, Hall MJ, Gibson LE 1992 Urticarial vasculitis: a histopathologic and clinical review of 72 cases. J Am Acad Dermatol 26: 441.
Monroe EW 1981 Urticarial vasculitis: an updated review. J Am Acad Dermatol 5: 88.
Monroe EW, Jones HE 1977 Urticaria: an updated review. Arch Dermatol 113: 80.

Varicella

The **varicella-zoster virus** (VZV) is a member of the human herpesvirus group. It undergoes latency and reactivation as do other herpesviruses.

Varicella is a highly communicable illness, with an incubation period of 11–20 days following droplet or direct contact. The virus is carried by the white blood cells to the skin and viscera.

> - A vesiculating rash appears in successive crops, especially on the face and trunk. This resolves over 7–10 days. There is associated fever, headache and malaise.
> - In adults, a diffuse reticulonodular pneumonitis may occur, which can eventually calcify. There is cough, tachypnoea and prolonged abnormality of gas exchange.
> - Rarely, arthritis, encephalitis, myocarditis, nephritis, orchitis and thrombocytopenia may occur.
> - Disseminated disease occurs chiefly in the presence of associated malignancy.
> - Reinfection does not occur, except in immunocompromised hosts when it is usually mild.

Zoster (shingles) arises from reactivation and is thus usually seen in older patients and especially in the immunocompromised.

Varicella does not lead to zoster in another person, though vice versa applies.

The diagnosis is made by virus isolation or positive serology.

The chief differential diagnosis is disseminated herpes simplex infection.

Treatment is with **acyclovir** *(q.v.).*

- **Isolation** *is recommended to prevent nosocomial transmission to susceptible patients. Patients so exposed should receive prophylactic immune globulin.*

- *Varicella* **vaccine** *is now available and is recommended for universal use, though it is not yet known if such vaccination influences the incidence or severity of any later shingles.*

Bibliography

Strassels, SA, Sullivan SD 1997 Clinical and economic considerations of vaccination against varicella. Pharmacotherapy 17: 133.

Straus SE, Ostrove JM, Inchauspe G et al 1988 Varicella-zoster virus infections: biology, natural history, treatment, and prevention. Ann Intern Med 108: 221.

Vasculitis

Vasculitis refers to inflammation of the blood vessels and comprises a group of conditions of variable aetiology, clinical features and outcome.

> Most cases of generalized or systemic vasculitis are of unknown aetiology but presumably have an immune pathogenesis.
>
> - Clinical features include fever, weight loss, malaise, myalgia, arthropathy and neuropathy.
> - There is anaemia, thrombocytosis, raised ESR and hypoalbuminaemia.
> - The most specific and sensitive test is biopsy of an affected area.
> - The diagnosis can often be difficult.
> - **Corticosteroids** *are the mainstay of treatment.*

Vasculitis may also be

- **secondary** to systemic autoimmune inflammatory conditions, such as
  - rheumatoid arthritis;
  - Sjögren's syndrome;

- **organ-specific**, such as

  - primary angiitis or arteritis of the central nervous system;
  - neutrophilic dermatoses (e.g. Behçet's syndrome – q.v.);
  - chronic lymphocytic vasculitis (e.g. pyoderma gangrenosum – q.v.).

There a number of specific types of vasculitis, including those:

- affecting mostly large vessels;
- affecting primarily medium-sized vessels;
- affecting primarily small vessels;
- associated with thrombosis;
- associated with spasm;
- associated with vessel wall degeneration.

1. Vasculitis affecting mostly large vessels

- **Takayasu's arteritis**, or pulseless disease. This particularly affects the upper extremities of young Asian women. The aortic intima becomes thickened and inflamed. The condition may respond to corticosteroids.

- giant cell arteritis or temporal arteritis (q.v.). This is often associated with polymyalgia rheumatica (q.v.).

- aortitis (see Endarteritis). This may sometimes be secondary to rheumatoid arthritis, ankylosing spondylitis or syphilis.

- primary angiitis of the central nervous system (see Cerebral arteritis)

2. Vasculitis affecting primarily medium-sized vessels

- polyarteritis nodosa (PAN) (q.v.)

- **microscopic polyangiitis**. This was formerly considered a variant of PAN but is now recognized to be one of the ANCA-associated systemic necrotizing vasculitides.

- granulomatous arteritis (Wegener's granulomatosis)(q.v.). In addition, vessels as small as capillaries may also be involved in this condition.

- Churg–Strauss syndrome (q.v.)

- Behçet's disease (q.v.)

- Kawasaki disease

- vasculitis due to hepatitis B

- vasculitis due to HIV infection

3. Vasculitis affecting primarily small vessels

- **hypersensitivity angiitis**. This term, which may now be outdated though it is still commonly used, refers usually to drug-related vasculitis. It can be associated with crops of palpable purpura or even Henoch–Schönlein purpura. Although small vessels are primarily involved, all cutaneous vessels may be affected. There may be associated renal, gut, lung or neurological involvement. *It responds to corticosteroids*.

- Goodpasture's syndrome (q.v.) and cryoglobulinaemia (q.v.). These can be associated with a similar picture.

- **leukocytoclastic vasculitis**. This comprises necrosis of the walls of vessels up to arterioles with extravasation of formed blood elements. It is more commonly considered among the Urticarias (q.v.).

- vasculitis due to

  - meningococcaemia,
  - hepatitis B or C infection (sometimes),
  - other bacterial, rickettsial or viral infections (occasionally)

- drug-induced cutaneous necrotizing vasculitis, due to

  - antimicrobials (beta-lactams, cotrimoxazole, quinolones, sulfonamides)
  - non-steroidal anti-inflammatory agents
  - diuretics
  - granulocyte colony stimulating factor (G-CSF)
  - insulin
  - phenytoin
  - quinine
  - streptokinase

- cutaneous necrotizing vasculitis due to miscellaneous immunological, inflammatory, connective tissue and neoplastic conditions

4. Vasculitis associated with thrombosis

- antiphospholipid syndrome with anti-cardiolipin antibody (q.v.)

- livedo vasculitis (see Livedo reticularis)

5. Vasculitis associated with spasm

- Raynaud's disease (q.v.)

- migraine

- eclampsia

- ergotism

6. **Vasculitis associated with vessel wall degeneration**

- atherosclerosis
- connective tissue disorders

Bibliography

Arend WP, Michel BA, Bloch DA et al 1990 The American College of Rheumatology 1990 criteria for the classification of Takayasu arteritis. Arthritis Rheum 33: 1129.

Calabrese L, Dune G, Lie J 1997 Vasculitis in the central nervous system. Arthritis Rheum 40: 1189.

Coffman JD 1991 Raynaud's phenomenon: an update. Hypertension 17: 593.

Conn DL 1989 Update on systemic necrotizing vasculitis. Mayo Clin Proc 64: 535.

Gatenby PA 1999 Vasculitis – diagnosis and treatment. Aust NZ J Med 29: 662.

Gibson LE 1990 Cutaneous vasculitis: approach to diagnosis and systemic associations. Mayo Clin Proc 65: 221.

Hamilton CR, Shelley WM, Tumulty PA 1971 Giant cell arteritis: including temporal arteritis and polymyalgia rheumatica. Medicine 50: 1.

Hunder GG, Bloch DA, Michel BA et al 1990 The American College of Rheumatology 1990 criteria for the classification of giant cell arteritis. Arthritis Rheum 33: 1122.

Jayne DRW, Davies MJ, Cox CJV et al 1991 Treatment of systemic vasculitis with pooled intravenous immunoglobulin. Lancet 337: 1137.

Jennette JC, Falk RJ 1997 Small-vessel vasculitis. N Engl J Med 337: 1512.

Jennette JC, Falk RJ, Andrassy K et al 1994 Nomenclature of systemic vasculitides: proposal of an international consensus conference. Arthritis Rheum 37: 187.

Kerr GS, Hallahan CW, Giordano J et al 1994 Takayasu arteritis. Ann Intern Med 120: 919.

Lie JT 1988 Classification and immunodiagnosis of vasculitis: a new solution or promises unfulfilled? J Rheumatol 15: 728.

Lupi-Herrera E, Sanchez-Torres G, Marcushamer J et al 1997 Takayasu's arteritis: clinical study of 107 cases. Am Heart J 93: 94.

Mehregan RD, Hall MJ, Gibson LE 1992 Urticarial vasculitis: a histopathologic and clinical review of 72 cases. J Am Acad Dermatol 26: 441.

Moore PM 1989 Diagnosis and management of isolated angiitis of the central nervous system. Neurology 39: 167.

Oz MC, Brener BJ, Buda JA et al 1989 A ten-year experience with bacterial aortitis. J Vasc Surg 10: 439.

Royle J, Williams K, Elliott E et al 1998 Kawasaki disease in Australia, 1993–95. Arch Dis Child 78: 33.

Savage COS, Harper L, Adu D 1997 Primary systemic vasculitis. Lancet 349: 553.

Szer I 1996 Henoch–Schonlein purpura: when and how to treat. J Rheumatol 23: 1661.

Zilko PJ 1996 Polymyalgia rheumatica and giant cell arteritis. Med J Aust 165: 438.

Vasopressin (see Desmopressin and Pituitary)

Vertigo

Vertigo is the distressing symptom of a spinning or revolving sensation. While it may be due to the same conditions as cause tinnitus (q.v.), the most common causes are:

- vestibular neuronitis;
- trauma;
- a recurrent condition called benign positional vertigo.

Bibliography

Harrison MS 1962 "Epidemic vertigo" – "vestibular neuronitis": a clinical study. Brain 85: 613.

Vesiculobullous diseases

Vesiculobullous diseases compromise a large and heterogeneous group of blistering disorders. They include:

- **pemphigus vulgaris** and its variants (q.v.);
- **dermatitis herpetiformis** (see Dermatitis);
- **erythema multiforme** (q.v.);
- **epidermolysis bullosa** (q.v.);
- **other conditions**, such as contact dermatitis, drug eruptions, heat rash, herpes infections, scabies and SLE, which may sometimes produce blistering.

Bibliography
Katz SI, Hall RP, Lawlwy TJ et al 1980 Dermatitis
herpetiformis: the skin and the gut. Ann Intern
Med 93: 857.
Sehgal VN, Gangwani OP 1987 Fixed drug
eruption: current concepts. Int J Dermatol 26:
67.

VIPoma (see Diarrhoea)

Viral haemorrhagic fever (see Ebola
haemorrhagic fever)

Vitamin deficiency

It has long been known that certain foods are required for health. In 1906, Hopkins found that in addition to protein, carbohydrate, fat, minerals and water, there were certain essential 'accessory factors'. In 1912, Frank showed that the anti-beriberi fraction in unpolished rice was an amine, which he therefore called a vital amine or vitamine. This name was then applied to all 'accessory factors', though later the 'e' was dropped off, as the substances were found to be chemically very different and not many were in fact amines.

Later in the same year, Hopkins and Frank proposed the theory of diseases due to vitamin deficiency, and the individual vitamins were subsequently discovered, being given letters according to their perceived function. As with trace elements, deficiency of any one of these substances gives rise to clinical disease, and the major deficiencies are discussed elsewhere in relation to the individual vitamins.

As with trace elements, there have been recently published guidelines for the appropriate iv dosage of vitamins in critical illness, with particular emphasis on prevention of deficiency. However, unlike those for trace elements, the guidelines for vitamins re-emphasize previous knowledge and practice. The recommended daily iv doses of vitamins for this purpose are listed in the table below.

Vitamin requirements

Vitamin	Dosage
A	1 mg (3000 IU)
C	100 mg
D	5 µg (200 IU)
E	10 mg (10 IU)
K	–
Thiamine	3 mg
Riboflavin	3.6 mg
Pyridoxine	4 mg
Niacin	40 mg
Biotin	60 µg
Pantothenic acid	15 mg
Folic acid	400 µg
B$_{12}$	5 µg

Doses are in µg or mg per day for iv administration in patients receiving a total parenteral nutrition (TPN). They may be conveniently obtained by adding a commercial multi-vitamin preparation (such as MVI-12 or Cernevit) to the TPN solution. The dose requirements for vitamin K vary greatly between individual patients and may be conveniently assessed by measurement of the prothrombin time, since this test is largely determined by the plasma levels of the vitamin K-dependent coagulation factors (see Vitamin K deficiency).

Bibliography
Anderson JJB, Toverud SU 1994 Diet and vitamin
D: a review with an emphasis on human function.
J Nutr Biochem 5: 58.
Chandra RK 1992 Effect of vitamin and trace-
element supplementation on immune responses
and infection in elderly patients. Lancet 340:
1124.
DeLuca HF 1978 Vitamin D metabolism and
function. Arch Intern Med 138: 836.
Shearer MJ 1995 Vitamin K Lancet 345: 229.
Shenkin A 1986 Vitamin and essential trace element
recommendations during intravenous therapy:
theory and practice. Proc Nutr Soc 45: 383.

Vitamin B$_{12}$ deficiency (see
Megaloblastic anaemia and Pernicious anaemia)

Vitamin K deficiency

Vitamin K deficiency was until recently thought to cause solely decreased plasma levels of four coagulation factors or clotting proteins, namely prothrombin (factor II) and factors VII, IX and X. This coagulation abnormality is most readily demonstrated by an increased prothrombin time.

Although vitamin K was discovered in 1929 (and later named K for 'koagulation'), it was not until 1974 that its unique mechanism of action was elucidated and this in turn has led to the recognition of other vitamin-K dependent proteins. When precursor proteins (PIVKA) bind to vitamin K-dependent γ-carboxylase, several glutamic acid residues (Glu) are converted to γ-carboxyglutamic acid residues (Gla). Gla residues are essential for the vitamin K-dependent proteins to form active complexes able to bind calcium and attach to phospholipids, so that in vitamin K deficiency only inactive proteins are produced.

The other, more recently discovered vitamin K–dependent proteins include:

- the anticoagulant factors, protein C (q.v.) and protein S (q.v.);
- bone Gla protein (osteocalcin) and matrix Gla protein;
- other less well defined proteins in lung, liver, kidney, pancreas, and placenta.

The action of vitamin K is manganese-dependent, so that manganese deficiency is in turn one of the uncommon causes of vitamin K deficiency (see Manganese).

Bibliography

Dam H 1935 The antihaemorrhagic vitamin of the chick: occurrence and chemical nature. Nature 135: 652.

Dowd P, Ham S-W, Naganathan S et al 1995 The mechanism of action of vitamin K. Annu Rev Nutr 15: 419.

Shearer MJ 1995 Vitamin K. Lancet 345: 229.

Stenflo J, Fernlund P, Egan W et al 1974 Vitamin K dependent modifications of glutamic acid residues in prothrombin. Proc Natl Acad Sci 71: 2730.

Vitiligo (see Pigmentation disorders)

Von Recklinghausen's disease (see Neurofibromatosis)

Von Willebrand's disease

Von Willebrand's disease or perhaps preferably disorder (vWD either way) is the most common congenital coagulation abnormality, with a heterozygous incidence of about 1%. It was first described in 1926 in Helsinki by Professor Erik von Willebrand. The disease arises because of either deficient or defective von Willebrand's factor, vWF, a plasma protein coded for by a gene on chromosome 12.

Von Willebrand's factor circulates as variable multimers from $0.5–20 \times 10^3$ kd. Its haemostatic function is to carry and protect factor VIII: C and assist platelet adhesion by associating platelet receptors with subendothelial structures, such as collagen. This it achieves because it has specific binding sites for factor VIII:C, platelet glycoprotein receptors and collagen. Very large multimers are stored in the endothelial cells as Weibel–Palade bodies, from where they are released in response to injury.

Von Willebrand's disease may be classified as follows.

- **Type I**, the classical type

This is inherited as an autosomal dominant and is usually seen in its heterozygous form, with mild to moderate disease. There is a quantitative abnormality of vWF.

- **Type II**

This consists of several sub-types of abnormal multimer patterns. There is normal total vWF but a qualitative abnormality.

- **Type III**

This is the severe and homozygous form of type I.

> Clinical features often commence only in adult life and comprise bleeding, either spontaneously or in excess after surgery or trauma.

There is commonly a spontaneous improvement during pregnancy.

The diagnosis is suspected from screening tests, which show with a prolonged APTT, together with a normal platelet count and an increased bleeding time. The vWF quantity is measured immunologically (as VWF:Ag), and vWF function is commonly measured via impaired ristocetin-induced platelet aggregation.

Treatment is with **cryoprecipitate***, which contains large and functionally active vWF multimers. Typically, 10 bags may be given 12 hourly until bleeding ceases.*

DDAVP *(desmopressin – q.v.) causes release of vWF from endothelial cells and is usually given in a dose of 20 μg iv, which may be repeated in 6 h. DDAVP is most suitable for preoperative prophylaxis, although sometimes tachycardia, headache, flushing and water retention may result. Since DDAVP may stimulate fibrinolysis, concomitant epsilon aminocaproic acid (EACA, 4 g 4 hourly) should be used as a fibrinolytic inhibitor in those cases where local fibrinolysis may be enhanced (e.g. dental extraction).*

Aspirin should be avoided.

Bibliography

Bloom AL 1991 Von Willebrand factor: clinical features of inherited and acquired disorders. Mayo Clin Proc 66: 743.

Sadler JE, Mannucci PM, Berntorp E et al 2000 Impact, diagnosis and treatment of von Willebrand disease. Thromb Haemost 84: 160.

Veyradier A, Jenkins CSP, Fressinaud E et al 2000 Acquired von Willebrand syndrome: from pathophysiology to management. Thromb Haemost 84: 175.

Waldenstrom's macroglobulinaemia (see Multiple myeloma)

Warfare Agents (see also Germ warfare)

Chemical warfare agents are substances which cause nausea, asphyxia, blindness, paralysis or burns. They may or may not be fatal. The term usually includes defoliants but not smoke. They were first used in the First World War, in the form of chlorine, phosgene and mustard gas. Because of public outrage and because they usually had minimal military efficacy, these agents became banned and though available were not used in the Second World War. However, some of these agents remain stocked and have even been used in recent years. Tear gas continues to be widely available for civilian riot control.

The different agents may be classified as follows.

1. Nerve agents

These most commonly are organophosphates, related to insecticides. They are thus easy to manufacture and can be possessed by 'rogue' military regimes or terrorist groups. They are potent inhibitors of acetylcholinesterase and are lethal at about 1 mg (G agents). One of the most toxic of such compounds is sarin (isopropyl methylphosphonofluoridate).

Nerve agents produce a cholinergic crisis (q.v.) with dramatic muscarinic and nicotinic effects.

- The former include sweating, lacrimation, bronchospasm, diarrhoea and bradycardia.
- The latter include weakness, fasciculation and paralysis.

Coma and fits are seen, and death occurs from respiratory failure.

Survivors may suffer permanent neurological defects.

Treatment is with **atropine** *in large doses, i.e. 2–6 mg iv and up to 15 mg in the first 30 min. Dosage should be doubled every 5–10 min until muscarinic symptoms are relieved. A continuous iv infusion of 6 mg/h may be used for maintenance, since in severe cases prolonged treatment may be required, with hundreds of mg given over days or even weeks.*

The most effective antidote is an oxime, such as **pralidoxime***, which complexes with the agent and thus removes it from acetylcholinesterase (see Anticholinergic agents). It should be given promptly and is used in a dose of 1–2 g iv in 100 mL saline over 15 min. If there is continued absorption or if muscle weakness persists, the dose may be repeated once or twice hourly or a continuous iv infusion of 0.5 g/h given.*

Diazepam *up to 10 mg iv may be concomitantly useful, especially for fits.*

Pyridostigmine *is paradoxically effective as a prophylactic agent, because it binds reversibly to cholinesterase and thus protects it.*

2. Mustards

These act as vesicants.

They are chiefly treated locally and **symptomatically***, though iv fluids and possibly sodium thiosulfate may be useful.*

3. Lewisite

This is a vesicant arsenical.

It requires treatment as for the mustards, with the addition of **BAL** *parenterally (q.v.) and also as an eye ointment.*

4. Phosgene

This is carbonyl chloride, a colourless but reactive and toxic gas with a smell of musty hay. It is denser than air and becomes a liquid at 8°. Carbonyl is a polar chemical unit of carbon and oxygen and is a reactive constituent in many organic compounds, including aldehydes, ketones, esters, amides, quinines and carboxylic acids. Phosgene is thus widely used industrially in chemical processes. It was first prepared in 1811 from carbon monoxide and chlorine, but it dissolves in water to give arbon dioxide and hydrochloric acid. It is thus a potent respiratory irritant with a progressive effect over several hours.

*Its effects are treated **symptomatically** and with intravenous and inhaled **corticosteroids**.*

5. **Cyanide** (q.v.)

6. **Incapacitating agents**

These are usually anticholinergics (q.v.).

*They are treated with **physostigmine**.*

7. **Local irritants and nauseants**

These require no specific treatment and spontaneous recovery occurs.

Bibliography

Bardin PG, Van Eeden SF, Moolman JA et al 1994 Organophosphate and carbamate poisoning. Ann Intern Med 154: 1433.

Dunn MA, Sidell FR 1989 Progress in medical defense against nerve agents. JAMA 262: 649.

Emad A, Rezaian GR 1997 The diversity of the effects of sulfur mustard gas inhalation on respiratory system 10 years after a single heavy exposure. Chest 112: 734.

Marrs TC 1993 Organophosphate poisoning. Pharmacol Ther 58: 51.

Nozaki H, Aikawa N, Shinozawa Y et al 1995 Sarin poisoning in Tokyo subway. Lancet 345: 980.

Rickett DL, Glenn JF, Houston WE 1987 Medical defense against nerve agents: new directions. Milit Med 152: 35.

Sidell FR, Borak J 1992 Chemical warfare agents. Ann Emerg Med 21: 865.

Tafuri J, Roberts J 1987 Organophosphate poisoning. Ann Emerg Med 16: 193.

Vedder EB 1925 The Medical Aspects of Chemical Warfare. Baltimore: Williams & Wilkins.

Wasp stings (see Bites and stings)

Water-related accidents (see Bathing, Diving and Drowning)

Waterhouse–Friderichsen syndrome

The Waterhouse–Friderichsen syndrome refers to acute fulminant meningococcaemia with resultant shock.

This form of severe septicaemia is seen in about 10% of cases of meningococcaemia and presents as typical endotoxaemia. It is commonly complicated by:

- myocarditis;
- disseminated intravascular coagulation;
- acute adrenal failure;
- acute oliguric renal failure;
- adult respiratory distress syndrome.

Although typically caused by meningococcaemia, it is not distinguishable from similar conditions caused by other Gram-negative bacteria (including *H. influenzae* type b in children) and also by *S. pneumoniae* in asplenic patients.

*Treatment is with **resuscitation** and supportive therapy, high-dose parenteral **antibiotics**, **corticosteroids** and possibly **heparin** if DIC if severe.*

***Plasmapheresis** and **monoclonal antibodies to endotoxin** have been reported to be helpful.*

Prevention is important for contacts and for patients at risk. Although there is a high mortality, there are usually no long-term sequelae for survivors.

WDHA syndrome (see Diarrhoea)

Weil's disease (see Leptospirosis)

Wegener's granulomatosis

Wegener's granulomatosis is the most common form of pulmonary vasculitis. It consists of a necrotizing granulomatous vasculitis of the upper respiratory tract (nose, sinuses), lungs and kidneys. A limited form may affect the lungs only.

The aetiology is unknown, but the pathogenesis appears immunological since it is associated with the presence of a specific antibody.

The patient may be of either sex and any age but is most typically a middle-aged man. Clinical features are very variable, but they commonly comprise cough, pleuritic pain and haemoptysis. Upper respiratory tract involvement is manifest by rhinorrhoea, ulcers, pain and purulent drainage.

There may be symptoms of multi-organ involvement, especially affecting the kidneys, but also skin, joints and eyes.

Blood examination typically shows anaemia, leukocytosis, thrombocytosis and raised ESR.

Serology is positive for rheumatoid factor but not ANA. The presence of antineutrophil cytoplasmic autoantibodies (ANCAs) is nearly 100% specific and about 70% sensitive for the condition. The particular ANCA in Wegener's granulomatosis is directed against cytoplasmic proteinase-3, which is present in the lysosomes of neutrophils and monocytes. This autoantibody is therefore called c-ANCA or anti-PR3. BAL is also positive for ANCA and generally has about 50% neutrophils and a few eosinophils. Some other vasculitides are also ANCA-associated (e.g. Churg–Strauss syndrome, microscopic polyangiitis, renal-limited vasculitis), but these conditions are generally positive for p-ANCA (i.e. the antigenic target is myeloperoxidase, MPO, which is perinuclear).

The chest X-ray shows single or multiple densities of varying size, often with cavitation, but sometimes there is a more general infiltration.

The condition is often initially misdiagnosed as pulmonary malignancy, but histological examination establishes the diagnosis.

Treatment is with **corticosteroids** *and* **cytotoxics** *(usually cyclophosphamide).*

The illness is fatal within one year if untreated, but long-term remission is now usual with treatment.

Variants of Wegener's granulomatosis probably include the following.

1. **Lymphomatoid granulomatosis** is an uncommon condition with histological features resembling both Wegener's granulomatosis and lymphoma. There is a pulmonary infiltrate which is angiocentric, destructive and lymphoreticular, with atypical cells showing mitoses. Similar lesions may be found in other organs, especially skin and sometimes the mouth.

Respiratory symptoms include cough, sputum and dyspnoea.

The chest X-ray shows bilateral infiltrates, rounded lesions similar to metastases and cavitation.

No consistently effective treatment is available, although combined **corticosteroid** *and* **cytotoxic** *therapy is usually given.*

There is a high mortality, often with progression to malignant lymphoma.

2. **Bronchocentric granulomatosis** is a destructive condition similar to Wegener's granulomatosis, except that the lesions are centred on bronchi and not on blood vessels. The distinction is important because its prognosis is much better.

Many patients have asthma, eosinophilia, mucus plugs and hypersensitivity to *Aspergillus fumigatus*. In these patients, the condition may represent a variant of 'mucoid impaction'.

Bibliography

Cordier JF, Valeyre D, Gullevin L et al 1990 Pulmonary Wegener's granulomatosis. Chest 97: 906.

European Vasculitis Study Group 1999 A multicenter randomized trial of cyclophosphamide versus azathioprine during remission in ANCA-associated systemic vasculitis. Arthritis Rheum 42 (suppl): 225.

Falk RJ, Jennett JC 1991 Wegener's granulomatosis, systemic vasculitis, and antineutrophil cytoplasmic autoantibodies. Annu Rev Med 42: 459.

Fauci AS, Haynes BF, Costa J et al 1982

Lymphomatoid granulomatosis. N Engl J Med 306: 68.

Hagen EC, Ballieux BEPB, van Es LA et al 1993 Antineutrophil cytoplasmic autoantibodies: a review of the antigens involved, the assays, and the clinical and possible pathogenetic consequences. Blood 81: 1996.

Hoffman G 1997 Treatment of Wegener's granulomatosis: time to change the standard of care? Arthritis Rheum 40: 2099.

Hoffman GS, Specks U 1998 Antineutrophil cytoplasmic antibodies. Arthritis Rheum 41: 1521.

Kallenberg C, Brouwer E, Weening J et al 1994 Anti-neutrophil cytoplasmic antibodies: current diagnostic and pathophysiological potential. Kidney Int 46: 1.

Ricketti AJ, Greenberger PA, Mintzer RA et al 1983 Allergic bronchopulmonary aspergillosis. Arch Intern Med 143: 1553.

Salama AD 1999 Pathogenesis and treatment of ANCA-associated systemic vasculitis. J R Soc Med 92: 456.

Schuyler MR 1983 Allergic bronchopulmonary aspergillosis. Clin Chest Med 4: 15.

Wernicke–Korsakoff syndrome

Wernicke–Korsakoff syndrome is the name given to the encephalopathy caused by thiamine deficiency. It is seen in:

- alcoholism;
- hyperemesis gravidarum;
- malnutrition;
- starvation;
- AIDS.

The **Wernicke** component comprises:

- acute delirium,
- with associated ophthalmoplegia, nystagmus and ataxia.

It responds to **thiamine** *100 mg iv daily.*

Glucose should not be administered without concomitant thiamine.

The **Korsakoff** component of the syndrome refers to a state of chronic and usually permanent dementia.

Bibliography

Harper CG, Giles M, Finlay-Jones R 1986 Clinical signs in the Wernicke–Korsakoff complex. J Neurol Neurosurg Psychiatry 49: 341.

Kopelman MD 1995 The Korsakoff syndrome. Br J Psychiatry 166: 154.

Reuler JB, Girard DE, Cooney TG 1985 Wernicke's encephalopathy. N Engl J Med 312: 1035.

Whipple's disease

Whipple's disease is a rare systemic disorder presumed to be due to infection with a recently described Gram-positive actinomycete, *Tropheryma whippelii*. While it chiefly affects the small bowel, arthritis is also common, as in inflammatory bowel disease.

Clinical features are seen mainly in men and comprise fever, weakness, weight loss, malabsorption and increased pigmentation. Seronegative spondylarthropathy and lymphadenopathy resembling sarcoidosis is common. There may also be digital clubbing, aortic and mitral valve disease, and a slow dementia, manifest by confusion and loss of memory. The patient is typically anergic.

PCR identification of the specific organism is now available.

Treatment is with a prolonged course of **antibiotics**, *usually penicillin, amoxycillin or tetracycline, for 12–18 months. For neurological involvement,* **cotrimoxazole** *is used together with* **corticosteroids**.

Whipple's disease was previously fatal, but antibiotic treatment now produces long remissions.

Bibliography

Relman DA, Schmidt TM, MacDermott RP et al 1992 Identification of the uncultured bacillus of Whipple's disease. N Engl J Med 327: 293.

Swartz MN 2000 Whipple's disease: past, present and future. N Engl J Med 342: 648.

Wilson's disease (see Copper)

Woolsorter's disease (see Anthrax)

Yellow fever

Yellow fever is one of the viral zoonoses. It is caused by a group B arborvirus or flavivirus, which is morphologically indistinguishable from other members of the togavirus family which cause encephalitis in the Americas. The disease occurs mainly in South America and sub-Saharan Africa. Typically, there is a tropical reservoir in monkeys and a mosquito vector (A. aegypti), though in urban areas the reservoir is in humans.

After an incubation period of 3–6 days, there are non-specific symptoms of fever, malaise, weakness, nausea, vomiting and back pain. The patient is highly infectious during this time.

These clinical features subside after 1–7 days. The patient then appears well for up to a day or so, only to relapse with:

- jaundice (due to acute fulminant hepatitis);
- shock;
- renal failure;
- coma;
- generalized bleeding tendency (due to disseminated intravascular coagulation).

Diagnosis is made by viral isolation or serologically. A PCR method has recently become available. Characteristic inclusion (Councilman) bodies and midzonal necrosis are seen on liver histology, usually however examined only postmortem.

*Treatment is **supportive**, though early **ribavirin** administration has shown promise in experimental studies.*

*The disease is best controlled by vector elimination, because although **immunization** is available it is given chiefly to travellers.*

The average mortality is 5% in endemic cases but about 40% in epidemics and 50% in severe cases. In those who survive, there is a prolonged convalescence.

Bibliography

Monath TP 1987 Yellow fever: a medically neglected disease. Rev Infect Dis 9: 165.

Robertson SE, Hull BP, Tomori O et al 1996 Yellow fever: a decade of reemergence. JAMA 276: 1157.

Zinc

Zinc (Zn, atomic number 30, atomic weight 65) is a metal with a low melting point and related to cadmium and mercury. It has been a widely used metal since antiquity, primarily as an alloy, and it was first isolated as a separate substance in India in the 13th century.

Zinc is essential for many forms of life. It is present in carbonic anhydrase (and thus in high concentration in red blood cells) and in a number of gastrointestinal enzymes. It takes the place of iron in snails' blood. In addition to its presence in many enzymes, it is also needed for growth and tissue repair. It is thus an essential trace element.

The normal sources are meat and seafood, and deficient zinc intake is therefore common in situations of protein malnutrition. The normal daily requirement is 2.5–4 mg orally and the recommended iv dose is 50–100 µmol/day. These doses should be increased if there are excessive gastrointestinal losses.

> Marked losses can occur in serious illness, especially from gastrointestinal fistulae.
>
> The most obvious clinical feature of zinc deficiency is an eczematous rash, especially of the nasolabial folds on the face, but also in the perineum and on the extensor surfaces.
>
> Alopecia, diarrhoea, ileus, tremor, apathy and depression can also be produced.

Zinc overdose has been reported to cause nausea, vomiting, hypothermia, hypotension, pulmonary oedema, oliguria, jaundice, coma and raised serum amylase.

Bibliography
Berger MM, Cavadini C, Chiolero R et al 1996 Copper, selenium and zinc status and balances after major trauma. J Trauma 40: 103.

McClain C, Soutor C, Zieve L 1980 Zinc deficiency: a complication of Crohn's disease. Gastroenterology 78: 272.

Prasad AS 1988 Clinical spectrum and diagnostic aspects of human zinc deficiency. In: Prasad AS, (ed) Essential and Toxic Trace Elements in Human Health and Disease. New York: Liss. p 3.

Zollinger–Ellison syndrome

The Zollinger–Ellison syndrome refers to the condition of refractory, painful and often multiple peptic ulceration and diarrhoea associated with a gastrinoma or gastrin-secreting tumour.

The tumour arises either in the duodenal wall or more particularly in the pancreas, with about 25% of cases having other additional endocrine tumours. These include especially pancreatic insulinoma, but also adrenal, parathyroid and thyroid adenomas and pituitary chromophobe adenoma (see Multiple endocrine neoplasia). Two thirds of cases are malignant.

The diagnosis is based on increased basal gastric acid secretion (>15 mmol/h) and increased fasting serum gastrin (always >200 ng/L and often up to 1000 ng/L, though similar levels can also be seen in renal failure or after omeprazole).

> The serum bicarbonate is typically high, often >40 mmol/L.

Since the tumour is often small, it can be difficult to locate even with sophisticated imaging.

*Treatment is with **resection** if possible, though the tumour cannot be located in 25% of cases or has metastasized in 50% of cases.*

*Medical treatment is with high-dose **H₂ antagonists** or better with **omeprazole** if the tumour cannot be resected.*

Bibliography
Wolfe MM, Jensen RT 1987 Zollinger–Ellison syndrome: current concepts in diagnosis and management. N Engl J Med 317: 1200.

Zoonoses (see Rabies)

Zoster (see Varicella)